# Iron Deficiency and Overload

# Nutrition and Health

Adrianne Bendich, PhD, FACN, Series Editor

For other titles published in this series, go to
www.springer.com/series/7659

# IRON DEFICIENCY AND OVERLOAD

## From Basic Biology to Clinical Medicine

*Edited by*
SHLOMO YEHUDA, PhD
*Department of Psychology, Bar-Ilan University, Ramat Gan, Israel*

*and*

DAVID I. MOSTOFSKY, PhD
*Department of Psychology, Boston University, Boston, MA, USA*

Humana Press

*Editors*
Shlomo Yehuda
Department of Psychology
Psychopharmacology Lab
Bar-Ilan University
52900 Ramat Gan, Israel
syehuda31@gmail.com

David I. Mostofsky
Department of Psychology
Boston University
64 Cummington St.
Boston MA 02215-2407
USA
david.mostofsky@gmail.com

*Series Editor*
Adrianne Bendich
GlaxoSmithKline Consumer Healthcare
Parsippany, NJ

ISBN 978-1-61779-665-4
e-ISBN 978-1-59745-462-9
DOI 10.1007/978-1-59745-462-9



Printed on acid-free paper

springer.com

# Series Editor Introduction

The Nutrition and Health series of books have, as an overriding mission, to provide health professionals with texts that are considered essential because each includes (1) a synthesis of the state of the science, (2) timely, in-depth reviews by the leading researchers in their respective fields, (3) extensive, up-to-date fully annotated reference lists, (4) a detailed index, (5) relevant tables and figures, (6) identification of paradigm shifts and the consequences, (7) virtually no overlap of information between chapters, but targeted inter-chapter referrals, (8) suggestions of areas for future research, and (9) balanced data-driven answers to patient /health professionals questions that are based upon the totality of evidence rather than the findings of any single study.

The series volumes are not the outcome of a symposium. Rather, each editor has the potential to examine a chosen area with a broad perspective, both in subject matter as well as in the choice of chapter authors. The international perspective, especially with regard to public health initiatives, is emphasized where appropriate. The editors, whose trainings are both research- and practice-oriented, have the opportunity to develop a primary objective for their book, define the scope and focus, and then invite the leading authorities from around the world to be part of their initiative. The authors are encouraged to provide an overview of the field, discuss their own research, and relate the research findings to potential human health consequences. Because each book is developed de novo, the chapters are coordinated so that the resulting volume imparts greater knowledge than the sum of the information contained in the individual chapters.

*Iron Deficiency and Overload: From Basic Biology to Clinical Medicine*, edited by Shlomo Yehuda and David I. Mostofsky, fully exemplifies the Nutrition and Health Series' goals. Iron, an essential micronutrient for humans, is critical for the synthesis of DNA and proteins and serves as a co-factor for numerous enzymes involved in energy metabolism and brain biochemical functions, as well as being required for the transfer of oxygen to all cells in the body. Iron is also the most abundant transition metal in the human body. Yet, many nutritionists are more aware of the adverse effects of iron overload than its critical role in brain development. This volume is very timely as there is currently no up-to-date volume for professionals concerning the role of iron in nutrition and clinical medicine. Moreover, the fastest growing population in the United States as well as globally is those over 60 years of age and especially the oldest-old, those over 80 years of age; and iron status, both deficiencies as well as iron overload, becomes more of a medical issue as we age. This important text provides a timely review of the latest science concerning iron metabolism as well as practical, data-driven options to manage at-risk populations with the best accepted therapeutic nutritional interventions. The overarching goal of the editors is to provide fully referenced information to health professionals so they may enhance the nutritional welfare and overall health of clients and patients who are at risk for less than optimal iron status. This excellent, up-to-date volume will add great value to the practicing health professional as well as those professionals and students who have an interest in the latest information on the science behind iron requirements during the lifespan, and the potential for iron to modulate the effects of chronic diseases and conditions that are widely seen in the majority of patient populations.

Drs. Yehuda and Mostofsky, who have edited two other volumes in the Nutrition and Health Series, *Fatty Acids* and *Nutrients, Stress and Medical Disorders*, are internationally recognized leaders in the field of bioactive nutrients that affect the brain and nervous system. Both editors are excellent communicators and they have worked tirelessly to develop a book on iron that will be the benchmark in the field because of its extensive, in-depth chapters covering the most important aspects of the complex interactions between cellular functions, diet and iron requirements, and their impact on the chronic diseases as well as the acute conditions that can adversely affect the quality of life and health of both men and women. The introductory chapters provide readers with the newly recognized basics of the complexities involved in assuring that iron is absorbed and moves from the absorptive surface to the intestinal cell, then to the blood, and then to target organs and organelles without oxidizing the vital molecules that are nearby. The chapters in the first part of the volume concerned with iron biochemistry and metabolism provide the reader with a clear understanding of the state of the science and where gaps in knowledge still remain so that the clinically related chapters can be more easily understood. Chapters include clear explanations of the importance of serum ferritin as the best measure of body iron stores. The value of other, less sensitive measures of body iron stores, including serum iron, total iron-binding capacity, and transferrin saturation, are explained. Of importance to patient care, normal values for the more common iron status measures that are not directly related to body iron stores, including hemoglobin, hematocrit, and erythrocyte protoporphyrin, are provided in informative tables.

There is an important update on the genetics of iron metabolism and the role of mutations in the discoveries of critical ligands responsible for import and export of iron from cells. Moreover, the authors have provided excellent diagrams that help the reader to visualize the movement of iron within the cellular compartments, especially the mitochondria. The final chapter in this part reviews the administration of iron and provides practical information about the myriad of compounds that can be given to reduce iron deficiency, including oral as well as parenteral choices. Detailed information about dosing and potential drug/iron interactions is tabulated. Additionally, therapy for iron overload from either primary or secondary hemochromatoses is described in detail. Thus, in the first part of the volume, the reader is provided with valuable information about the basics of iron metabolism as well as its use to prevent deficiencies, and also the treatment of iron overload.

The second part of the volume contains seven chapters that examine the effects of iron overload and deficiency in depth. Specific emphasis is placed on the importance of iron in brain function. Iron is required for the optimal functioning of the enzymes responsible for the synthesis and degradation of the major brain neuropeptides, including dopamine, serotonin, and noradrenalin. Iron is found in specific sites within the brain, and the activity of neurotransmitters that require iron and the site of iron within the brain have been correlated with behavioral effects seen with iron deficiency, especially in the youngest children that are affected. Iron is also required for the synthesis of myelin, and the consequences of low iron status in the neonatal brain may be the result of lower than normal formation of the protective myelin sheath covering critical brain neurons. Important new studies that examine the interaction between zinc and iron in the brain are described and provide further evidence of the complexity of nutrient–nutrient interactions. In addition to the adverse effects of low iron status in children, excess iron within the brain has been associated with a number of neurodegenerative diseases, some of which are also associated with aging. These include Parkinson's disease, Alzheimer's disease, Friedreich's ataxia, Wilson's disease, and others. Additionally, as we age, there is an accumulation of iron in the brain that may participate in oxidative damage to neural tissues. Enhanced synthesis of enzymes that result in increased iron in mitochondria and concomitant increased oxidative damage have been seen in the brain tissues from animal models of human neurodegenerative diseases as well as in the tissues from affected human brains. Separate chapters examine the importance of iron to the synthesis of brain neuromodulators including dopamine. Dopamine is required for the processing of environmental information involved in forming perceptions and also for movement. Iron is required for the synthesis of dopamine, and the recent data on the effects of dietary deficiency on brain dopamine secretion and function are well described. Impairment of the dopamine system in the brain is associated with psychotic and psychoaffective disorders including illicit drug use. Attention-deficit hyperactivity disorder (ADHD) may also be related to low iron in the brain although further research is needed to determine if the association is linked to cause and effect. The depth of information in this volume is clearly exemplified by the chapter that looks at the distribution of iron in the neurons and oligodendrocytes that are responsible for synthesizing myelin during iron deficiency, normal iron intake, as well as iron overload. Under normal conditions, cellular iron concentrations in the brain are tightly controlled. When iron is lacking, brain neurons alter their metabolism and less myelin is formed. Dietary iron deficiency is associated with a decrease in IQ and depression in mood; there is a concomitant decrease in dopamine levels. As in animal models, duration and magnitude of iron deficiency determines the extent of cognitive deficits. Neonatal iron deficiency can adversely affect hearing, the endocrine system, and the immune system.

When iron levels are abnormally high, the brain reduces the level of iron taken into the brain and is resistant to the adverse effects of iron overload initially, but peripheral changes may result in secondary damage to the brain that results in oxidative damage. Aging is also associated with progressive increases in brain iron levels. Neurodegenerative diseases seen in aging can be characterized by their impaired iron homeostasis; however, it is not clear if this is a cause-and-effect relationship or that the iron excess occurs after some initiating event.

The essentiality of iron for hemoglobin production and the consequences of iron deficiency as well as iron deficiency anemia are described in detail in Chapter 10 concerning the peripheral effects of iron deficiency. In addition to the adverse effects of iron deficiency on oxygen-carrying capacity of the blood, there are many non-hematological clinical manifestations of iron deficiency. Often, the skin color will be reduced and this may be due to vasoconstriction in the skin; there may be increased cardiac output and breathing may be labored; muscle fatigue and cramping are often seen. Endurance is lessened and may be the consequence of reduction in iron-requiring enzymes. Detailed descriptions of the peripheral effects of human iron deficiency are tabulated for the reader. The final chapter in the second part reviews the newest research on the interactions between the brain and the immune system and how iron status affects these interactions, mainly through the effects of cytokines on cerebral neurons.

Part III includes chapters that examine the newest diagnostic tools that can be used to detect iron in the brain and also chapters that describe the clinical aspects of iron-associated central nervous system disorders. High-field magnetic resonance imaging scanners can identify iron deposits in distinct parts of the brain. MRIs can distinguish between iron in the form of hemoglobin, iron released in a hemorrhagic stroke or small hemorrhages, and endogenous iron within brain cells. Because MRIs are non-invasive, these have become a critically important tool in diagnosing the genetic defects associated with increased brain iron; the disorders are tabulated in the chapter. The next clinically focused chapter provides extensive information concerning the association of iron levels in specific areas in the brain with the development of Alzheimer's disease and, in the next chapter, the potential role of iron metabolism in brain mitochondria and the physical manifestations of the most common genetically inherited disorders of the central nervous system. A number of genetic defects result in abnormal accumulation of iron in certain cerebral areas whereas iron accumulation appears to be secondary in other inherited disorders. The adverse consequences of reactive iron on brain tissue and cells, and even the subcellular compartments, are described in detail. Valuable explanations for differential diagnoses and treatment of defects in iron handling in the genetic disorders discussed, including Friedreich's ataxia and hemochromatosis, are included.

The final part of the volume addresses the public health issues of iron status (both overload and deficiency) in populations around the globe. The first chapter in this part reviews the survey data that examine the association of iron overload with cardiovascular disease risk and finds no clear, consistent association between these two factors in studies that have looked in populations across the world. This chapter includes unique tables containing heretofore unpublished analyses from the Center for Disease Control that compare serum transferrin to ferritin levels and these biomarkers in different age groups and sexes. With regard to iron deficiency, low iron status is a critical risk factor for optimal development of the growing fetus and young child and the health of women especially during pregnancy. Globally, it has been recognized for nearly 50 years that iron deficiency and the more severe iron deficiency anemia are the most common nutritionally related deficiencies seen throughout the world. The chapter on the global consequences of iron deficiency includes a comprehensive review of the history, World Health Organization (WHO) activities, and biological effects of this deficiency, especially in women of childbearing potential and young children in developing as well as in the developed nations. Because of the clinical importance of iron status in young children and women of childbearing potential, each of these population groups is examined in depth in subsequent separate chapters. We are reminded in the chapter on children that there remains no "gold standard" test for iron deficiency anemia and thus the criteria used by nations differ. Yet, it is agreed that iron deficiency alone can result in reduced cognitive function and other mental deficits that may not be reversible. Low birth weight and premature birth are the risk factors for neonatal iron deficiency as there was insufficient time for iron storage. Other physiological factors as well as nutritional factors that increase risk are outlined along with suggestions for reducing the risk of iron deficiency in childhood. The following chapter outlines the factors that increase the risk of iron deficiency in women of childbearing potential as well as the consequences of iron deficiency, the alterations in iron measures during pregnancy and lactation and their relevance to actual iron status, the association of low iron status and infertility, and the effects of low iron status on overall women's health.

The editors of this comprehensive volume have chosen 29 of the most well-recognized and respected authors who are internationally distinguished researchers, clinicians, and epidemiologists who provide a broad foundation for understanding the role of iron in the molecular, genetic, cellular, and clinical aspects of nutritional and therapeutic management of iron status. Hallmarks of all of the 19 chapters include complete explanations of terms with the abbreviations fully defined for the reader and consistent use of terminology between chapters. Key features of the volume include informative bulleted summary points and key words that are at the beginning of each chapter, and appendices that include a detailed list of food sources of iron as well as an up-to-date compilation of the normal values for blood levels for iron constituents Recommendations and practice guidelines are included at the end of relevant chapters. The volume contains more than 65 detailed tables and informative figures, an extensive, detailed index, and more than 2000 up-to-date references that provide the reader with excellent sources of worthwhile information about nutrition options to help maintain optimal iron status.

In conclusion, *Iron Deficiency and Overload: From Basic Biology to Clinical Medicine*, edited by Shlomo Yehuda and David I. Mostofsky, provides health professionals in many areas of research and practice with the most up-to-date, well-referenced volume on the importance of iron status in determining the potential for optimal human development, especially in the central nervous system. This volume will serve the reader as the benchmark in this complex area of interrelationships between the essentiality of iron; its functions throughout the body including the biochemistry of iron-containing enzymes and other active molecules involved in iron absorption, transport, metabolism, and excretion; the importance of optimal iron status on immune function, the function of the heart, blood, lungs, kidney, muscle, bone, and the brain. Moreover, the interactions between genetic and environmental factors and the numerous co-morbidities seen with both iron deficiency and iron overload in the most at-risk populations are clearly delineated so that students as well as practitioners can better understand the complexities of these interactions. Drs. Yehuda and Mostofsky are applauded for their efforts to develop the most authoritative resource in the field to date, and this excellent text is a very welcome addition to the Nutrition and Health Series.

***Adrianne Bendich, PhD, FACN***

# Preface

In Shakespeare's *The Twelfth Night*, the story is told of a young woman who became severely depressed because she was in love with somebody and could not tell anyone about it, not even the beloved himself. She is described as suffering from a "green and yellow melancholy," a green sickness resulting from the teenager having fallen in love. It is a fact that iron deficiency commonly occurs after a few menstrual periods and imparts a green color to the complexion, while the yellow is no doubt due to jaundice and liver disease that will often cause a person to become depressed.

Iron deficiency is ever-present among all populations throughout the world, irrespective of race, culture, or ethnic background. Even with the latest advances in medicine, improved nutrition, and the ready availability of cheap oral iron, there is still no satisfactory explanation for the widespread occurrence of iron deficiency or for the absence of effective treatment. Several thousand years ago, human societies changed with the advent of the agrarian revolution, when humans turned to agriculture and to eat more fruits and vegetables than meat. The diet became iron-deficient and new epidemic infections emerged due to the stressors of crowding and lifestyle changes. This change of diet increased the frequency of iron deficiency. Some historians go so far as to claim that nutritional deficiency and iron deficiency, in particular, were the major factors responsible for the disappearance of the Maya culture.

The old notion that iron deficiency effects are mediated by the hemoglobin system and its corresponding decrease in oxygen supply to the tissues has been replaced by the findings that, in addition to the impact on the oxygen system, iron plays a major role in brain neurochemistry (e.g., neurotransmitters) and brain structure (e.g., myelin). Recent studies indicate that overload of iron might be linked to severe CNS age-related disorders, not least because iron is a substrate for free radicals. The story is unfolding, and clearly multidisciplinary approaches are needed to study the integrated effects of iron and brain and behavior and health disorders.

*Iron Deficiency and Overload: From Biology to Clinical Medicine* represents our attempt to present a sampling of the major issues in iron research, from the most basic research level to human applications. We have assembled chapters whose topics reflect the excitement in current theoretical development and laboratory activity in this area. The distinguished authors who contributed to this volume address their presentations to professionals and graduate students from diverse areas, disciplines, who need to be better informed about the concepts, methodologies, and current status of the field. Such information is all too often to be found only in the specialized scientific literature of some neighboring discipline and not likely to be routinely consulted by all. We leave the reader to forge the individual integration of the information provided in this volume.

We are most appreciative of the support provided by Humana Press in bringing this book to publication. We are especially grateful to Paul Dolgert, Editorial Director, and to Dr. Adrianne Bendich, Series Editor, for their constant guidance and help. We hope that this book will encourage more scientists and researchers to focus on issues in the topic of iron deficiency and iron overload, in order to gain a better understanding of the problems and to devise better methods to overcome those problems.

***Shlomo Yehuda***
***David I. Mostofsky***

# Contents

Series Editor Introduction .................... v
Preface .................... xi
Contributors .................... xv

PART I: IRON BIOCHEMISTRY AND METABOLISM

1 The Cellular Physiology of Iron .................... 3
***Gregory J. Anderson and Christopher D. Vulpe***

2 Regulation of Iron Absorption and Distribution .................... 31
***Gladys Oluyemisi Latunde-Dada and Robert J. Simpson***

3 The Role of Hepcidin in Iron Homeostasis .................... 51
***Tomas Ganz***

4 Iron as Nutrient: Strategies for Iron Acquisition and Usage by Pathogenic Microorganisms .................... 65
***Eric Massé and Peter D. Pawelek***

5 Iron as a Drug and Drug–Drug Interactions .................... 77
***Tracy M. Hagemann and Teresa V. Lewis***

PART II: IRON OVERLOAD AND DEFICIENCY PATHOLOGIES

6 Iron Deficiency and Excess in the Brain: Implications for Cognitive Impairment and Neurodegeneration .................... 95
***Moussa B.H. Youdim, Manfred Gerlach, and Peder Riederer***

7 Brain Iron Deposition in Aging and Disease: Role of HO-1 .................... 125
***Hyman M. Schipper***

8 Iron Deficiency and Neuropharmacology .................... 141
***Laura Bianco, Erica Unger, and John Beard***

9 Peripheral Effects of Iron Deficiency .................... 159
***Daniel B. Costa and Reed E. Drews***

10 Iron-Metabolism in Neurons of the Motor System of the Central Nervous System: Lessons from Iron Deficiency and Overloading Pathologies .................... 181
***Torben Moos***

**11** The Effects of Brain Iron Deficiency on Cognitive and Behavioral Aspects ......... 195
***S. Yehuda, S. Rabinovitz, R.L. Carasso, and D.I. Mostofsky***

**12** Stress, Immunology, and Cytokines ........................................ 207
***Dvora Sredni-Kenigsbuch***

**Part III: Diagnostic and Clinical Aspects in CNS Disorders**

**13** MRI of Brain Iron and Neurodegenerative Diseases: A Potential Biomarker ........ 223
***John F. Schenck***

**14** Alzheimer's Dementia ........................................ 241
***Seema Gulyani and Mark P. Mattson***

**15** Inherited Disorders of Brain Iron Homeostasis ........................................ 251
***Hyman M. Schipper and Prem Ponka***

**Part IV: Public Health Issues**

**16** Iron and Heart Disease: A Review of the Epidemiologic Data.................... 279
***Christopher T. Sempos, Anne C. Looker, Daniel L. McGee, and Jürgen Rehm***

**17** Global Concept of Iron Deficiency ........................................ 299
***S.M. Lewis and J.C. Emmanuel***

**18** Nutritional Iron Deficiency in Early Childhood ........................................ 313
***Robert J.D. Moy***

**19** Iron and Women's Health ........................................ 327
***Adrianne Bendich and Ronit Zilberboim***

Appendix A: *Reference Ranges for Common Laboratory Assays of Iron Metabolism* ....... 351
***Anthony N. Sireci and Alexander Kratz***

Appendix B: *Nutritional Sources of Iron*........................................ 355
***Anthony N. Sireci and Alexander Kratz***

Subject Index ........................................ 359

# Contributors


GREGORY J. ANDERSON*, PHD • *Iron Metabolism Laboratory, Queensland Institute of Medical Research, P.O. Royal Brisbane Hospital, Brisbane, Queensland, Australia*

JOHN BEARD*, PHD • *Department of Nutritional Sciences, College of Health and Human Development, The Pennsylvania State University, University Park, PA*

ADRIANNE BENDICH*, PHD • *GSK Consumer Health Care, 1500 Littleton Road, Parsippany, NJ*

LAURA BIANCO, PHD • *Department of Nutritional Sciences, The Pennsylvania State University, University Park, PA*

R.L. CARASSO • *Department of Neurology, Hillel Yaffe Medical Center, Hadera, Israel*

DANIEL B. COSTA*, MD • *Division of Hematology/Oncology, Harvard Medical School, Beth Israel Deaconess Medical Center, Boston, MA*

REED E. DREWS, MD • *Division of Hematology/Oncology, Harvard Medical School, Beth Israel Deaconess Medical Center, Boston, MA*

JEAN EMMANUEL, MB, CHB • *WHO Department of Blood Safety and Clinical Technologies, New Delhi, India; Blood Transfusion Medicine Consultant, Borrowdale, Zimbabwe*

TOMAS GANZ*, PHD, MD • *Department of Medicine, UCLA David Geffen School of Meldicine, Los Angeles, CA*

MANFRED GERLACH • *Laboratory of Clinical Neurochemistry, Department of Psychiatry, University of Wurzburg, Wurzbrug, Germany*

SEEMA GULYANI*, PHD, RN • *Laboratory of Neurosciences, National Institute on Aging Intramural Research Program, Baltimore, MD*

TRACY M. HAGEMANN*, PHARMD • *University of Oklahoma Health Sciences Center, College of Pharmacy, Oklahoma City, OK,*

ALEXANDER KRATZ*, MD, PHD • *Core Laboratory, Columbia University Medical Center, New York Presbyterian Hospital, New York*

GLADYS O. LATUNDE-DADA*, PHD • *Nutrition Research Division, Department of Biochemistry, King's College London, London, UK*

TERESA V. LEWIS*, PHARMD, BCPS • *University of Oklahoma Health Sciences Center, College of Pharmacy, Oklahoma City, OK*

ANNE C. LOOKER, PHD, RD • *National Center for Health Statistics, Centers for Disease Control and Prevention, Hyattsville, MD*

ERIC MASS*, PHD • *RNA Group, Departement de Biochimie, Universite de Sherbrooke, Sherbrooke, QC, Canada*

* Senior Authors

Mark P. Mattson, PhD • *Laboratory of Neurosciences, National Institute on Aging Intramural Research Program, Baltimore, MD*
Daniel L. McGee Sr, PhD • *Department of Statistics, College of Arts and Sciences, Florida State University, Tallahassee, FL*
S. Mitchell Lewis BSc, MD, DCP, FRCPath, FIMBMS • *Department of Haematology, Imperial College Faculty of Medicine, Hammersmith Hospital, London*
Torben Moos*, MD, PhD, DMSc • *Section of Neurobiology, Department of Health Science & Technology, Aalborg University, Denmark*
D.I. Mostofsky • *Boston University, Psychology Department, Boston, MA*
Robert J. D. Moy*, MD • *Institute of Child Health, University of Birmingham, Birmingham, UK*
Peter D. Pawelek, PhD • *Department of Chemistry and Biochemistry, Concordia University, Montreal, QC, Canada*
Prem Ponka, MD, PhD • *Department Neurology & Neurosurgery, Lady Davis Institute for Medical Research, Centre for Neurotranslational Research, Sir Mortimer B. Davis- Jewish General Hospital, McGill University, Montreal, Quebec, Canada*
S. Rabinovitz • *Departments of Psychology and Criminology, Bar Ilan University, Ramat Gan, Israel*
Jürgen Rehm, PhD • *Centre for Addiction and Mental Health, Toronto, Ontario, Canada*
Peter Riederer • *Laboratory of Clinical Neurochemistry, Department of Psychiatry, University of Wurzburg, Wurzbrug, Germany*
John Schenck*, MD, PhD • *General Electric Global Research Center, Niskayuna, NY*
Hyman M. Schipper*, MD, PhD FRPC • *Department Neurology &Neurosurgery, Lady Davis Institute for Medical Research, Centre for Neurotranslational Research, Sir Mortimer B. Davis-Jewish General Hospital, McGill University, Montreal, Quebec, Canada*
Christopher T. Sempos*, PhD • *Office of Dietary Supplements, National Institutes of Health, Bethesda, MD*
Robert J. Simpson*, DPhil • *Nutrition Sciences Division, Department of Biochemistry, King's College London, London, UK*
Anthony N. Sireci, MD • *New York Presbyterian Hospital, New York, NY*
Dvora Sredni-Kenigsbuch • *Interdisciplinary Department, Bar Ilan University, Ramat Gan, Israel*
Erica Unger, PhD • *Department of Nutritional Sciences, The Pennsylvania State University, University Park, PA*
Christopher D. Vulpe, MD, PhD • *Department of Nutritional Sciences and Toxicology, University of California, Berkeley, Berkeley, CA*
S. Yehuda • *Bar-Ilan University, Department of Psychology, Ramat Gan, Israel*
Moussa B.H. Youdim*, PhD • *Eve Topf and National Parkinson Foundation, Faculty of Medicine, Centers for Excellence for Neurodegenerative Diseases Technion, Haifa, Israel; Department of Pharmacology, Technion-Faculty of Medicine, Rappaport Family Research Institute, Haifa, Israel*
Ronit Zilberboim, PhD • *GSK Consumer Health Care, 1500 Littleton Road, Parsippany, NJ*

# I

# Iron Biochemistry and Metabolism

# 1 The Cellular Physiology of Iron

*Gregory J. Anderson and Christopher D. Vulpe*

**Summary**

- Most iron is delivered to cells bound to the plasma protein transferrin.
- Mitochondria are a major sink for cellular iron due to their key role on heme and Fe—S cluster synthesis.
- Iron not required immediately for biochemical processes is stored within ferritin.
- Iron is exported from cells via the plasma membrane transporter ferroportin.
- Cellular iron uptake and storage are regulated via the IRE/IRP system at the post-transcriptional level.
- Hepcidin has emerged as a central regulator of body iron homeostasis.

**Key Words:** Iron homeostasis; iron transport; iron storage; hepcidin; systemic regulation

## 1. INTRODUCTION

Iron is an essential component of virtually all living cells, and it certainly is a necessity for all human cells. The ability of iron to convert between two thermodynamically stable oxidation states, the $Fe^{3+}$ or ferric form and the $Fe^{2+}$ or ferrous form, under physiological conditions makes it ideally suited to the catalysis of biochemical reactions, and a large number of enzymes depend on iron for their biological function. These very characteristics that make iron so valuable for living systems also mean that the metal is able to catalyze reactions leading to the production of toxic oxygen radicals, particularly when it is present in excess. To deal with this dual nature of iron, individual cells and the body as a whole have evolved sophisticated mechanisms for regulating iron influx and efflux. It is important to supply enough iron to cells to meet their metabolic requirements, but equally important to prevent excess iron delivery as this could place the cell under oxidative stress. In recent years our understanding of iron metabolism, both at the cellular level and at the level of the whole organism, has advanced enormously and these developments will be summarized in this chapter. While emphasis will be placed on how iron is taken up and utilized by individual cells, it is not possible to cover this area without briefly considering systemic iron homeostasis as this ultimately drives what happens at the cellular level.

A summary of some of the main proteins involved in cellular iron homeostasis is provided in Table 1. Many of these proteins were identified originally by searching for the source of the genetic abnormality in various inherited disorders of iron metabolism, and the role of most has been confirmed by disruption of the relevant gene in murine models. In view of the importance of

From: *Nutrition and Health: Iron Deficiency and Overload*
Edited by: S. Yehuda and D.I. Mostofsky, DOI 10.1007/978-1-59745-462-9_1

Table 1
**Some Proteins of Cellular Iron Homeostasis and Their Functions**

| *Protein* | *Protein Abbrev.* | *Gene Symbol*[a] | *Function/Role in Iron Metabolism* | *Human Disease* | *Animal Model* | *Main Phenotype* |
|---|---|---|---|---|---|---|
| *Iron Uptake* | | | | | | |
| Transferrin | Tf | *TF* | Plasma iron transport | Atransferrinemia | *hpx* mouse | Iron deficiency anemia with tissue iron overload |
| Transferrin receptor 1 | TfR1 | *TFRC* | Internalization of diferric transferrin | None known | *Tfrc*$^{-/-}$ mouse | Embryonic lethality in homozygote. Mild anemia in heterozygotes. |
| Divalent metal-ion transporter 1 | DMT1 | *SLC11A2* | Ferrous iron importer | Refractory hypochromic, microcytic anemia | Belgrade rat<br>*mk* mouse<br>*Slc11a2*$^{-/-}$ mouse | Iron deficiency anemia |
| Six-transmembrane epithelial antigen of prostate protein 3 | STEAP3 | *STEAP3* | Iron reductase of erythroid cells | None known | *nm1054* mouse | Iron deficiency anemia |
| Exocyst complex component 6 | SEC15L1 | *EXOC6* | Vesicle trafficking | None known | *hbd* mouse | Iron deficiency anemia |
| Duodenal cytochrome b | DCYTB | *CYBRD1* | Enterocyte brush border reductase | None known | *Cybrd1*$^{-/-}$ mouse | No overt phenotype |
| *Iron Storage* | | | | | | |
| H-ferritin | H-Ft | *FTH1* | Iron storage | None known definitively | *Fth1*$^{-/-}$ mouse | Embryonic lethality |
| L-ferritin | L-Ft | *FTL* | Iron storage | Hereditary hyperferritinemia cataract syndrome | None known | Bilateral cataracts |

| | | | | | | |
|---|---|---|---|---|---|---|
| *Iron Export* | | | | | | |
| Ferroportin | FPN | *SLC40A1* | Ferrous iron exporter | Hemochromatosis type 4 | *Slc40a1*$^{-/-}$ mouse | Iron overload in heterozygous state; embryonic lethality in homozygotes |
| Ceruloplasmin | Cp | *CP* | Iron oxidase | Aceruloplasminemia | *Cp*$^{-/-}$ mouse | Iron overload; CNS dysfunction |
| Hephaestin | Hp | *HEPH* | Iron oxidase (gut and CNS) | None known | *sla* mouse | Iron deficiency anemia |
| *Mitochondrial Iron Metabolism* | | | | | | |
| Mitoferrin | MFRN | *SLC25A37* | Mitochondrial iron importer | None known | *frascati* zebrafish | Iron deficiency anemia; erythroid maturation arrest |
| Frataxin | FXN | *FXN* | Mitochondrial iron utilization | Friedreich ataxia | *Fxn*$^{-/-}$ mouse Several others | Neuromuscular and cardiac dysfunction in humans; embryonic lethality in mice |
| Mitochondrial ferritin | MtF | *FTMT* | Mitochondrial iron storage | None known | None known | |
| *Cellular Regulation* | | | | | | |
| Iron-regulatory protein 1 | IRP1 | *ACO1* | Iron-dependent RNA binding protein | None known | *Aco1*$^{-/-}$ mouse | Negligible. Some abnormalities in brown fat and kidney. |
| Iron-regulatory protein 2 | IRP2 | *IREB2* | Iron-dependent RNA binding protein | None known | *Ireb*$^{-/-}$ mouse | Anemia; CNS abnormalities of varying severity |
| *Systemic Regulation* | | | | | | |
| Hepcidin | HEPC | *HAMP* | Regulator of iron release into plasma | Hemochromatosis type 2B | *Hamp1*$^{-/-}$ mouse | Severe iron overload |

**Table 1**
(continued)

| *Protein* | *Protein Abbrev.* | *Gene Symbol*[a] | *Function/Role in Iron Metabolism* | *Human Disease* | *Animal Model* | *Main Phenotype* |
|---|---|---|---|---|---|---|
| Hemochromatosis protein | HFE | *HFE* | Regulator of hepcidin | Hemochromatosis type 1 | *Hfe*$^{-/-}$ mouse | Iron overload |
| Transferrin receptor 2 | TfR2 | *TFR2* | Regulator of hepcidin | Hemochromatosis type 3 | *Tfr2*$^{-/-}$ mouse | Iron overload |
| Hemojuvelin | HJV | *HFE2* | Regulator of hepcidin | Hemochromatosis type 2A | *Hjv*$^{-/-}$ mouse | Severe iron overload |

[a]Human Genome Organization approved symbol.

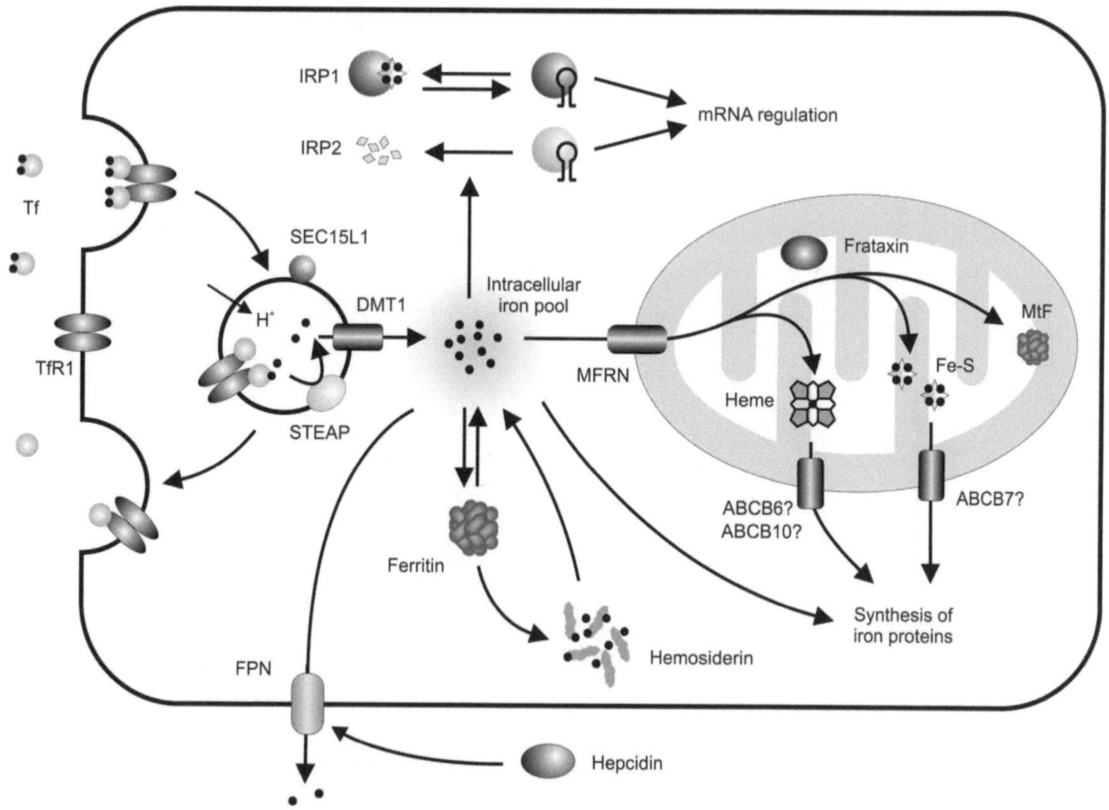


**Fig. 1. Basic iron trafficking and regulation in the cell.** Diferric transferrin is the main source of iron for most types of cells. It binds to TfR1 on the plasma membrane and the complex is taken up by receptor-mediated endocytosis. Acidification of the endosome and reduction of the iron (likely by one of the STEAP proteins) facilitate iron release from Tf and it is subsequently transported via DMT1 into the cytoplasm. The TfR1–apoTf complex is recycled to the cell surface where Tf is released to bind more iron. Iron in the cytoplasm is thought to be present in a poorly characterized, low molecular weight pool. Iron from this pool can be used for incorporation into proteins either in the cytoplasm or in mitochondria. Mitochondria play a particularly important role in the synthesis of heme and Fe—S clusters. Iron in excess of metabolic needs is stored within ferritin; and when large amounts of iron are present, hemosiderin may form from aggregated, degraded ferritin. Iron in the intracellular pool will also determine the activity of the regulatory proteins IRP1 and IRP2. High iron will lead to the degradation of IRP2 and the assembly of an Fe—S cluster in the active site of IRP1, converting it to an aconitase. Under low iron conditions the IRPs bind to stem-loop structures (IREs) in the mRNAs encoding key iron proteins and regulate their expression. Iron is released from the cell through the plasma membrane protein FPN, the expression of which responds to extracellular hepcidin.

these inherited conditions, they are also summarized in Table 1. The role of the proteins mentioned in the text is shown schematically in Figs. 1 and 2. Figure 1 shows a "generic" cell, while Fig. 2 shows several specific cell types that play specialized roles in iron physiology.

## 2. WHAT IS IRON USED FOR IN THE CELL?

Iron is incorporated into a large number of cellular proteins. Many are involved in enzyme catalysis and electron transport, whereas others are involved in carrying oxygen or storing and transporting iron itself. Major classes of such proteins include those with heme centers

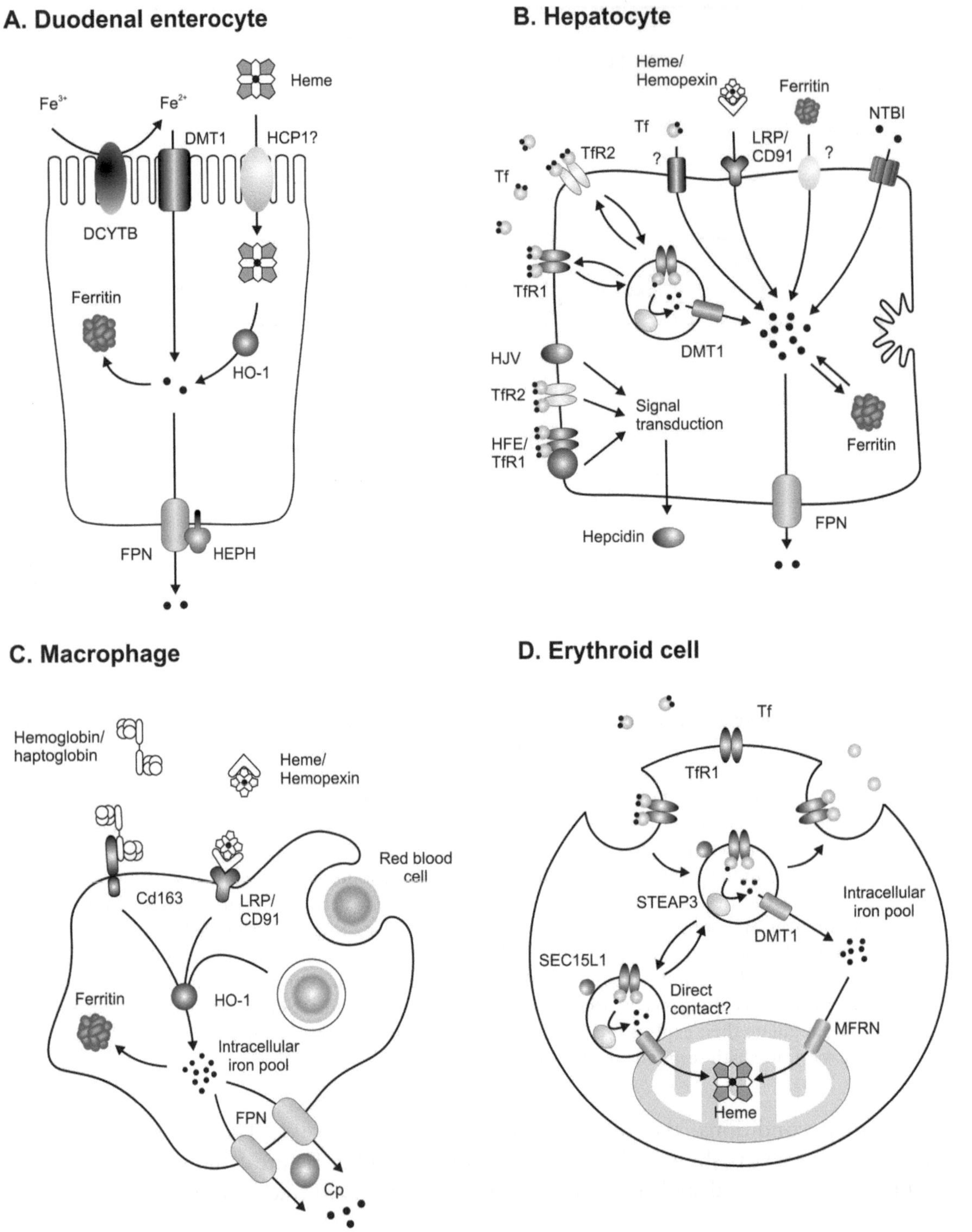


**Fig. 2. Some characteristics of iron metabolism in specific cell types.** While most body cells share some similarities in iron homeostasis, different types of cells have particular specialized functions. Several examples are shown here. **(A)** The duodenal enterocyte plays an essential role in transporting iron from the intestinal lumen across the brush border and basolateral membranes into the circulation. Heme and non-heme iron are taken across the brush border by separate mechanisms, but appear to share the same basolateral efflux step **(B)** The hepatocyte

(hemoproteins) and those with iron–sulfur clusters, but many proteins utilize the coordination chemistry of iron in quite different ways and the list of non-heme, non-iron–sulfur proteins is growing steadily. A comprehensive overview of the biology of iron-containing proteins is beyond the scope of this chapter, but excellent online resources exist to explore this area further (e.g., http://metallo.scripps.edu/promise/; http://pfam.sanger.ac.uk/).

Quantitatively, the most abundant iron-containing proteins in the body are the hemoproteins hemoglobin and myoglobin (Wilson & Reeder, 2008). These proteins carry the oxygen required for cellular respiration and are produced in large amounts by specialized cells and tissues – immature erythroid cells in the case of hemoglobin and myocytes in the case of myoglobin. The synthesis of many other hemoproteins is more widely distributed as they play central roles in basic cellular metabolism. Examples include the cytochromes (*a*, *b*, and *c*) that play essential roles in electron transfer, e.g., in the electron transport chain of mitochondria, while yet others such as the catalases, cytochrome oxidase, and cytochrome P450 s play important catalytic roles.

Another major class of iron-containing proteins is those involving iron–sulfur (Fe—S) clusters (Rouault & Tong, 2005; Lill & Mühlenhoff, 2006). The iron–sulfur centers can either be simple (containing varying, yet defined, proportions of iron and sulfur atoms) or complex (containing other moieties such as flavins and heme in addition to iron and sulfur). Iron–sulfur proteins play important roles in electron transport and catalysis. Examples include the mitochondrial respiratory complexes I–III, ferrochelatase, and xanthine oxidase. From the cellular iron physiologist's point of view, perhaps the best known iron–sulfur protein is cytosolic aconitase. In its iron-bound form it has aconitase activity, but when the Fe—S cluster is lost it becomes an mRNA-binding protein (IRP1) that plays a major role in the regulation of cellular iron homeostasis (Eisenstein, 2000). This will be considered in greater detail below.

The non-heme, non Fe—S proteins are a diverse group containing a range of different iron centres. Most have enzymatic activity, but under this banner also fall the iron storage and transport proteins, the ferritins and transferrin, respectively. These will be covered more thoroughly below. Proteins with mononuclear iron centers include the lipoxygenases and amino acid hydroxylases, whereas the best known of the proteins with dinuclear iron centers is ribonucleotide reductase, the rate-limiting enzyme in DNA synthesis.

## 3. CELLULAR IRON UPTAKE

Iron can be delivered to cells in a number of different ways. Under normal conditions, the great majority of iron circulating in the blood is bound to transferrin (Tf), and diferric Tf is the dominant source of iron for most cells (Trinder & Morgan, 2001; Chua, Graham, Trinder, & Olynyk, 2007). However, in certain pathological states, notably iron-loading disorders, when the capacity of plasma Tf to bind iron is exceeded, non-transferrin-bound iron (NTBI) can make a major contribution to cellular iron uptake (Parkes & Templeton, 2001; Hider, 2002). Iron from

**Fig. 2.** (continued) plays an important role in iron storage and it can handle iron in a range of forms (diferric Tf, NTBI, heme/hemopexin, ferritin). It is also the main site of synthesis of hepcidin, and thus plays a central role in the regulation of systemic iron metabolism. (**C**) Macrophages scavenge senescent red blood cells and various iron-containing proteins and recycle the iron to the plasma. They also have an important role to play in iron storage. (**D**) Immature erythroid cells are specifically adapted for producing large amounts of hemoglobin and express high levels of TfR1 on their plasma membrane. Macrophages, enterocytes, and hepatocytes are major contributors to the plasma iron pool and are all particularly responsive to the regulatory peptide hepcidin.

circulating heme, hemoglobin, and ferritin can also be utilized by some cells, but these do not usually deliver physiologically significant amounts of iron and they become relevant under pathological conditions only, e.g., with hemolysis or tissue damage. Under normal conditions the levels of these potential iron sources are very low in plasma.

### *3.1. Transferrin-Bound Iron Delivery to Cells*

Transferrin delivers its iron to cells by binding with high affinity to the plasma membrane protein transferrin receptor 1 (TfR1) (Enns, 2001; Aisen, 2004). TfR1 is a disulfide-bonded, homodimeric receptor that traffics between the plasma membrane and various intracellular vesicular compartments. TfR1 binds diferric Tf with 10-fold higher affinity than monoferric Tf at physiological pH and 2,000-fold higher affinity than apotransferrin. After diferric Tf binds to its receptor, the complex is endocytosed through clathrin-coated pits. The resulting vesicles are then uncoated to become endosomes and are acidified by a proton-pumping ATPase. At a pH of around 5.5, iron is released from Tf, a process that also likely requires reduction (Watkins et al., 1992) and takes advantage of a conformational change in Tf which accompanies its binding to TfR1 (Bali, Zak, & Aisen, 1991). The iron released from Tf (now in its reduced or ferrous form) makes its way across the endosomal membrane and into the cytoplasm through the ferrous iron transporter divalent metal-ion transporter 1 (DMT1) (Fleming et al., 1998), which will be considered in more detail below. At the low pH of the endosome, the affinity of TfR1 for apoTf is much higher than at physiological pH and the two proteins remain bound as the endosome is recycled to the plasma membrane. Apotransferrin is then released into the extracellular milieu where it can participate in another round of iron binding and uptake.

While the basic aspects of the delivery of Tf-bound iron to cells have been known for some time, the recent analysis of two mouse strains with inherited disturbances in iron homeostasis has revealed further details. The *nm1054* mouse is characterized by a hypochromic, microcytic anemia, consistent with iron deficiency anemia (Ohgami, Campagna, & Antiochos, et al., 2005). The gene mutated in these mice has been identified as *STEAP3*, and subsequent studies have shown it to encode a candidate endosomal ferric iron reductase (Ohgami, Campagna, & Greer, et al., 2005). STEAP3 is expressed at high levels in immature erythroid cells, thus implicating it in the delivery of Tf-bound iron for hemoglobin production, but is also found in a wide range of other tissues where it might be expected to play a similar role. A number of homologs of STEAP3 have been identified, which have varying tissue expression patterns so there could be some functional redundancy in the STEAP system, particularly in non-erythroid tissues (Ohgami, Campagna, McDonald, & Fleming, 2006; Knutson, 2007). Another inherited microcytic, hypochromic anemia is found in hemoglobin-deficit (*hbd*) mice, and the defective gene in these animals has been identified as the exocyst protein *Sec15l1* (Lim et al., 2005). Sec15l1 has been co-localized with TfR1 in recycling endosomes (Zhang, Xiong, Tsukamoto, & Enns, 2004), and it is proposed that when Sec15l1 levels are reduced more rapid recycling of iron/Tf/TfR1-containing endosomes reduces the time available for iron delivery to the cytoplasm (Lim et al., 2005). It is long been known that the recycling of Tf-containing endosomes is defective in the immature erythroid cells of *hbd* mice (Garrick, Edwards, Hoke, & Bannerman, 1987; Zhang, Sheftel, & Ponka, 2006), but whether this is indeed the function of Sec15l1 remains unresolved. The apparent erythroid specificity of the *hbd* mutation suggests that the role of Sec15l1 may be performed by other proteins in non-erythroid tissues.

Since TfR1 represents the main avenue of iron uptake by most cells, the expression of the protein is highly regulated (Aisen, 2004). When cellular iron requirements are high, TfR1 levels decrease, and the opposite is seen when cells are iron replete. For example, immature erythroid cells have a particularly high iron requirement due to their synthesis of hemoglobin, so they express very high amounts of TfR1 on their surface. The mechanism by which TfR1 is regulated in response to changes in cellular iron demand will be considered in more detail below.

While the iron uptake of immature erythroid cells is dominated by the high-affinity uptake of diferric transferrin by TfR1, this is not the case for all cells. Many cell types, for example, hepatocytes and intestinal enterocytes, are able to utilize Tf-bound iron by both high- and low-affinity processes (Anderson, Powell, & Halliday, 1994; Chua et al., 2007). The molecular basis of the low-affinity process has long proved elusive. Reducing TfR1 expression (by antisense mRNA) (Trinder, Zak, & Aisen, 1996) or its ability to bind Tf (using antibodies) (Trinder, Morgan, & Baker, 1988) does not block the low-affinity process in hepatocytes and hepatoma cells, indicating that TfR1 is not involved. Recent studies suggest that the low-affinity process may be mediated by the TfR1 homolog transferrin receptor 2 (TfR2) (Kawabata et al., 1999; Lee, Oates, & Trinder, 2003; Robb, Ericsson, & Wessling-Resnick, 2004). TfR2, like TfR1, is a plasma membrane Tf-binding protein, but its affinity for diferric Tf is 25-fold lower than that of TfR1, making it a strong candidate for the low-affinity binding site. TfR2 also differs from TfR1 in its expression pattern. While TfR1 is expressed on all nucleate cells of the body, TfR2 has a much more restricted tissue distribution. High levels of expression are found on hepatic parenchymal cells (Fleming et al., 2000; Deaglio et al., 2002), with lower levels in immature erythroid cells, spleen, lung, skeletal muscle, and prostate. Immunohistochemistry has demonstrated TfR2 on the cell surface, although a considerable proportion is located at intracellular sites (Deaglio et al., 2002; Robb et al., 2004). This is consistent with earlier studies of the low-affinity process, indicating that diferric Tf is endocytosed and returned to the plasma membrane after iron delivery (Morgan, Smith, & Peters, 1986; Trinder, Morgan, & Baker, 1986; Trinder et al., 1996), although there is evidence in a hepatoma cell line that much of the Tf taken up by TfR2 remains intracellularly in multivesicular bodies (Robb et al., 2004). Also, unlike TfR1, TfR2 does not contain any iron-regulatory elements in its mRNA (see below) and the expression of the message is not regulated by cellular iron content (Fleming et al., 2000).

While TfR2 appears to be a strong candidate for the low-affinity uptake of transferrin-bound iron, other evidence suggests that this may not be the case. As noted above, TfR2 has a limited tissue distribution and some cell types that show low-affinity uptake of Tf, such as the crypt enterocytes in the small intestine, do not express TfR2. In addition, human patients with mutations in *TFR2*, or mice in which the *Tfr2* gene has been deleted, develop a form of iron-loading disease (or hemochromatosis) (Camaschella et al., 2000; Fleming et al., 2002). In this case, iron is very effectively delivered to tissues in the absence of TfR2. These lines of evidence suggest that TfR2 is not the sole pathway for the low-affinity uptake of transferrin-bound iron and may not be the major one. Other studies have suggested that iron-loaded Tf can be taken up by hepatocytes via proteoglycans or fluid-phase endocytosis and this could also be relevant in other cell types, but whether these represent quantitatively significant pathways is unclear (Trinder & Morgan, 2001).

Although it appears that most of the Tf-bound iron is taken up by cells via processes that involve the endocytosis of Tf, there is also evidence that Tf-bound iron can be released at the cell surface. This process has been described for several cell types, but is most prominent in hepatocytes (Thorstensen & Romslo, 1990). Membrane-impermeant iron chelators are able to reduce the uptake of iron from Tf, suggesting iron release at the cell surface (Cole & Glass, 1983; Thorstensen & Romslo, 1988). There is also evidence for a cell surface ferric iron reductase activity that may facilitate iron release from Tf (Thorstensen & Romslo, 1988). Furthermore, NTBI can reduce the uptake of Tf-bound iron and vice versa (Trinder & Morgan, 1997; Graham, Morgan, & Baker,

1998). NTBI alters neither the rate of Tf endocytosis nor iron uptake through the TfR-mediated pathways, suggesting it acts at the cell surface. The surface uptake of Tf-derived iron could involve DMT1, which recycles in the cell via the plasma membrane.

### *3.2. Iron Movement Across the Endosomal and Plasma Membranes – Divalent Metal-Ion Transporter 1*

Once Tf-bound iron has been delivered to the lumen of the endosome, it must still cross the endosomal membrane to reach the cytoplasm. This is achieved via the ferrous iron transporter divalent metal-ion transporter 1 (DMT1). DMT1 is a multi-spanning membrane protein that is widely distributed in body tissues (Gunshin et al., 1997; Courville, Chaloupka, & Cellier, 2006). While it is able to efficiently transport ferrous iron, as its name suggests it can also handle a wide range of other divalent metal ions including $Cu^{2+}$, $Zn^{2+}$, $Co^{2+}$, and $Cd^{2+}$. The major function of DMT1 in most cells appears to be the delivery of Tf-derived iron from the endosome to the cytoplasm (Bowen & Morgan, 1987; Fleming et al., 1998), but it also has a specialized role in the transport of iron across the brush border membrane of intestinal epithelial cells (Mackenzie & Garrick, 2005), a process that does not require Tf. Particularly high levels of DMT1 are found in duodenal enterocytes, immature erythroid cells, kidney, and brain, but at least some expression is found in all tissues examined (Courville et al., 2006). In addition to being involved in the uptake of Tf-bound iron through the TfR1 pathway, DMT1 is also likely to participate in iron uptake through the TfR2-mediated endocytosis of Tf and may contribute to the uptake of NTBI or Tf-derived iron at the cell surface (Trinder & Morgan, 1997; Trinder & Morgan, 2001).

Since DMT1 is involved in cellular iron acquisition, its expression is generally, but not always, increased when iron demand increases (Gunshin et al., 1997; Mims & Prchal, 2005). The basis of this regulation is only partially understood. *DMT1* mRNA has two 3′ splice variants, one of which, like TfR1, contains an iron-responsive element that regulates the stability of mRNA in an iron-dependent manner (see below). When cellular iron levels decline, the mRNA is stabilized and more protein is produced. However, DMT1 is not regulated solely at the level of message stability as the non-IRE splice variant also is upregulated by iron deficiency (e.g., Frazer et al., 2001), presumably at the level of transcription. The IRE-containing splice variant is particularly abundant in the duodenum, while in other tissues, such as the liver, the two splice forms are expressed at comparable levels (Tchernitchko, Bourgeois, Martin, & Beaumont, 2002). While the expression of DMT1 is increased substantially under iron-deficient conditions in some tissues and many cell lines (Mims & Prchal, 2005), in other tissues such as the kidney and liver there is either no change or even an increase in the presence of iron. For example, in the liver and in hepatoma cells, DMT1 levels are enhanced by iron loading (Trinder, Oates, Thomas, Sadlier, & Morgan, 2000; Scheiber-Mojdehkar, Sturm, Plank, Kryzer, & Goldenberg, 2003). The mechanism underlying this increase in DMT1 expression is unknown, as is the physiological significance of such a response. However, it may help reduce the level of potentially toxic NTBI in the circulation when the body iron load is high.

### *3.3. Non-transferrin-Bound Iron Uptake*

Under normal conditions the vast majority of iron in the plasma is bound to Tf, but a very small proportion is present as NTBI. In iron-loading syndromes, however, particularly those associated with elevated intestinal iron absorption such as HFE-associated hemochromatosis, the amount of iron in the plasma can increase to such an extent that the capacity of Tf to sequester it is exceeded. Under these conditions the level of NTBI can reach 10–15 μM, whereas it is essentially undetectable under normal conditions (Breuer, Shvartsman, & Cabantchik, 2008; Parkes

& Templeton, 2001). The precise form of NTBI has not been fully defined. Much is thought to be chelated by small organic acids such as citrate, but smaller amounts could be bound loosely to proteins such as albumin (Hider, 2002).

NTBI can be taken up very efficiently by various tissues, but particularly by the liver. This is well demonstrated in rare instances of congenital Tf deficiency in humans (atransferrinemia) and mice (Bernstein, 1987; Hayashi, Wada, Suzuki, & Shimizu, 1993). Despite lacking Tf, the affected individuals absorb iron from their diet very efficiently and large amounts are deposited in the liver and other tissues. In another study, wild-type mice were first given sufficient intravenous iron to saturate their circulating Tf, and a subsequent dose of radioactive NTBI was given either orally or intravenously (Craven et al., 1987). Most of the radioactive iron (and over 70% in the case of gastrointestinal administration) was taken up by the liver, irrespective of the route of administration, indicating how effective this process is. A significant amount was also directed to the pancreas. Studies in isolated perfused livers have also shown very efficient extraction of NTBI (Wright, Brissot, Ma, & Weisinger, 1986).

The molecular basis of NTBI uptake has not been fully resolved. Early studies indicated that reduction of ferric iron may be required prior to uptake (Randell, Parkes, Olivieri, & Templeton, 1994), and the uptake itself has the characteristics of a carrier-mediated process (Baker, Baker, & Morgan, 1998; Trinder & Morgan, 2001). Candidates for the carrier include DMT1, SFT (stimulator of Fe transport), ZIP14 (Zrt-Irt-like protein 14), and L-type voltage-dependent calcium channels, but apart from DMT1 the role of other proteins in iron transport remains relatively poorly understood. SFT was isolated as a membrane iron transporter from the erythroid leukemia cell line K562 by expression cloning in *Xenopus* oocytes (Gutierrez, Yu, Rivera, & Wessling-Resnick, 1997), while the zinc transporter ZIP14 has been shown to facilitate NTBI uptake in hepatocytes (Liuzzi, Aydemir, Nam, Knutson, & Cousins, 2006). Calcium channel blockers will inhibit iron uptake in cardiac myocytes, implying that such channels are involved in NTBI transport in these cells (Oudit et al., 2003). One interesting characteristic of NTBI uptake is that it is greater under iron-loading conditions than in iron deficiency (Randell et al., 1994; Parkes & Templeton, 2001; Chua, Olynyk, Leedman, & Trinder, 2004), and it has been proposed that this represents a protective response to remove potentially damaging NTBI from the circulation. In keeping with this, DMT1 expression is increased on the hepatocyte plasma membrane with iron loading (Trinder et al., 2000) and the expression of SFT is increased in the liver of iron-loaded hemochromatosis patients (J. Yu, Z. K. Yu, & Wessling-Resnick, 1998).

### *3.4. The Uptake of Other Forms of Iron*

Under certain, usually pathological, conditions, iron can appear in the circulation in the form of heme, hemoglobin, or ferritin. These proteins can be cleared efficiently and the iron reutilized. Hemoglobin released into the circulation is readily bound stoichiometrically by the liver-derived plasma protein haptoglobin (Wassell, 2000) and the hemoglobin/haptoglobin complex is taken up by macrophages via receptor-mediated endocytosis (Moestrup & Moller, 2004). CD163, a member of the SRCR scavenger receptor family, acts as a receptor for hemoglobin/haptoglobin complexes and is expressed on the surface of macrophages throughout the body (Kristiansen et al., 2001; Fabriek, Dijkstra, & van den Berg, 2005). These cells normally play a major role in the recycling of iron from senescent red blood cells, so they are well adapted to catabolizing hemoglobin (Knutson & Wessling-Resnick, 2003). Any free heme released into the circulation is rapidly sequestered by the liver-derived protein hemopexin (Tolosano & Altruda, 2002). The heme/hemopexin complex is removed from the circulation by low-density lipoprotein receptor-related protein (LRP)/CD91, a heterodimeric complex found on the surface of hepatocytes, macrophages, and some other cell types (Herz & Strickland, 2001; Hvidberg et al., 2005). While earlier work suggested that hemopexin was recycled to the extracellular medium following endocytosis and the delivery of heme (Smith et al., 1991), studies with the LRP/CD91 receptor indicate that hemopexin is degraded in lysosomes (Hvidberg et al., 2005), so this area requires further investigation. Irrespective of the mechanism of uptake, it is expected that iron from internalized heme is released from the porphyrin ring via heme oxygenases (HO-1 and HO-2) (Maines, 2005). Mice in which the *haptoglobin* or *hemopexin* genes have been inactivated do not have overt disturbances in iron metabolism (Lim et al., 1998; Tolosano et al., 1999), and an adverse phenotype is seen only when the animals are hemolyzed. This confirms that these proteins play a significant role in the detoxifying/scavenging response to a pathological insult, rather than a role in normal iron metabolism.

One physiological situation where the cellular uptake of heme is important is in the duodenum. Heme derived from hemoproteins in the diet can make a significant contribution to body iron intake, and the presence of an enterocyte brush border heme transporter has long been proposed (Latunde-Dada, Simpson, & McKie, 2006). A candidate heme transporter, HCP1, was described recently (Shayeghi et al., 2005), but subsequent investigations have shown that this protein transports folate more efficiently than heme (Qiu et al., 2006), so whether it is the major enterocyte heme transporter remains unclear. This subject is covered in more detail in Chapter 2.

Another potential iron source, but again only likely to become significant under pathological conditions, is the iron storage protein ferritin. Under normal conditions, small amounts of glycosylated ferritin are secreted into the circulation (Harrison & Arosio, 1996), but this contains little iron and is unlikely to make any significant contribution to iron traffic around the body. However, cellular damage can lead to the release of ferritin containing larger quantities of iron. Such tissue ferritin can be rapidly removed from the plasma by the liver (Mack, Cooksley, Ferris, Powell, & Halliday, 1981). The nature of the ferritin-binding protein has remained elusive for many years, but recent studies have indicated that the plasma membrane protein TIM-2 is able to bind ferritin and mediate its internalization (Chen et al., 2005). TIM-2 is expressed on the bile canaliculi of hepatocytes, bile duct epithelial cells, and B cells and binds H- but not L-ferritin, so whether it is the scavenging receptor for tissue ferritin is unclear. How ferritin-derived iron is recovered for reutilization is unknown, but presumably the protein shell is degraded in lysosomes.

## 4. INTRACELLULAR IRON UTILIZATION

Irrespective of its source, iron that enters the cell ultimately appears to enter the same intracellular pool although the size and relative importance of this pool may vary between cell types. Iron from this central source may be used for metabolic functions, may be stored within ferritin, or may contribute to the regulation of cellular iron metabolism by influencing the activity of IRPs and likely other factors. Most, if not all, cells appear to have such an intracellular pool of iron, but its physical nature is poorly defined. It is possible that specific iron chaperone proteins are present, as is the case for copper (Prohaska & Gybina, 2004), but to date none have been identified. It is more likely that iron is bound to low molecular weight organic acids such as citrate or attached to a variety of intracellular proteins through low-affinity interactions (Kruszewski, 2003).

A major sink for iron within the cell is the mitochondrion (Napier, Ponka, & Richardson, 2005). This organelle is the site of heme synthesis and is the major site of synthesis of iron–sulfur clusters, so the iron homeostasis of mitochondria is intimately related to the iron homeostasis of the entire cell. Details of heme and Fe—S protein synthesis are beyond the scope of this chapter, but they have been reviewed extensively elsewhere (e.g., Ajioka, Phillips, & Kushner, 2006; Rouault & Tong, 2005).

How mitochondria take up iron is still relatively poorly understood, but the protein mitoferrin (Mfrn) appears to play a major role in this process in erythroid cells (Shaw et al., 2006). A homolog, Mfrn2, is proposed to play the same role in non-erythroid tissues. Disruption of the *mitoferrin* gene leads to reduced mitochondrial iron uptake and heme synthesis, but is not lethal, suggesting that other pathways for iron entry into mitochondria exist. An intriguing possibility, at least in immature erythroid cells, is that much of the iron entering mitochondria comes not from the intracellular iron pool but from the direct apposition of Tf-containing endocytic vesicles with the mitochondrial outer membrane. This was proposed some time ago, but recent more detailed cell biology studies lend support to the proposal (Sheftel et al., 2007).

Some important insights into mitochondrial iron homeostasis have come from the analysis of Fe—S cluster biogenesis and from the observation that disruption of Fe—S cluster synthesis leads to significant mitochondrial iron overload. One of the lines of evidence supporting this comes from studies of the progressive neurodegenerative disorder Friedrich's ataxia, in which the gene encoding the mitochondrial protein frataxin is mutated (Lodi et al., 2006). The precise function of frataxin is not known, but lowered levels of the protein lead to reduced Fe-S cluster assembly and subsequent mitochondrial iron accumulation (Puccio et al., 2001; Pandolfo, 2003). This observation suggests that Fe—S cluster formation may act as a sensor of mitochondrial iron status (Rouault & Tong, 2005). Low Fe—S levels may be perceived by the mitochondrial iron-regulatory machinery as an inadequate iron supply and, in response, mitochondrial iron uptake may be increased and/or iron efflux decreased. Alternatively, iron may need to be incorporated into Fe—S clusters before it can be exported from mitochondria. If cluster synthesis was disrupted, iron would accumulate in the organelle. The inner mitochondrial membrane protein ABCB7 has been proposed to play a role in the efflux of Fe—S clusters (Pondarré et al., 2006), and mutations in this gene in humans lead to X-linked sideroblastic anemia, which is characterized by extensive iron deposits in mitochondria (Bekri et al., 2000). Together, these observations indicate that the assembly and transport of Fe—S clusters are fundamental to regulating mitochondrial iron homeostasis, although the precise functions of the key proteins involved have yet to be fully defined. Indeed, another proposal is that frataxin acts as a sensor for protoporphyrin IX, the penultimate intermediate in the heme biosynthetic pathway (Napier et al., 2005), thus linking mitochondrial iron levels to both Fe—S and heme synthesis.

Both heme and Fe—S clusters can be utilized not only in mitochondria but also in the cytoplasm, implying that export from the mitochondrion is involved. As noted above, ABCB7 contributes to Fe—S cluster export, but its precise role has yet to be defined. Likewise, how heme exits the mitochondrion is not well understood. Potential candidates include the mitochondrial ABC transporters ABCB6 and ABCB10 (Krishnamurthy, Xie, & Schuetz, 2007). Other heme transport proteins that are expressed on the plasma membrane but could potentially also contribute to mitcochondrial heme transport include ABCG2 (BRCP) (Krishnamurthy & Schuetz, 2006) and FLVCR (Keel et al., 2008).

While considerable information is available on heme and Fe—S cluster biosynthesis, our understanding of how other types of iron centres are synthesized and how iron is utilized outside the mitochondrion remains in its infancy.

## 5. INTRACELLULAR IRON STORAGE

Since iron is able to catalyze reactions leading to the production of toxic oxygen radicals, free iron concentrations within cells must be kept at very low levels. The great majority of intracellular iron that is not required for metabolic purposes is stored within the ubiquitously expressed protein ferritin (Harrison & Arosio, 1996; Koorts & Viljoen, 2007). Ferritin is a large protein consisting of 24 subunits of two types – H (heavy) and L (light) (Koorts & Viljoen, 2007). These subunits assemble to create a roughly spherical protein shell that surrounds a cavity in which up to 4,500 atoms of iron can be deposited. Ferritins from different tissues have different proportions of the two subunits. In tissues where longer-term storage of iron occurs, such as the liver, L-ferritin subunits predominate (e.g., H:L ratio of 1:10–1:20 in human liver ferritin). These subunits contain nucleation sites for ferrihydrite crystal formation on their internal (cavity) face and are well suited to this task. Cells that turn over iron rapidly, such as macrophages or cardiac myocytes, express more H subunits (Harrison & Arosio, 1996; Koorts & Viljoen, 2007). Ferrous iron enters ferritin by passing through hydrophilic channels in the protein shell (Theil, Matzapetakis, & Liu, 2006). Dinuclear ferroxidase sites on the H subunits oxidize the ferrous iron to the ferric form, which then moves to the L-chain nucleation sites. Once ferrihydrite crystals have formed, any additional iron accretion occurs on the crystal surface.

The level of ferritin within the cell is positively correlated with cellular iron content, a physiologically important response if ferritin is to sequester potentially cytotoxic iron in times of excess (Hintze & Theil, 2006). Subunit synthesis is controlled in an iron-dependent manner predominantly at the translational level through the IRE/IRP system (Harrison & Arosio, 1996; Arosio & Levi, 2001), which will be described in more detail below. This is not the only mechanism by which ferritin synthesis is controlled in response to iron, and transcriptional regulation is also likely to play a role (Arosio & Levi, 2001; Hintze & Theil, 2006). Under normal circumstances, iron is the major factor influencing ferritin expression, but it is also an acute phase protein and its synthesis is enhanced by inflammatory stimuli and various cytokines.

More recent studies have demonstrated that mitochondria have their own type of ferritin (Levi & Arosio, 2004). This mitochondrial ferritin (MtF) is encoded by a nuclear gene and has considerable homology to the H-ferritin subunit, although its biochemical properties differ (Bou-Abdallah, Santambrogio, Levi, Arosio, & Chasteen, 2005) and it does not possess an IRE in its 5′ UTR. MtF has a restricted tissue distribution (Santambrogio et al., 2007) and has been proposed to act as an iron sink to protect mitochondria in cells with a high metabolic activity from iron-mediated oxidative damage.

As cells become more heavily iron loaded, another form of storage iron known as hemosiderin appears (Iancu, 1990; Iancu, Deugnier, Halliday, Powell, & Brissot, 1997; Koorts & Viljoen, 2007). Unlike ferritin, which is a discrete protein, hemosiderin is an insoluble amorphous deposit containing ferric hydroxide polymers and degraded protein (Iancu, 1990; Ringeling et al., 1990). Hemosiderin is derived from the proteolytic degradation of ferritin aggregates (Andrews, Treffry, & Harrison, 1987; Miyazaki et al., 2002). As intracellular storage increases, ferritin forms aggregates that are engulfed by smooth endoplasmic reticulum to form structures known as autophagic vacuoles. These in turn fuse with lysosomes to form secondary lysosomes, and it is within these that the ferritin protein shell is degraded.

One particularly vexing problem in understanding the biology of storage iron is how it is released into the circulation when it is required by the body. That stored iron can be mobilized very efficiently is the basis for phlebotomy therapy for the iron-overload disease hemochromatosis, but whether iron is released from intact ferritin, whether the protein needs to be degraded prior to cellular efflux, or whether both processes are operating has not been resolved (Koorts & Viljoen, 2007). Some in vitro studies have been able to demonstrate iron mobilization from ferritin, but these have used conditions that are not found in vivo, so their applicability to living cells is questionable. However, recent molecular studies have shown that iron can be mobilized from intact cells before the protein is ubiquitinated and degraded by the proteasome (De Domenico et al., 2006). The same study showed that ferritin can be degraded by the lysosome, and the authors suggest that this pathway becomes more important when the cell is placed under stress.

## 6. CELLULAR IRON RELEASE

Iron release from cells and tissues is an important component of iron homeostasis. Humans have a very limited capacity to excrete iron (McCance & Widdowson, 1937), so the iron that is in the body is continually being recycled. The vast majority of this recycling occurs through the reticuloendothelial system, where macrophages phagocytose senescent red blood cells, degrade their hemoglobin, and export the iron to plasma transferrin. However, it is likely that most cells are able to release stored iron in times of metabolic need. This is again well illustrated during phlebotomy therapy of the common iron-overload disease HFE-associated hemochromatosis. Affected patients store large quantities of iron in their liver and other tissues, but this iron is released into the circulation to cater for the synthesis of new hemoglobin that is required following blood removal (O'Neil & Powell, 2005).

The major protein responsible for iron efflux across the plasma membrane is ferroportin 1 (FPN) (also known as IREG1 or MTP1) (McKie et al., 2000; Donovan et al., 2000; Abboud & Haile, 2000). FPN was initially identified as the protein responsible for iron efflux from intestinal enterocytes, but it is expressed in most tissues in the body and at particularly high levels in cells that must export large quantities of iron. Macrophages fall into the latter category as they must divest themselves of large quantities of erythrocyte-derived iron (Knutson & Wessling Resnick, 2003), but cells involved in iron storage such as hepatocytes also express considerable amounts of the protein (Zhang et al., 2004). Disruption of FPN through mutations in humans or by deletion of the gene in mice has verified that the protein plays an essential role in cellular iron release (Pietrangelo, 2004; Donovan et al., 2005). Affected individuals have impaired iron absorption as duodenal enterocytes are unable to effectively export iron derived from the diet into the circulation. Iron accumulation is also seen in the liver and other tissues. In the liver, iron loading is initially seen in the resident macrophages (Kupffer cells), but becomes more prominent in hepatocytes with age. FPN regulation appears to be quite complex. Its mRNA contains an IRE in its 5′ UTR, like the ferritin genes, and its expression in the liver is increased with iron loading, suggesting that it is under iron-dependent translational control through the IRE/IRP system (Abboud & Haile, 2000). It is suspected that this increase may represent a form of protective mechanism, serving to limit iron accumulation in this organ in times of iron excess. In the duodenum, however, FPN expression declines with body iron loading, an appropriate physiological response to prevent the accumulation of iron when it is not required by the body. This direction of regulation makes it unlikely that the IRE/IRP system is regulating FPN mRNA in the gut.

The plasma protein ceruloplasmin (Cp) plays an important role in iron release from many tissues (Hellman & Gitlin, 2002). Patients with congenital Cp deficiency or mice in which the Cp gene has been inactivated have reduced plasma iron concentrations but increased tissue iron stores (Harris, Durley, Man, & Gitlin, 1999; Xu, Pin, Gathinji, Fuchs, & Harris, 2004). Cp possesses a ferroxidase activity (the ability to oxidize ferrous iron to ferric iron) and this activity is required for its function (Hellman & Gitlin, 2002), but precisely how the protein facilitates iron efflux from cells is unclear. Recent data have indicated that a GPI-linked form of Cp can stabilize FPN on the cell surface, thus facilitating iron release (De Domenico, Ward, di Patti, et al., 2007). The membrane-bound ceruloplasmin homolog hephaestin (HEPH) is expressed predominantly in the small intestine and clearly plays a role in iron release from enterocytes (Vulpe et al., 1999; Anderson, Frazer, McKie, & Vulpe, 2002). Hephaestin is also found in the CNS and disruption of both Cp and Heph leads to greater iron accumulation in the brain than deletion of Cp alone (Hadziahmetovic et al., 2008). Another Cp homolog has been demonstrated in the placenta and is thought to facilitate iron transfer to the fetus (McArdle, Andersen, Jones, & Gambling, 2008).

Since the release of iron from cells is normally determined by the iron requirements of the erythroid system, it is not surprising that systemic factors are able to regulate iron release. The most important of these is the hepatocyte-derived peptide hepcidin. Hepcidin has been shown to inhibit iron release from a number of cell types, including macrophages, enterocytes, and hepatocytes (Ganz, 2005; Rivera et al., 2005), and the peptide has recently been demonstrated to bind to FPN and facilitate its internalization and degradation (Nemeth et al., 2004; De Domenico, Ward, Langelier, et al., 2007), thus removing it from the cell surface so that it can no longer participate in iron release. The role of hepcidin in the regulation of systemic iron homeostasis will be considered briefly below and in more detail in Chapter 3.

## 7. REGULATION OF CELLULAR IRON METABOLISM

Cellular iron levels are tightly regulated. The cell requires enough iron for metabolic processes, but because excess iron is toxic it needs to limit the intake of unneeded iron and to ensure that iron in excess of metabolic requirements is effectively sequestered. In most cells this is largely achieved by the coordinate regulation of TfR1 and ferritin. In times of iron need, TfR1 levels are increased while levels of ferritin are low. When iron is plentiful, however, TfR1 expression is reduced and ferritin synthesis is increased.

This coordinate regulation is achieved through the IRP/IRE system (Pantopoulos, 2004; Rouault, 2006; Cairo & Recalcati, 2007). IRPs (iron-regulatory proteins) are iron-dependent RNA-binding proteins. Two such proteins are known, IRP1 and IRP2. IRP1 is a bifunctional protein containing an Fe—S cluster. When iron is plentiful, the cluster is fully assembled and the protein has aconitase activity. Indeed, before its role as a regulatory protein was identified, it was known solely as a cytosolic aconitase. However, when the supply of iron is insufficient, the Fe—S cluster disassembles and IRP1 is then able to bind to stem-loop structures (iron-responsive elements or IREs) in the mRNAs encoding TfR1, ferritin, and several other proteins. IRP2 does not contain an Fe—S cluster and is regulated by iron in a different manner. When iron is plentiful, the protein is ubiquitinated and degraded via the proteasome, but in the absence of iron it is stabilized and is able to bind to target mRNAs.

The physiological importance of the IRPs has been demonstrated by the targeted deletion of these proteins in mice. Since IRP1 is widely distributed in body tissues, it was expected that Irp1 null mice would have a significant phenotype. However, this did not prove to be the case. Irp1 knockouts have a surprisingly mild phenotype, with abnormalities found only in brown fat and kidney, tissues rich in Irp1 (Meyron-Holtz, Ghosh, Iwai, et al., 2004). In contrast, when Irp2 is disrupted, mice show a much more severe phenotype, developing anemia and progressive neurological disease (LaVaute et al., 2001; Galy et al., 2005). These findings suggest that, under normal conditions, IRP2 plays the major role in regulating cellular iron homeostasis in vivo. It has been pointed out that under the low tissue oxygen concentrations, typically found in vivo, IRP1 likely functions mainly as an aconitase as the critical Fe—S cluster is relatively stable under these conditions (Meyron-Holtz, Ghosh, & Rouault, 2004). Under the same oxygen tensions, IRP2 remains relatively stable and can respond to changes in intracellular iron levels (Rouault, 2006).

The H and L-ferritin mRNAs contain a single IRE in their 5′ untranslated region (UTR) (Ponka et al., 1998; Koorts & Viljoen, 2007). When iron is scarce, the IRPs are able to bind to the mRNA and effectively block translation. Consequently, ferritin synthesis is reduced. This is an appropriate response of the cell as there is no need to synthesize large amounts of ferritin when there is little iron that requires storage. When iron is plentiful, the IRPs no longer bind to the mRNA and translation is able to proceed. This provides the cell with a rapidly inducible system that is able to synthesize iron-sequestering ferritin in times of need. TfR1 is regulated in a somewhat different manner. The TfR1 mRNA contains five IREs in its 3′ UTR (Ponka et al., 1998; Aisen, 2004). These bind IRPs under iron-deficient conditions as is the case with the ferritin message, but in this situation the mRNA is stabilized by being protected from endonuclease digestion. Thus more TfR1 protein can be translated at a time when the cell needs to maximize its capacity to acquire iron. When iron is plentiful, the IRPs no longer bind to the TfR1 mRNA and it is degraded. This serves to limit iron intake in times of iron sufficiency. The capacity of this system to confer different directions of regulation depending on either the 5′ or the 3′ UTR location of IREs explains why ferritin and TfR1 are regulated coordinately but in different directions.

IREs are also found in the mRNAs encoding several other proteins including DMT1, ferroportin, and the erythroid form of ALA synthase (eALAS). One of the 3′ splice variants of *DMT1* mRNA contains an IRE and its expression is regulated in the same direction as TfR1, being increased in iron deficiency and decreased with iron loading (Gunshin et al., 1997; Gunshin et al., 2001). In *FPN* mRNA, the IRE is in the 5′ UTR and the regulation seen is ferritin-like, being increased with iron loading (Abboud & Haile, 2000). However, this is the case only in some tissues such as the liver. In the small intestine, FPN expression is increased under iron-deficient conditions and decreased with iron loading. This suggests that a different regulatory mechanism is operating in this tissue. The *eALAS* transcript also has a 5′ IRE, thus facilitating translation of the protein when iron is available for heme synthesis (Melefors et al., 1993).

Although the best described mechanism for the iron-dependent regulation of some of the key proteins of cellular iron homeostasis is at the post-transcriptional level through the IRP/IRE system, most of the genes encoding these proteins also appear to be regulated by iron at the transcriptional level to some extent. This has been observed for the ferritin (Hintze & Theil, 2006) and TfR1 (Casey, Di Jeso, Rao, Klausner, & Harford, 1988) genes, although the effects are small. One of the 3′ splice variants of DMT1 does not possess an IRE and is still regulated by iron, albeit also over a smaller range than that of the IRE-containing variant (Frazer et al., 2001). The mRNA encoding the enterocyte iron oxidase DCYTB does not possess an IRE, yet its expression is increased in response to iron deficiency, so again transcriptional regulation is implicated (McKie et al., 2001). In none of these cases has the molecular basis of the transcriptional control been well described. However, the expression of many of these genes is increased at the transcriptional level by inflammatory cytokines (Weiss, 2005) and hypoxia (Peyssonnaux et al., 2008), and the mechanisms here are better understood.

In addition to transcriptional and post-transcriptional control, in some situations the post-translational regulation of important iron-related proteins has been recognized. In recent years the best described of these has been the internalization of plasma membrane FPN following the binding of hepcidin (Nemeth et al., 2004). This occurs when body hepcidin levels are increased in response to iron loading or inflammation. The iron-dependent internalization of DMT1 from the enterocyte brush border to intracellular sites has also been described (Yeh et al., 2000), but the mechanisms involved are poorly understood. A third example is the stabilization of TfR2 in the presence of diferric Tf and its redirection to recycling endosomes (Johnson et al., 2007). As our understanding of the regulation of cellular iron homeostasis improves, no doubt other examples of post-translational control will be revealed.

## 8. SYSTEMIC IRON METABOLISM

### *8.1. Systemic Iron Transport*

As noted earlier, under normal conditions the vast majority of iron is bound to Tf in the plasma and other extracellular fluids. Tf binds iron that is newly absorbed from the diet or which has been released from macrophages and other types of cells and distributes it to tissues where it is required for metabolic purposes. Since Tf binds iron with a particularly high affinity (Aisen, Leibman, & Zweier, 1978), the concentration of potentially cytotoxic NTBI is kept very low. Under normal conditions, the iron-binding sites of Tf are only about 30% saturated with iron, thus there is a protective buffering capacity to cater for increases in iron entry into the plasma. Transferrin is one of the most abundant plasma proteins and is produced largely by the hepatocytes of the liver (Ponka et al., 1998). Its synthesis and secretion remain reasonably constant under a wide range of physiological conditions, which is not surprising considering its central role in the delivery of essential iron to the tissues. Somewhat more transferrin is produced in response to iron deficiency, but iron loading has little effect on synthesis. A number of other factors affect Tf production, including cytokines, hormones, and hypoxia (Ponka et al., 1998; Cairo, 2001). Most regulation of Tf appears to occur at the level of transcription, although there may be some regulation at the translational level (Lok & Loh, 1998). Where there are physiological barriers that prevent the free movement of plasma proteins, such as the blood–brain barrier and the blood–testis barrier, Tf is also synthesized by the isolated organs. Thus cells in the CNS and the Sertoli cells of the testis also produce Tf (Zakin, 1992; Sylvester & Griswold, 1994).

### *8.2. Regulation of Systemic Iron Homeostasis*

The tight regulation of iron homeostasis by individual cells is integrated with a similarly tight regulation at the whole body level. The high iron requirements of the erythroid marrow combined with the smaller, yet essential, iron requirements of all other body cells are what drives the systemic regulation of iron metabolism. Central to this homeostatic process is the passage of iron through plasma Tf, as Tf delivers iron to the tissues where it is required. The supply of iron to plasma Tf is met from two main sources: (1) the recycling of hemoglobin-derived iron from senescent red blood cells and (2) through intestinal iron absorption. The former is part of the tight conservation of existing body iron, whereas the latter comes into play when body iron levels drop below those required for normal metabolic purposes. Iron absorption is considered in detail in Chapter 2.

How the body communicates its iron needs to the reticuloendothelial system and small intestine has long been a puzzle, but in recent years it has been revealed that the liver-derived peptide hepcidin plays a central role in this process. Hepcidin in its mature form is a 25 amino acid peptide that is secreted by hepatocytes (Pigeon et al., 2001) (and possibly in smaller amounts by some other cell types) into the circulation where it acts as an inhibitor of iron release from a variety of cells, including duodenal enterocytes, macrophages, and hepatocytes (Ganz, 2005; Nicolas et al., 2001; Nicolas, Bennoun, et al., 2002). As noted above, it achieves this by interacting with FPN and facilitating the internalization and degradation of the complex (Nemeth et al., 2004). Thus hepcidin acts as a repressor of cellular iron release. Consistent with this role, hepcidin synthesis is decreased when iron demands are high [e.g., during iron deficiency (Pigeon et al., 2001), during pregnancy (Millard et al., 2004), and with increased erythropoiesis (Nicolas, Chauvet, et al., 2002)], allowing stored iron to be released, and increased when the body is iron replete (Pigeon et al., 2001), resulting in the storage of excess iron in macrophages and hepatocytes. Hepcidin expression is also stimulated by inflammation and hypoxia, and its synthesis has been shown to be responsible for the hypoferremia that accompanies an inflammatory insult (Nicolas, Chauvet, et al., 2002). The importance of hepcidin in maintaining body iron balance is demonstrated by patients with mutations in the *HAMP* (*hepcidin*) gene (Roetto et al., 2003). Such patients develop an early onset, severe iron-loading disorder (juvenile hemochromatosis) as a result of an uncontrolled high level of intestinal iron absorption.

How hepcidin itself is regulated is currently an area of intense interest, but studies of inherited disorders of iron homeostasis have shed considerable light on this topic. Mutations in three genes that are associated with iron loading in humans, *HFE*, *TfR2*, and *hemojuvelin* (*HJV*), are characterized by reduced hepcidin expression (Ahmad et al., 2002; Bridle et al., 2003; Fleming, Britton, Waheed, Sly, & Bacon, 2004; Papanikolaou et al., 2004; Nemeth, Roetto, Garozzo, Ganz, & Camaschella, 2005). In each of these cases, intestinal iron absorption is inappropriately high and this is what leads to the increased body iron load. Data from these studies suggest that HFE, TfR2, and HJV are upstream regulators of hepcidin expression. How HFE and TfR2 might regulate hepcidin is still unclear, but recent data have shown that HJV can influence hepcidin expression by acting through the BMP/SMAD signaling pathway (Wang et al., 2005; Babitt et al., 2006; Anderson & Frazer, 2006). Equally interesting is how HFE, TfR2, and HJV might respond to signals that relay information about body iron requirements. The level of diferric transferrin has been suggested as one possible signal (Frazer & Anderson, 2003; Wilkins et al., 2006), but hypoxia or other factors such as the erythroid-derived protein GDF15 (Tanno et al., 2007) could also be involved.

A more detailed coverage of the role of hepcidin in body iron homeostasis is provided in Chapter 3.

## 9. CONCLUSION

Cellular iron metabolism has been under investigation for many years, but for much of that time only a limited number of the main players could be studied, either because of their high abundance or because of their relative stability. However, with the advent of molecular techniques, the availability of tractable experimental systems, such as knockout mice and yeast, and the analysis of inherited disorders of iron homeostasis, that situation has changed and we are now beginning to understand the complexity of cellular iron traffic and its regulation. Despite this, our understanding in many areas remains in its infancy. A particularly poorly understood area is how iron that is delivered to the cytoplasm is handled and directed to where it is required for protein synthesis. In contrast, our appreciation of how the body responds to alterations in iron demand has progressed rapidly in recent years with the discovery of hepcidin and its regulators.

While this chapter has concentrated on how a "generic" cell might handle iron, in reality there is no such thing. There are some fundamental aspects of iron handling that are shared by most cells, but superimposed upon this, each cell type handles iron in its own specific way that is appropriate for its function. Some cells turn over iron rapidly, others store it readily, and yet others, such as immature erythroid cells, utilize most of their iron for a single specific function i.e., heme synthesis. Deciphering how these cell-specific functions are encoded and regulated adds yet another dimension to this fascinating area of cellular physiology.

**Acknowledgment** GJA is the recipient of a Senior Research Fellowship from the National Health and Medical Research Council of Australia.

## ABBREVIATIONS

| | |
|---|---|
| ABCB7 | ATP-binding cassette protein B7 |
| BMP | bone morphogenetic protein |
| Cp | ceruloplasmin |
| DCYTB | duodenal cytochrome b |
| DMT1 | divalent metal-ion transporter 1 |
| eALAS | erythroid aminolevulinic acid synthase |
| Fe–S | iron–sulfur |
| FLVCR | feline leukemia virus subgroup c receptor |
| FPN | ferroportin 1 |
| GDF15 | growth differentiation factor 15 |
| HAMP | hepcidin antimicrobial peptide |
| HCP1 | heme carrier protein 1 |
| HEPH | hephaestin |
| HFE | gene mutated in commonest form of hemochromatosis |
| HJV | hemojuvelin |
| HO | heme oxygenase |
| IRE | iron-responsive element |
| IRP | iron-regulatory protein |
| LRP | low-density lipoprotein receptor-related protein |
| MFRN | mitoferrin |
| NTBI | non-transferrin-bound iron |
| SFT | stimulator of Fe (iron) transport |
| STEAP | six-transmembrane epithelial antigen of prostate protein 3 |
| Tf | transferrin |
| TfR1 | transferrin receptor 1 |
| TfR2 | transferrin receptor 2 |
| TIM-2 | T-cell immunoglobulin-domain and mucin-domain protein 2 |
| UTR | untranslated region |
| ZIP14 | Zrt-Irt-like protein 14 |

## REFERENCES

Abboud, S., & Haile, D. J. (2000). A novel mammalian iron-regulated protein involved in intracellular iron metabolism. *Journal of Biological Chemistry, 275*, 19906–19912.

Ahmad, K. A., Ahmann, J. R., Migas, M. C., Waheed, A., Britton, R. S., Bacon, B. R., et al. (2002). Decreased liver hepcidin expression in the Hfe knockout mouse. *Blood Cells Molecules and Disease, 29*, 361–366.

Aisen, P. (2004). Transferrin receptor 1. *International Journal of Biochemistry and Cell Biology, 36*, 2137–2143.

Aisen, P., Leibman, A., & Zweier, J. (1978). Stoichiometric and site characteristics of the binding of iron to human transferrin. *Journal of Biological Chemistry, 253*, 1930–1937.

Ajioka, R. S., Phillips, J. D., & Kushner, J. P. (2006). Biosynthesis of heme in mammals. *Biochimica et Biophysica Acta, 1763*, 723–736.

Anderson, G. J., & Frazer, D. M. (2006). Iron metabolism meets signal transduction. *Nature Genetics, 38*, 503–504.

Anderson, G. J., Frazer, D. M., McKie, A. T., & Vulpe, C. D. (2002). The ceruloplasmin homolog hephaestin and the control of intestinal iron absorption. *Blood Cells Molecules and Disease, 29*, 367–375.

Anderson, G. J., Powell, L. W., & Halliday, J. W. (1994). The endocytosis of transferrin by rat intestinal epithelial cells. *Gastroenterology, 106*, 414–422.

Andrews, S. C., Treffry, A., & Harrison, P. M. (1987). Siderosomal ferritin. The missing link between ferritin and haemosiderin? *Biochemical Journal, 245*, 439–446.

Arosio, P., & Levi, S. (2001). Ferritins: Structural and functional aspects. In D. M. Templeton (Ed.), *Molecular and cellular iron transport* (pp. 125–154). New York: Marcel Dekker Inc.

Babitt, J. L., Huang, F. W., Wrighting, D. M., Xia, Y., Sidis, Y., Samad, T. A., et al. (2006). Bone morphogenetic protein signaling by hemojuvelin regulates hepcidin expression. *Nature Genetics, 38*, 531–539.

Baker, E., Baker, S. M., & Morgan, E. H. (1998). Characterisation of non-transferrin-bound iron (ferric citrate) uptake by rat hepatocytes in culture. *Biochimica et Biophysica Acta, 1380*, 21–30.

Bali, P. K., Zak, O., & Aisen, P. (1991). A new role for the transferrin receptor in the release of iron from transferrin. *Biochemistry, 30*, 324–328.

Bekri, S., Kispal, G., Lange, H., Fitzsimons, E., Tolmie, J., Lill, R., et al. (2000). Human ABC7 transporter: Gene structure and mutation causing X-linked sideroblastic anemia with ataxia with disruption of cytosolic iron-sulfur protein maturation. *Blood, 96*, 3256–3264.

Bernstein, S. E. (1987). Hereditary hypotransferrinemia with hemosiderosis, a murine disorder resembling human atransferrinemia. *Journal of Laboratory and Clinical Medicine, 110*, 690–705.

Bou-Abdallah, F., Santambrogio, P., Levi, S., Arosio, P., & Chasteen, N. D. (2005). Unique iron binding and oxidation properties of human mitochondrial ferritin: A comparative analysis with Human H-chain ferritin. *Journal of Molecular Biology, 347*, 543–554.

Bowen, B. J., & Morgan, E. H. (1987). Anemia of the Belgrade rat: Evidence for defective membrane transport of iron. *Blood, 70*, 38–44.

Breuer, W., Shvartsman, M., & Cabantchik, Z. I. (2008). Intracellular labile iron. *International Journal of Biochemistry and Cell Biology, 40*, 350–354.

Bridle, K. R., Frazer, D. M., Wilkins, S. J., Dixon, J. L., Purdie, D. M., Crawford, D. H., et al. (2003). Disrupted hepcidin regulation in HFE-associated haemochromatosis and the liver as a regulator of body iron homoeostasis. *Lancet, 361*, 669–673.

Cairo, G. (2001). Regulation of liver iron metabolism. In D. M. Templeton (Ed.), *Molecular and cellular iron transport* (pp. 613–641). New York: Marcel Dekker Inc.

Cairo, G., & Recalcati, S. (2007). Iron-regulatory proteins: Molecular biology and pathophysiological implications. *Expert Reviews in Molecular Medicine, 9*, 1–13.

Camaschella, C., Roetto, A., Cali, A., De Gobbi, M., Garozzo, G., Carella, M., et al. (2000). The gene TFR2 is mutated in a new type of haemochromatosis mapping to 7q22. *Nature Genetics, 25*, 14–15.

Casey, J. L., Di Jeso, B., Rao, K., Klausner, R. D., & Harford, J. B. (1988). Two genetic loci participate in the regulation by iron of the gene for the human transferrin receptor. *Proceedings of the National Academy of Sciences, USA, 85*, 1787–1791.

Chen, T. T., Li, L., Chung, D. H., Allen, C. D., Torti, S. V., Torti, F. M., et al. (2005). TIM-2 is expressed on B cells and in liver and kidney and is a receptor for H-ferritin endocytosis. *Journal of Experimental Medicine, 202*, 955–965.

Chua, A. C., Graham, R. M., Trinder, D., & Olynyk, J. K. (2007). The regulation of cellular iron metabolism. *Critical Reviews in Clinical Laboratory Science, 44*, 413–459.

Chua, A. C., Olynyk, J. K., Leedman, P. J., & Trinder, D. (2004). Nontransferrin-bound iron uptake by hepatocytes is increased in the Hfe knockout mouse model of hereditary hemochromatosis. *Blood, 104*, 1519–1525.

Cole, E. S., & Glass, J. (1983). Transferrin binding and iron uptake in mouse hepatocytes. *Biochimica et Biophysica Acta, 762*, 102–110.

Courville, P., Chaloupka, R., & Cellier, M. F. (2006). Recent progress in structure-function analyses of Nramp proton-dependent metal-ion transporters. *Biochemistry and Cell Biology, 84*, 960–978.

Craven, C. M., Alexander, J., Eldridge, M., Kushner, J. P., Bernstein, S., & Kaplan, J. (1987). Tissue distribution and clearance kinetics of non-transferrin-bound iron in the hypotransferrinemic mouse: A rodent model for hemochromatosis. *Proceedings of the National Academy of Sciences, USA, 84*, 3457–3461.

Deaglio, S., Capobianco, A., Cali, A., Bellora, F., Alberti, F., Righi, L., et al. (2002). Structural, functional, and tissue distribution analysis of human transferrin receptor-2 by murine monoclonal antibodies and polyclonal antiserum. *Blood, 100*, 3782–3789.

De Domenico, I., Vaughn, M. B., Li, L., Bagley, D., Musci, G., Ward, D. M., et al. (2006). Ferroportin-mediated mobilization of ferritin iron precedes ferritin degradation by the proteasome. *EMBO Journal, 25*, 5396–5404.

De Domenico, I., Ward, D. M., di Patti, M. C., Jeong, S. Y., David, S., Musci, G., et al. (2007). Ferroxidase activity is required for the stability of cell surface ferroportin in cells expressing GPI-ceruloplasmin. *EMBO Journal, 26*, 2823–2831.

De Domenico, I., Ward, D. M., Langelier, C., Vaughn, M. B., Nemeth, E., Sundquist, W. I., et al. (2007). The molecular mechanism of hepcidin-mediated ferroportin down-regulation. *Molecular Biology of the Cell, 18*, 2569–2578.

Donovan, A., Brownlie, A., Zhou, Y., Shepard, J., Pratt, S. J., Moynihan, J., et al. (2000). Positional cloning of zebrafish ferroportin1 identifies a conserved vertebrate iron exporter. *Nature, 403*, 776–781.

Donovan, A., Lima, C. A., Pinkus, J. L., Pinkus, G. S., Zon, L. I., Robine, S., et al. (2005). The iron exporter ferroportin/Slc40a1 is essential for iron homeostasis. *Cell Metabolism, 1*, 191–200.

Eisenstein, R. S. (2000). Iron regulatory proteins and the molecular control of mammalian iron metabolism. *Annual Review of Nutrition, 20*, 627–662.

Enns, C. A. (2001). The transferrin receptor. In D. M. Templeton (Ed.), *Molecular and cellular iron transport* (pp. 71–94). New York: Marcel Dekker Inc.

Fabriek, B. O., Dijkstra, C. D., & van den Berg, T. K. (2005). The macrophage scavenger receptor CD163. *Immunobiology, 210*, 153–160.

Fleming, R. E., Ahmann, J. R., Migas, M. C., Waheed, A., Koeffler, H. P., Kawabata, H., et al. (2002). Targeted mutagenesis of the murine transferrin receptor-2 gene produces hemochromatosis. *Proceedings of the National Academy of Sciences, USA, 99*, 10653–10658.

Fleming, R. E., Britton, R. S., Waheed, A., Sly, W. S., & Bacon, B. R. (2004). Pathogenesis of hereditary hemochromatosis. *Clinics in Liver Disease, 8*, 755–773.

Fleming, R. E., Migas, M. C., Holden, C. C., Waheed, A., Britton, R. S., Tomatsu, S., et al. (2000). Transferrin receptor 2: Continued expression in mouse liver in the face of iron overload and in hereditary hemochromatosis. *Proceedings of the National Academy of Sciences, USA, 97*, 2214–2219.

Fleming, M. D., Romano, M. A., Su, M. A., Garrick, L. M., Garrick, M. D., & Andrews, N. C. (1998). NRAMP2 is mutated in the anemic Belgrade (b) rat: Evidence of a role for Nramp2 in endosomal iron transport. *Proceedings of the National Academy of Sciences, USA, 95*, 1148–1153.

Frazer, D. M., & Anderson, G. J. (2003). The orchestration of body iron intake: How and where do enterocytes receive their cues? *Blood Cells Molecules and Disease, 30*, 288–297.

Frazer, D. M., Vulpe, C. D., McKie, A. T., Wilkins, S. J., Trinder, D., Cleghorn, G. J., et al. (2001). Cloning and gastrointestinal expression of rat hephaestin: Relationship to other iron transport proteins. *American Journal of Physiology, Gastrointestinal and Liver Physiology, 281*, G931–G939.

Galy, B., Ferring, D., Minana, B., Bell, O., Janser, H. G., Muckenthaler, et al. (2005). Altered body iron distribution and microcytosis in mice deficient in iron regulatory protein 2 (IRP2). *Blood, 106*, 2580–2589.

Ganz, T. (2005). Hepcidin – A regulator of intestinal iron absorption and iron recycling by macrophages. *Best Practice and Research in Clinical Haematology, 18*, 171–182.

Garrick, L. M., Edwards, J. A., Hoke, J. E., & Bannerman, R. M. (1987). Diminished acquisition of iron by reticulocytes from mice with hemoglobin deficit. *Experimental Hematology, 15*, 671–675.

Graham, R. M., Morgan, E. H., & Baker, E. (1998). Ferric citrate uptake by cultured rat hepatocytes is inhibited in the presence of transferrin. *European Journal of Biochemistry, 253*, 139–145.

Gunshin, H., Allerson, C. R., Polycarpou-Schwarz, M., Rofts, A., Rogers, J. T., Kishi, F., et al. (2001). Iron-dependent regulation of the divalent metal ion transporter. *FEBS Letters, 509*, 309–316.

Gunshin, H., Mackenzie, B., Berger, U. V., Gunshin, Y., Romero, M. F., Boron, W. F., et al. (1997). Cloning and characterization of a mammalian proton-coupled metal-ion transporter. *Nature, 388*, 482–488.

Gutierrez, J. A., Yu, J., Rivera, S., & Wessling-Resnick, M. (1997). Functional expression cloning and characterization of SFT, a stimulator of Fe transport. *Journal of Cell Biology, 139*, 895–905.

Hadziahmetovic, M., Dentchev, T., Song, Y., Haddad, N., He, X., Hahn, P., et al. (2008). Ceruloplasmin/Hephaestin knockout mice model morphologic and molecular features of AMD. *Investigative Ophthalmology and Visual Science, March 7*, [Epub ahead of print]

Harris, Z. L., Durley, A. P., Man, T. K., & Gitlin, J. D. (1999). Targeted gene disruption reveals an essential role for ceruloplasmin in cellular iron efflux. *Proceedings of the National Academy of Sciences, USA, 96*, 10812–10817.

Harrison, P. M., & Arosio, P. (1996). The ferritins: Molecular properties, iron storage function and cellular regulation. *Biochimica et Biophysica Acta, 1275*, 161–203.

Hayashi, A., Wada, Y., Suzuki, T., & Shimizu, A. (1993). Studies on familial hypotransferrinemia: Unique clinical course and molecular pathology. *American Journal of Human Genetics, 53*, 201–213.

Hellman, N. E., & Gitlin, J. D. (2002). Ceruloplasmin metabolism and function. *Annual Review of Nutrition, 22*, 439–458.

Herz, J., & Strickland, D. K. (2001). LRP: A multifunctional scavenger and signaling receptor. *Journal of Clinical Investigation, 108*, 779–784.

Hider, R. C. (2002). Nature of nontransferrin-bound iron. *European Journal of Clinical Investigation, 32*(Suppl. 1), 50–54.

Hintze, K. J., & Theil, E. C. (2006). Cellular regulation and molecular interactions of the ferritins. *Cellular and Molecular Life Sciences, 63*, 591–600.

Hvidberg, V., Maniecki, M. B., Jacobsen, C., Hojrup, P., Moller, H. J., & Moestrup, S. K. (2005). Identification of the receptor scavenging hemopexin-heme complexes. *Blood, 106*, 2572–2579.

Iancu, T. C. (1990). Biological and ultrastructural aspects of iron overload: An overview. *Pediatric Pathology, 10*, 281–296.

Iancu, T. C., Deugnier, Y., Halliday, J. W., Powell, L. W., & Brissot, P. (1997). Ultrastructural sequences during liver iron overload in genetic hemochromatosis. *Journal of Hepatology, 27*, 628–638.

Johnson, M. B., Chen, J., Murchison, N., Green, F. A., & Enns, C. A. (2007). Transferrin receptor 2: Evidence for ligand-induced stabilization and redirection to a recycling pathway. *Molecular Biology of the Cell, 18*, 743–754.

Kawabata, H., Yang, R., Hirama, T., Vuong, P. T., Kawano, S., Gombart, A. F., et al. (1999). Molecular cloning of transferrin receptor 2: A new member of the transferrin receptor-like family. *Journal of Biological Chemistry, 274*, 20826–20832.

Keel, S. B., Doty, R. T., Yang, Z., Quigley, J. G., Chen, J., Knoblaugh, S., et al. (2008). A heme export protein is required for red blood cell differentiation and iron homeostasis. *Science, 319*, 825–828.

Knutson, M. D. (2007). Steap proteins: Implications for iron and copper metabolism. *Nutrition Reviews, 65*, 335–340.

Knutson, M., & Wessling-Resnick, M. (2003). Iron metabolism in the reticuloendothelial system. *Critical Reviews in Biochemistry and Molecular Biology, 38*, 61–88.

Koorts, A. M., & Viljoen, M. (2007). Ferritin and ferritin isoforms I: Structure-function relationships, synthesis, degradation and secretion. *Archives of Physiology and Biochemistry, 113*, 30–54.

Krishnamurthy, P., & Schuetz, J. D. (2006). Role of ABCG2/BCRP in biology and medicine. *Annual Review of Pharmacology and Toxicology, 46*, 381–410.

Krishnamurthy, P., Xie, T., & Schuetz, J. D. (2007). The role of transporters in cellular heme and porphyrin homeostasis. *Pharmacology and Therapeutics, 114*, 345–358.

Kristiansen, M., Graversen, J. H., Jacobsen, C., Sonne, O., Hoffman, H. J., Law, S. K., et al. (2001). Identification of the haemoglobin scavenger receptor. *Nature, 409*, 198–201.

Kruszewski, M. (2003). Labile iron pool: The main determinant of cellular response to oxidative stress. *Mutation Research*, 531, 81–92.

Latunde-Dada, G. O., Simpson, R. J., & McKie, A. T. (2006). Recent advances in mammalian haem transport. *Trends in Biochemical Sciences, 31*, 182–188.

LaVaute, T., Smith, S., Cooperman, S., Iwai, K., Land, W., Meyron-Holtz, E., et al. (2001). Targeted deletion of the gene encoding iron regulatory protein-2 causes misregulation of iron metabolism and neurodegenerative disease in mice. *Nature Genetics, 27*, 209–214.

Lee, A. W., Oates, P. S., & Trinder, D. (2003). Effects of cell proliferation on the uptake of transferrin-bound iron by human hepatoma cells. *Hepatology, 38*, 967–977.

Levi, S., & Arosio, P. (2004). Mitochondrial ferritin. *International Journal of Biochemistry and Cell Biology, 36*, 1887–1889.

Lill, R., & Mühlenhoff, U. (2006). Iron-sulfur protein biogenesis in eukaryotes: Components and mechanisms. *Annual Review of Cell and Developmental Biology, 22*, 457–486.

Lim, J. E., Jin, O., Bennett, C., Morgan, K., Wang, F., Trenor, C. C., et al. (2005). A mutation in Sec15l1 causes anemia in hemoglobin deficit (hbd) mice. *Nature Genetics, 37*, 1270–1273.

Lim, S. K., Kim, H., Lim, S. K., bin Ali, A., Lim, Y. K., Wang, Y., et al. (1998). Increased susceptibility in Hp knockout mice during acute hemolysis. *Blood, 92*, 1870–1877.

Liuzzi, J. P., Aydemir, F., Nam, H., Knutson, M. D., & Cousins, R. J. (2006). Zip14 (Slc39a14) mediates non-transferrin-bound iron uptake into cells. *Proceedings of the National Academy of Sciences USA, 103*, 13612–13617.

Lodi, R., Tonon, C., Calabrese, V., & Schapira, A. H. (2006). Friedreich's ataxia: From disease mechanisms to therapeutic interventions. *Antioxidants and Redox Signaling, 8*, 438–443.

Lok, C. N., & Loh, T. T. (1998). Regulation of transferrin function and expression: Review and update. *Biological Signals and Receptors, 7*, 157–178.

McCance, R. A., & Widdowson, E. M. (1937). Absorption and excretion of iron. *Lancet, 2*, 680–684.

McArdle, H. J., Andersen, H. S., Jones, H., & Gambling, L. (2008). Copper and iron transport across the placenta: Regulation and interactions. *Journal of Neuroendocrinology, 20*, 427–431.

Mackenzie, B., & Garrick, M. D. (2005). Iron Imports. II. Iron uptake at the apical membrane in the intestine. *American Journal of Physiology, Gastrointestinal and Liver Physiology, 289*, G981–G986.

McKie, A. T., Barrow, D., Latunde-Dada, G. O., Rolfs, A., Sager, G., Mudaly, E., et al. (2001). An iron-regulated ferric reductase associated with the absorption of dietary iron. *Science, 291*, 1755–1759.

McKie, A. T., Marciani, P., Rolfs, A., Brennan, K., Wehr, K., Barrow, D., et al. (2000). A novel duodenal iron-regulated transporter, IREG1, implicated in the basolateral transfer of iron to the circulation. *Molecular Cell, 5*, 299–309.

Mack, U., Cooksley, W. G., Ferris, R. A., Powell, L. W., & Halliday, J. W. (1981). Regulation of plasma ferritin by the isolated perfused rat liver. *British Journal of Haematology, 47*, 403–412.

Maines, M. D. (2005). The heme oxygenase system: Update 2005. *Antioxidants and Redox Signaling, 7*, 1761–1766.

Melefors, O., Goossen, B., Johansson, H. E., Stripecke, R., Gray, N. K., & Hentze, M. W. (1993). Translational control of 5-aminolevulinate synthase mRNA by iron-responsive elements in erythroid cells. *Journal of Biological Chemistry, 268*, 5974–5978.

Meyron-Holtz, E. G., Ghosh, M. C., Iwai, K., LaVaute, T., Brazzolotto, X., Berger, U. V., et al. (2004). Genetic ablations of iron regulatory proteins 1 and 2 reveal why iron regulatory protein 2 dominates iron homeostasis. *EMBO Journal, 23*, 386–395.

Meyron-Holtz, E. G., Ghosh, M. C., & Rouault, T. A. (2004). Mammalian tissue oxygen levels modulate iron-regulatory protein activities in vivo. *Science, 306*, 2087–2090.

Millard, K. N., Frazer, D. M., Wilkins, S. J., & Anderson, G. J. (2004). Changes in the expression of intestinal iron transport and hepatic regulatory molecules explain the enhanced iron absorption associated with pregnancy in the rat. *Gut, 53*, 655–660.

Mims, M. P., & Prchal, J. T. (2005). Divalent metal transporter 1. *Hematology, 10*, 339–345.

Miyazaki, E., Kato, J., Kobune, M., Okumura, K., Sasaki, K., Shintani, N., et al. (2002). Denatured H-ferritin subunit is a major constituent of haemosiderin in the liver of patients with iron overload. *Gut, 50*, 413–419.

Moestrup, S. K., & Moller, H. J. (2004). CD163: A regulated hemoglobin scavenger receptor with a role in the anti-inflammatory response. *Annals of Medicine, 36*, 347–354.

Morgan, E. H., Smith, G. D., & Peters, T. J. (1986). Uptake and subcellular processing of 59Fe-125I-labelled transferrin by rat liver. *Biochemical Journal, 237*, 163–173.

Napier, I., Ponka, P., & Richardson, D. R. (2005). Iron trafficking in the mitochondrion: Novel pathways revealed by disease. *Blood, 105*, 1867–1874.

Nemeth, E., Roetto, A., Garozzo, G., Ganz, T., & Camaschella, C. (2005). Hepcidin is decreased in TFR2 hemochromatosis. *Blood, 105*, 1803–1806.

Nemeth, E., Tuttle, M. S., Powelson, J., Vaughn, M. B., Donovan, A., Ward, D. M., et al. (2004). Hepcidin regulates cellular iron efflux by binding to ferroportin and inducing its internalization. *Science, 306*, 2090–2093.

Nicolas, G., Bennoun, M., Devaux, I., Beaumont, C., Grandchamp, B., Kahn, A., et al. (2001). Lack of hepcidin gene expression and severe tissue iron overload in upstream stimulatory factor 2 (USF2) knockout mice. *Proceedings of the National Academy of Sciences, USA, 98*, 8780–8785.

Nicolas, G., Bennoun, M., Porteu, A., Mativet, S., Beaumont, C., Grandchamp, B., et al. (2002). Severe iron deficiency anemia in transgenic mice expressing liver hepcidin. *Proceedings of the National Academy of Sciences, USA, 99*, 4596–4601.

Nicolas, G., Chauvet, C., Viatte, L., Danan, J. L., Bigard, X., Devaux, I., et al. (2002). The gene encoding the iron regulatory peptide hepcidin is regulated by anemia, hypoxia, and inflammation. *Journal of Clinical Investigation, 110*, 1037–1044.

Ohgami, R. S., Campagna, D. R., Antiochos, B., Wood, E. B., Sharp, J. J., Barker, J. E., et al. (2005). nm1054: A spontaneous, recessive, hypochromic, microcytic anemia mutation in the mouse. *Blood, 106*, 3625–3631.

Ohgami, R. S., Campagna, D. R., Greer, E. L., Antiochos, B., McDonald, A., Chen, J., et al. (2005). Identification of a ferrireductase required for efficient transferrin-dependent iron uptake in erythroid cells. *Nature Genetics, 37*, 1264–1269.

Ohgami, R. S., Campagna, D. R., McDonald, A., & Fleming, M. D. (2006). The Steap proteins are metalloreductases. *Blood, 108*, 1388–1394.

O'Neil, J., & Powell, L. (2005).Clinical aspects of hemochromatosis. *Seminars in Liver Disease, 25*, 381–391.

Oudit, G. Y., Sun, H., Trivieri, M. G., Koch, S. E., Dawood, F., Ackerley, C., et al. (2003). L-type Ca2+ channels provide a major pathway for iron entry into cardiomyocytes in iron-overload cardiomyopathy. *Nature Medicine, 9*, 1187–1194.

Pandolfo, M. (2003). Friedreich ataxia. *Seminars in Pediatric Neurology, 10*, 163–172.

Pantopoulos, K. (2004). Iron metabolism and the IRE/IRP regulatory system: An update. *Annals of the New York Academy of Sciences, 1012*, 1–13.

Papanikolaou, G., Samuels, M. E., Ludwig, E. H., MacDonald, M. L., Franchini, P. L., Dube, M. P., et al. (2004). Mutations in HFE2 cause iron overload in chromosome 1q-linked juvenile hemochromatosis. *Nature Genetics, 36*, 77–82.

Parkes, J. G., & Templeton, D. M. (2001). Transport of non-transferrin-bound iron by hepatocytes. In D. M. Templeton (Ed.), *Molecular and cellular iron transport* (pp. 451–466). New York: Marcel Dekker Inc.

Peyssonnaux, C., Nizet, V., & Johnson, R. S. (2008). Role of the hypoxia inducible factors HIF in iron metabolism. *Cell Cycle, 7*, 28–32.

Pietrangelo, A. (2004). Non-HFE hemochromatosis. *Hepatology, 39*, 21–29.

Pigeon, C., Ilyin, G., Courselaud, B., Leroyer, P., Turlin, B., Brissot, P., et al. (2001). A new mouse liver-specific gene, encoding a protein homologous to human antimicrobial peptide hepcidin, is overexpressed during iron overload. *Journal of Biological Chemistry, 276*, 7811–7819.

Pondarré, C., Antiochos, B. B., Campagna, D. R., Clarke, S. L., Greer, E. L., Deck, K. M., et al. (2006). The mitochondrial ATP-binding cassette transporter Abcb7 is essential in mice and participates in cytosolic iron-sulfur cluster biogenesis. *Human Molecular Genetics, 15*, 953–964.

Ponka, P., Beaumont, C., & Richardson, D. R. (1998). Function and regulation of transferrin and ferritin. *Seminars in Hematology, 35*, 35–54.

Prohaska, J. R., & Gybina, A. A. (2004). Intracellular copper transport in mammals. *Journal of Nutrition, 134*, 1003–1006.

Puccio, H., Simon, D., Cossée, M., Criqui-Filipe, P., Tiziano, F., Melki, J., et al. (2001). Mouse models for Friedreich ataxia exhibit cardiomyopathy, sensory nerve defect and Fe—S enzyme deficiency followed by intramitochondrial iron deposits. *Nature Genetics, 27*, 181–186.

Qiu, A., Jansen, M., Sakaris, A., Min, S. H., Chattopadhyay, S., Tsai, E., et al. (2006). Identification of an intestinal folate transporter and the molecular basis for hereditary folate malabsorption. *Cell, 127*, 917–928.

Randell, E. W., Parkes, J. G., Olivieri, N. F., & Templeton, D. M. (1994). Uptake of non-transferrin-bound iron by both reductive and nonreductive processes is modulated by intracellular iron. *Journal of Biological Chemistry, 269*, 16046–16053.

Ringeling, P. L., Cleton, M. I., Huijskes-Heins, M. I., Seip, M. J., de Bruijn, W. C., & van Eijk, H. G. (1990). Analysis of iron-containing compounds in different compartments of the rat liver after iron loading. *Biology of Metals, 3*, 176–182.

Rivera, S., Liu, L., Nemeth, E., Gabayan, V., Sorensen, O. E., & Ganz, T. (2005). Hepcidin excess induces the sequestration of iron and exacerbates tumor-associated anemia. *Blood, 105*, 1797–1802.

Robb, A. D., Ericsson, M., & Wessling-Resnick, M. (2004). Transferrin receptor 2 mediates a biphasic pattern of transferrin uptake associated with ligand delivery to multivesicular bodies. *American Journal of Physiology, Cellular Physiology, 287*, C1769–C1775.

Roetto, A., Papanikolaou, G., Politou, M., Alberti, F., Girelli, D., Christakis, J., et al. (2003). Mutant antimicrobial peptide hepcidin is associated with severe juvenile hemochromatosis. *Nature Genetics, 33*, 21–22.

Rouault, T. A. (2006). The role of iron regulatory proteins in mammalian iron homeostasis and disease. *Nature Chemical Biology, 2*, 406–414.

Rouault, T. A., & Tong, W. H. (2005). Iron-sulphur cluster biogenesis and mitochondrial iron homeostasis. *Nature Reviews Molecular Cell Biology, 6*, 345–351.

Santambrogio, P., Biasiotto, G., Sanvito, F., Olivieri, S., Arosio, P., & Levi, S. (2007). Mitochondrial ferritin expression in adult mouse tissues. *Journal of Histochemistry and Cytochemistry, 55*, 1129–1137.

Scheiber-Mojdehkar, B., Sturm, B., Plank, L., Kryzer, I., & Goldenberg, H. (2003). Influence of parenteral iron preparations on non-transferrin bound iron uptake, the iron regulatory protein and the expression of ferritin and the divalent metal transporter DMT-1 in HepG2 human hepatoma cells. *Biochemical Pharmacology, 65*, 1973–1978.

Shaw, G. C., Cope, J. J., Li, L., Corson, K., Hersey, C., Ackermann, G. E., et al. (2006). Mitoferrin is essential for erythroid iron assimilation. *Nature, 440*, 96–100.

Shayeghi, M., Latunde-Dada, G. O., Oakhill, J. S., Laftah, A. H., Takeuchi, K., Halliday, N., et al. (2005). Identification of an intestinal heme transporter. *Cell, 122*, 789–801.

Sheftel, A. D., Zhang, A. S., Brown, C., Shirihai, O. S., & Ponka, P. (2007). Direct interorganellar transfer of iron from endosome to mitochondrion. *Blood, 110*, 125–132.

Smith, A., Farooqui, S. M., & Morgan, W. T. (1991). The murine haemopexin receptor. Evidence that the haemopexin-binding site resides on a 20 kDa subunit and that receptor recycling is regulated by protein kinase C. *Biochemical Journal, 276*, 417–425.

Sylvester, S. R., & Griswold, M. D. (1994). The testicular iron shuttle: A "nurse" function of the Sertoli cells. *Journal of Andrology, 15*, 381–385.

Tanno, T., Bhanu, N. V., Oneal, P. A., Goh, S. H., Staker, P., Lee, Y. T., et al. (2007). High levels of GDF15 in thalassemia suppress expression of the iron regulatory protein hepcidin. *Nature Medicine, 13*, 1096–1101.

Tchernitchko, D., Bourgeois, M., Martin, M.-E., & Beaumont, C. (2002). Expression of the two mRNA isoforms of the iron transporter Nramp2/DMT1 in mice and function of the iron responsive element. *Biochemical Journal, 363*, 449–455.

Theil, E. C., Matzapetakis, M., & Liu, X. (2006). Ferritins: Iron/oxygen biominerals in protein nanocages. *Journal of Biological Inorganic Chemistry, 11*, 803–810.

Thorstensen, K., & Romslo, I. (1988). Uptake of iron from transferrin by isolated rat hepatocytes. A redox-mediated plasma membrane process? *Journal of Biological Chemistry, 263*, 8844–8850.

Thorstensen, K., & Romslo, I. (1990). The role of transferrin in the mechanism of cellular iron uptake. *Biochemical Journal, 271*, 1–10.

Tolosano, E., & Altruda, F. (2002). Hemopexin: Structure, function, and regulation. *DNA and Cell Biology, 21*, 297–306.

Tolosano, E., Hirsch, E., Patrucco, E., Camaschella, C., Navone, R., Silengo, L., et al. (1999). Defective recovery and severe renal damage after acute hemolysis in hemopexin-deficient mice. *Blood, 94*, 3906–3914.

Trinder, D., & Morgan, E. (1997). Inhibition of uptake of transferrin-bound iron by human hepatoma cells by nontransferrin-bound iron. *Hepatology, 26*, 691–698.

Trinder, D., & Morgan, E. (2001). Uptake of transferrin-bound iron by mammalian cells. In D. M. Templeton (Ed.), *Molecular and cellular iron transport* (pp. 427–449). New York: Marcel Dekker Inc.

Trinder, D., Morgan, E. H., & Baker, E. (1986). The mechanisms of iron uptake by fetal rat hepatocytes in culture. *Hepatology, 6*, 852–858.

Trinder, D., Morgan, E. H., & Baker, E. (1988). The effects of an antibody to the rat transferrin receptor and of rat serum albumin on the uptake of diferric transferrin by rat hepatocytes. *Biochimica et Biophysica Acta, 943*, 440–446.

Trinder, D., Oates, P. S., Thomas, C., Sadlier, J., & Morgan, E. H. (2000). Localisation of divalent metal transporter 1 (DMT1) to the microvillus membrane of rat duodenal enterocytes in iron deficiency, but to hepatocytes in iron overload. *Gut, 46*, 270–276.

Trinder, D., Zak, O., & Aisen, P. (1996). Transferrin receptor-independent uptake of differic transferrin by human hepatoma cells with antisense inhibition of receptor expression. *Hepatology, 23*, 1512–1520.

Vulpe, C. D., Kuo, Y. M., Murphy, T. L., Cowley, L., Askwith, C., Libina, N., et al. (1999). Hephaestin, a ceruloplasmin homologue implicated in intestinal iron transport, is defective in the sla mouse. *Nature Genetics, 21*, 195–199.

Wang, R. H., Li, C., Xu, X., Zheng, Y., Xiao, C., Zerfas, P., et al. (2005). A role of SMAD4 in iron metabolism through the positive regulation of hepcidin expression. *Cell Metabolism, 2*, 399–409.

Wassell, J. (2000). Haptoglobin: Function and polymorphism. *Clinical Laboratory, 46*, 547–552.

Watkins, J. A., Altazan, J. D., Elder, P., Li, C.-Y., Nunez, M.-T., Cui, X.-X., et al. (1992). Kinetic characterization of reductant dependent processes in iron mobilization from endocytic vesicles. *Biochemistry, 31*, 5820–5830.

Weiss, G. (2005). Modification of iron regulation by the inflammatory response. *Best Practice and Research Clinical Haematology, 18*, 183–201.

Wilkins, S. J., Frazer, D. M., Millard, K. N., McLaren, G. D., & Anderson, G. J. (2006). Iron metabolism in the hemoglobin-deficit mouse: Correlation of diferric transferrin with hepcidin expression. *Blood, 107*, 1659–1664.

Wilson, M. T., & Reeder, B. J. (2008). Oxygen-binding haem proteins. *Experimental Physiology, 93*, 128–132.

Wright, T. L., Brissot, P., Ma, W.-L., & Weisinger, R. A. (1986). Characterization of non-transferrin-bound iron clearance by rat liver. *Journal of Biological Chemistry, 261*, 10909–10914.

Xu, X., Pin, S., Gathinji, M., Fuchs, R., & Harris, Z. L. (2004). Aceruloplasminemia: An inherited neurodegenerative disease with impairment of iron homeostasis. *Annals of the New York Academy of Sciences, 1012*, 299–305.

Yeh, K. Y., Yeh, M., Watkins, J. A., Rodriguez-Paris, J., & Glass, J. (2000). Dietary iron induces rapid changes in rat intestinal divalent metal transporter expression. *American Journal of Physiology, Gastrointestinal and Liver Physiology, 279*, G1070–G1079.

Yu, J., Yu, Z. K., & Wessling-Resnick, M. (1998). Expression of SFT (stimulator of Fe transport) is enhanced by iron chelation in HeLa cells and by hemochromatosis in liver. *Journal of Biological Chemistry, 273*, 34675–34678.

Zakin, M. M. (1992). Regulation of transferrin gene expression. *FASEB Journal, 6*, 3253–3258.

Zhang, A. S., Sheftel, A. D., & Ponka, P. (2006). The anemia of "haemoglobin-deficit" (hbd/hbd) mice is caused by a defect in transferrin cycling. *Experimental Hematology, 34*, 593–598.

Zhang, X. M., Ellis, S., Sriratana, A., Mitchell, C. A., & Rowe, T. (2004). Sec15 is an effector for the Rab11 GTPase in mammalian cells. *Journal of Biological Chemistry, 279*, 43027–43034.

Zhang, A.-N., Xiong, S., Tsukamoto, H., & Enns, C. A. (2004). Localization of iron metabolism-related mRNAs in rat liver indicate that HFE is expressed predominantly in hepatocytes. *Blood, 103*, 1509–1514.

[illegible]

[illegible]

[illegible]

[illegible]

[illegible]

[illegible]

[illegible]

# 2 Regulation of Iron Absorption and Distribution

*Gladys Oluyemisi Latunde-Dada and Robert J. Simpson*

**Summary**

- Iron absorption and distribution are determined by the activities of iron transport and storage proteins.
- Absorption of iron by the epithelial cells of the proximal gastrointestinal tract is a highly regulated physiological process that maintains body iron homeostasis.
- Iron efflux from cells occurs through the transporter ferroportin.
- Hepcidin is a plasma peptide that regulates plasma iron levels by controlling the iron export function of ferroportin and thereby also regulates iron absorption and distribution.
- Other mechanisms exist within cells to modulate the activity of iron transport and storage systems in response to cellular iron levels.
- Disordered iron distribution in the body occurs in chronic inflammatory conditions.

**Key Words:** DMT1; iron overload; iron turnover; ferroportin; transferrin receptor 1; transferrin receptor 2; Dcytb; HCP1; hephaestin; ceruloplasmin; transferrin; ferritin; IRP1; IRP2; erythropoiesis; hepcidin

## 1. INTRODUCTION AND SCOPE OF REVIEW

Iron absorption and distribution are determined by the activities of iron transport and storage proteins. Early work identified transferrin (Tf), transferrin receptor (TFR1), ferritin and haemosiderin as the major transport and storage proteins, while the past decade has seen the discovery of an additional series of proteins (DMT1, ferroportin, hephaestin, Dcytb, HCP1 and STEAP3) that provide a framework for explaining the molecular basis for iron absorption and cell iron uptake and release (Dunn, Rahmanto, & Richardson, 2007; Latunde-Dada, Simpson, & Mckie, 2006).

The regulation of iron metabolism was initially understood at a cellular level by the discovery of the effects of iron regulatory proteins IRP1 and IRP2 and their action in controlling the levels of transferrin receptor and ferritin (Rouault, 2006). Our understanding of whole body iron metabolism has been revolutionised by the discovery of hepcidin, a plasma peptide that regulates plasma iron levels by controlling the iron export function of ferroportin (Ganz & Nemeth, 2006). These discoveries have been extensively reviewed by others (see references below), and this chapter brings together key features of these findings and suggests some areas where more work is needed.

From: *Nutrition and Health: Iron Deficiency and Overload*
Edited by: S. Yehuda and D.I. Mostofsky, DOI 10.1007/978-1-59745-462-9_2

## 2. IRON UPTAKE AND RELEASE BY CELLS

Cellular iron movements in mammals are explained by membrane transport steps which are coupled to oxidation or reduction of iron ions. The latter is necessary as proteins that hold iron tightly (transferrin in plasma or ferritin inside cells) bind the more stable oxidised iron ion, Fe(III) (ferric or $Fe^{3+}$), while iron seems to move around within cells and across membranes as the more soluble but unstable, reduced Fe(II) (ferrous or $Fe^{2+}$) ion. Iron enters cells via DMT1 [for divalent metal transporter 1, also called Slc11a2, DCT1 or nramp2 (Andrews, Fleming, & Gunshin, 1999)] and a single electron reduction step is associated with this process [catalysed by STEAP3 in reticulocytes (Ohgami et al., 2005) and Dcytb (also called Cybrd1) (Mckie et al., 2001) in duodenal epithelial cells (see later)]. The influx of iron into cells is driven by a proton gradient as DMT1 is a coupled co-transporter of $H^+$ and $Fe^{2+}$ (Courville, Chaloupka, & Cellier, 2006; Gunshin et al., 1997). Iron leaves cells via ferroportin (IREG1, MTP1), a process that is coupled to oxidation to $Fe^{3+}$ catalysed by hephaestin (in the gut) or ceruloplasmin in plasma.

Iron outside cells is normally tightly bound to the plasma iron transport protein, transferrin. This protein is bound at the cell surface by transferrin receptor, then internalised via clathrin-coated pits to endosomes where acidification of the endosomal lumen leads to dissociation of iron from transferrin (VanEijk & deJong, 1992), allowing reduction by STEAP3 and then transport by DMT1. Iron can also enter cells via fluid-phase internalisation (pinocytosis; Richardson, Chua, & Baker, 1999) of transferrin or by uptake of non-transferrin-bound plasma iron. The latter is important in iron-overload conditions. The finding that DMT1 knockout mice can still take up iron into certain tissues (Gunshin et al., 2005) suggests other transporters for iron exist. There is some evidence that iron can be transported into cells via transporters for other metals, e.g. Zn or Ca transporters [(Liuzzi, Aydemir, Nam, Knutson, & Cousins, 2006; Oudit, Trivieri, Khaper, Liu, & Backx, 2006), although the latter is controversial (Ludwiczek et al., 2007; Savigni, Wege, Cliff, Meesters, & Morgan, 2003)], or by other transporters (Mwanjewe & Grover, 2004) and these may be important in iron-overload conditions. A second transferrin receptor has been found (TFR2; Kawabata et al., 1999); however, this protein seems to be mainly involved in the regulation of iron metabolism as its loss leads to iron overload rather than iron deficiency (Wallace, Summerville, Lusby, & Subramaniam, 2005) (see below). Phagocytic cells can take up iron via internalisation of particles, bacteria or cells, e.g. senescent red cells, and phagocytic cells have both DMT1 and an additional iron transporter, nramp1 (SLC11a1; Blackwell, Searle, Mohamed, & White, 2003; Nevo & Nelson, 2006). This latter transporter is thought to reduce the viability and growth of phagocytosed microorganisms by transporting metals across the phagosome membrane (Courville, Chaloupka, & Cellier, 2006; Nevo & Nelson, 2006). The exact direction of metal transport by nramp1 (into or out of the phagosome) is disputed (Nevo & Nelson, 2006); thus there is uncertainty about the precise function of nramp1. There are, however, many reports of association between genetic variants of nramp1 and susceptibility to infections and autoimmune disease (Blackwell, Searle, Mohamed, & White, 2003); thus this transporter is important in immune function.

Iron efflux from cells occurs through the transporter ferroportin (Abboud & Haile, 2000; Donovan et al., 2000; Mckie et al., 2000). This is thought to be a passive transport (i.e. down the concentration gradient) (McGregor, 2006); however, the strong binding of iron by extracellular transferrin means that iron will tend to leave cells if ferroportin is active. Ferroportin expression is confined to cells with a specific iron efflux function, i.e. placenta, duodenum, macrophages, hepatocytes and brain endothelial cells (Rouault & Cooperman, 2006). Loss of ferroportin leads to severe anaemia and death in unborn mice or zebrafish (Donovan et al., 2005), emphasising the importance of this protein in placental iron transfer. Tissue-specific knockout of ferroportin confirmed that this protein is essential for intestinal iron absorption (Donovan et al., 2005). Efflux is linked to oxidation as ferroportin seems to transport $Fe^{2+}$ ions (McGregor, 2006) while extracellular iron is $Fe^{3+}$ bound to transferrin. Hephaestin and ceruloplasmin are both important for this oxidation as shown by the effects of mutation or loss of these genes in mice (Harris, Durley, Man, & Gitlin, 1999; Wallace, Summerville, Lusby, & Subramaniam, 2005) and aceruloplasminemia in humans (Harris et al., 1995; Yoshida et al., 1995). Loss of hephaestin leads to anaemia due to reduced export of iron from the gut (Vulpe et al., 1999) while loss of ceruloplasmin leads to build up of iron in macrophages due to inefficient efflux of iron from these cells (Harris, Durley, Man, & Gitlin, 1999). Thus there is some tissue specificity in the utilisation of these two proteins for the oxidation step.

Excess iron within cells is stored as $Fe^{3+}$ ions within the storage protein ferritin. Cellular iron uptake from, and release as, ferritin has been reported (Gelvan, Fibach, MeyronHoltz, & Konijn, 1996; Sibille, Kondo, & Aisen, 1988); however, this is not likely to be a major pathway for cellular iron transport in the normal situation (see Konijn, Gelvan, MeyronHoltz, & Fibach, 1997; Ponka & Richardson, 1997).

## 3. MECHANISMS OF IRON ABSORPTION AND LOSS BY MAMMALS

Absorption of iron by the epithelial cells of the proximal gastrointestinal tract is a highly regulated physiological process that maintains body iron homeostasis (Miret, Simpson, & Mckie, 2003). The intestine therefore attunes enterocyte apical iron influx, storage, transcellular transit and/or basolateral efflux in response to systemic requirements. Absorption of iron, therefore, correlates with the body's iron status or requirements under normal physiological conditions (Cox & Peters, 1980; Finch, 1994). Thus, while iron absorption is elevated during depletion (Finch, 1994), hypoxia (Simpson, 1996), development (Anderson, Walsh, Powell, & Halliday, 1991) and pregnancy (Gambling et al., 2001; Millard, Frazer, Wilkins, & Anderson, 2004), it is depressed in secondary iron-overload conditions (Gavin, McCarthy, & Garry, 1994). However, aberrations such as anaemia of inflammation and mutations of iron metabolism genes exert diverse consequences on the magnitude of iron absorption (Fleming, et al., 1997, 1998; Pietrangelo, 2006; Vulpe et al., 1999). The molecular mechanisms underlying these processes and the expression and regulation of the genes and proteins involved have been deciphered to a considerable extent in the past decade.

Dietary iron is broadly classified into haem and non-haem, and each has a separate and distinct mode of uptake by the enterocytes (Carpenter & Mahoney, 1992). Haem is organically bound to the porphyrin moiety of haemoglobin and myoglobin in meat and is believed to be absorbed intact as a metalloporphyrin complex (Wyllie & Kaufman, 1982) after proteolytic cleavage of globin. Haem is highly bioavailable, it is less influenced by dietary constituents, and meals with high haem content (i.e. high meat content) confer an enhancing influence on non-haem iron sources in a composite meal (Carpenter & Mahoney, 1992). Advances in recent years have revealed the molecular mechanism of non-haem iron absorption while that for haem is still emerging.

Earlier evidence showed the presence of a haem receptor in the intestine of pig (Grasbeck, Majuri, Kouvonen, & Tenhunen, 1982) and humans (Worthington, Cohn, Miller, Luo, & Berg, 2001). Furthermore, electron microscopy revealed apical uptake of haem and its subsequent endocytosis in pits at the base of the microvilli, before transit into lysosomes (Parmley, Barton, Conrad, Austin, & Holland, 1981). Temperature-dependent and saturable-specific uptake of haem or haem analogues has been shown in cultured cells such as Caco-2, K562 and HepG2 (Uc, Stokes, & Britigan, 2004; Worthington, Cohn, Miller, Luo, & Berg, 2001). Absorbed haem is catabolised by haem oxygenase 1 (HO-1) to release inorganic iron that enters the cytosolic pool. Haem carrier protein 1 (HCP1) was cloned and characterised (Shayeghi et al., 2005) as a putative haem transport protein (Fig. 1), but recent evidence shows that it is more active as a transporter of folate (Qiu et al., 2006). Breast cancer resistance protein (BCRP/ABCG2) and Feline leukemic virus protein C (FLVCR) recently reported (Krishnamurthy et al., 2004; Quigley et al., 2004) as haem efflux proteins are also localised in the intestine. These haem transport proteins exhibit a broad substrate spectrum and their specific functions in the gut are not fully characterised; however, they function to export excess haem or other dietary porphyrins or structurally similar compounds (Fig. 1). Non-haem iron, on the other hand, consists of mostly ferric ion and its absorption is subject to a synergism of enhancers and inhibitory components of diets and gut secretions (Cox, Mazurier, Spik, Montreuil, & Peters, 1979; Fairweather-Tait, 1989; Miret, Simpson, & Mckie, 2003).

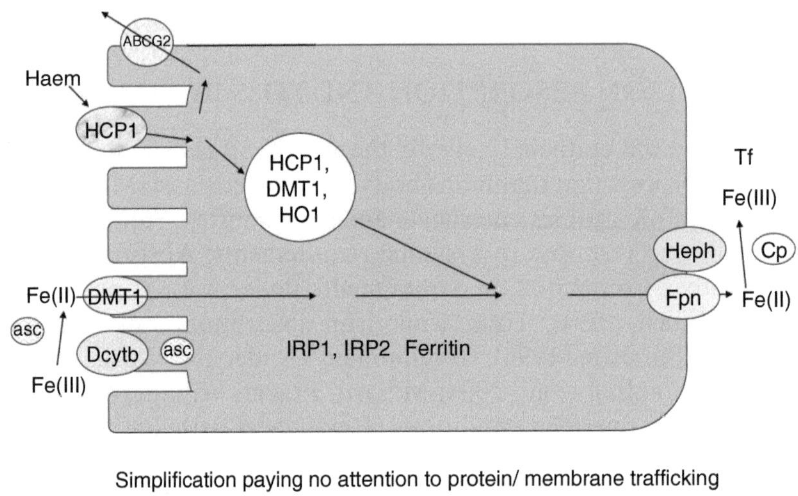


**Fig. 1. Enterocyte iron transport mechanisms.** HO1, haem oxygenase 1; HCP1, haem carrier protein 1; Cp, ceruloplasmin; Heph, hephaestin; Fpn, ferroportin; DMT1, divalent metal transporter 1; asc, ascorbate.

Lumenal factors (particularly ascorbic acid) from the diet or secretions, along with DcytB or Cybrd1, reduce ferric ions to ferrous for uptake at the apical surface of the enterocytes (Fairweather-Tait, 1989; Mckie et al., 2001) (Fig. 1). Ferric reductase redundancy reported (Gunshin et al., 2005) in DcytB knockout mice might not represent the situation in scorbutic species such as guinea pigs and humans or in conditions of high iron demands. STEAP metal ion reductases have also been localised in the intestine (Ohgami et al., 2005). Ferrous ion is driven by proton-coupled electrogenic transport into the cytosol of enterocytes by DMT1 (Fig. 1). In addition to $Fe^{2+}$ transport, DMT1 has been functionally implicated in the mucosal proton-dependent uptake of other divalent metals including $Co^{2+}$, $Mn^{2+}$, $Cd^{2+}$, $Cu^{2+}$, $Ni^{2+}$ and $Pb^{2+}$ (Gunshin et al., 1997). DMT1 has four mRNA splice variants, differing in the presence or absence of the 3′ iron-response element (IRE), regulatory exon at the 5′ end, tissue and functional specificities (Mackenzie, Takanaga, Hubert, Rolfs, & Hediger, 2007). Mutations in the DMT1 gene (G185R) cause microcytic anaemia (Fleming et al., 1997, 1998) respectively in mouse (mk) and rat (Belgrade), and the latter is also reported to show liver iron loading (Thompson, Molina, Brain, & Wessling-Resnick, 2006). In man, mutations in DMT1 leading to loss of active protein from the plasma membrane cause microcytic anaemia with liver iron loading (Beaumont et al., 2006; Iolascon et al., 2005; Lam-Yuk-Tseung, Touret, Grinstein, & Gros, 2005). While the global knockout of DMT1 in mice is lethal due to its specific roles in the intestine and erythropoiesis, selective ablation revealed it is non-essential in the hepatocytes and placenta (Gunshin et al., 2005). Selective knockout of intestinal DMT1 confirms that this transporter is essential for intestinal iron absorption in adult mice (Gunshin et al., 2005).

Absorbed iron enters an uncharacterised pool in the cytosol and its fate is thence subject to systemic regulation. When the body is iron-replete, significant amounts of iron are retained and deposited as ferritin in the cytosol and this is sloughed off into the gut lumen during exfoliation of mature enterocytes. However, in situations of high systemic iron demands or depletion, absorbed iron is trafficked into the circulation through the coordinating actions of the efflux protein ferroportin (Ireg 1, MTP1) and the ferroxidase, hephaestin, a homologue of ceruloplasmin (Vulpe et al., 1999) (Fig. 1). The transit of exogenous iron into circulation (basolateral iron transfer) represents a regulatory set-point involving ferroportin–hepcidin interaction and this is expounded further below. Several mutations in the iron efflux protein ferroportin have been described (Pietrangelo, 2006) and the phenotype generally is tissue iron loading often coupled with hypoferremia (DeDomenico et al., 2005). Similarly, hephaestin-mutant mice (sla) exhibit duodenal iron loading with defective transfer of iron to the body, which results in anaemia (Vulpe et al, 1999). It has been reported that this defect in iron transfer can be overcome by feeding iron-deficient diets (Edwards, Ursillo, & Hoke, 1975), showing that an alternative oxidation mechanism exists in duodenum and this could be explained by ceruloplasmin which was found to contribute to intestinal iron transfer in circumstances of increased iron demand (Cherukuri et al., 2005). Plasma ceruloplasmin can be increased by iron deficiency (Mukhopadhyay, Mazumder, & Fox, 2000).

Intestinal absorption of both dietary forms (haem and non-haem) of iron occurs principally in the duodenum (Forth & Rummel, 1973), and absorption declines progressively down the gastrointestinal tract in parallel with the expression of key proteins involved in the transport machinery, especially Dcytb and Fpn (Gunshin et al., 1997; LatundeDada et al., 2002; Mckie et al., 2000). Moreover, the expression of these proteins is remarkably adaptive and responsive to local and systemic regulation. Early reports have shown biphasic kinetics of iron uptake into mucosal cells and transfer to the body (Forth & Rummel, 1973). An initial rapid phase of iron uptake and basolateral transfer precedes a slower serosal transfer period lasting about 6–24 h following ingestion of iron (Forth & Rummel, 1973). Recent molecular studies have reinforced this idea as the repression of the rapid phase is due in part to the local downregulation of the genes involved in the uptake process (Frazer et al., 2003), while the lag phase corresponds in duration with the time taken to respond to systemic signal. Efflux of iron from the intestine was suggested (Marx, 1979) as the rate-determining step in the absorption process and this has now been ascribed to the regulation of ferroportin in the basolateral enterocyte (Chen et al., 2003).

## 4. IRON TRANSPORT ROUND THE BODY AND TISSUE UPTAKE

Absorbed iron binds to transferrin (Fig. 2) and this, as well as non-transferrin-bound iron (NTBI), which is seen in pathological conditions of iron overload such as haemochromatosis, transfusional siderosis and in hypotransferrinemic (Hpx) mice, enters the circulation where excess is deposited in the liver. Diferric-Tf forms a complex with transferrin receptors, which can be

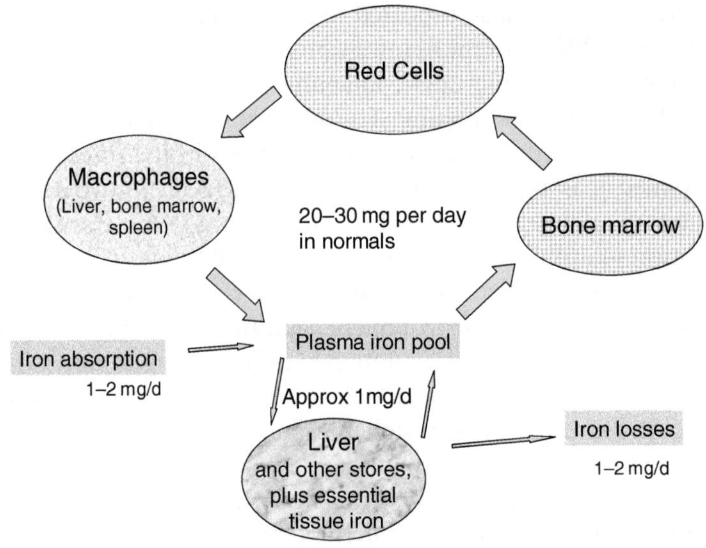


**Fig. 2.** Body iron compartments and fluxes.

endocytosed into hepatocytes where iron is released through DMT1 in acidified endosomes and the receptor is recycled back to the cell surface. This pathway is, however, insignificant as targeted mutation of the DMT1 gene did not obliterate iron uptake in the hepatocyte (Gunshin et al., 2005). Liver also takes up plasma (including iron) by fluid-phase pinocytosis and this can contribute to overall rates of liver iron uptake. NTBI is taken into the hepatocyte by unknown mechanisms although calcium channels, zinc transporters, e.g. ZIP 14, and transient receptor canonical protein TRPC have been proposed as candidates (Liuzzi, Aydemir, Nam, Knutson, & Cousins, 2006; Mwanjewe & Grover, 2004; Oudit et al., 2003). These channels contribute to massive iron loading of the liver in some pathological conditions (Chua, Olynyk, Leedman, & Trinder, 2004; van der et al., 2006) and also cardiomyopathy and endocrinopathy of iron overload. Excess haem in the circulation is similarly endocytosed in the liver by the CD91 haemopexin receptor on hepatocytes and macrophages (Hvidberg et al., 2005). This, as well as haemoglobin-CD163 (haptoglobin receptor on macrophages) endocytosis, represents an acute-phase response to offset elevated levels of free haem in the circulation under pathological conditions such as haemorrhage, haemolysis and rhabdomyolysis.

The liver is the central organ that controls iron storage and release by ferroportin into circulation through the regulation of hepcidin expression (discussed below). Iron release encompasses quantitatively large amounts of iron (about 20–25 mg in man) entering the circulation via reticuloendothelial erythrophagocytosis of senescent red blood cells (Fig. 2). Iron released from macrophages binds to transferrin and supplies the high demand for iron by developing erythroid progenitor cells via the TFR1/STEAP3/DMT1 mechanism. An adequate amount of new erythrocytes is therefore produced to replenish depletion by senescence and prevent anaemia. A minor uptake of Tf-bound iron probably occurs in the polarised epithelial cells of the kidney through megalin-dependent, cubilin-mediated endocytosis (Kozyraki et al., 2001). The dynamic and high turnover rate of Tf-bound iron emphasizes the importance of the regulation of tissue iron distribution and kinetics in maintaining homeostatic equilibrium (Gehrke et al., 2003; Uchida et al., 1983). Systemic iron circulation therefore precisely supplies metabolic and physiological requirements while averting excessive tissue deposition. Consequently, plasma iron concentration is kept within a narrow range in spite of variable fluxes within body compartments (Fig. 2). The maintenance of plasma iron levels through efflux from macrophages of the RES and absorption from the intestine is regulated by ferroportin through its interaction with hepcidin (Nemeth, Tuttle, et al., 2004) (see below). A summary of the proteins involved in iron absorption and regulation is shown in Table 1.

**Table 1**
**Summary of Putative Functions of Proteins Involved in Intestinal Iron Absorption and Regulation**

| *Proteins* | *Localisation* | *Function* |
|---|---|---|
| *Mucosa Iron Uptake* | | |
| Duodenal cytochrome b (Dcytb) | Brush border apical membrane | Ferrireductase, supplies $Fe^{2+}$ to DMT1 |
| Divalent metal transporter (DMT1) | Brush border apical membrane, particularly during enhanced uptake | Uptake of iron and other divalent metals into enterocytes |
| Iron-responsive protein (IRP1, IRP2) | Cytosol | Regulate mRNA expression of DMT1, TFR1 and ferritin |
| HCP1 | Brush border apical membrane | Putative haem transporter/folate transporter |
| ABCG2 | Brush border apical membrane | Possibly apical haem efflux protein |
| *Intracellular Processing* | | |
| Ferritin | Cytosol | Enterocyte storage of excess iron |
| Haem oxygenase 1 (HO1) | Microsomes (lysosomes) | Haem degradation and iron release and recycling of Hb iron |
| *Basolateral Transfer* | | |
| Ferroportin | Basolateral membrane | Iron export from enterocytes and cells |
| Hephaestin | Basolateral/supranuclear region | Basolateral membrane-bound ferroxidase |
| Ceruloplasmin | Serosal side | Cu-binding-plasma ferroxidase |
| *Regulation of Iron Absorption* | | |
| HFE (Hfe) | Liver/crypt enterocyte | Senses iron status, interacts with TfR1 and TfR2 |
| Transferrin receptor 1 (TfR1) | Liver/crypt enterocyte | Membrane receptor for Tf. May be involved with HFE in the regulation of hepcidin expression |
| Transferrin receptor 2 (TfR2) | Liver/crypt enterocyte (?) | Membrane receptor for Tf. May be involved with HFE in the regulation of hepcidin expression |
| Haemojuvelin | Liver, heart, muscle, haematopoietic cells | Membrane and soluble forms associate with bone morphogenic protein in regulating hepcidin expression |
| Hepcidin | Liver, heart? | Antimicrobial peptide that inhibit iron absorption from the enterocytes and efflux in macrophages and placenta |

Disordered iron distribution in the body occurs in chronic inflammatory conditions as iron is sequestered in macrophages and the enterocyte to induce hypoferremia (Nemeth, Rivera, et al., 2004). This situation is believed to be part of the host defence strategy against microbial infection. This acute-phase response elicits expression of inflammatory cytokines to induce hepcidin production (inhibition of iron release through hepcidin–ferroportin interaction is discussed below). In iron overload, specific tissues and even specific cells within tissues are affected. In the most common types of genetic haemochromatosis, some epithelial cells (pancreatic acinar cells and hepatocytes) become very highly iron-loaded while some muscles (especially smooth muscle including heart) show a lower loading, but this can be clinically significant. Other cells are relatively spared from iron loading for reasons that are not well understood. The differential distribution of transferrin receptors or DMT1 between cells is likely to be important as is the presence of ferroportin in some cells. The presence of iron uptake via non-DMT1 pathways may also be significant.

## 5. REGULATION AT THE CELLULAR LEVEL

Iron uptake and release by cells are controlled locally by post-transcriptional regulation of the levels of TFR1, DMT1, ferritin and ferroportin. The mechanism of this regulation is by iron-dependent activity of IRP1 and IRP2. IRP1 binds messenger RNAs (mRNAs) for these proteins only when cellular iron levels are low. When iron is abundant, IRP1 has a complete iron–sulphur centre bound to it and functions as cytoplasmic aconitase. IRP2 also binds mRNAs when iron levels are low; however, when iron is abundant, IRP2 is targeted for degradation by an iron-dependent mechanism (Rouault, 2006). Thus both IRPs bind mRNAs for key cellular iron proteins when iron levels are low. The effect of this binding is to block translation of mRNAs for proteins that remove iron from the cytosol, i.e. the storage protein ferritin, the efflux protein ferroportin, or in erythroid cells the rate-limiting enzyme for haem biosynthesis, delta amino laevulinic acid synthase (ALAS) which indirectly promotes iron removal from the cytosol for incorporation into haem. The effect of IRP binding to mRNAs is different for uptake proteins which deliver iron to the cytosol, i.e. TFR1 or DMT1. Whereas the ferritin and ferroportin mRNAs have IRP-binding sites (called iron-responsive elements or IREs) in their 5′ end near the initiation codons for translation, the TFR1 and DMT1 IREs are in the 3′ untranslated region of the mRNA, where the effect of IRP binding is to prevent degradation of the mRNA, thus elevating the levels available for translation and leading to increased levels of DMT1 and TFR1.

This mechanism allows cells some degree of direct control over their own iron levels and allows them to make ferritin to store away excess iron in a relatively non-toxic form. In erythroid cells the control of ALAS by iron levels helps to ensure coupling of iron supply to haem biosynthesis (Ponka, 2002).

IRPs can also be affected by reactive oxygen and nitrogen species (ROS, RNS) and their activity can be altered by kinase/phosphatase-mediated phosphorylation–dephosphorylation reactions (Wallander, Leibold, & Eisenstein, 2006); thus indirect responses to iron levels and an integration of cellular defence mechanisms are possible (see also below). Note that DMT1 exists in alternately spliced forms, only some of which have IREs. These forms have specific tissue distributions (Hubert & Hentze, 2002); thus iron-dependent control of DMT1 activity varies between tissues. The best understood tissue is the gut and this is described in detail below.

Loss of IRP1 by gene knockout leads to changes only in kidney and brown fat, and it seems that IRP2 is more generally important in regulating iron metabolism in vivo (Meyron-Holtz et al., 2004). Loss of IRP2 leads to more widespread alterations in iron metabolism, with a mild deficit in erythron iron uptake and altered iron distribution between storage compartments in the liver and spleen (Galy et al., 2005) and a late-onset neurodegeneration (LaVaute et al., 2001) implying an important role for IRP2 in the brain. Loss of IRP2 combined with reduction in IRP1 results in anaemia with a more severe neurodegeneration (Smith et al., 2004). Overall total body iron appears to be approximately normal in IRP2 KO mice [R Simpson estimate from data in (Galy et al., 2005)] and radio-iron absorption was found to be normal, despite local increased iron storage in the absorptive enterocytes (Galy et al., 2005). Mutations in IREs within single mRNAs highlight the relatively subtle and tissue-specific roles of the IRE/IRP system; thus hereditary cataracts result from mutations in the L-ferritin IRE in humans, while in mice loss of the ferroportin IRE results in a complex series of changes in tissue iron accumulation, which are not yet fully understood (Mok, Mlodnicka, Hentze, Muckenthaler, & Schumacher, 2006).

There must be other mechanisms for control of protein levels and activity by iron; however, these are not as well understood as the IRP/IRE system. One system that has been well studied is the hypoxia gene response system which is controlled by Hifs (hypoxia-inducible factors) (Metzen & Ratcliffe, 2004). Hifs are transcription factors that activate transcription of genes with appropriate promoter-response elements. The levels of Hifs are controlled by a complex signalling system that responds to cellular levels of oxygen, iron and ascorbate (Jones, Trowbridge, & Harris, 2006; Metzen & Ratcliffe, 2004; Pan et al., 2007). On the other hand, genes with hypoxia-response elements in their promoters (including TFR1 and hepcidin) can potentially respond to oxygen levels; thus there is a regulatory mechanism operating at the cellular level that can integrate control of oxygen and iron-responsive genes. Calreticulin is reported to be an iron-binding protein (Conrad, Umbreit, & Moore, 1993) whose levels are altered by iron (Nunez, Osorio, Tapia, Vergara, & Mura, 2001). Calreticulin has also been reported to alter synthesis of the transcription factor C/EBPalpha (Timchenko, Iakova, Welm, Cai, & Timchenko, 2002) which controls transcription of a variety of genes including hepcidin (Courselaud et al., 2002). There is also evidence that the redox-responsive transcription factor, NfkappaB, can respond to cellular iron levels (Templeton & Liu, 2003); thus NfkappaB-responsive genes may also respond to iron levels. Thus iron levels can potentially control transcription of a wide range of genes, while several signalling pathways may also affect iron metabolism.

Specifically, iron-sensitive transcription factors remain elusive in mammals, and until they are identified, transcriptional control of genes by iron remains poorly understood and seems to be somewhat indirect, operating via transcription factors that have other duties and potentially integrate several diverse signalling pathways.

A third level at which control exists is the cellular localisation of proteins, such as DMT1, being controlled by iron. This has been shown to occur in intestinal enterocytes, with the amounts of DMT1 at the brush border membrane decreasing in response to oral iron dosing (K. Y. Yeh, M. Yeh, Watkins, RodriguezParis, & Glass, 2000). Different DMT1 isoforms also recycle between the cell surface and the intracellular sites with distinctive kinetics, thus allowing differential expression of DMT1 at the cell surface depending on tissue-specific alternate splicing of the mRNA (Thomson, Rogers, & Leedman, 1999).

## 6. REGULATION OF WHOLE BODY IRON STATUS

Total body iron levels are maintained primarily by controlling duodenal iron absorption from the diet. Iron is lost from the body via uncontrolled blood losses (mainly gastrointestinal in men, with menstrual losses also significant in women of child-bearing age), epithelial cell losses (mainly gastrointestinal tract, skin and kidney epithelial cells) and via secretions (tears, sweat and gastrointestinal secretions). Figure 3 shows the relative importance of these losses. Body iron losses vary somewhat in proportion to body iron levels, e.g. blood iron losses will presumably be less in anaemia and epithelial cell iron losses may be greater in iron overload; however, there is no close linkage of body iron losses to the levels of iron stores or tissue iron requirements. Absorption of dietary iron is, on the other hand, closely linked to iron stores and iron requirement and is therefore the main way the body controls its iron content (Hallberg, Hulten, & Gramatkovski, 1997). Iron losses are seen as obligatory, uncontrolled losses and these are balanced by the regulation of iron absorption by duodenum. The mechanisms by which this regulation is brought about are now being understood at the molecular level (see hepcidin section below). There is some evidence that re-absorption of intestinal iron losses in the colon can be important; however, this has been little studied (Takeuchi et al., 2005).

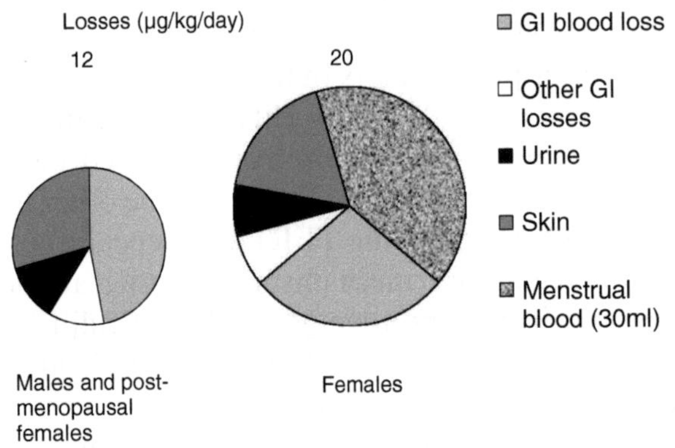


**Fig. 3. Body iron losses**. The charts indicate the relative size of iron losses from the body; the numbers show the total losses in µg/kg body weight/day.

Regulation of body iron levels therefore requires a sensing mechanism that can regulate iron absorption in response to decreased iron levels in critical compartments, thereby maintaining homeostasis. The key compartments appear to be the erythroid compartment, plasma transferrin and tissue iron stores. Production of hepcidin is thought to be regulated in response to decreased iron stores or plasma diferric transferrin (Steele, Frazer, & Anderson, 2005), thereby providing a homeostatic loop that regulates plasma iron and iron stores by its blocking effect on iron efflux from enterocytes, hepatocytes and macrophages. Deranged body iron homeostasis occurs in several diseases, all of which seem to affect hepcidin production, and this is discussed in detail below. Mutations in ferroportin can lead to loss of sensitivity to hepcidin (DeDomenico et al., 2005; Schimanski et al., 2005) or loss of ferroportin activity (McGregor et al., 2005; Sham et al., 2005), leading to inappropriate iron accumulation in iron stores. Mutations that directly affect hepcidin levels are described below.

Inappropriate body iron losses occur mainly through increased bleeding as losses through sweat and urine are relatively small (Beard & Tobin, 2000). These can result from gastrointestinal diseases (e.g. cancer, ulcers, Annibale et al., 2001), parasites (Crompton & Nesheim, 2002), post operatively (Wallis, Wells, Whitehead, & Brewster, 2005), NSAID treatment (Ferrara, Coppola, Coppola, & Capozzi, 2006) or from increased menstrual losses (Ferrara, Coppola, Coppola, & Capozzi, 2006; Hallberg, Hulthen, Bengtsson, Lapidus, & Lindstedt, 1995). These can rapidly lead to iron deficiency when the body's normal homeostatic mechanism of increased duodenal iron absorption fails to compensate, either because of lack of sufficient dietary iron in a suitably available form (Ferrara, Coppola, Coppola, & Capozzi, 2006) or because of a failure to absorb sufficient iron due to gastrointestinal disease (e.g. gastritis & or IBD (Annibale et al., 2001; Gasche & Kulnigg, 2006)) or chronic inflammation (Ganz & Nemeth, 2006). In these conditions the underlying cause of iron loss has to be addressed. Iron deficiency can arise over a long period where there is a chronic condition that reduces iron absorption, e.g. a chronic inflammatory condition as noted above or poor dietary iron supply. Rapid growth rates or pregnancy combined with poor supply of dietary iron can lead to more rapid onset of iron deficiency (Milman, 2006).

## 7. HEPCIDIN IN THE REGULATION OF IRON ABSORPTION AND DISTRIBUTION

Hepcidin (hepatic bactericidal protein) is a liver-expressed antimicrobial peptide (LEAP1) found in the blood (Krause et al., 2000) and in urine (Park, Valore, Waring, & Ganz, 2001). Hepcidin gene is called HAMP (hepcidin antimicrobial peptide (OMIM)) and is expressed predominantly in the liver (Nicolas et al., 2002; Park, Valore, Waring, & Ganz, 2001; Pigeon et al., 2001). It is also expressed in the heart, pancreas, lungs and haematopoietic cells (Peyssonnaux et al., 2006). The bioactive 25 amino acid hepcidin peptide is rich in β-sheet which is stabilized by conserved disulfide bonds in a hairpin configuration (Kemna, Tjalsma, Podust, & Swinkels, 2007). Hepcidin's role in iron metabolism was serendipitously discovered in USF knockout mice that displayed a massive iron overload phenotype, characteristic of haemochromatosis (Nicolas et al., 2001). In contrast, however, transgenic mice over-expressing hepcidin developed a severe iron-deficient phenotype (Nicolas, Bennoun, et al., 2002). Furthermore, hepcidin expression is increased after the administration of large oral doses of iron (Frazer et al., 2003) when iron stores are elevated (Pigeon et al., 2001) or in inflammation (Nemeth, Rivera, et al., 2004; Nicolas, Chauvet, et al., 2002) and decreased under conditions of anaemia (Nicolas, Chauvet, et al., 2002), iron deficiency (Frazer et al., 2002) and hypotransferrinemia (Weinstein et al., 2002). Compelling direct evidence revealed that the injection of hepcidin into mice resulted in decreased absorption of iron (Laftah et al., 2004), while a hepcidin-secreting tumour was found to cause anaemia (Weinstein et al., 2002).

Substantive evidence has accrued to implicate hepcidin as a peptide that inhibits the release of iron into circulation from the intestine, hepatic and splenic macrophages and the placenta (Rivera et al., 2005). Hepcidin was found to interact with ferroportin at the apical surface of HEK 293 cells causing its internalization and degradation (Nemeth, Tuttle, et al., 2004) in endolysosomes, thus providing a mechanism whereby cellular iron efflux by ferroportin is inhibited by hepcidin. This direct interaction of hepcidin with ferroportin mediates in vivo iron absorption in the duodenum as well as iron efflux from hepatocytes and macrophages (DeDomenico et al., 2005; Njajou et al., 2001). Hepcidin is therefore a negative regulator of iron efflux in these tissues. In the case of enterocytes, decreased ferroportin could lead to iron build up in enterocytes, which in turn downregulates iron uptake from the intestinal lumen; however, a more direct effect of hepcidin on enterocyte iron uptake is also possible (Yamaji, Sharp, Ramesh, & Srai, 2004).

The mechanism by which hepcidin production is regulated in hepatocytes in response to the iron requirements of the whole organism is the subject of intense ongoing investigation. Delineation of the regulatory mechanisms of hepcidin expression has been achieved from studies of iron-loading phenotypes in humans and mice (see above). However, compelling evidence indicates that the BMP/Smad, STAT3 and ERK/p38 MAP kinase signal transduction pathways are involved in the transcriptional regulation of hepcidin expression (Babitt et al., 2006; Calzolari et al., 2006; Verga Falzacappa et al., 2007; Wrighting & Andrews, 2006).

Advances in understanding the regulation of hepcidin induction seem to be progressing faster than knowledge of signals that repress its expression as seen in iron depletion, hypoxia or increased erythropoiesis (Gardenghi et al., 2007; Latunde-Dada, Vulpe, Anderson, Simpson, & Mckie, 2004; Nicolas, Chauvet, et al., 2002). Anaemia (decreased circulating haemoglobin) leads to increased erythropoiesis, which also seems to regulate hepcidin production to increase iron absorption. The mechanism of this link between the bone marrow (site of erythropoiesis) and the liver (site of hepcidin production) is unclear but may involve plasma diferric transferrin levels or some other factor (e.g. 5-amino laevulinic acid (Laftah, Raja, Simpson, & Peters, 2003; Laftah et al., 2003, 2004) or erythropoietic factors such as GDF15 (Tanno et al., 2007)). While the mechanism of the erythropoietic signal is still unknown, it overrides the iron-sensing regulation in certain iron-loading conditions such as thalassemia intermedia. It seems apparent therefore that a signal which modulates iron absorption originates in the bone marrow as a result of ineffective erythropoiesis and causes the suppression of hepcidin expression. This is perhaps the reason why anaemia that involves peripheral destruction of mature red blood cells, e.g. sickle cell, hereditary spherocytosis or autoimmune haemolytic anaemia, does not enhance iron absorption.

Oxygen delivery to liver also seems to regulate hepcidin production (Nicolas, Chauvet, et al., 2002), thereby providing a mechanism whereby hypoxia increases iron absorption (Laftah et al., 2005). Moreover, a recent study in cultured HepG2 cells showed that reactive oxygen species (ROS) repress hepcidin gene expression by inhibiting C/EBPα and STAT3 binding to hepcidin promoter during hypoxia (Choi, Cho, Kim, & Park, 2007), while a study of the Hif (hypoxia-inducible factor) pathway suggested this may also regulate hepcidin synthesis (Peyssonnaux et al., 2007). Other factors that can regulate iron absorption include gender-related factors (e.g. sex hormones, Hershko & Eilon, 1974), pregnancy and inflammation. These all affect hepcidin levels (Courselaud et al., 2004; Millard, Frazer, Wilkins, & Anderson, 2004; Nicolas, Chauvet, et al., 2002), which in turn controls iron absorption.

## 8. CONCLUDING OVERVIEW AND UNKNOWNS

The model for iron regulation of iron absorption and distribution described above remains qualitative but seems to contain mechanisms that can explain most of the observed features of these processes. The main gaps are the identity of the 'erythroid factor' that can stimulate iron absorption even in the face of iron loading and possible gender-specific factors and minor genetic factors which could combine with known components to modulate body iron levels and distribution. Details of the signalling pathways that regulate hepcidin are still emerging. The reasons why only specific cells load up with iron in iron-overload diseases and the reasons why some cells seem to be more susceptible to damage by iron are poorly understood. Other challenges are quantitative – there is no widely available quantitative assay for hepcidin, and when one becomes available, measurements of this key regulator need to be combined with measurements of other parameters of iron metabolism (many of which have ceased to be widely measured, e.g. plasma iron turnover, plasma/serum diferric transferrin levels, iron absorption rates). The resulting data will then allow the plasma iron-hepcidin-iron absorption regulation model to be tested thoroughly, in particular to explain the high variability in reported hepcidin levels (even within normal groups) and the poor correlation between plasma iron levels or transferrin saturation and iron absorption (e.g. Walters, Jacobs, Worwood, Trevett, & Thomson, 1975). Only then will the adequacy of our knowledge be apparent.

## REFERENCES


Abboud, S., & Haile, D. J. (2000). A novel mammalian iron-regulated protein involved in intracellular iron metabolism. *The Journal of Biological Chemistry, 275*, 19906–19912.

Anderson, G. J., Walsh, M. D., Powell, L. W., & Halliday, J. W. (1991). Intestinal transferrin receptors and iron absorption in the neonatal rat. *British Journal of Haematology, 77*, 229–236.

Andrews, N. C., Fleming, M. D., & Gunshin, H. (1999). Iron transport across biologic membranes. *Nutrition Reviews, 57*, 114–123.

Annibale, B., Capurso, G., Chistolini, A., D'Ambra, G., DiGiulio, E., Monarca, B., et al. (2001). Gastrointestinal causes of refractory iron deficiency anemia in patients without gastrointestinal symptoms. *The American Journal of Medicine, 111*, 439–445.

Babitt, J. L., Huang, F. W., Wrighting, D. M., Xia, Y., Sidis, Y., Samad, T. A., et al. (2006). Bone morphogenetic protein signaling by hemojuvelin regulates hepcidin expression. *Nature Genetics, 38*, 531–539.

Beard, J., & Tobin, B. (2000). Iron status and exercise. *The American Journal of Clinical Nutrition, 72*, 594S–597S.

Beaumont, C., Delaunay, J., Hetet, G., Grandchamp, B., de Montalembert, M., & Tchernia, G. (2006). Two new human DMT1 gene mutations in a patient with microcytic anemia, low ferritinemia, and liver iron overload. *Blood, 107*, 4168–4170.

Blackwell, J. M., Searle, S., Mohamed, H., & White, J. K. (2003). Divalent cation transport and susceptibility to infectious and autoimmune disease: Continuation of the Ity/Lsh/Bcg/Nramp1/Slc11a1 gene story. *Immunology Letters, 85*, 197–203.

Calzolari, A., Raggi, C., Deaglio, S., Sposi, N. M., Stafsnes, M., Fecchi, K., et al. (2006). TfR2 localizes in lipid raft domains and is released in exosomes to activate signal transduction along the MAPK pathway. *Journal of Cell Science, 119*, 4486–4498.

Carpenter, C. E., & Mahoney, A. W. (1992). Contributions of heme and nonheme iron to human nutrition. *Critical Reviews in Food Science and Nutrition, 31*, 333–367.

Chen, H., Su, T., Attieh, Z. K., Fox, T. C., Mckie, A. T., Anderson, G. J., et al. (2003). Systemic regulation of HEPHAESTIN and IREG1 revealed in studies of genetic and nutritional iron deficiency. *Blood, 102*, 1893–1899.

Cherukuri, S., Potla, R., Sarkar, J., Nurko, S., Harris, Z. L., & Fox, P. L. (2005). Unexpected role of ceruloplasmin in intestinal iron absorption. *Cell Metabolism, 2*, 309–319.

Choi, S. O., Cho, Y. S., Kim, H. L., & Park, J. W. (2007). ROS mediate the hypoxic repression of the hepcidin gene by inhibiting C/EBPalpha and STAT-3. *Biochemical and Biophysical Research Communications, 356*, 312–317.

Chua, A. C., Olynyk, J. K., Leedman, P. J., & Trinder, D. (2004). Nontransferrin-bound iron uptake by hepatocytes is increased in the Hfe knockout mouse model of hereditary hemochromatosis. *Blood, 104*, 1519–1525.

Conrad, M. E., Umbreit, J. N., & Moore, E. G. (1993). Rat duodenal iron-binding protein mobilferrin is a homologue of calreticulin. *Gastroenterology, 104*, 1700–1704.

Courselaud, B., Pigeon, C., Inoue, Y., Inoue, J., Gonzalez, F. J., Leroyer, P., et al. (2002). C/EBPalpha regulates hepatic transcription of hepcidin, an antimicrobial peptide and regulator of iron metabolism. Cross-talk between C/EBP pathway and iron metabolism. *The Journal of Biological Chemistry, 277*, 41163–41170.

Courselaud, B., Troadec, M. B., Fruchon, S., Ilyin, G., Borot, N., Leroyer, P., et al. (2004). Strain and gender modulate hepatic hepcidin 1 and 2 mRNA expression in mice. *Blood Cells, Molecules & Diseases, 32*, 283–289.

Courville, P., Chaloupka, R., & Cellier, M. F. (2006). Recent progress in structure-function analyses of Nramp proton-dependent metal-ion transporters. *Biochemistry and Cell Biology, 84*, 960–978.

Cox, T. M., Mazurier, J., Spik, G., Montreuil, J., & Peters, T. J. (1979). Iron binding proteins and influx of iron across the duodenal brush border. Evidence for special lactotransferrin receptors in human intestine. *Biochimica et Biophysica Acta, 588*, 120–128.

Cox, T. M., & Peters, T. J. (1980). Cellular mechanisms in the regulation of iron absorption: Studies in deficiency before and after treatment. *British Journal of Haematology, 44*, 75–86.

Crompton, D. W., & Nesheim, M. C. (2002). Nutritional impact of intestinal helminthiasis during the human life cycle. *Annual Review of Nutrition, 22*, 35–59.

DeDomenico, I., Ward, D. M., Nemeth, E., Vaughn, M. B., Musci, G., Ganz, T., et al. (2005). The molecular basis of ferroportin-linked hemochromatosis. *Proceedings of the National Academy of Sciences USA, 102*, 8955–8960.

Donovan, A., Brownlie, A., Zhou, Y., Shepard, J., Pratt, S. J., Moynihan, J., et al. (2000). Positional cloning of zebrafish ferroportin1 identifies a conserved vertebrate iron exporter. *Nature, 403*, 776–781.

Donovan, A., Lima, C. A., Pinkus, J. L., Pinkus, G. S., Zon, L. I., Robine, S., et al. (2005). The iron exporter ferroportin/Slc40a1 is essential for iron homeostasis. *Cell Metabolism, 1*, 191–200.

Dunn, L. L., Rahmanto, Y. S., & Richardson, D. R. (2007). Iron uptake and metabolism in the new millennium. *Trends in Cell Biology, 17*, 93–100.

Edwards, J. A., Ursillo, R. C., & Hoke, J. E. (1975). Effect of dietary iron manipulation and phenobarbitone treatment on in vivo intestinal absorption of iron in mice with sex-linked anaemia. *The American Journal of Clinical Nutrition, 28*, 140–145.

Fairweather-Tait, S. J. (1989). Iron in food and its availability. *Acta Paediatrica Scandinavica. Supplement, 361*, 12–20.

Ferrara, M., Coppola, L., Coppola, A., & Capozzi, L. (2006). Iron deficiency in childhood and adolescence: Retrospective review. *Hematology, 11*, 183–186.

Finch, C. (1994). Regulators of iron balance in humans. *Blood, 84*, 1697–1702.

Fleming, M. D., Michelle, A., Romano, M. A., Su, L. M., Garrick, M. D., & Andrews, N. C. (1998). Nramp2 is mutated in the anemic Belgrade (b) rat: Evidence of a role for Nramp2 in endosomal iron transport. *Proceedings of the National Academy of Sciences USA, 95*, 1148–1153.

Fleming, M. D., Trenor, C. C., Su, M. A., Foernzler, D., Beier, D. R., Deitrich, W. F., et al. (1997). Microcytic anaemia mice have a mutation in Nramp2, a candidate iron transporter gene. *Nature Genetics, 16*, 383–386.

Forth, W., & Rummel, W. (1973). Iron absorption. *Physiological Reviews*, 53, 724–792.

Frazer, D. M., Wilkins, S. J., Becker, E. M., Murphy, T. L., Vulpe, C. D., Mckie, A. T., et al. (2003). A rapid decrease in the expression of DMT1 and Dcytb but not Ireg1 or hephaestin explains the mucosal block phenomenon of iron absorption. *Gut, 52*, 340–346.

Frazer, D. M., Wilkins, S. J., Becker, E. M., Vulpe, C. D., Mckie, A. T., Trinder, D., et al. (2002). Hepcidin expression inversely correlates with the expression of duodenal iron transporters and iron absorption in rats. *Gastroenterology, 123*, 835–844.

Galy, B., Ferring, D., Minana, B., Bell, O., Janser, H. G., Muckenthaler, M., et al. (2005). Altered body iron distribution and microcytosis in mice deficient in iron regulatory protein 2 (IRP2). *Blood, 106*, 2580–2589.

Gambling, L., Danzeisen, R., Gair, S., Lea, R. G., Charania, Z., Solanky, N., et al. (2001). Effect of iron deficiency on placental transfer of iron and expression of iron transport proteins in vivo and in vitro. *The Biochemical Journal, 356*, 883–889.

Ganz, T., & Nemeth, E. (2006). Regulation of iron acquisition and iron distribution in mammals. *Biochimica et Biophysica Acta, 1763*, 690–699.

Gardenghi, S., Marongiu, M. F., Ramos, P., Guy, E., Breda, L., Chadburn, A., et al. (2007). Ineffective erythropoiesis in {beta}-thalassemia is characterized by increased iron absorption mediated by down-regulation of hepcidin and up-regulation of ferroportin. *Blood, 109*, 5027–5035.

Gasche, C., & Kulnigg, S. (2006). Intravenous iron in inflammatory bowel disease. *Seminars in Hematology, 43*, S18–S22.

Gavin, M. W., McCarthy, D. M., & Garry, P. J. (1994). Evidence that iron stores regulate iron absorption – A setpoint theory. *The American Journal of Clinical Nutrition, 59*, 1376–1380.

Gehrke, S. G., Kulaksiz, H., Herrmann, T., Riedel, H. D., Bents, K., Veltkamp, C., et al. (2003). Expression of hepcidin in hereditary hemochromatosis: Evidence for a regulation in response to serum transferrin saturation and non-transferrin-bound iron. Regulation of human hepcidin expression. *Blood, 102*, 371–376.

Gelvan, D., Fibach, E., MeyronHoltz, E. G., & Konijn, A. M. (1996). Ferritin uptake by human erythroid precursos is a regulated iron uptake pathway. *Blood, 88*, 3200–3207.

Grasbeck, R., Majuri, R., Kouvonen, I., & Tenhunen, R. (1982). Spectral and other studies on the intestinal haem receptor of the pig. *Biochimica et Biophysica Acta, 700*, 137–142.

Gunshin, H., Fujiwara, Y., Custodio, A. O., Direnzo, C., Robine, S., & Andrews, N. C. (2005). Slc11a2 is required for intestinal iron absorption and erythropoiesis but dispensable in placenta and liver. *The Journal of Clinical Investigation, 115*, 1258–1266.

Gunshin, H., Mackenzie, B., Berger, U., Gunshin, Y., Romero, M. F., Boron, W. F., et al. (1997). Cloning and characterization of a mammalian proton coupled metal ion transporter. *Nature, 388*, 482–488.

Gunshin, H., Starr, C. N., Direnzo, C., Fleming, M. D., Jin, J., Greer, E. L., et al. (2005). Cybrd1 (duodenal cytochrome b) is not necessary for dietary iron absorption in mice. *Blood, 106*, 2879–2883.

Hallberg, L., Hulten, L., & Gramatkovski, E. (1997). Iron absorption from the whole diet in men: How effective is the regulation of iron absorption? *The American Journal of Clinical Nutrition, 66*, 347–356.

Hallberg, L., Hulthen, L., Bengtsson, C., Lapidus, L., & Lindstedt, G. (1995). Iron balance in menstruating women. *European Journal of Clinical Nutrition, 49*, 200–207.

Harris, Z. L., Durley, A. P., Man, T. K., & Gitlin, J. D. (1999). Targeted gene disruption reveals an essential role for ceruloplasmin in cellular iron efflux. *Proceedings of the National Academy of Sciences USA, 96*, 10812–10817.

Harris, Z. L., Takahashi, Y., Miyajima, H., Serizawa, M., MacGillivray, R. T., & Gitlin, J. D. (1995). Aceruloplasminemia: Molecular characterization of this disorder of iron metabolism. *Proceedings of the National Academy of Sciences USA, 92*, 2539–2543.

Hershko, C., & Eilon, L. (1974). The effect of sex difference on iron exchange in the rat. *British Journal of Haematology, 28*, 471–482.

Hubert, N., & Hentze, M. W. (2002). Previously uncharacterized isoforms of divalent metal transporter (DMT)-1: Implications for regulation and cellular function. *Proceedings of the National Academy of Sciences USA*, September 3 [epub ahead of print].

Hvidberg, V., Maniecki, M. B., Jacobsen, C., Hojrup, P., Moller, H. J., & Moestrup, S. K. (2005). Identification of the receptor scavenging hemopexin-heme complexes. *Blood, 106*, 2572–2579.

Iolascon, A., d'Apolito, M., Servedio, V., Cimmino, F., Piga, A., & Camaschella, C. (2005). Microcytic anemia and hepatic iron overload in a child with compound heterozygous mutations in DMT1. *Blood, 107*, 349–354.

Jones, D. T., Trowbridge, I. S., & Harris, A. L. (2006). Effects of transferrin receptor blockade on cancer cell proliferation and hypoxia-inducible factor function and their differential regulation by ascorbate. *Cancer Research, 66*, 2749–2756.

Kawabata, H., Yang, R., Hirama, T., Vuong, P. T., Kawano, S., Gombart, A. F., et al. (1999). Molecular cloning of transferrin receptor 2. A new member of the transferrin receptor-like family. *The Journal of Biological Chemistry, 274*, 20826–20832.

Kemna, E. H., Tjalsma, H., Podust, V. N., & Swinkels, D. W. (2007). Mass spectrometry-based hepcidin measurements in serum and urine: Analytical aspects and clinical implications. *Clinical Chemistry, 53*, 620–628.

Konijn, A. M., Gelvan, D., MeyronHoltz, E., & Fibach, E. (1997). Can ferritin provide iron for hemoglobin synthesis-response. *Blood, 89*, 2612.

Kozyraki, R., Fyfe, J., Verroust, P. J., Jacobsen, C., Dautry-Varsat, A., Gburek, J., et al. (2001). Megalin-dependent cubilin-mediated endocytosis is a major pathway for the apical uptake of transferrin in polarized epithelia. *Proceedings of the National Academy of Sciences USA, 98*, 12491–12496.

Krause, A., Neitz, S., Magert, H. J., Schulz, A., Forssmann, W. G., SchulzKnappe, P., et al. (2000). LEAP-1, a novel highly disulfide-bonded human peptide, exhibits antimicrobial activity. *FEBS Letters, 480*, 147–150.

Krishnamurthy, P., Ross, D. D., Nakanishi, T., Bailey-Dell, K., Zhou, S., Mercer, K. E., et al. (2004). The stem cell marker Bcrp/ABCG2 enhances hypoxic cell survival through interactions with heme. *The Journal of Biological Chemistry, 279*, 24218–24225.

Laftah, A. H., Raja, K., Simpson, R. J., & Peters, T. J. (2003). Effect of Tin-mesoporphyrin, an inhibitor of haem catabolism, on intestinal iron absorption. *British Journal of Haematology, 122*, 298–304.

Laftah, A. H., Raja, K. B., Beaumont, N., Simpson, R. J., Deacon, A., Solanky, N., et al. (2004). The effects of inhibition of haem biosynthesis by griseofulvin on intestinal iron absorption. *Basic and Clinical Pharmacology and Toxicology, 94*, 161–168.

Laftah, A. H., Raja, K. B., Latunde-Dada, G. O., Vergi, T., Mckie, A. T., Simpson, R. J., et al. (2005). Effect of altered iron metabolism on markers of haem biosynthesis and intestinal iron absorption in mice. *Annals of Hematology, 84*, 177–182.

Laftah, A. H., Ramesh, B., Simpson, R. J., Solanky, N., Bahram, S., Schumann, K., et al. (2004). Effect of hepcidin on intestinal iron absorption in mice. *Blood, 103*, 3940–3944.

Laftah, A. H., Simpson, R. J., Beaumont, N., Bahram, S., Schumann, K., & Srai, S. K. S. (2003). Hypoxic response of iron absorption is not affected by Hfe gene knock-out in mice. *British Journal of Haematology, 123*, 170–172.

Lam-Yuk-Tseung, S., Touret, N., Grinstein, S., & Gros, P. (2005). Carboxyl-terminus determinants of the iron transporter DMT1/SLC11A2 isoform II (-IRE/1B) mediate internalization from the plasma membrane into recycling endosomes. *Biochemistry, 44*, 12149–12159.

Latunde-Dada, G. O., Simpson, R. J., & Mckie, A. T. (2006). Recent advances in mammalian haem transport. *Trends in Biochemical Sciences, 31*, 182–188.

Latunde-Dada, G. O., Vulpe, C. D., Anderson, G. J., Simpson, R. J., & Mckie, A. T. (2004). Tissue-specific changes in iron metabolism genes in mice following phenylhydrazine-induced haemolysis. *Biochimica et Biophysica Acta, 1690*, 169–176.

LatundeDada, G. O., Van Der Westhuizen, J. P., Vulpe, C. D., Anderson, G., Simpson, R. J., & Mckie, A. T. (2002). Molecular and functional roles of duodenal cytochrome B (Dcytb) in iron metabolism. *Blood Cells Molecules and Diseases, 29*, 356–360.

LaVaute, T., Smith, S., Cooperman, S., Iwail, K., Land, W., MeyronHoltz, E., et al. (2001). Targeted deletion of the gene encoding iron regulatory proteins causes misregulation of iron metabolism and neurodegenerative disease in mice. *Nature Genetics, 27*, 209–214.

Liuzzi, J. P., Aydemir, F., Nam, H., Knutson, M. D., & Cousins, R. J. (2006). Zip14 (Slc39a14) mediates non-transferrin-bound iron uptake into cells. *Proceedings of the National Academy of Sciences USA, 103*, 13612–13617.

Ludwiczek, S., Theurl, I., Muckenthaler, M. U., Jakab, M., Mair, S. M., Theurl, M., et al. (2007). Ca(2+) channel blockers reverse iron overload by a new mechanism via divalent metal transporter-1. *Nature Medicine, 13*, 448–454.

Mackenzie, B., Takanaga, H., Hubert, N., Rolfs, A., & Hediger, M. A. (2007). Functional properties of multiple isoforms of human divalent metal-ion transporter 1 (DMT1). *The Biochemical Journal, 403*, 59–69.

Marx, J. J. M. (1979). Mucosal uptake, mucosal transfer and retention of iron measured by whole-body counting. *Scandinavian Journal of Haematology, 23*, 293–302.

McGregor, J. A. (2006). *The genetic and functional characterisation of iron metabolism genes in health and disease*. London: University of London.

McGregor, J. A., Shayeghi, M., Vulpe, C. D., Anderson, G. J., Pietrangelo, A., Simpson, R. J., et al. (2005). Impaired iron transport activity of ferroportin 1 in hereditary iron overload. *The Journal of Membrane Biology, 206*, 3–7.

Mckie, A. T., Barrow, D., LatundeDada, G. O., Rolfs, A., Sager, G., Mudaly, E., et al. (2001). An iron-regulated ferric reductase associated with the absorption of dietary iron. *Science, 291*, 1755–1759.

Mckie, A. T., Marcani, P., Rolfs, A., Brennan, K., Wehr, K., Barrow, D., et al. (2000). A novel duodenal iron-regulated transporter (Iregl) implicated in the basolateral transfer of iron to the circulation. *Molecular Cell, 5*, 299–309.

Metzen, E., & Ratcliffe, P. J. (2004). HIF hydroxylation and cellular oxygen sensing. *Biological Chemistry, 385*, 223–230.

Meyron-Holtz, E. G., Ghosh, M. C., Iwai, K., LaVaute, T., Brazzolotto, X., Berger, U. V., et al. (2004). Genetic ablations of iron regulatory proteins 1 and 2 reveal why iron regulatory protein 2 dominates iron homeostasis. *EMBO Journal, 23*, 386–395.

Millard, K. N., Frazer, D. M., Wilkins, S. J., & Anderson, G. J. (2004). Changes in the expression of intestinal iron transport and hepatic regulatory molecules explain the enhanced iron absorption associated with pregnancy in the rat. *Gut, 53*, 655–660.

Milman, N. (2006). Iron and pregnancy – A delicate balance. *Annals of Hematology, 85*, 559–565.

Miret, S., Simpson, R. J., & Mckie, A. T. (2003). Physiology and molecular biology of dietary iron absorption. *Annual Review of Nutrition, 23*, 283–301.

Mok, H., Mlodnicka, A. E., Hentze, M. W., Muckenthaler, M., & Schumacher, A. (2006). The molecular circuitry regulating the switch between iron deficiency and overload in mice. *The Journal of Biological Chemistry, 281*, 7946–7951.

Mukhopadhyay, C. K., Mazumder, B., & Fox, P. L. (2000). Role of hypoxia-inducible factor-1 in transcriptional activation of ceruloplasmin by iron deficiency. *The Journal of Biological Chemistry, 275*, 21048–21054.

Mwanjewe, J., & Grover, A. K. (2004). Role of transient receptor potential canonical 6 (TRPC6) in non-transferrin-bound iron uptake in neuronal phenotype PC12 cells. *The Biochemical Journal, 378*, 975–982.

Nemeth, E., Rivera, S., Gabayan, V., Keller, C., Taudorf, S., Pedersen, B. K., et al. (2004). IL-6 mediates hypoferremia of inflammation by inducing the synthesis of the iron regulatory hormone hepcidin. *The Journal of Clinical Investigation, 113*, 1271–1276.

Nemeth, E., Tuttle, M. S., Powelson, J., Vaughn, M. B., Donovan, A., Ward, D. M., et al. (2004). Hepcidin regulates iron efflux by binding to ferroportin and inducing its internalization. *Science, 306*, 2090–2093.

Nevo, Y., & Nelson, N. (2006). The NRAMP family of metal-ion transporters. *Biochimica et Biophysica Acta, 1763*, 609–620.

Nicolas, G., Bennoun, M., Devaux, I., Beaumont, C., Grandchamp, B., Kahn, A., et al. (2001). Lack of hepcidin gene expression and severe tissue iron overload in upstream stimulatory factor 2 (USF2) knockout mice. *Proceedings of the National Academy of Sciences USA, 98*, 8780–8785.

Nicolas, G., Bennoun, M., Porteu, A., Mativet, S., Beaumont, C., Grandchamp, B., et al. (2002). Severe iron deficiency anemia in transgenic mice expressing liver hepcidin. *Proceedings of the National Academy of Sciences USA, 99*, 4596–4601.

Nicolas, G., Chauvet, C., Viatte, L., Danan, J. L., Bigard, X., Devaux, I., et al. (2002). The gene encoding the iron regulatory peptide hepcidin is regulated by anemia, hypoxia, and inflammation. *The Journal of Clinical Investigation, 110*, 1037–1044.

Nicolas, G., Viatte, L., Bennoun, M., Beaumont, C., Kahn, A., & Vaulont, S. (2002). Hepcidin, a new iron regulatory peptide. *Blood Cells, Molecules and Diseases, 29*, 327–335.

Njajou, O. T., Vaessen, N., Joosse, M., Berghuis, B., Van Dongen, J. W., Breuning, M. H., et al. (2001). A mutation in SLC11A3 is associated with autosomal dominant hemochromatosis. *Nature Genetics, 28*, 213–214.

Nunez, M. T., Osorio, A., Tapia, V., Vergara, A., & Mura, C. V. (2001). Iron-induced oxidative stress up-regulates calreticulin levels in intestinal epithelial (Caco-2) cells. *Journal of Cellular Biochemistry, 82*, 660–665.

Ohgami, R. S., Campagna, D. R., Greer, E. L., Antiochos, B., McDonald, A., Chen, J., et al. (2005). Identification of a ferrireductase required for efficient transferrin-dependent iron uptake in erythroid cells. *Nature Genetics, 37*, 1264–1269.

Oudit, G. Y., Sun, H., Trivieri, M. G., Koch, S. E., Dawood, F., Ackerley, C., et al. (2003). L-type Ca2+ channels provide a major pathway for iron entry into cardiomyocytes in iron-overload cardiomyopathy. *Nature Medicine, 9*, 1187–1194.

Oudit, G. Y., Trivieri, M. G., Khaper, N., Liu, P. P., & Backx, P. H. (2006). Role of L-type Ca2+ channels in iron transport and iron-overload cardiomyopathy. *Journal of Molecular Medicine, 84*, 349–364.

Pan, Y., Mansfield, K. D., Bertozzi, C. C., Rudenko, V., Chan, D. A., Giaccia, A. J., et al. (2007). Multiple factors affecting cellular redox status and energy metabolism modulate hypoxia-inducible factor prolyl hydroxylase activity in vivo and in vitro. *Molecular and Cellular Biology, 27*, 912–925.

Park, C. H., Valore, E. V., Waring, A. J., & Ganz, T. (2001). Hepcidin, a urinary antimicrobial peptide synthesized in the liver. *The Journal of Biological Chemistry, 276*, 7806–7810.

Parmley, R. T., Barton, J. C., Conrad, M. E., Austin, R. L., & Holland, R. M. (1981). Ultrastructural cytochemistry and autoradiography of hemoglobin-iron absorption. *Experimental and Molecular Pathology, 34*, 131–144.

Peyssonnaux, C., Zinkernagel, A. S., Datta, V., Lauth, X., Johnson, R. S., & Nizet, V. (2006). TLR4-dependent hepcidin expression by myeloid cells in response to bacterial pathogens. *Blood, 107*, 3727–3732.

Peyssonnaux, C., Zinkernagel, A. S., Schuepbach, R. A., Rankin, E., Vaulont, S., Haase, V. H., et al. (2007). Regulation of iron homeostasis by the hypoxia-inducible transcription factors (HIFs). *The Journal of Clinical Investigation, 117*, 1926–1932.

Pietrangelo, A. (2006). Hereditary hemochromatosis. *Biochimica et Biophysica Acta, 1763*, 700–710.

Pigeon, C., Ilyin, G., Courselaud, B., Leroyer, P., Turlin, B., Brissot, P., et al. (2001). A new mouse liver-specific gene, encoding a protein homologous to human antimicrobial peptide hepcidin, is overexpressed during iron overload. *The Journal of Biological Chemistry, 276*, 7811–7819.

Ponka, P. (2002). Iron utilization in erythrocyte formation and hemoglobin synthesis. In D. M. Templeton (Ed.), *Molecular and cellular iron transport* (pp. 643–677). New York: Marcel Dekker Inc.

Ponka, P., & Richardson, D. R. (1997). Can ferritin provide iron for hemoglobin synthesis. *Blood, 89*, 2611–2612.

Qiu, A., Jansen, M., Sakaris, A., Min, S. H., Chattopadhyay, S., Tsai, E., et al. (2006). Identification of an intestinal folate transporter and the molecular basis for hereditary folate malabsorption. *Cell, 127*, 917–928.

Quigley, J. G., Yang, Z., Worthington, M. T., Phillips, J. D., Sabo, K. M., Sabath, D. E., et al. (2004). Identification of a human heme exporter that is essential for erythropoiesis. *Cell, 118*, 757–766.

Richardson, D. R., Chua, A. C., & Baker, E. (1999). Activation of an iron uptake mechanism from transferrin in hepatocytes by small-molecular-weight iron complexes: Implications for the pathogenesis of iron-overload disease. The *Journal of Laboratory and Clinical Medicine, 133*, 144–151.

Rivera, S., Nemeth, E., Gabayan, V., Lopez, M. A., Farshidi, D., & Ganz, T. (2005). Synthetic hepcidin causes rapid dose-dependent hypoferremia and is concentrated in ferroportin-containing organs. *Blood, 106*, 2196–2199.

Rouault, T. A. (2006). The role of iron regulatory proteins in mammalian iron homeostasis and disease. *Nature Chemical Biology, 2*, 406–414.

Rouault, T. A., & Cooperman, S. (2006). Brain iron metabolism. *Seminars in Pediatric Neurology, 13*, 142–148.

Savigni, D. L., Wege, D., Cliff, G. S., Meesters, M. L., & Morgan, E. H. (2003). Iron and transition metal transport into erythrocytes mediated by nifedipine degradation products and related compounds. *Biochemical Pharmacology, 65*, 1215–1226.

Schimanski, L. M., Drakesmith, H., Merryweather-Clarke, A. T., Viprakasit, V., Edwards, J. P., Sweetland, E., et al. (2005). In vitro functional analysis of human ferroportin (FPN) and hemochromatosis-associated FPN mutations. *Blood, 105*, 4096–4102.

Sham, R. L., Phatak, P. D., West, C., Lee, P., Andrews, C., & Beutler, E. (2005). Autosomal dominant hereditary hemochromatosis associated with a novel ferroportin mutation and unique clinical features. *Blood Cells, Molecules and Diseases, 34*, 157–161.

Shayeghi, M., Latunde-Dada, G. O., Oakhill, J. S., Laftah, A. H., Takeuchi, K., Halliday, N., et al. (2005). Identification of an intestinal heme transporter. *Cell, 122*, 789–801.

Sibille, J. C., Kondo, H., & Aisen, P. (1988). Interactions between isolated hepatocytes and Kupffer cells in iron metabolism: A possible role for ferritin as an iron carrier protein. *Hepatology, 8*, 296–301.

Simpson, R. J. (1996). Dietary iron levels and hypoxia independently affect iron absorption in mice. *The Journal of Nutrition, 126*, 1858–1864.

Smith, S. R., Cooperman, S., LaVaute, T., Tresser, N., Ghosh, M., Meyron-Holtz, E., et al. (2004). Severity of neurodegeneration correlates with compromise of iron metabolism in mice with iron regulatory protein deficiencies. *Annals of the New York Academy of Sciences, 1012*, 65–83.

Steele, T. M., Frazer, D. M., & Anderson, G. J. (2005). Systemic regulation of intestinal iron absorption. *IUBMB Life, 57*, 499–503.

Takeuchi, K., Bjarnason, I., Laftah, A. H., Latunde-Dada, G. O., Simpson, R. J., & Mckie, A. T. (2005). Expression of iron absorption genes in mouse large intestine. *Scandinavian Journal of Gastroenterology, 40*, 169–177.

Tanno, T., Bhanu, N. V., Oneal, P. A., Goh, S. H., Staker, P., Lee, Y. T., et al. (2007). High levels of GDF15 in thalassemia suppress expression of the iron regulatory protein hepcidin. *Nature Medicine, 13*, 1096–1101.

Templeton, D. M., & Liu, Y. (2003). Genetic regulation of cell function in response to iron overload or chelation. *Biochimica et Biophysica Acta, 1619*, 113–124.

Thompson, K., Molina, R. M., Brain, J. D., & Wessling-Resnick, M. (2006). Belgrade rats display liver iron loading. *The Journal of Nutrition, 136*, 3010–3014.

Thomson, A. M., Rogers, J. T., & Leedman, P. J. (1999). Iron-regulatory proteins, iron-responsive elements and ferritin mRNA translation. The *International Journal of Biochemistry and Cell Biology, 31*, 1139–1152.

Timchenko, L. T., Iakova, P., Welm, A. L., Cai, Z. J., & Timchenko, N. A. (2002). Calreticulin interacts with C/EBPalpha and C/EBPbeta mRNAs and represses translation of C/EBP proteins. *Molecular and Cellular Biology, 22*, 7242–7257.

Uc, A., Stokes, J. B., & Britigan, B. E. (2004). Heme transport exhibits polarity in caco-2 cells: Evidence for an active and membrane protein-mediated process. *American Journal of Physiology. Gastrointestinal and Liver Physiology, 287*, G1150–G1157.

Uchida, T., Akitsuki, T., Kimura, H., Tanaka, T., Matsuda, S., & Kariyone, S. (1983). Relationship among plasma iron, plasma iron turnover, and reticuloendothelial iron release. *Blood, 61*, 799–802.

van der, A. D., Marx, J. J., Grobbee, D. E., Kamphuis, M. H., Georgiou, N. A., van Kats-Renaud, J. H., et al. (2006). Non-transferrin-bound iron and risk of coronary heart disease in postmenopausal women. *Circulation, 113*, 1942–1949.

VanEijk, H. G., & deJong, G. (1992). The physiology of iron, transferrin, and ferritin. *Biological Trace Element Research, 35*, 13–24.

Verga Falzacappa, M. V., Vujic, S. M., Kessler, R., Stolte, J., Hentze, M. W., & Muckenthaler, M. U. (2007). STAT3 mediates hepatic hepcidin expression and its inflammatory stimulation. *Blood, 109*, 353–358.

Vulpe, C. D., Kuo, Y. M., Murphy, T. L., Cowley, L., Askwith, C., Libina, N., et al. (1999). Hephaestin, a ceruloplasmin homologue implicated in intestinal iron transport, is defective in the sla mouse. *Nature Genetics, 21*, 195–199.

Wallace, D. F., Summerville, L., Lusby, P. E., & Subramaniam, V. N. (2005). First phenotypic description of transferrin receptor 2 knockout mouse, and the role of hepcidin. *Gut, 54*, 980–986.

Wallander, M. L., Leibold, E. A., & Eisenstein, R. S. (2006). Molecular control of vertebrate iron homeostasis by iron regulatory proteins. *Biochimica et Biophysica Acta, 1763*, 668–689.

Wallis, J. P., Wells, A. W., Whitehead, S., & Brewster, N. (2005). Recovery from post-operative anaemia. *Transfusion Medicine, 15*, 413–418.

Walters, G. O., Jacobs, A., Worwood, M., Trevett, D., & Thomson, W. (1975). Iron absorption in normal subjects and patients with idiopathic haemochromatosis: Relationship with serum ferritin concentration. *Gut, 16*, 188–192.

Weinstein, D. A., Roy, C. N., Fleming, M. D., Loda, M. F., Wolfsdorf, J. I., & Andrews, N. C. (2002). Inappropriate expression of hepcidin is associated with iron refractory anemia: Implications for the anemia of chronic disease. *Blood, 100*, 3776–3781.

Worthington, M. T., Cohn, S. M., Miller, S. K., Luo, R. Q., & Berg, C. L. (2001). Characterization of a human plasma membrane heme transporter in intestinal and hepatocyte cell lines. *American Journal of Physiology. Gastrointestinal and Liver Physiology, 280*, G1172–G1177.

Wrighting, D. M., & Andrews, N. C. (2006). Interleukin-6 induces hepcidin expression through STAT3. *Blood, 108*, 3204–3209.

Wyllie, J. C., & Kaufman, N. (1982). An electron microscopic study of heme uptake by rat duodenum. *Laboratory Investigation, 47*, 471–476.

Yamaji, S., Sharp, P., Ramesh, B., & Srai, S. K. (2004). Inhibition of iron transport across human intestinal epithelial cells by hepcidin. *Blood, 104*, 2178–2180.

Yeh, K. Y., Yeh, M., Watkins, J. A., RodriguezParis, J., & Glass, J. (2000). Dietary iron induces rapid changes in rat intestinal divalent metal transporter expression. *American Journal of Physiology. Gastrointestinal and Liver Physiology, 279*, G1070–G1079.

Yoshida, K., Furihata, K., Takeda, S., Nakamura, A., Yamamoto, K., Morita, H., et al. (1995). A mutation in the ceruloplasmin gene is associated with systemic hemosiderosis in humans. *Nature Genetics, 9*, 267–272.

# 3 The Role of Hepcidin in Iron Homeostasis

*Tomas Ganz*

**Summary**

- Hepcidin is the principal iron-regulatory hormone that controls the absorption of dietary iron and its distribution between stores and extracellular fluid.
- Hepcidin acts by binding to the sole known cellular iron efflux channel, ferroportin, and inducing its internalization and degradation, and thereby inhibits the efflux of iron from cells.
- Hepcidin synthesis and release are induced by iron loading or inflammation and inhibited by increased erythropoietic activity or hypoxia.
- Hereditary hemochromatosis is due to the deficiency of hepcidin or rarely due to resistance to the effects of hepcidin.
- Increased hepcidin concentrations from inflammation, genetic diseases, or tumor production lead to iron-restricted anemia refractory to oral iron.

**Key Words:** Iron overload; iron deficiency; anemia; inflammation

## 1. INTRODUCTION

Iron concentrations in extracellular fluid and plasma are regulated so that plasma iron remains within the 10–30 μM range, despite the variability of iron supply from dietary sources and erythrocyte destruction and changing demands for iron for erythropoiesis and tissue regeneration and growth. Mechanisms that adjust iron absorption and recycling to keep extracellular iron concentrations constant also effectively match iron supply to iron demand but would not assure stable iron reserves. Additional control mechanisms must regulate iron absorption to maintain iron stores in the liver that help buffer surges in iron demand. Based on studies of iron absorption in animals and humans, it has long been known that a homeostatic system for the regulation of extracellular iron concentrations and iron stores must exist (Bothwell & Finch, 1962), but the specific molecular mechanisms were identified only recently.

From: *Nutrition and Health: Iron Deficiency and Overload*
Edited by: S. Yehuda and D.I. Mostofsky, DOI 10.1007/978-1-59745-462-9_3

## 2. THE INTERACTION OF THE HORMONE HEPCIDIN AND ITS RECEPTOR FERROPORTIN REGULATES SYSTEMIC IRON METABOLISM

### 2.1. *Hepcidin*

Hepcidin is a 25 amino acid (2.7 kD) peptide containing four disulfide bridges (Krause et al., 2000; Park, Valore, Waring, & Ganz, 2001; Pigeon et al., 2001). It is synthesized in hepatocytes as an 84 amino acid prepropeptide that undergoes rapid intracellular processing to mature hepcidin, followed by secretion (Valore & Ganz, 2008). Hepcidin is an amphipathic cationic peptide that structurally resembles antimicrobial peptides such as defensins and protegrins and displays weak antimicrobial activity in vitro (Krause et al., 2000; Park et al., 2001). It differs from antimicrobial peptides by greater evolutionary conservation (Park et al., 2001) indicative of strict functional constraints. The involvement of hepcidin in iron metabolism was suggested by its overexpression in the livers of iron-overloaded mice (Pigeon et al., 2001), and its essential iron-regulatory role was established by the rapidly progressive iron overload of mice and humans with genetic hepcidin deficiency (Nicolas et al., 2001; Roetto et al., 2003), and the development of severe iron deficiency refractory to oral iron in mice and human overexpressing hepcidin (Nicolas, Bennoun, et al., 2002; Weinstein et al., 2002). The administration of synthetic hepcidin peptide to mice produced profound hypoferremia (Rivera, Nemeth, et al., 2005), demonstrating the in vivo iron-regulatory activity of the 25 amino acid hepcidin peptide.

### 2.2. *Ferroportin*

Ferroportin (Abboud & Haile, 2000; McKie et al., 2000; Donovan et al., 2000) is also known as solute carrier family 40 (iron-regulated transporter), member 1 (SLC40A1); iron regulated gene 1 (IREG1); solute carrier family 11 (proton-coupled divalent metal ion transporters), member 3 (SLC11A3); and metal transport protein 1 (MTP1). Ferroportin is a 571 amino acid membrane protein thought to have 10 or 12 transmembrane domains and cytoplasmic amino and carboxy termini (Liu, Yang, & Haile, 2005; De Domenico et al., 2005), but the details of its structure have not yet been established. Based on biochemical studies and the dominant-negative effect of clinically significant ferroportin mutations, ferroportin is dimeric or multimeric (De Domenico, Ward, Musci, & Kaplan, 2007), but this interpretation is contested (Goncalves et al., 2006; Schimanski et al., 2008; Pignatti et al., 2006). Ferroportin constructs expressed in *Xenopus* oocytes or mammalian cells cause iron efflux (Donovan et al., 2005; McKie et al., 2000; Abboud & Haile, 2000). Moreover, the mRNA and protein are found in all the cell types that export iron: duodenal enterocytes, placental syncytiotrophoblast, hepatocytes, and macrophages. The iron export function of ferroportin is essential as shown by the embryonic lethal systemic iron deficiency in mice and zebrafish that lack ferroportin (Donovan et al., 2005, 2000). Mice with inactivation of ferroportin in the embryo but not the maternal–fetal interface survive to birth but rapidly become iron-deficient and anemic and manifest abnormal iron accumulation in iron-exporting tissues, including duodenal enterocytes, macrophages, and hepatocytes (Donovan et al., 2005). These findings confirm the essential cellular iron export function of ferroportin.

### 2.3. *Regulation of Ferroportin by Hepcidin*

Hepcidin regulates cellular iron export by an elegantly simple mechanism dependent on hepcidin-induced ferroportin internalization and degradation (Nemeth, Tuttle, et al., 2004). The molecular mechanism of ferroportin internalization is similar to that of other receptors internalized by their ligands and involves hepcidin-induced serial phosphorylation and ubiquitination of ferroportin (De Domenico, Ward, Langelier, et al., 2007). The large cytoplasmic loop containing residues 229–306 contains the motifs that undergo ligand-induced modification. It has been reported that tyrosine phosphorylation is required for ferroportin internalization, as revealed by the resistance of Y302F, Y303F double mutants to tyrosine phosphorylation, and hepcidin-induced internalization. Subsequent lysine ubiquitination on K253 is required for efficient ferroportin degradation, as the K253A mutant (but not other lysine mutants) is not ubiquitinated and its degradation is very slow. The effect of all these mutations is specific for internalization as they do not impair the iron-exporting function of ferroportin.

### 2.4. *Structure–Function Analysis of Hepcidin*

Evolutionary analysis of mammalian hepcidin sequences indicates a strong conservation of the disulfide bridge structure and the N-terminal six amino acids. The N-terminus differs in fish and amphibian hepcidins, but the substitutions are quite conservative. Deletion of amino acids from the N-terminus causes progressive loss of activity (Nemeth et al., 2006) so that the 20 amino acid form of hepcidin, also naturally found in urine and serum (Krause et al., 2000; Park et al., 2001), is inactive in cellular ferroportin internalization assays (Nemeth, Tuttle, et al., 2004; Nemeth et al., 2006) and in vivo (Rivera, Nemeth, et al., 2005). In contrast, the hepcidin structure retains bioactivity in cellular assays when amino acids in the rest of the structure, including the disulfide bonds, are altered (Nemeth et al., 2006) although the stability of the molecule may be decreased.

### 2.5. *Hepcidin Catabolism*

Fluorescently tagged hepcidin is taken up by ferroportin-expressing cells in culture and colocalizes in lysosomes with GFP-ferroportin (G. Preza et al., 2009). When radiolabeled hepcidin is given to mice, the tracer is predominantly found in urine but is also taken up by ferroportin-rich tissues (Rivera, Nemeth, et al., 2005), indicating that both renal excretion and uptake and degradation in ferroportin-rich tissues could contribute to hepcidin clearance from plasma.

### 2.6. *Cellular Regulation of Ferroportin*

Hepcidin is not the only signal that regulates ferroportin. Each macrophage that ingests senescent erythrocytes faces a large load of iron that must be stored or exported, depending on systemic requirements for iron. Whereas the systemic regulation of macrophage iron export is mediated by plasma hepcidin, which internalizes and degrades membrane-associated ferroportin (Knutson, Oukka, Koss, Aydemir, & Wessling-Resnick, 2005), ferroportin is also subject to independent cellular regulation by macrophage heme and iron levels (Knutson & Wessling-Resnick, 2003; Delaby et al., 2008; Delaby, Pilard, Goncalves, Beaumont, & Canonne-Hergaux, 2005). Cellular iron and heme increase ferroportin mRNA and protein and induce the translocation of ferroportin from intracellular vesicles to the cellular membrane. The increase in ferroportin is mediated by both transcriptional and translational mechanisms, the latter involving the 5′ iron regulatory element (IRE) located in the ferroportin mRNA (Liu et al., 2002). The amount of ferroportin on the membrane and therefore the ability of macrophages to export iron are thus closely linked to the iron and heme content of each macrophage. In combination, the cellular and systemic regulators deliver iron to extracellular fluid and plasma when iron is required for systemic needs, obtaining it preferentially from those macrophages that contain abundant iron and heme.

## 3. REGULATION OF HEPCIDIN SYNTHESIS BY IRON

### *3.1. Hereditary Hemochromatosis Proteins Are Hepcidin Regulators*

Analysis of hepcidin expression in patients with hereditary hemochromatosis (Roetto et al., 2003; Gehrke et al., 2003; Bridle et al., 2003; Papanikolaou et al., 2004; Nemeth, Roetto, Garozzo, Ganz, & Camaschella, 2005) and in mouse models (Nicolas et al., 2001; Ahmad et al., 2002; Bridle et al., 2003; Nicolas et al., 2003; Muckenthaler et al., 2003; Kawabata et al., 2005; Niederkofler, Salie, & Arber, 2005; Huang, J. L. Pinkus, G. S. Pinkus, Fleming, & Andrews, 2005) revealed that the major forms of juvenile and adult hereditary hemochromatosis are due to the deficiency of hepcidin that allows excessive iron absorption. Iron overload develops most rapidly and is most severe in the juvenile form of hemochromatosis, which manifests the lowest hepcidin expression, usually caused by homozygous disruption of hepcidin (HAMP) or hemojuvelin (HJV) genes. The adult forms are less hepcidin-deficient and are caused by homozygous disruption of the genes encoding transferrin receptor 2 (TfR2) or, most commonly, the hemochromatosis gene *HFE*. Two siblings with phenotypically juvenile form of hereditary hemochromatosis were found to have both homozygous Q317X TfR2 mutations and compound heterozygous C282Y/H63D HFE mutations, suggesting an additive effect of HFE and TfR2 disruption. The simplest explanation of the genotype–phenotype relationships is that HFE, TfR2, and hemojuvelin are regulators of hepcidin and that HFE and TfR2 are partially redundant and perhaps operating on parallel pathways that converge on hepcidin or hemojuvelin.

### *3.2. Hemojuvelin*

Hemojuvelin was identified as a hepcidin regulator through positional cloning of the gene mutated in most cases of juvenile hemochromatosis (Papanikolaou et al., 2004). The gene encodes a GPI-linked membrane protein with homology to repulsive guidance molecules (RgmA and RgmB) involved in the development of the central nervous system. Suppression of hemojuvelin by siRNAs proportionally decreased hepcidin mRNA in hepatic cell lines, indicating that hemojuvelin, unlike other Rgm (Lin, Goldberg, & Ganz, 2005), directly regulates hepcidin synthesis and is not principally a developmental mediator. In addition to the membrane-associated GPI-linked form, hemojuvelin also exists as a soluble protein that acts as a suppressor of hepcidin synthesis by hepatocytes in cell culture (Lin et al., 2005) and in vivo in the mouse (Babitt et al., 2007). The prohormone convertase furin is responsible for the release of soluble hemojuvelin and may act in the Golgi or on the membrane (Silvestri, Pagani, & Camaschella, 2008; Lin et al., 2008). The shedding or secretion of hemojuvelin is suppressed by iron (Lin et al., 2005) through an as yet undefined mechanism and stimulated by hypoxia and iron deficiency in part through increased synthesis of the prohormone convertase furin (Silvestri et al., 2008). Other Rgms act at least in part through their interactions with the receptor neogenin and, indeed, such an interaction may modulate the effect of hemojuvelin as well (Zhang, West, Wyman, Bjorkman, & Enns, 2005; Zhang et al., 2007), probably through the regulation of hemojuvelin shedding. However, the predominant effect of hemojuvelin on hepcidin synthesis is mediated by its interactions with BMP2, BMP4, BMP6, and BMP receptor (Babitt et al., 2006), where hemojuvelin acts as a BMP co-receptor to greatly potentiate BMP signaling. The BMP-dependent effect of hemojuvelin is required for the regulation of hepcidin synthesis by iron–transferrin in primary hepatocytes (Lin et al., 2007).

### 3.3. *The Bone Morphogenetic Protein (BMP) Pathway in Hepcidin Regulation*

With the exception of hepcidin itself, all the genes disrupted in hereditary hemochromatosis encoded proteins whose function was not known. An important insight into how these proteins may fit together came from the phenotype of a liver-specific SMAD4 knockout mouse (Wang et al., 2005) which manifested systemic iron overload and nearly complete deficiency of hepcidin. SMAD4 is a transcription factor used by the BMP and TGFβ pathways, and the phenotype of the SMAD4 knockout implicated both pathways in iron regulation. In unrelated studies (Babitt et al., 2005), RgmB (Dragon) was shown to act as a co-receptor for the BMP receptor and to enhance its signaling, and subsequently, hemojuvelin (RgmC) was also found to act as a co-receptor for the BMP receptor (Babitt et al., 2006) and BMP2, 4, and 9 were shown to be strong inducers of hepcidin synthesis (Babitt et al., 2006; Truksa, Peng, Lee, & Beutler, 2006).

The BMP signaling pathway is activated by dimeric ligands that bring together type I and type II receptor serine/threonine kinases on the cell membrane. The constitutively active type II receptor kinase phosphorylates and activates the kinase activity of type I receptor, which in turn phosphorylates the receptor-regulated Smads, Smad 1, 5, and 8. Upon phosphorylation, these Smad proteins form a complex with the common mediator Smad-4. The activated Smad complex translocates into the nucleus and regulates transcription of its target genes. The BMP receptor heterodimers are formed by combining one of three type II receptors (BMPRII, ActRIIA, and ActRIIB) with one of three type I receptors (ALK3, ALK6, and ALK2). Specific combinations of type I and type II receptors are preferentially utilized by different BMP ligands, and additional co-receptors can modify this preference and the intensity of signaling (Xia et al., 2007). Multiple BMPs and other potential ligands are expressed in the liver (Babitt et al., 2007), but only a few appear to be involved in the regulation of hepcidin by iron. Although BMP2, BMP4 and BMP6 interact with hemojuvelin and appear to function in the pathway by which iron regulates hepcidin (Lin et al., 2007), BMP9 does not interact with hemojuvelin and uses a different BMP receptor heterodimer not involved in iron-related signaling (Lin et al., 2007; Babitt et al., 2007). The dramatic effect of the BMP pathway on hepcidin transcription and the strong phenotype of the hemojuvelin-deficient mice and humans put them at the center of the current models of hepcidin and iron regulation. However, neither hemojuvelin nor the BMPs and their receptors are iron-binding molecules and so they must interact with other molecules that bind iron and can "sense" iron concentrations.

### 3.4. *Transferrin and Transferrin Receptors 1 and 2*

#### 3.4.1. TfR1

Transferrin receptors 1 and 2 bind holotransferrin (diferric transferrin) as well as monoferric transferrin, and both can mediate the cellular uptake of iron. TfR1 is expressed abundantly on erythropoietic precursors and present in most other cell types while TfR2 is hepatocyte specific. Homozygous ablation of TfR1 is embryonic lethal, producing severe anemia and malformation of the central nervous system (Levy, Jin, Fujiwara, Kuo, & Andrews, 1999). TfR1$^{+/-}$ heterozygotes have iron-deficient erythropoiesis despite iron reserves in macrophages, indicating a defect in iron uptake by erythrocyte precursors (Levy et al., 1999). Despite the lack of involvement of TfR1 in intestinal iron uptake, iron stores in TfR1$^{+/-}$ mice are diminished, indicating that the receptor could play a role in iron regulation.

### 3.4.2. TfR2

The effects of TfR1 deficiency on iron regulation contrast with the effects of TfR2 or transferrin deficiency. Deficiency of TfR2 in mice or humans causes systemic iron overload (Camaschella et al., 2000; Fleming et al., 2002; Wallace, Summerville, Lusby, & Subramaniam, 2005) and liver-specific deficiency of TfR2 is sufficient for iron overload, clearly indicating TfR2 involvement in iron regulation (Wallace, Summerville, & Subramaniam, 2007). Hepcidin is very low in TfR2-deficient humans (Nemeth et al., 2005) and mice (Kawabata et al., 2005; Wallace et al., 2005), indicating that TfR2 defects cause iron overload through the lack of hepcidin.

### 3.4.3. Holotransferrin

Genetic deficiency of transferrin is associated with a very severe form of iron overload in humans (summarized in Knisely, Gelbart, & Beutler, 2004) and in mice (Trenor, III, Campagna, Sellers, Andrews, & Fleming, 2000), indicating that transferrin is required for systemic homeostatic regulation of iron. After a test dose of iron, transient increases in transferrin saturation elicit proportional changes in urinary hepcidin concentrations (Lin et al., 2007). Holotransferrin, but not elemental iron, induces hepcidin mRNA in freshly isolated hepatocytes (Lin et al., 2007). These observations suggest that holotransferrin is an important form of iron sensed by the systemic homeostatic mechanisms.

### 3.4.4. Iron Sensing

In the aggregate, genetic studies of transferrin and its receptors suggest that all three are involved in iron regulation, acting by regulating hepcidin synthesis, with TfR2/holotransferrin complex stimulating hepcidin synthesis and TfR1/holotransferrin complex possibly inhibiting it.

## *3.5. HFE*

Mutations in the gene *HFE* are responsible for most cases of hereditary hemochromatosis in patients of European descent. Patients with HFE hemochromatosis carry homozygous or compound heterozygous mutations and manifest hepcidin protein levels that are either lower than normal or normal but inadequate for the high iron load and transferrin saturation (Piperno et al., 2007). Moreover, patients with HFE hemochromatosis lack the acute hepcidin response to iron ingestion, but the chronic response to iron loading is at least partially preserved (Piperno et al., 2007). Both humans and mice with HFE hemochromatosis are deficient in hepcidin mRNA (Ahmad et al., 2002; Bridle et al., 2003), suggesting decreased hepcidin gene transcription (or less likely, mRNA instability). The gene encodes a membrane protein that forms a heterodimer with β2-microglobulin and is similar to proteins of the type I major histocompatibility complex.

The HFE ectodomain competes with holotransferrin for binding to the TfR1 ectodomain, and the binding sites of the two TfR1 ligands overlap (Lebron, West, & Bjorkman, 1999; Bennett, Lebron, & Bjorkman, 2000). Moreover, complete TfR1 and holotransferrin compete for HFE in cellular models (Giannetti & Bjorkman, 2004). Although the TfR2 ectodomain was reported not to bind to the HFE ectodomain, in cellular models with overexpressed whole proteins TfR2 competed with TfR1 for binding to HFE (Goswami & Andrews, 2006). Unlike the interaction of TfR1 with HFE, the interaction of TfR2 with HFE was not diminished by holotransferrin. In fact, holotransferrin stabilized TfR2 (Johnson & Enns, 2004; Robb & Wessling-Resnick, 2004) enabling it to compete more effectively for HFE. Based on the phenotypes of mice with a deficiency of transferrin or TfR1 or TfR2, both transferrin receptors could act as sensors for holotransferrin, acting synergistically and using HFE as a signaling intermediary.

Holotransferrin would release HFE from its association with TfR1 and make more HFE available to bind to the holotransferrin-stabilized TfR2. The TfR2–HFE complex would then stimulate hepcidin synthesis.

### 3.6. *A Model of Hepcidin Regulation*

A comprehensive model of hepcidin regulation must account for the effects of known genetic lesions on iron metabolism, and must provide a plausible scheme by which iron is sensed and its concentrations affect the synthesis of the iron-regulatory hormone. A current model of hepcidin regulation is built around the regulatory complex of hemojuvelin, BMP2/4/6, and the BMP receptor regulating the transcription of hepcidin via the SMAD pathway. The activity or assembly of this complex is regulated by its association with TfR2 and HFE, with their effects synergistic. The availability of TfR2 and HFE is in turn determined by the concentration of holotransferrin which stabilizes TfR2 and releases HFE from TfR1.

## 4. REGULATION OF SYSTEMIC IRON METABOLISM AND HEPCIDIN SYNTHESIS BY HYPOXIA-INDUCIBLE TRANSCRIPTION FACTORS

### 4.1. *Gene Regulation by Hypoxia*

Hypoxia is a potent regulator of cellular and systemic processes, and has a particularly strong effect on erythropoiesis where it acts as a dominant inducer of the production of erythropoietin. Hypoxia regulates the transcription of erythropoietin and dozens of other hypoxia-regulated genes through heterodimeric hypoxia-inducible transcription factors (HIF) that bind to hypoxia-responsive elements (HRE) in the promoters of target genes (Semenza, 2007). HIF consist of one of three tissue-specific cytoplasmic HIF1α, HIF2α, or HIF3α that can combine with the constitutive HIF1β subunit. During hypoxia, HIFα subunits accumulate, translocate into the nucleus, and interact with HIF1β and other transcription factors. When oxygen is abundant, HIFα subunits are subjected to hydroxylation on one or two of their prolines, and this modification targets the HIFα for interaction with the von Hippel-Lindau tumor-suppressor protein (VHL) and for degradation. Another oxygen-sensing hydroxylase, FIH-1 (factor inhibiting HIF-1), hydroxylates a specific asparagine on HIFα, thereby inhibiting the interaction of HIF with other transcription factors. Both types of hydroxylases contain an essential iron and their activity is inhibited by iron chelators.

### 4.2. *Iron and Hepcidin Regulation by Hypoxia*

Mice and rats subjected to hypoxia respond by increased production of erythropoietin, enhanced erythropoiesis, and increased iron absorption. The increase in iron absorption is at least in part independent of the effect of increased erythropoiesis, as revealed by early experiments in which the erythropoietic response is suppressed by nephrectomy or by a combination of irradiation of the bone marrow by radioactive strontium and splenectomy (Mendel, 1961; Raja, Simpson, Pippard, & Peters, 1988). More recent studies suggest that the increased iron absorption is due to suppression of hepcidin by hypoxia. Mice made hypoxic by exposure to oxygen pressures found at 5,500 m manifested gradually decreasing hepcidin mRNA but the effect appears to be relatively slow, peaking at 4 days (Nicolas, Chauvet, et al., 2002), suggesting that the effect on hepcidin included indirect, erythropoiesis-mediated effects of hypoxia. Direct effects of hypoxia on hepatocytes were deduced from hypoxia-exposed hepatocyte cell lines that showed a decrease in hepcidin mRNA within 24–48 hours (Nicolas, Chauvet, et al., 2002; Leung,

Srai, Mascarenhas, Churchill, & Debnam, 2005). In the aggregate, these studies suggest that hepcidin is subject to direct regulation by hepatic hypoxia, but the relative contribution of direct and indirect effects remains to be demonstrated.

### *4.3. HIF Involvement in Hepcidin Suppression During Iron Deficiency*

Systemic iron deficiency was shown to suppress hepcidin in humans (Nemeth et al., 2003). In mice, the suppression of hepcidin by iron deprivation appears to be partially dependent on HIF1α because HIF1α-deficient mice suppress hepcidin mRNA less than do wild-type mice (Peyssonnaux et al., 2007). The suppressive effect of HIF1α on hepcidin takes place in hepatocytes as iron depletion suppressed hepcidin mRNA 10-fold more in wild-type mice than in mice with hepatocyte-specific ablation of HIF1α. Nevertheless, hepcidin suppression still takes place even in HIF1α-deficient mice, indicating that other pathways may also regulate hepcidin during iron deficiency. Although the specific HREs in the hepcidin promoter differ in number and location between mice and humans, both promoters were found to bind HIF (Peyssonnaux et al., 2007). The HIF-dependent mechanism of hepcidin regulation would be expected to be responsive to hepatocyte iron stores rather than holotransferrin concentration, and thus could complement the effect of the BMP/hemojuvelin/TfR pathway that senses holotransferrin.

## 5. REGULATION OF PLASMA IRON AND OF HEPCIDIN SYNTHESIS BY INFLAMMATION

### *5.1. Hepcidin and the Acute Hypoferremia of Inflammation*

Hypoferremia develops within hours of acute infections and persists in states of chronic infection or inflammation. Recent studies indicate that hepcidin is the key mediator of this hypoferremic response. In humans, hepcidin is induced by inflammation within hours and increased hepcidin is followed by hypoferremia a few hours later (Kemna, Pickkers, Nemeth, van der, & Swinkels, 2005). The hypoferremic response to turpentine-induced inflammation is lost in hepcidin-deficient mice, indicating that the increased hepcidin concentrations mediate the hypoferremia of inflammation (Nicolas, Chauvet, et al., 2002). Injection of hepcidin produces hypoferremia within 1 hour (Rivera, Nemeth, et al., 2005), in agreement with the time course of the development of hypoferremia in acute infections in humans and in mice. Thus, the role of circulating hepcidin in acute hypoferremia of inflammation is well supported by evidence. Additional mechanisms may contribute to local or systemic hypoferremia. Autocrine secretion of hepcidin by macrophages (Theurl et al., 2008) may act locally to reduce macrophage ferroportin, cause macrophage iron retention, and decrease the local extracellular iron concentrations. In addition, transcriptional suppression of ferroportin by inflammatory stimuli may also contribute to iron retention in macrophages (Yang et al., 2002; Liu, Nguyen, Marquess, Yang, & Haile, 2005).

### *5.2. Hepcidin and Anemia of Inflammation*

Mice and humans chronically overexpressing hepcidin develop not only hypoferremia but also an iron-restricted anemia (Nicolas, Bennoun, et al., 2002; Weinstein et al., 2002; Rivera, Liu, et al., 2005; Roy et al., 2007). Urinary hepcidin is increased in patients with anemia of inflammation (Nemeth et al., 2003), suggesting that the overproduction of hepcidin accounts for the defining features of anemia of inflammation: iron-restricted anemia with hypoferremia.

### 5.3. *Regulation of Hepcidin During Infection and Inflammation*

The induction of hepcidin by infection or microbial products has been demonstrated in humans (Nemeth et al., 2003; Kemna et al., 2005), mice (Pigeon et al., 2001; Nicolas, Chauvet, et al., 2002), and fish (Shike et al., 2002). Infection or microbial products induce hepcidin mRNA directly in primary hepatocytes (Pigeon et al., 2001) and in monocytes and macrophages (Liu, Nguyen, et al., 2005; Peyssonnaux et al., 2006; Nguyen, Callaghan, Ghio, Haile, & Yang, 2006; Sow et al., 2007; Theurl et al., 2008; Nemeth, Rivera, et al., 2004). Moreover, media conditioned by lipopolysaccharide-treated blood monocytes induce hepcidin synthesis in isolated hepatocytes and hepatocyte-derived cell lines (Nemeth et al., 2003) and this effect is neutralized by anti-IL-6 antibody, indicating that IL-6 is an important macrophage-derived mediator of hepcidin regulation. Unlike wild-type C57Bl6 mice, IL-6-deficient mice injected with turpentine do not acutely increase their hepcidin mRNA, and do not develop hypoferremia, supporting the role of IL-6 in acute hypoferremia of inflammation (Nemeth, Rivera, et al., 2004). Moreover, human volunteers infused with moderate amounts of IL-6 develop increased hepcidin and hypoferremia within hours of infusion (Nemeth, Rivera, et al., 2004). The transcriptional induction of hepcidin by IL-6 is dependent on the STAT3 pathway (Wrighting & Andrews, 2006; Pietrangelo et al., 2007; Verga Falzacappa et al., 2007). Other inflammatory mediators and the direct effect of bacterial substances on hepatocytes and macrophages can also induce hepcidin (Pigeon et al., 2001; Kemna et al., 2005; Liu, Nguyen, et al., 2005; Lee, Peng, Gelbart, & Beutler, 2004; Rivera, Gabayan, & Ganz, 2004), and IL-6-independent pathways may be especially important in the chronic setting.

### 5.4. *Regulation of Hemojuvelin by Inflammation*

Inflammation not only exerts a stimulatory effect on hepcidin synthesis but also affects the iron-regulatory pathway by suppressing hemojuvelin mRNA (Krijt, Vokurka, Chang, & Necas, 2004; Niederkofler et al., 2005; Constante, Wang, Raymond, Bilodeau, & Santos, 2007; Sheikh, Dudas, & Ramadori, 2007). Although this remains to be demonstrated experimentally, the suppression of hemojuvelin would be expected to uncouple the iron-regulatory pathway so that the effect of the inflammatory stimuli on hepcidin synthesis would not be outweighed by the opposing effects of iron restriction.

## 6. REGULATION OF HEPCIDIN SYNTHESIS BY ERYTHROPOIETIC ACTIVITY

### 6.1. *Erythropoiesis Suppresses Hepcidin Synthesis*

It is well established that increased erythropoietic activity leads to increased intestinal iron absorption (Krantz, Goldwasser, & Jacobson, 1959; Mendel, 1961). Again, the ultimate mediator is apparently hepcidin, as both hemolytic anemia and hemorrhage suppress hepcidin synthesis (Nicolas, Chauvet, et al., 2002; Vokurka, Krijt, Sulc, & Necas, 2006; Pak, Lopez, Gabayan, Ganz, & Rivera, 2006). However, as anticipated by earlier iron absorption studies, anemia does not suppress hepcidin synthesis in the absence of active erythropoiesis (Vokurka, Krijt, Sulc, & Necas, 2006; Pak et al., 2006), suggesting that a bone marrow–derived factor affects hepcidin synthesis. The nature of the factor that signals from the bone marrow to the liver to modulate hepcidin is not yet known.

### 6.2. *Hepcidin Suppression in Expanded but Ineffective Erythropoiesis*

β-Thalassemia major and intermedia represent extreme examples of increased erythropoiesis compounded by the premature death of erythroid precursors. Hepcidin is very low in untransfused patients with β-thalassemia intermedia (Papanikolaou et al., 2005; Origa et al., 2007) and in the mouse models of β-thalassemia (Adamsky et al., 2004; Breda et al., 2005; Gardenghi et al., 2007). Hepcidin is higher in transfused patients with β-thalassemia but still inappropriately low for the degree of iron overload (Papanikolaou et al., 2005; Kattamis et al., 2006; Kearney et al., 2007; Origa et al., 2007). A hepcidin-regulating humoral factor present in β-thalassemia was implicated by the observation that sera from patients with β-thalassemia suppressed hepcidin production in hepatocyte cell lines (Weizer-Stern et al., 2006). GDF15, a member of the TGFβ/BMP family of ligands, is produced by erythrocyte precursors and is present at very high concentrations in the plasma of patients with β-thalassemia (Tanno et al., 2007). At these high concentrations, GDF15 suppressed hepcidin production by primary human hepatocytes and by hepatocyte cell lines and emerged as a strong candidate for bone marrow-derived humoral factor in β-thalassemia. It is not yet clear whether GDF15 contributes to hepcidin regulation in situations where erythroid precursor expansion and apoptosis are less extreme.

## 7. SUMMARY

Systemic iron homeostasis is mediated predominantly by the interaction of the iron-regulatory hormone hepcidin with the cellular iron efflux channel, ferroportin. In the efferent arm of iron homeostasis, hepcidin binds to ferroportin, causing its internalization and degradation and thereby inhibiting cellular iron export into extracellular fluid. In the afferent arm of the homeostatic arc, extracellular iron, hepatic iron stores, and inflammation stimulate hepcidin synthesis, and hypoxia and erythropoietic activity suppress it. Direct effects of many of these stimuli on ferroportin synthesis have also been observed and may contribute to iron regulation.

## REFERENCES


Abboud, S., & Haile, D. J. (2000). A novel mammalian iron-regulated protein involved in intracellular iron metabolism. *Journal of Biological Chemistry, 275*, 19906–19912.

Adamsky, K., Weizer, O., Amariglio, N., Breda, L., Harmelin, A., Rivella, S., et al. (2004). Decreased hepcidin mRNA expression in thalassemic mice. *British Journal of Haematology, 124*, 123–124.

Ahmad, K. A., Ahmann, J. R., Migas, M. C., Waheed, A., Britton, R. S., Bacon, B. R., et al. (2002). Decreased liver hepcidin expression in the HFE knockout mouse. *Blood Cells, Molecules, and Diseases, 29*, 361–366.

Babitt, J. L., Huang, F. W., Wrighting, D. M., Xia, Y., Sidis, Y., Samad, T. A., et al. (2006). Bone morphogenetic protein signaling by hemojuvelin regulates hepcidin expression. *Nature Genetics, 38*, 531–539.

Babitt, J. L., Huang, F. W., Xia, Y., Sidis, Y., Andrews, N. C., & Lin, H. Y. (2007). Modulation of bone morphogenetic protein signaling in vivo regulates systemic iron balance. *Journal of Clinical Investigation, 117*, 1933–1939.

Babitt, J. L., Zhang, Y., Samad, T. A., Xia, Y., Tang, J., Campagna, J. A., et al. (2005). Repulsive guidance molecule (RGMa), a DRAGON homologue, is a bone morphogenetic protein co-receptor. *Journal of Biological Chemistry, 280*, 29820–29827.

Bennett, M. J., Lebron, J. A., & Bjorkman, P. J. (2000). Crystal structure of the hereditary haemochromatosis protein HFE complexed with transferrin receptor. *Nature, 403*, 46–53.

Bothwell, T. H., & Finch, C. A. (1962). *Iron metabolism* (1st ed.). Boston: Little, Brown.

Breda, L., Gardenghi, S., Guy, E., Rachmilewitz, E. A., Weizer-Stern, O., Adamsky, K., et al. (2005). Exploring the role of hepcidin, an antimicrobial and iron regulatory peptide, in increased iron absorption in {beta}-thalassemia. *Annals of the New York Academy of Sciences, 1054*, 417–422.

Bridle, K. R., Frazer, D. M., Wilkins, S. J., Dixon, J. L., Purdie, D. M., Crawford, D. H. G., et al. (2003). Disrupted hepcidin regulation in *HFE*-associated haemochromatosis and the liver as a regulator of body iron homoeostasis. *Lancet, 361*, 669–673.

Camaschella, C., Roetto, A., Cali, A., De Gobbi, M., Garozzo, G., Carella, M., et al. (2000). The gene TFR2 is mutated in a new type of haemochromatosis mapping to 7q22. *Nature Genetics, 25*, 14–15.

Constante, M., Wang, D., Raymond, V. A., Bilodeau, M., & Santos, M. M. (2007). Repression of repulsive guidance molecule C during inflammation is independent of HFE and involves tumor necrosis factor-alpha. *American Journal of Pathology, 170*, 497–504.

De Domenico, I., Ward, D. M., Musci, G., & Kaplan, J. (2007). Evidence for the multimeric structure of ferroportin. *Blood, 109*, 2205–2209.

De Domenico, I., Ward, D. M., Nemeth, E., Vaughn, M. B., Musci, G., Ganz, T., et al. (2005). The molecular basis of ferroportin-linked hemochromatosis. *Proceedings of the National Academy of Sciences, 102*, 8955–8960.

De Domenico, I., Ward, D. M., Langelier, C., Vaughn, M. B., Nemeth, E., Sundquist, W. I., et al. (2007). The molecular mechanism of hepcidin-mediated ferroportin down-regulation. *Molecular Biology of the Cell, 18*, 2569–2578.

Delaby, C., Pilard, N., Goncalves, A. S., Beaumont, C., & Canonne-Hergaux, F. (2005). Presence of the iron exporter ferroportin at the plasma membrane of macrophages is enhanced by iron loading and down-regulated by hepcidin. *Blood, 106*, 3979–3984.

Delaby, C., Pilard, N., Puy, H., & Canonne-Hergaux, F. (2008). Sequential regulation of ferroportin expression after erythrophagocytosis in murine macrophages: Early mRNA induction by heme followed by iron-dependent protein expression. *Biochemical Journal, 411*, 123–131.

Donovan, A., Brownlie, A., Zhou, Y., Shepard, J., Pratt, S. J., Moynihan, J., et al. (2000). Positional cloning of zebrafish ferroportin1 identifies a conserved vertebrate iron exporter. *Nature, 403*, 776–781.

Donovan, A., Lima, C. A., Pinkus, J. L., Pinkus, G. S., Zon, L. I., Robine, S., et al. (2005). The iron exporter ferroportin/Slc40a1 is essential for iron homeostasis. *Cell Metabolism, 1*, 191–200.

Fleming, R. E., Ahmann, J. R., Migas, M. C., Waheed, A., Koeffler, H. P., Kawabata, H. et al. (2002). Targeted mutagenesis of the murine transferrin receptor-2 gene produces hemochromatosis. *Proceedings of the National Academy of Sciences, 99*, 10653–10658.

Gardenghi, S., Marongiu, M. F., Ramos, P., Guy, E., Breda, L., Chadburn, A., et al. (2007). Ineffective erythropoiesis in β-thalassemia is characterized by increased iron absorption mediated by down-regulation of hepcidin and up-regulation of ferroportin. *Blood, 109*, 5027–5035.

Gehrke, S. G., Kulaksiz, H., Herrmann, T., Riedel, H. D., Bents, K., Veltkamp, C., et al. (2003). Expression of hepcidin in hereditary hemochromatosis: Evidence for a regulation in response to the serum transferrin saturation and to non-transferrin-bound iron. *Blood, 102*, 371–376.

Giannetti, A. M., & Bjorkman, P. J. (2004). HFE and transferrin directly compete for transferrin receptor in solution and at the cell surface. *Journal of Biological Chemistry, 279*, 25866–25875.

Goncalves, A. S., Muzeau, F., Blaybel, R., Hetet, G., Driss, F., Delaby, C., et al. (2006). Wild-type and mutant ferroportins do not form oligomers in transfected cells. *Biochemical Journal, 396*, 265–275.

Goswami, T., & Andrews, N. C. (2006). Hereditary hemochromatosis protein, HFE, interaction with transferrin receptor 2 suggests a molecular mechanism for mammalian iron sensing. *Journal of Biological Chemistry, 281*, 28494–28498.

Huang, F. W., Pinkus, J. L., Pinkus, G. S., Fleming, M. D., & Andrews, N. C. (2005). A mouse model of juvenile hemochromatosis. *Journal of Clinical Investigation, 115*, 2187–2191.

Johnson, M. B., & Enns, C. A. (2004). Diferric transferrin regulates transferrin receptor 2 protein stability. *Blood, 104*, 4287–4293.

Kattamis, A., Papassotiriou, I., Palaiologou, D., Apostolakou, F., Galani, A., Ladis, V., et al. (2006). The effects of erythropoetic activity and iron burden on hepcidin expression in patients with thalassemia major. *Haematologica, 91*, 809–812.

Kawabata, H., Fleming, R. E., Gui, D., Moon, S. Y., Saitoh, T., O'Kelly, J., et al. (2005). Expression of hepcidin is down-regulated in TfR2 mutant mice manifesting a phenotype of hereditary hemochromatosis. *Blood, 105*, 376–381.

Kearney, S. L., Nemeth, E., Neufeld, E. J., Thapa, D., Ganz, T., Weinstein, D. A., et al. (2007). Urinary hepcidin in congenital chronic anemias. *Pediatric Blood & Cancer, 48*, 57–63.

Kemna, E., Pickkers, P., Nemeth, E., van der, H. H., & Swinkels, D. (2005). Time-course analysis of hepcidin, serum iron, and plasma cytokine levels in humans injected with LPS. *Blood, 106*, 1864–1866.

Knisely, A. S., Gelbart, T., & Beutler, E. (2004). Molecular characterization of a third case of human atransferrinemia. *Blood, 104*, 2607.

Knutson, M., & Wessling-Resnick, M. (2003). Iron metabolism in the reticuloendothelial system. *Critical Reviews in Biochemistry and Molecular Biology, 38*, 61–88.

Knutson, M. D., Oukka, M., Koss, L. M., Aydemir, F., & Wessling-Resnick, M. (2005). Iron release from macrophages after erythrophagocytosis is up-regulated by ferroportin 1 overexpression and down-regulated by hepcidin. *Proceedings of the National Academy of Sciences, 102*, 1324–1328.

Krantz, S. B., Goldwasser, E., & Jacobson, L. O. (1959). Studies on erythropoiesis. XIV. The relationship of humoral stimulation to iron absorption. *Blood, 14*, 654–661.

Krause, A., Neitz, S., Magert, H. J., Schulz, A., Forssmann, W. G., Schulz-Knappe, P., et al. (2000). LEAP-1, a novel highly disulfide-bonded human peptide, exhibits antimicrobial activity. *FEBS Letters, 480*, 147–150.

Krijt, J., Vokurka, M., Chang, K. T., & Necas, E. (2004). Expression of Rgmc, the murine ortholog of hemojuvelin gene, is modulated by development and inflammation, but not by iron status or erythropoietin. *Blood, 104*, 4308–4310.

Lebron, J. A., West, J., & Bjorkman, P. J. (1999). The hemochromatosis protein HFE competes with transferrin for binding to the transferrin receptor. *Journal of Molecular Biology, 294*, 239–245.

Lee, P., Peng, H., Gelbart, T., & Beutler, E. (2004). The IL-6- and lipopolysaccharide-induced transcription of hepcidin in HFE-, transferrin receptor 2-, and {beta}2-microglobulin-deficient hepatocytes. *Proceedings of the National Academy of Sciences, 101*, 9263–9265.

Leung, P. S., Srai, S. K., Mascarenhas, M., Churchill, L. J., & Debnam, E. S. (2005). Increased duodenal iron uptake and transfer in a rat model of chronic hypoxia is accompanied by reduced hepcidin expression. *Gut, 54*, 1391–1395.

Levy, J. E., Jin, O., Fujiwara, Y., Kuo, F., & Andrews, N. C. (1999). Transferrin receptor is necessary for development of erythrocytes and the nervous system. *Nature Genetics, 21*, 396–399.

Lin, L., Goldberg, Y. P., & Ganz, T. (2005). Competitive regulation of hepcidin mRNA by soluble and cell-associated hemojuvelin. *Blood, 106*, 2884–2889.

Lin, L., Nemeth, E., Goodnough, J. B., Thapa, D. R., Gabayan, V., & Ganz, T. (2008). Soluble hemojuvelin is released by proprotein convertase-mediated cleavage at a conserved polybasic RNRR site. *Blood Cells, Molecules, and Diseases, 40*, 122–131.

Lin, L., Valore, E. V., Nemeth, E., Goodnough, J. B., Gabayan, V., & Ganz, T. (2007). Iron transferrin regulates hepcidin synthesis in primary hepatocyte culture through hemojuvelin and BMP2/4. *Blood, 110*, 2182–2189.

Liu, X. B., Hill, P., & Haile, D. J. (2002). Role of the ferroportin iron-responsive element in iron and nitric oxide dependent gene regulation. *Blood Cells, Molecules, and Diseases, 29*, 315–326.

Liu, X. B., Nguyen, N. B., Marquess, K. D., Yang, F., & Haile, D. J. (2005). Regulation of hepcidin and ferroportin expression by lipopolysaccharide in splenic macrophages. *Blood Cells, Molecules, and Diseases, 35*, 47–56.

Liu, X. B., Yang, F., & Haile, D. J. (2005). Functional consequences of ferroportin 1 mutations. *Blood Cells, Molecules, and Diseases, 35*, 33–46.

McKie, A. T., Marciani, P., Rolfs, A., Brennan, K., Wehr, K., Barrow, D., et al. (2000). A novel duodenal iron-regulated transporter, IREG1, implicated in the basolateral transfer of iron to the circulation. *Molecular Cell, 5*, 299–309.

Mendel, G. A. (1961). Studies on iron absorption. I. The relationships between the rate of erythropoiesis, hypoxia and iron absorption. *Blood, 18*, 727–736.

Muckenthaler, M., Roy, C. N., Custodio, A. O., Minana, B., deGraaf, J., Montross, L. K. et al. (2003). Regulatory defects in liver and intestine implicate abnormal hepcidin and Cybrd1 expression in mouse hemochromatosis. *Nature Genetics, 34*, 102–107.

Nemeth, E., Preza, G. C., Jung, C. L., Kaplan, J., Waring, A. J., & Ganz, T. (2006). The N-terminus of hepcidin is essential for its interaction with ferroportin: Structure-function study. *Blood, 107*, 328–333.

Nemeth, E., Rivera, S., Gabayan, V., Keller, C., Taudorf, S., Pedersen, B. K., et al. (2004). IL-6 mediates hypoferremia of inflammation by inducing the synthesis of the iron regulatory hormone hepcidin. *Journal of Clinical Investigation, 113*, 1271–1276.

Nemeth, E., Roetto, A., Garozzo, G., Ganz, T., & Camaschella, C. (2005). Hepcidin is decreased in TFR2 hemochromatosis. *Blood, 105*, 1803–1806.

Nemeth, E., Tuttle, M. S., Powelson, J., Vaughn, M. B., Donovan, A., Ward, D. M., et al. (2004). Hepcidin regulates cellular iron efflux by binding to ferroportin and inducing its internalization. *Science, 306*, 2090–2093.

Nemeth, E., Valore, E. V., Territo, M., Schiller, G., Lichtenstein, A., & Ganz, T. (2003). Hepcidin, a putative mediator of anemia of inflammation, is a type II acute-phase protein. *Blood, 101*, 2461–2463.

Nguyen, N. B., Callaghan, K. D., Ghio, A. J., Haile, D. J., & Yang, F. (2006). Hepcidin expression and iron transport in alveolar macrophages. *American Journal of Physiology Lung Cell and Molecular Physiology, 291*, L417–L425.

Nicolas, G., Bennoun, M., Devaux, I., Beaumont, C., Grandchamp, B., Kahn, A., et al. (2001). Lack of hepcidin gene expression and severe tissue iron overload in upstream stimulatory factor 2 (USF2) knockout mice. *Proceedings of the National Academy of Sciences, 98*, 8780–8785.

Nicolas, G., Bennoun, M., Porteu, A., Mativet, S., Beaumont, C., Grandchamp, B., et al. (2002). Severe iron deficiency anemia in transgenic mice expressing liver hepcidin. *Proceedings of the National Academy of Sciences, 99*, 4596–4601.

Nicolas, G., Chauvet, C., Viatte, L., Danan, J. L., Bigard, X., Devaux, I., et al. (2002). The gene encoding the iron regulatory peptide hepcidin is regulated by anemia, hypoxia, and inflammation. *Journal of Clinical Investigation, 110*, 1037–1044.

Nicolas, G., Viatte, L., Lou, D. Q., Bennoun, M., Beaumont, C., Kahn, A., et al. (2003). Constitutive hepcidin expression prevents iron overload in a mouse model of hemochromatosis. *Nature Genetics, 34*, 97–101.

Niederkofler, V., Salie, R., & Arber, S. (2005). Hemojuvelin is essential for dietary iron sensing, and its mutation leads to severe iron overload. *Journal of Clinical Investigation, 115*, 2180–2186.

Origa, R., Galanello, R., Ganz, T., Giagu, N., Maccioni, L., Faa, G., et al. (2007). Liver iron concentrations and urinary hepcidin in beta-thalassemia. *Haematologica, 92*, 583–588.

Pak, M., Lopez, M. A., Gabayan, V., Ganz, T., & Rivera, S. (2006). Suppression of hepcidin during anemia requires erythropoietic activity. *Blood, 108*, 3730–3735.

Papanikolaou, G., Samuels, M. E., Ludwig, E. H., MacDonald, M. L., Franchini, P. L., Dube, M. P., et al. (2004). Mutations in HFE2 cause iron overload in chromosome 1q-linked juvenile hemochromatosis. *Nature Genetics, 36*, 77–82.

Papanikolaou, G., Tzilianos, M., Christakis, J. I., Bogdanos, D., Tsimirika, K., MacFarlane, J., et al. (2005). Hepcidin in iron overload disorders. *Blood, 105*, 4103–4105.

Park, C. H., Valore, E. V., Waring, A. J., & Ganz, T. (2001). Hepcidin, a urinary antimicrobial peptide synthesized in the liver. *Journal of Biological Chemistry, 276*, 7806–7810.

Peyssonnaux, C., Zinkernagel, A. S., Datta, V., Lauth, X., Johnson, R. S., & Nizet, V. (2006). TLR4-dependent hepcidin expression by myeloid cells in response to bacterial pathogens. *Blood, 107*, 3727–3732.

Peyssonnaux, C., Zinkernagel, A. S., Schuepbach, R. A., Rankin, E., Vaulont, S., Haase, V. H., et al. (2007). Regulation of iron homeostasis by the hypoxia-inducible transcription factors (HIFs). *Journal of Clinical Investigation, 117*, 1926–1932.

Pietrangelo, A., Dierssen, U., Valli, L., Garuti, C., Rump, A., Corradini, E., et al. (2007). STAT3 is required for IL-6-gp130-dependent activation of hepcidin in vivo. *Gastroenterology, 132*, 294–300.

Pigeon, C., Ilyin, G., Courselaud, B., Leroyer, P., Turlin, B., Brissot, P., et al. (2001). A new mouse liver-specific gene, encoding a protein homologous to human antimicrobial peptide hepcidin, is overexpressed during iron overload. *Journal of Biological Chemistry, 276*, 7811–7819.

Pignatti, E., Mascheroni, L., Sabelli, M., Barelli, S., Biffo, S., & Pietrangelo, A. (2006). Ferroportin is a monomer in vivo in mice. *Blood Cells, Molecules, and Diseases, 36*, 26–32.

Piperno, A., Girelli, D., Nemeth, E., Trombini, P., Bozzini, C., Poggiali, E., et al. (2007). Blunted hepcidin response to oral iron challenge in HFE-related hemochromatosis. *Blood, 110*, 4096–4100.

Raja, K. B., Simpson, R. J., Pippard, M. J., & Peters, T. J. (1988). In vivo studies on the relationship between intestinal iron ($Fe3+$) absorption, hypoxia and erythropoiesis in the mouse. *British Journal of Haematology, 68*, 373–378.

Rivera, S., Liu, L., Nemeth, E., Gabayan, V., Sorensen, O. E., & Ganz, T. (2005). Hepcidin excess induces the sequestration of iron and exacerbates tumor-associated anemia. *Blood, 105*, 1797–1802.

Rivera, S., Nemeth, E., Gabayan, V., Lopez, M. A., Farshidi, D., & Ganz, T. (2005). Synthetic hepcidin causes rapid dose-dependent hypoferremia and is concentrated in ferroportin-containing organs. *Blood, 106*, 2196–2199.

Rivera, S., Gabayan, V., & Ganz, T. (2004). In chronic inflammation, there exists an IL-6 independent pathway for the induction of hepcidin. *ASH Annual Meeting Abstracts, 104*, 3205.

Robb, A., & Wessling-Resnick, M. (2004). Regulation of transferrin receptor 2 protein levels by transferrin. *Blood, 104*, 4294–4299.

Roetto, A., Papanikolaou, G., Politou, M., Alberti, F., Girelli, D., Christakis, J., et al. (2003). Mutant antimicrobial peptide hepcidin is associated with severe juvenile hemochromatosis. *Nature Genetics, 33*, 21–22.

Roy, C. N., Mak, H. H., Akpan, I., Losyev, G., Zurakowski, D., & Andrews, N. C. (2007). Hepcidin antimicrobial peptide transgenic mice exhibit features of the anemia of inflammation. *Blood, 109*, 4038–4044.

Schimanski, L. M., Drakesmith, H., Talbott, C., Horne, K., James, J. R., Davis, S. J., et al. (2008). Ferroportin: Lack of evidence for multimers. *Blood Cells, Molecules, and Diseases, 40*, 360–369.

Semenza, G. L. (2007). Hypoxia-inducible factor 1 (HIF-1) pathway. *Science's Signal Transduction Knowledge Environment, 2007*, cm8.

Sheikh, N., Dudas, J., & Ramadori, G. (2007). Changes of gene expression of iron regulatory proteins during turpentine oil-induced acute-phase response in the rat. *Laboratory Investigation, 87*, 713–725.

Shike, H., Lauth, X., Westerman, M. E., Ostland, V. E., Carlberg, J. M., Van Olst, J. C. et al. (2002). Bass hepcidin is a novel antimicrobial peptide induced by bacterial challenge. *European Journal of Biochemistry, 269*, 2232–2237.

Silvestri, L., Pagani, A., & Camaschella, C. (2008). Furin mediated release of soluble hemojuvelin: A new link between hypoxia and iron homeostasis. *Blood, 111*, 924–931.

Sow, F. B., Florence, W. C., Satoskar, A. R., Schlesinger, L. S., Zwilling, B. S., & Lafuse, W. P. (2007). Expression and localization of hepcidin in macrophages: A role in host defense against tuberculosis. *Journal of Leukocyte Biology, 82*, 934–945.

Tanno, T., Bhanu, N. V., Oneal, P. A., Goh, S. H., Staker, P., Lee, Y. T., et al. (2007). High levels of GDF15 in thalassemia suppress expression of the iron regulatory protein hepcidin. *Nature Medicine, 13*, 1096–1101.

Theurl, I., Theurl, M., Seifert, M., Mair, S., Nairz, M., Rumpold, H., et al. (2008). Autocrine formation of hepcidin induces iron retention in human monocytes. *Blood, 111*, 2392–2399.

Trenor, C. C., III, Campagna, D. R., Sellers, V. M., Andrews, N. C., & Fleming, M. D. (2000). The molecular defect in hypotransferrinemic mice. *Blood, 96*, 1113–1118.

Truksa, J., Peng, H., Lee, P., & Beutler, E. (2006). Bone morphogenetic proteins 2, 4, and 9 stimulate murine hepcidin 1 expression independently of HFE, transferrin receptor 2 (Tfr2), and IL-6. *Proceedings of the National Academy of Sciences, 103*, 10289–10293.

Valore, E. V., & Ganz, T. (2008). Posttranslational processing of hepcidin in human hepatocytes is mediated by the prohormone convertase furin. *Blood Cells, Molecules, and Diseases, 40*, 132–138.

Verga Falzacappa, M. V., Vujic, S. M., Kessler, R., Stolte, J., Hentze, M. W., & Muckenthaler, M. U. (2007). STAT3 mediates hepatic hepcidin expression and its inflammatory stimulation. *Blood, 109*, 353–358.

Vokurka, M., Krijt, J., Sulc, K., & Necas, E. (2006). Hepcidin mRNA levels in mouse liver respond to inhibition of erythropoiesis. *Physiological Research, 55*, 667–674.

Wallace, D. F., Summerville, L., Lusby, P. E., & Subramaniam, V. N. (2005). First phenotypic description of transferrin receptor 2 knockout mouse, and the role of hepcidin. *Gut, 54*, 980–986.

Wallace, D. F., Summerville, L., & Subramaniam, V. N. (2007). Targeted disruption of the hepatic transferrin receptor 2 gene in mice leads to iron overload. *Gastroenterology, 132*, 301–310.

Wang, R. H., Li, C., Xu, X., Zheng, Y., Xiao, C., Zerfas, P., et al. (2005). A role of SMAD4 in iron metabolism through the positive regulation of hepcidin expression. *Cell Metabolism, 2*, 399–409.

Weinstein, D. A., Roy, C. N., Fleming, M. D., Loda, M. F., Wolfsdorf, J. I., & Andrews, N. C. (2002). Inappropriate expression of hepcidin is associated with iron refractory anemia: Implications for the anemia of chronic disease. *Blood, 100*, 3776–3781.

Weizer-Stern, O., Adamsky, K., Amariglio, N., Levin, C., Koren, A., Breuer, W., et al. (2006). Downregulation of hepcidin and haemojuvelin expression in the hepatocyte cell-line HepG2 induced by thalassaemic sera. *British Journal of Haematology, 135*, 129–138.

Wrighting, D. M., & Andrews, N. C. (2006). Interleukin-6 induces hepcidin expression through STAT3. *Blood, 108*, 3204–3209.

Xia, Y., Yu, P. B., Sidis, Y., Beppu, H., Bloch, K. D., Schneyer, A. L., et al. (2007). Repulsive guidance molecule RGMa alters utilization of bone morphogenetic protein (BMP) type II receptors by BMP2 and BMP4. *Journal of Biological Chemistry, 282*, 18129–18140.

Yang, F., Liu, X. B., Quinones, M., Melby, P. C., Ghio, A., & Haile, D. J. (2002). Regulation of reticuloendothelial iron transporter MTP1 (Slc11a3) by inflammation. *Journal of Biological Chemistry, 277*, 39786–39791.

Zhang, A. S., Anderson, S. A., Meyers, K. R., Hernandez, C., Eisenstein, R. S., & Enns, C. A. (2007). Evidence that inhibition of hemojuvelin shedding in response to iron is mediated through neogenin. *Journal of Biological Chemistry, 282*, 12547–12556.

Zhang, A. S., West, A. P., Jr., Wyman, A. E., Bjorkman, P. J., & Enns, C. A. (2005). Interaction of hemojuvelin with neogenin results in iron accumulation in human embryonic kidney 293 cells. *Journal of Biological Chemistry, 280*, 33885–33894.

# 4 Iron as Nutrient: Strategies for Iron Acquisition and Usage by Pathogenic Microorganisms

*Eric Massé and Peter D. Pawelek*

**Summary**

- Many bacteria utilize low molecular weight molecules known as siderophores to obtain scarce iron nutrient from their extracellular environment.
- Siderophores and the molecular mechanisms required to synthesize, secrete, and ultimately import them are known virulence factors in many pathogenic bacteria.
- Extraintestinal pathogenic *Escherichia coli* as well as *Salmonella* possess a five-gene apparatus to modify siderophores in order to overcome the host's innate immune system.
- Siderophore modification systems present an ideal target for the development of novel antimicrobial agents that could potentially result in "virulence disarmament".
- Once the iron is inside the cell, it is directed to the most critical functions, especially during iron starvation.
- The small regulatory RNA RyhB reduces the cell's requirements in iron, which allows adaptation during iron starvation.

**Key Words:** Iron uptake; iron starvation; siderophores; enterobactin; pathogenic bacteria; small regulatory RNAs; RyhB

## 1. IRON AS NUTRIENT

### *1.1. The Importance of Fe Metabolism*

For a long time, the relationship between the mammalian host and the naturally occurring bacteria has been overlooked. Today, however, the importance of intestinal bacterial ecology has been recognized. While bacteria are involved in normal intestinal tract functions, such as protection against infections, production of vitamins, and degradation of otherwise indigestible components (Sonnenburg et al., 2005), they are also associated with obesity (Turnbaugh et al., 2006) and many forms of cancer (Vogelmann & Amieva, 2007). Although bacterial growth in the intestine can be flourishing, the ecological niches offered by the host are plagued with environmental stresses to which the bacteria need to adapt rapidly and continuously. This is especially true of extraintestinal environments in which many pathogenic bacteria must survive in order to be virulent. These environmental insults include thermal, acid, osmotic, and nutritional shocks. One such nutritional shock is iron (Fe) starvation. Indeed, Fe is one of the most important metals

From: *Nutrition and Health: Iron Deficiency and Overload*
Edited by: S. Yehuda and D.I. Mostofsky, DOI 10.1007/978-1-59745-462-9_4

for nearly all prokaryotes and eukaryotes (Outten & O'Halloran, 2001). It is found in the active site of numerous metallo-enzymes, which play essential functions in metabolic pathways such as the tricarboxylic acid (TCA) cycle, respiration, synthesis of organic compounds, and DNA synthesis and repair (Andrews, Robinson, & Rodriguez-Quinones, 2003). Because of the universal use of Fe, its acquisition and utilization are critical steps for successful establishment of most pathogens into a mammalian host.

### *1.2. Fe and Pathogenic Bacteria*

Infections from pathogenic extraintestinal *Escherichia coli* represent a serious challenge to our medical system. Uropathogenic *E. coli* (UPEC) accounts for approximately 90% of the reported annual cases of acute cystitis in the United States, as well as a quarter of a million cases of pyelonephritis (Welch et al., 2002). In order to colonize and thrive in the extraintestinal environment of the urinary tract, which has an alkaline rather than acidic pH, UPEC has adapted its Fe transport processes to tolerate a broader range of chemical environments in comparison to intestinal *E. coli* strains (Valdebenito, Bister, Reissbrodt, Hantke, & Winkelmann, 2005). The molecular mechanisms that UPEC have adapted to thrive in the mammalian urinary tract, to confer virulence, and to allow this pathogen to circumvent the mammalian immune system are the focus of this section of the chapter.

At physiological pH, Fe is mostly inaccessible to bacteria since it is either mostly insoluble in its ferric ($Fe^{3+}$) form or is bound to host proteins such as serum transferrin, which is the first line of defense of a host against bacterial pathogens (Barasch & Mori, 2004; Braun, 2005; Schaible & Kaufmann, 2004). To scavenge extracellular $Fe^{3+}$, bacteria have developed a high-affinity uptake strategy utilizing molecules known as siderophores. Because they are often critical to survival in the host, many siderophores synthesized by pathogenic bacteria are virulence factors (Fischbach, Lin, Zhou, Yu, Abergel, & Liu, 2006; Valdebenito, Crumbliss, Winkelmann, & Hantke, 2006). Iron-starved bacteria secrete siderophores to chelate low-abundance extracellular $Fe^{3+}$ with high affinity. Ferric siderophores are then taken up by a TonB-dependent signal transduction system found in the Gram-negative cell envelope (Pawelek et al., 2006; Wiener, 2005). While the $Fe^{3+}$-siderophore import mechanisms are well characterized, molecular mechanisms governing siderophore biosynthesis and export remain poorly characterized (Grass, 2006).

## 2. POST-SYNTHETIC MODIFICATION OF SIDEROPHORES IN PATHOGENIC BACTERIA

### *2.1. Enterobactin Biosynthesis and Secretion*

*Escherichia coli* K12 synthesizes and secretes a single catecholate siderophore known as enterobactin. This siderophore is composed of three 2,3-dihydroxybenzoyl serine (2,3-DHBS) groups linked as a trilactone (Fig. 1A). The arrangement of catechols from the 2,3-DHB groups enables it to chelate $Fe^{3+}$ in a hexadentate manner with extremely high affinity ($K_a \sim 10^{52}\ M^{-1}$). Enterobactin is hydrophobic and has been shown to partition into the ethyl acetate phase rather than the aqueous phase in vitro (Weitl, Harris, & Raymond, 1979), as well as being able to partition into membranes (Luo et al., 2006). The siderophore has also been shown to bind to serum albumin. Six enzymes synthesize enterobactin in the *E. coli* cytoplasm (Raymond, Dertz, & Kim, 2003). Three enzymes (EntC, EntB N-terminal (NT) domain, and EntA) function sequentially to synthesize the 2,3-DHB subunit. The EntB C-terminal (CT) domain, EntE, and EntF then function in a coordinated manner to link three 2,3-DHB subunits via non-ribosomal peptide synthesis (NRPS), thereby producing enterobactin. The NRPS activities have been described as

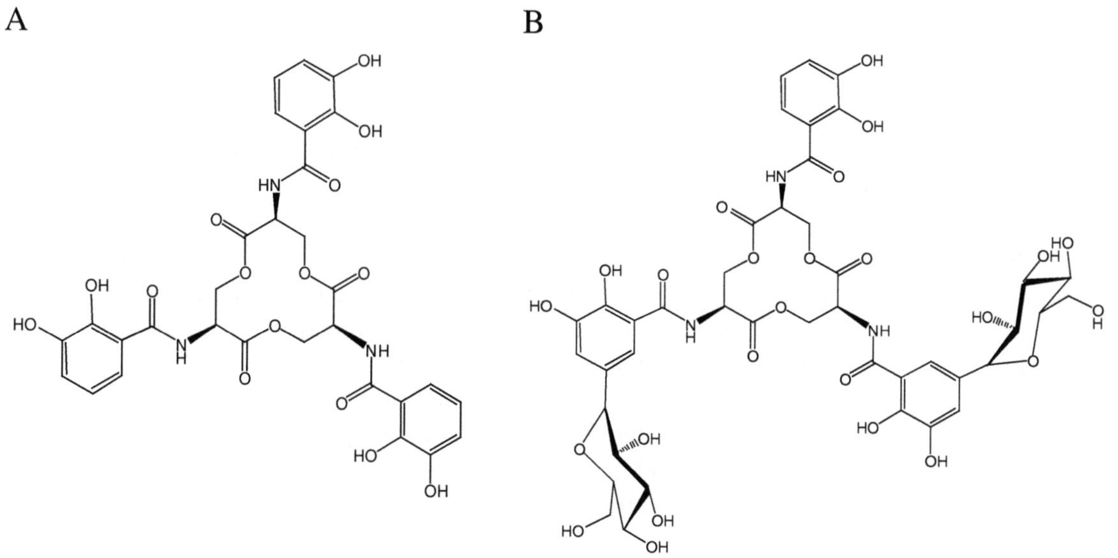


**Fig. 1.** Chemical structures of catecholate siderophores used by *Escherichia coli* K12 and UPEC. (**A**) enterobactin; (**B**) salmochelin S4.

operating within a "molecular assembly line" (Crosa & Walsh, 2002). Protein–protein interactions within the NRPS module have recently been identified [EntB–EntF (Lai, Fischbach, Liu, & Walsh, 2006), EntB–EntE (Drake, Nicolai, & Gulick, 2006)]. Recently, a seventh enzyme known as EntH has been identified as being essential for efficient enterobactin biosynthesis. The EntH thioesterase interacts with the EntB CT domain and appears to function as a quality-control factor in the NRPS process (Leduc, Battesti, & Bouveret, 2007).

Since enterobactin biosynthesis is cytoplasmic, the siderophore must cross the cell envelope for secretion into the extracellular environment. The *E. coli* cell envelope is composed of a cytoplasmic membrane (CM) and an outer membrane (OM) separated by the periplasmic space (PP). A 43-kDa protein, EntS, is an inner-membrane-embedded transporter involved in enterobactin secretion (Furrer, Sanders, Hook-Barnard, & McIntosh, 2002). The OM-embedded efflux pump TolC has also been shown to be involved in enterobactin secretion (Bleuel et al., 2005). The fate of the *apo* siderophore in transit within the periplasm from the CM-embedded EntS transporter to the TolC pore is currently unknown, although one or more periplasmic proteins are likely involved in delivering enterobactin to TolC (Grass, 2006). There is some evidence that the NRPS proteins co-fractionate with the cytoplasmic membrane (Hantash & Earhart, 2000). Although it is possible that an inner-membrane-proximal enterobactin biosynthetic machinery may co-localize with the efflux transporter EntS in order to mediate direct transfer of the enterobactin product to the transporter, this remains to be demonstrated.

### *2.2. Glucosylated Enterobactin Is a Virulence Factor in Pathogenic Bacteria*

Uropathogenic *E. coli* (UPEC), avian pathogenic *E. coli* (APEC), and *Salmonella typhimurium* possess a multi-protein apparatus that modifies enterobactin so that it can effectively circumvent the mammalian immune system, thereby allowing these pathogens to thrive in a host (Fischbach et al., 2006). These bacteria possess a five-gene cluster known as *IroA* that is located on a pathogenicity island. The *IroA* cluster contains five genes encoding the proteins IroB, IroC,

IroD, IroE, and IroN (Baumler et al., 1996). The enzyme IroB catalyzes the C-glucosylation of enterobactin in the cytoplasm (Fischbach, Lin, Liu, & Walsh, 2005). Glucosylated enterobactin, also known as salmochelin (Fig. 1B) (Bister et al., 2004; Hantke, Nicholson, Rabsch, & Winkelmann, 2003), is transported from the cytoplasm to the periplasm by the inner-membrane-embedded protein IroC. It is currently unknown how salmochelin is secreted from the cell via transport across the outer membrane. The periplasmic enzyme IroE catalyzes the linearization of salmochelin prior to its export (Lin, Fischbach, Liu, & Walsh, 2005); the precise role of this protein in salmochelin utilization remains enigmatic. It has been proposed that linearization may enhance secretion of the modified siderophore (Luo et al., 2006); such a mechanism could enhance salmochelin virulence. Salmochelin-secreting pathogenic bacteria then use IroN as an outer membrane receptor to uptake ferric salmochelin. IroN is TonB-dependent, similar to the OM receptor for ferric enterobactin, FepA (Hantke et al., 2003). The inner membrane transporter IroC has also been implicated in the transport of ferric salmochelin from the periplasm to the cytoplasm (Zhu, Valdebenito, Winkelmann, & Hantke, 2005). Upon import of ferric salmochelin to the cytoplasm, the Fes-like esterase IroD catalyzes the breakdown of salmochelin such that its Fe may be liberated for use in the cell (Zhu et al., 2005).

Why do pathogenic bacteria such as UPEC employ such an elaborate system for post-biosynthetic modification of enterobactin? A recent study reported that the mammalian innate immune system protein siderocalin (also known as lipocalin 2 (Flo et al., 2004)) specifically binds enterobactin (Fischbach et al., 2006) to prevent survival of pathogenic bacteria through sequestration of its essential Fe source. However, glucosylation of enterobactin by the IroA system in pathogenic bacteria results in the inability of siderocalin to bind the modified siderophore. This was demonstrated in a study involving immunodeficient mice that were injected with salmochelin-secreting *E. coli*. A high degree of mortality in the injected population was observed, effectively implicating salmochelin as a virulence factor (Fischbach et al., 2006). This elegant evasion of the mammalian immune system is a clear example of a bacterial anti-immunity mechanism (Finlay & McFadden, 2006).

At the molecular level, this evasion appears to occur due to the altered chemical nature of salmochelin. The addition of glucose molecules to the enterobactin backbone increases both the bulkiness and the hydrophilicity of the siderophore. This combination is sufficient to prevent salmochelin binding to the siderocalin-binding pocket (Fischbach et al., 2006). A recent study involving chemical modifications of enterobactin and enterobactin-like analogues showed that the addition of bulky methyl and *tert*-butyl groups to the carbon atoms that are glucosylated by IroB drastically reduces the binding affinity to siderocalin (Abergel, Moore, Strong, & Raymond, 2006).

Not all pathogenic bacteria circumvent our immune systems by siderophore modification. The pathogen *Bacillus anthracis* synthesizes two siderophores in order to survive and proliferate in the Fe-depleted host: bacillibactin and peterobactin (Cendrowski, MacArthur, & Hanna, 2004). Bacillibactin is a catecholate siderophore that structurally resembles enterobactin, but has methyl groups decorating the trilactone core; as well, the 2,3-DHB subunits extend further from this core by virtue of intervening glycine moieties. In contrast, petrobactin is an extended catecholate siderophore that contains two 3,4-DHB subunits. Chelation to $Fe^{3+}$ is hexadentate due to additional contributions from a citrate moiety in the spermidine backbone of the siderophore. Of the two siderophores, petrobactin appears to be the primary virulence factor. Petrobactin has been shown to be the sole siderophore synthesized by anthrax at physiological temperatures under Fe-depleted conditions (Koppisch et al., 2005). Also, binding studies have shown that while bacillibactin binds with high affinity to siderocalin, petrobactin is unable to bind. The altered arrangement of the catechol groups within the 3,4-DHB subunits of petrobactin appear to be sufficient to prevent binding to siderocalin (Abergel, Wilson, et al., 2006). Thus, anthrax can avoid mammalian immune surveillance through utilization of petrobactin to attain its Fe nutrient in the host, presumably from transferrin. This makes the petrobactin biosynthesis and secretion machinery an ideal target for the development of novel antibiotics to specifically target anthrax.

Taken together, these recent findings provide compelling justification to target virulence processes related to siderophore biosynthesis, modification, and secretion in order to develop a powerful new class of antibiotics. Recently, the paradigm of "virulence disarmament" has been proposed, in which a novel antimicrobial agent would function to attenuate one or more virulence factors while not necessarily killing the pathogens. Such agents could be used in combination therapy with more traditional antibiotics. This multivalent strategy could potentiate bacteriocidal efficacy while preventing the development of spontaneous mutations resulting in acquired antibiotic resistance (Baron & Coombes, 2007). This approach is especially valid in the case of siderophore-mediated Fe acquisition systems, since such agents could discriminate between commensal bacteria present in Fe-rich host environments and pathogenic bacteria that are struggling to survive and proliferate in Fe-starved extraintestinal host environments. These "conditionally essential" systems therefore provide a degree of selectivity desirable in drug development (Quadri, 2007).

## 3. INTRACELLULAR IRON HOMEOSTASIS IN BACTERIA

While the different strategies described above demonstrate how bacteria obtain Fe from the host, another important aspect is the intracellular management of Fe once it has entered the bacterium. Most bacteria have developed a precisely regulated system to maintain intracellular Fe within an optimal concentration range (Andrews et al., 2003). The intracellular Fe levels should be high enough to allow cellular functions, and yet low enough to prevent damage due to highly reactive hydroxyl radicals ($OH^{\cdot}$). These toxic radicals are formed through the Fenton reaction when intracellular Fe is abundant in the presence of oxygen, and they destroy DNA, RNA, proteins, and membranes (Imlay, 2003). In bacteria, when the intracellular Fe level is high, the protein Fur (Ferric uptake regulator) represses transcription initiation of Fe-uptake genes (Hantke, 1981). In addition, Fur represses a small RNA (sRNA) named RyhB, which induces the degradation of a large group of mRNAs encoding Fe-using proteins (Massé & Gottesman, 2002). Section 3.1 covers some general features of sRNA functions and mechanisms in bacteria.

### *3.1. Small Regulatory RNAs and Environmental Stresses*

Bacterial strategies developed to adapt to environmental stresses include the use of sRNAs, which are modulators of gene transcription, mRNA translation, as well as protein activity (Gottesman, 2005). These molecules are usually non-coding, smaller than 300 nucleotides, and found in both prokaryotic and eukaryotic organisms. About 30 years ago, the first sRNAs, 6S and Spot42, were discovered as abundant molecules in *E. coli*. Today, about 70 sRNA genes have been identified, located either on plasmid or the *E. coli* chromosome (Gottesman, 2005). Although no function has yet been attributed to most sRNAs, those characterized are involved in diverse cellular functions such as the initiation of DNA replication (RNAI; Eguchi, Itoh, & Tomizawa, 1991), regulation of transcription (6S; Wassarman & Storz, 2000), regulation of translation (OxyS, Spot42, DsrA, RprA, and MicA) (Altuvia, Zhang, Argaman, Tiwari, & Storz, 1998; Majdalani, Cunning, Sledjeski, Elliott, & Gottesman, 1998; Majdalani, Chen, Murrow, St John, & Gottesman, 2001; Moller, Franch, Udesen, Gerdes, & Valentin-Hansen,

2002; Udekwu et al., 2005), and mRNA stability (RyhB and SgrS) (Massé, Escorcia, & Gottesman, 2003; Morita, Maki, & Aiba, 2005). Each of these sRNAs is expressed in response to a specific stimulus that signals the cell of a possible threat to survival.

### *3.2. Role and Mechanism of the sRNA RyhB During Fe Starvation*

Recently, a novel cellular mechanism that is essential to redistribute scarce amounts of available Fe during Fe starvation has been characterized (Fig. 2) (Jacques et al., 2006; Massé & Arguin, 2005). This mechanism relies on the sRNA RyhB, which rapidly downregulates at least 18 mRNA transcripts encoding a total of 56 proteins (each transcript encodes at least one Fe-using protein) (Massé & Arguin, 2005). The speed at which the RyhB-mediated mRNA degradation occurs (within 2–3 min of RyhB induction) suggests that the target mRNAs have to be silenced as soon as possible under conditions where RyhB is expressed (low Fe). It has been demonstrated that in the first steps of this mechanism, RyhB functions in concert with the RNA chaperone Hfq to form a base-pairing complex with its target mRNAs (Geissmann & Touati, 2004). Following this, the RNA degradosome is recruited at the mRNA–RyhB complex to degrade both RNAs (Massé et al., 2003; Morita et al., 2005). The result of this regulation is the efficient silencing of an important group of genes in conditions of Fe starvation (Fig. 2) (Massé, Vanderpool, & Gottesman, 2005).

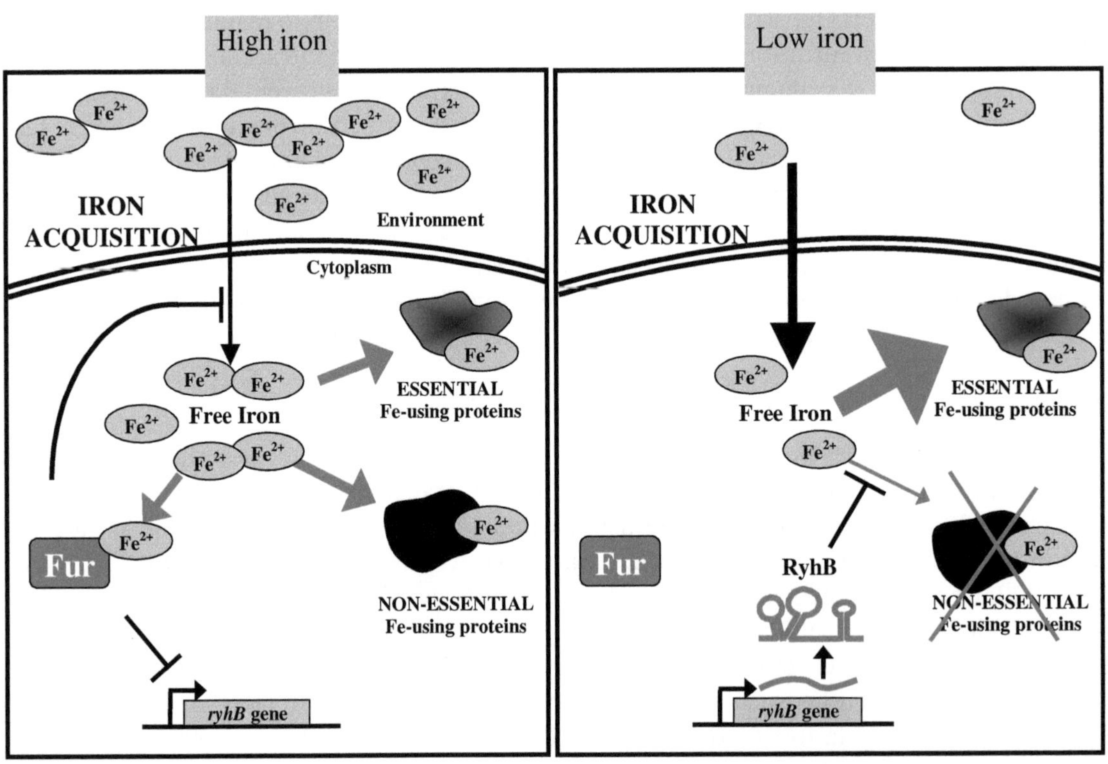


**Fig. 2.** Intracellular iron homeostasis during high iron level (*left panel*) and low iron level (*right panel*) in *Escherichia coli*. See text for details of the regulation.

While Fur and Fe directly regulate RyhB, there is strong evidence demonstrating that RyhB itself is sufficient to influence the level of free intracellular Fe (Massé et al., 2005). By cloning the *ryhB* gene downstream of an arabinose-inducible BAD promoter, induction of RyhB by a carbon source (and not an Fe chelator) resulted in unexpected outcomes. Under these conditions, even with Fe levels that are a priori unaltered, many genes specific to the Fur regulon become repressed. It was later demonstrated that expression of RyhB resulted in a significant increase in free intracellular Fe (Jacques et al., 2006). This increased level of free Fe activates Fur, which represses the transcription of many Fe acquisition genes. Further investigation demonstrated that this increase depends on newly acquired Fe and not on already internalized metal (Jacques et al., 2006). Thus, RyhB reduces the sequestration of newly acquired Fe by non-essential proteins, allowing only essential proteins to access the metal. This regulation also reinforces the idea that the concerted actions of Fur and RyhB adjust the intracellular pool of available Fe (Massé & Arguin, 2005).

It seems likely that RyhB activity allocates a minimum of accessible Fe for essential Fe-using proteins, such as ribonucleotide reductase and dihydroxyacid dehydratase. These two proteins, respectively involved in critical functions such as production of nucleic acids and amino acids, are not affected by RyhB. While much of the early work on RyhB was oriented to find new mRNA targets, the study of RyhB under different conditions indicated a significant growth delay of a *ryhB* mutant in the strict absence of Fe (Jacques et al., 2006). This observation suggests that the early phase of growth is most sensitive to Fe starvation, and that RyhB facilitates the cellular adaptation to this condition.

### *3.3. Roles of RyhB in Biofilms, Chemotaxis, and Acid Resistance*

As described in the first part of this chapter, adaptation to Fe starvation is critical for pathogenic bacteria to successfully infect a host. Because of its implication in Fe starvation, the sRNA RyhB has been the subject of many investigations in different pathogenic bacteria. The bacteria *Vibrio cholerae* and *E. coli* share a well-conserved sequence in the *ryhB* gene (Massé & Gottesman, 2002). While *V. cholerae ryhB* gene is also regulated by Fur and Fe, it is more than twice as long as the *ryhB* gene of *E. coli*. Investigation of the role of RyhB in *V. cholerae*, the cause of cholera, confirmed that it regulates transcripts encoding Fe-using proteins (Davis, Quinones, Pratt, Ding, & Waldor, 2005; Mey, Craig, & Payne, 2005). Interestingly, both studies report that RyhB is not essential for bacterial colonization of the mouse. Nevertheless, a *ryhB* mutant was demonstrated to be defective in both biofilm formation and chemotaxis. It was further shown that both phenotypes can be rescued by addition of excess Fe in the media (Mey et al., 2005). Thus, while RyhB itself is not essential for virulence of *V. cholerae*, it probably increases the available Fe necessary for biofilm formation and chemotaxis, both of which are virulence determinants.

An additional bacterial virulence determinant is acid resistance. Because it encounters acidic conditions in the stomach of its host, the causative agent of dysentery, *Shigella flexneri*, has developed resistance systems to survive these conditions. Recent experiments demonstrated that RyhB expression modulates the resistance to acid through *ydeP*, encoding a putative oxidoreductase that is essential for acid resistance of *Shigella* (Oglesby, Murphy, Iyer, & Payne, 2005). The suggested mechanism is that RyhB represses *evgA*, a transcriptional activator of *ydeP* (Oglesby et al., 2005). Notably, the authors demonstrated that RyhB overproduction in *Shigella* resulted in decreased acid resistance. According to these results, the resistance to acid is optimal in the presence of Fe. In an iron-rich intracellular environment, Fur represses RyhB, which allows activation of *ydeP* through *evgA*.

### *3.4. Similar Regulatory Mechanism in Other Species*

Following the discovery and characterization of RyhB, a very similar mechanism was described in another bacterium, *Pseudomonas aeruginosa* (Wilderman et al., 2004). While *E. coli* has only one copy of the *ryhB* gene, *P. aeruginosa* has two similar genes, *prrF1* and *prrF2*, located in tandem. As in *E. coli*, these two sRNAs repress specific mRNAs encoding Fe-using proteins in response to Fe depletion. Moreover, similar mechanisms were also unveiled in lower eukaryotes. For example, both the protein Cth2 in the budding yeast *Saccharomyces cerevisiae* and Php4 in the fission yeast *Schizosaccharomyces pombe* coordinate the repression of Fe-using proteins under conditions of low Fe (Mercier, Pelletier, & Labbé, 2006; Puig, Askeland, & Thiele, 2005). Contrary to bacteria, however, yeasts do not use sRNAs for regulation of Fe metabolism. These findings reinforce the idea that Fe is an essential factor that is carefully distributed among Fe-using proteins. This is likely why many organisms share a RyhB-like mechanism of Fe regulation (Massé & Arguin, 2005; Massé, Salvail, Desnoyers, & Arguin, 2007).

While the presence of a RyhB-like factor has not yet been demonstrated in many organisms, an increasing body of evidence points to a similar molecule (an sRNA or a protein) that represses genes encoding Fe-using proteins during Fe limitation. In the pathogenic bacterium *Staphylococcus aureus*, transcriptome studies performed during Fe starvation demonstrated the repression of many genes encoding Fe-using proteins (Allard et al., 2006; Friedman et al., 2006). In another pathogenic species, the bacterium *Campylobacter jejuni* exhibits a similar gene repression pattern under Fe starvation (Holmes et al., 2005).

Surprisingly, the human pathogen *Neisseria meningitidis* has developed a different approach to adapt to Fe starvation. Instead of regulating an sRNA, the protein Fur acts directly as a transcriptional activator of genes encoding Fe-using proteins when Fe concentration is high (Delany, Rappuoli, & Scarlato, 2004). Inversely, under low Fe conditions, Fur becomes inactive, which reduces the expression of Fe sequestration by Fe-using proteins. This seems to be a unique case since there is no evidence of such a similar Fur-activating mechanism in other species.

### *3.5. Siderophore Biosynthesis and RyhB*

As previously discussed, it appears that all the target mRNAs that base-pair with RyhB are eventually degraded through the RNA degradosome. Recently, however, a new family of target mRNAs has been shown to be positively regulated by RyhB (Prévost et al., 2007). Indeed, RyhB base-pairs with the *shiA* mRNA and activates its translation by eightfold. This is the first example of a positive regulation by an sRNA involved in sRNA-mediated mRNA degradation. It was demonstrated that RyhB base-pairs at the 5′-UTR of the *shiA* mRNA to unfold an inhibitory structure covering the ribosome-binding site and first codon (Prévost et al., 2007). The RyhB-activated gene, *shiA*, encodes for an inner-membrane-embedded permease that facilitates intake of extracellular shikimate, a compound that is used only by bacteria, protozoans, and plants. In these organisms, shikimate is essential for biosynthesis of aromatic amino acids and vitamins, as well as the *E. coli* siderophore enterobactin (Herrmann & Weaver, 1999). In addition to extracellular acquisition of shikimate, *E. coli* generates this compound through an internal biosynthesis pathway. It is thus very interesting that RyhB, which is expressed during Fe starvation, activates the acquisition machinery of extracellular shikimate, an Fe siderophore precursor. Indeed, the results demonstrate that shikimate corrects the defective adaptation of a *ryhB* mutant during Fe starvation (Prévost et al., 2007). Although the reason for this correction has not yet been discovered, it is likely that shikimate enhances siderophore synthesis by the bacteria.

### *3.6. Concluding Remarks*

Recent advances in bacterial Fe metabolism demonstrated that much of the regulation governing Fe uptake and usage is exquisitely sophisticated. Modification of bacterial siderophores to circumvent the host defence and thorough distribution of intracellular Fe are two striking examples of elegant strategies developed by bacteria to adapt to constantly varying environmental conditions. Still, many unanswered questions remain to be investigated. For example, what is the extent to which proteins involved in siderophore secretion and synthesis coordinate their activities through protein–protein interactions? Such interaction networks have been demonstrated to be critical for ferric-siderophore uptake mechanisms yet remain to be elucidated for synthesis and secretion mechanisms. Second, what are the regulatory mechanisms that govern siderophore modifications that confer virulence (e.g., enterobactin glycosylation)? Finally, the molecular mechanism of RyhB-mediated mRNA degradation is a key aspect of the gene regulation, which will be interesting to pursue in the next few years.

**Acknowledgments** We are grateful to Frederieke Brouwers and members of our laboratories for useful comments and discussions on the manuscript. Work in E.M. laboratory was funded by an operating grant MOP69005 from the Canadian Institute for Health Research (CIHR). E.M. is a Canadian Institutes for Health Research (CIHR) new investigator scholar. P.D.P. acknowledges financial support from the National Sciences and Engineering Research Council of Canada (NSERC) through a Discovery Grant (341983-07).

## REFERENCES

Abergel, R. J., Moore, E. G., Strong, R. K., & Raymond, K. N. (2006). Microbial evasion of the immune system: Structural modifications of enterobactin impair siderocalin recognition. *Journal of the American Chemical Society, 128*(34), 10998–10999.

Abergel, R. J., Wilson, M. K., Arceneaux, J. E., Hoette, T. M., Strong, R. K., Byers, B. R., et al. (2006). Anthrax pathogen evades the mammalian immune system through stealth siderophore production. *Proceedings of the National Academy of Sciences of the USA, 103*(49), 18499–18503.

Allard, M., Moisan, H., Brouillette, E., Gervais, A. L., Jacques, M., Lacasse, P., et al. (2006). Transcriptional modulation of some *Staphylococcus aureus* iron-regulated genes during growth in vitro and in a tissue cage model in vivo. *Microbes and Infection/Institut Pasteur, 8*(7), 1679–1690.

Altuvia, S., Zhang, A., Argaman, L., Tiwari, A., & Storz, G. (1998). The *Escherichia coli* OxyS regulatory RNA represses fhlA translation by blocking ribosome binding. *The EMBO Journal, 17*(20), 6069–6075.

Andrews, S. C., Robinson, A. K., & Rodriguez-Quinones, F. (2003). Bacterial iron homeostasis. *FEMS Microbiology Reviews, 27*(2–3), 215–237.

Barasch, J., & Mori, K. (2004). Cell biology: Iron thievery. *Nature, 432*(7019), 811–813.

Baron, C., & Coombes, B. (2007). Targeting bacterial secretion systems: Benefits of disarmament in the microcosm. *Infectious Disorders Drug Targets, 7*(1), 19–27.

Baumler, A. J., Tsolis, R. M., van der Velden, A. W., Stojiljkovic, I., Anic, S., & Heffron, F. (1996). Identification of a new iron regulated locus of *Salmonella typhi. Gene, 183*(1–2), 207–213.

Bister, B., Bischoff, D., Nicholson, G. J., Valdebenito, M., Schneider, K., Winkelmann, G., et al. (2004). The structure of salmochelins: C-glucosylated enterobactins of *Salmonella enterica. Biometals: An International Journal on the Role of Metal Ions in Biology, Biochemistry, and Medicine, 17*(4), 471–481.

Bleuel, C., Grosse, C., Taudte, N., Scherer, J., Wesenberg, D., Krauss, G. J., et al. (2005). TolC is involved in enterobactin efflux across the outer membrane of escherichia coli. *Journal of Bacteriology, 187*(19), 6701–6707.

Braun, V. (2005). Bacterial iron transport related to virulence. In W. Russell & H. Herwald (Eds.), *Concepts in bacterial virulence* (pp. 210–233). Basel, Switzerland: Karger.

Cendrowski, S., MacArthur, W., & Hanna, P. (2004). Bacillus anthracis requires siderophore biosynthesis for growth in macrophages and mouse virulence. *Molecular Microbiology, 51*(2), 407–417.

Crosa, J. H., & Walsh, C. T. (2002). Genetics and assembly line enzymology of siderophore biosynthesis in bacteria. *Microbiology and Molecular Biology Reviews: MMBR, 66*(2), 223–249.

Davis, B. M., Quinones, M., Pratt, J., Ding, Y., & Waldor, M. K. (2005). Characterization of the small untranslated RNA RyhB and its regulon in *Vibrio cholerae. Journal of Bacteriology, 187*(12), 4005–4014.

Delany, I., Rappuoli, R., & Scarlato, V. (2004). Fur functions as an activator and as a repressor of putative virulence genes in *Neisseria meningitidis*. *Molecular Microbiology, 52*(4), 1081–1090.

Drake, E. J., Nicolai, D. A., & Gulick, A. M. (2006). Structure of the EntB multidomain nonribosomal peptide synthetase and functional analysis of its interaction with the EntE adenylation domain. *Chemistry & Biology, 13*(4), 409–419.

Eguchi, Y., Itoh, T., & Tomizawa, J. (1991). Antisense RNA. *Annual Review of Biochemistry, 60*, 631–652.

Finlay, B. B., & McFadden, G. (2006). Anti-immunology: Evasion of the host immune system by bacterial and viral pathogens. *Cell, 124*(4), 767–782.

Fischbach, M. A., Lin, H., Liu, D. R., & Walsh, C. T. (2005). In vitro characterization of IroB, a pathogen-associated C-glycosyltransferase. *Proceedings of the National Academy of Sciences of the USA, 102*(3), 571–576.

Fischbach, M. A., Lin, H., Zhou, L., Yu, Y., Abergel, R. J., Liu, D. R., et al. (2006). The pathogen-associated iroA gene cluster mediates bacterial evasion of lipocalin 2. *Proceedings of the National Academy of Sciences of the USA, 103*(44), 16502–16507.

Flo, T. H., Smith, K. D., Sato, S., Rodriguez, D. J., Holmes, M. A., Strong, R. K., et al. (2004). Lipocalin 2 mediates an innate immune response to bacterial infection by sequestrating iron. *Nature, 432*(7019), 917–921.

Friedman, D. B., Stauff, D. L., Pishchany, G., Whitwell, C. W., Torres, V. J., & Skaar, E. P. (2006). Staphylococcus aureus redirects central metabolism to increase iron availability. *PLoS Pathogens, 2*(8), e87.

Furrer, J. L., Sanders, D. N., Hook-Barnard, I. G., & McIntosh, M. A. (2002). Export of the siderophore enterobactin in escherichia coli: Involvement of a 43 kDa membrane exporter. *Molecular Microbiology, 44*(5), 1225–1234.

Geissmann, T. A., & Touati, D. (2004). Hfq, a new chaperoning role: Binding to messenger RNA determines access for small RNA regulator. *The EMBO Journal, 23*(2), 396–405.

Gottesman, S. (2005). Micros for microbes: Non-coding regulatory RNAs in bacteria. *Trends in Genetics: TIG, 21*(7), 399–404.

Grass, G. (2006). Iron transport in escherichia coli: All has not been said and done. *Biometals: An International Journal on the Role of Metal Ions in Biology, Biochemistry, and Medicine, 19*(2), 159–172.

Hantash, F. M., & Earhart, C. F. (2000). Membrane association of the escherichia coli enterobactin synthase proteins EntB/G, EntE, and EntF. *Journal of Bacteriology, 182*(6), 1768–1773.

Hantke, K. (1981). Regulation of ferric iron transport in escherichia coli K12: Isolation of a constitutive mutant. *Molecular & General Genetics: MGG, 182*(2), 288–292.

Hantke, K., Nicholson, G., Rabsch, W., & Winkelmann, G. (2003). Salmochelins, siderophores of salmonella enterica and uropathogenic escherichia coli strains, are recognized by the outer membrane receptor IroN. *Proceedings of the National Academy of Sciences of the USA, 100*(7), 3677–3682.

Herrmann, K. M., & Weaver, L. M. (1999). The Shikimate pathway. *Annual Review of Plant Physiology and Plant Molecular Biology, 50*, 473–503.

Holmes, K., Mulholland, F., Pearson, B. M., Pin, C., McNicholl-Kennedy, J., Ketley, J. M., et al. (2005). *Campylobacter jejuni* gene expression in response to iron limitation and the role of fur. *Microbiology (Reading, England), 151*(Pt. 1), 243–257.

Imlay, J. A. (2003). Pathways of oxidative damage. *Annual Review of Microbiology, 57*, 395–418.

Jacques, J. F., Jang, S., Prévost, K., Desnoyers, G., Desmarais, M., Imlay, J., et al. (2006). RyhB small RNA modulates the free intracellular iron pool and is essential for normal growth during iron limitation in escherichia coli. *Molecular Microbiology, 62*(4), 1181–1190.

Koppisch, A. T., Browder, C. C., Moe, A. L., Shelley, J. T., Kinkel, B. A., Hersman, L. E., et al. (2005). Petrobactin is the primary siderophore synthesized by bacillus anthracis str. sterne under conditions of iron starvation. *Biometals: An International Journal on the Role of Metal Ions in Biology, Biochemistry, and Medicine, 18*(6), 577–585.

Lai, J. R., Fischbach, M. A., Liu, D. R., & Walsh, C. T. (2006). Localized protein interaction surfaces on the EntB carrier protein revealed by combinatorial mutagenesis and selection. *Journal of the American Chemical Society, 128*(34), 11002–11003.

Leduc, D., Battesti, A., & Bouveret, E. (2007). The hotdog thioesterase EntH (YbdB) plays a role in vivo in optimal enterobactin biosynthesis by interacting with the ArCP domain of EntB. *Journal of Bacteriology, 189*(19), 7112–7126.

Lin, H., Fischbach, M. A., Liu, D. R., & Walsh, C. T. (2005). In vitro characterization of salmochelin and enterobactin trilactone hydrolases IroD, IroE, and fes. *Journal of the American Chemical Society, 127*(31), 11075–11084.

Luo, M., Lin, H., Fischbach, M. A., Liu, D. R., Walsh, C. T., & Groves, J. T. (2006). Enzymatic tailoring of enterobactin alters membrane partitioning and iron acquisition. *ACS Chemical Biology, 1*(1), 29–32.

Majdalani, N., Chen, S., Murrow, J., St. John, K., & Gottesman, S. (2001). Regulation of RpoS by a novel small RNA: The characterization of RprA. *Molecular Microbiology, 39*(5), 1382–1394.

Majdalani, N., Cunning, C., Sledjeski, D., Elliott, T., & Gottesman, S. (1998). DsrA RNA regulates translation of RpoS message by an anti-antisense mechanism, independent of its action as an antisilencer of transcription. *Proceedings of the National Academy of Sciences of the USA, 95*(21), 12462–12467.

Massé, E., & Arguin, M. (2005). Ironing out the problem: New mechanisms of iron homeostasis. *Trends in Biochemical Sciences, 30*(8), 462–468.

Massé, E., Escorcia, F. E., & Gottesman, S. (2003). Coupled degradation of a small regulatory RNA and its mRNA targets in escherichia coli. *Genes & Development, 17*(19), 2374–2383.

Massé, E., & Gottesman, S. (2002). A small RNA regulates the expression of genes involved in iron metabolism in escherichia coli. *Proceedings of the National Academy of Sciences of the USA, 99*(7), 4620–4625.

Massé, E., Salvail, H., Desnoyers, G., & Arguin, M. (2007). Small RNAs controlling iron metabolism. *Current Opinion in Microbiology, 10*(2), 140–145.

Massé, E., Vanderpool, C. K., & Gottesman, S. (2005). Effect of RyhB small RNA on global iron use in escherichia coli. *Journal of Bacteriology, 187*(20), 6962–6971.

Mercier, A., Pelletier, B., & Labbé, S. (2006). A transcription factor cascade involving Fep1 and the CCAAT-binding factor Php4 regulates gene expression in response to iron deficiency in the fission yeast *Schizosaccharomyces pombe. Eukaryotic Cell, 5*(11), 1866–1881.

Mey, A. R., Craig, S. A., & Payne, S. M. (2005). Characterization of vibrio cholerae RyhB: The RyhB regulon and role of ryhB in biofilm formation. *Infection and Immunity, 73*(9), 5706–5719.

Moller, T., Franch, T., Udesen, C., Gerdes, K., & Valentin-Hansen, P. (2002). Spot 42 RNA mediates discoordinate expression of the E. coli galactose operon. *Genes & Development, 16*(13), 1696–1706.

Morita, T., Maki, K., & Aiba, H. (2005). RNase E-based ribonucleoprotein complexes: Mechanical basis of mRNA destabilization mediated by bacterial noncoding RNAs. *Genes & Development, 19*(18), 2176–2186.

Oglesby, A. G., Murphy, E. R., Iyer, V. R., & Payne, S. M. (2005). Fur regulates acid resistance in *Shigella flexneri* via RyhB and ydeP. *Molecular Microbiology, 58*(5), 1354–1367.

Outten, C. E., & O'Halloran, T. V. (2001). Femtomolar sensitivity of metalloregulatory proteins controlling zinc homeostasis. *Science, 292*(5526), 2488–2492.

Pawelek, P. D., Croteau, N., Ng-Thow-Hing, C., Khursigara, C. M., Moiseeva, N., Allaire, M., et al. (2006). Structure of TonB in complex with FhuA, E. coli outer membrane receptor. *Science (New York), 312*(5778), 1399–1402.

Prévost, K., Salvail, H., Desnoyers, G., Jacques, J. F., Phaneuf, E., & Massé, E. (2007). The small RNA RyhB activates the translation of *shiA* mRNA encoding a permease of shikimate, a compound involved in siderophore synthesis. *Molecular Microbiology, 64*, 1260–1273.

Puig, S., Askeland, E., & Thiele, D. J. (2005). Coordinated remodeling of cellular metabolism during iron deficiency through targeted mRNA degradation. *Cell, 120*(1), 99–110.

Quadri, L. E. (2007). Strategic paradigm shifts in the antimicrobial drug discovery process of the 21st century. *Infectious Disorders Drug Targets, 7*(3), 230–237.

Raymond, K. N., Dertz, E. A., & Kim, S. S. (2003). Enterobactin: An archetype for microbial iron transport. *Proceedings of the National Academy of Sciences of the USA, 100*(7), 3584–3588.

Schaible, U. E., & Kaufmann, S. H. (2004). Iron and microbial infection. *Nature Reviews. Microbiology, 2*(12), 946–953.

Sonnenburg, J. L., Xu, J., Leip, D. D., Chen, C. H., Westover, B. P., Weatherford, J., et al. (2005). Glycan foraging in vivo by an intestine-adapted bacterial symbiont. *Science, 307*(5717), 1955–1959.

Turnbaugh, P. J., Ley, R. E., Mahowald, M. A., Magrini, V., Mardis, E. R., & Gordon, J. I. (2006). An obesity-associated gut microbiome with increased capacity for energy harvest. *Nature, 444*(7122), 1027–1031.

Udekwu, K. I., Darfeuille, F., Vogel, J., Reimegard, J., Holmqvist, E., & Wagner, E. G. (2005). Hfq-dependent regulation of OmpA synthesis is mediated by an antisense RNA. *Genes & Development, 19*(19), 2355–2366.

Valdebenito, M., Bister, B., Reissbrodt, R., Hantke, K., & Winkelmann, G. (2005). The detection of salmochelin and yersiniabactin in uropathogenic escherichia coli strains by a novel hydrolysis-fluorescence-detection (HFD) method. *International Journal of Medical Microbiology: IJMM, 295*(2), 99–107.

Valdebenito, M., Crumbliss, A. L., Winkelmann, G., & Hantke, K. (2006). Environmental factors influence the production of enterobactin, salmochelin, aerobactin, and yersiniabactin in escherichia coli strain nissle 1917. *International Journal of Medical Microbiology: IJMM, 296*(8), 513–520.

Vogelmann, R., & Amieva, M. R. (2007). The role of bacterial pathogens in cancer. *Current Opinion in Microbiology, 10*(1), 76–81.

Wassarman, K. M., & Storz, G. (2000). 6S RNA regulates E. coli RNA polymerase activity. *Cell, 101*(6), 613–623.

Weitl, F. L., Harris, W. R., & Raymond, K. N. (1979). Sulfonated catecholamide analogues of enterobactin as iron sequestering agents. *Journal of Medicinal Chemistry, 22*(11), 1281–1283.

Welch, R. A., Burland, V., Plunkett, G., III, Redford, P., Roesch, P., Rasko, D., et al. (2002). Extensive mosaic structure revealed by the complete genome sequence of uropathogenic escherichia coli. *Proceedings of the National Academy of Sciences of the USA, 99*(26), 17020–17024.

Wiener, M. C. (2005). TonB-dependent outer membrane transport: Going for baroque? *Current Opinion in Structural Biology, 15*(4), 394–400.

Wilderman, P. J., Sowa, N. A., FitzGerald, D. J., FitzGerald, P. C., Gottesman, S., Ochsner, U. A., et al. (2004). Identification of tandem duplicate regulatory small RNAs in *Pseudomonas aeruginosa* involved in iron homeostasis. *Proceedings of the National Academy of Sciences of the USA, 101*(26), 9792–9797.

Zhu, M., Valdebenito, M., Winkelmann, G., & Hantke, K. (2005). Functions of the siderophore esterases IroD and IroE in iron-salmochelin utilization. *Microbiology (Reading, England), 151*(Pt. 7), 2363–2372.

# 5 Iron as a Drug and Drug–Drug Interactions

*Tracy M. Hagemann and Teresa V. Lewis*

**Summary**

- Bioavailabiltiy of oral iron may be enhanced in the presence of reducing agents such as ascorbic acid.
- All commercially available iron salts are effective in the treatment of iron deficiency.
- Administration of oral iron should be separated from other medications by at least 1–2 hours.
- The use of iron dextran is not attractive compared to other IV iron preparations because of its side effect profile.
- Infusion-related side effects such as hypotension can be alleviated by slowing the rate of administration of IV iron preparations.
- Acute iron toxicity should be treated promptly with gastric lavage and supportive care.
- Chronic iron toxicity can result in significant organ damage and is treated with chelation agents such as deferoxamine, deferiprone, and deferasirox.

**Key Words:** Iron salts; iron dextran; toxicity; administration; chelation; deferoxamine; deferiprone; deferasirox

Iron is a vital constituent of mammalian cells. Its major purpose is oxygen transport and it is a critical element of hemoglobin, myoglobin, and a number of proteins (Adamson, 1999). Nutritional iron deficiency can lead to depletion of iron stores. Untreated deficiency may progress into iron deficiency anemia and impaired oxygen delivery. Iron deficiency can affect immune function, muscle metabolism, heat production, and catecholamine metabolism (Beard, 2001). This condition is especially of concern in children because it can adversely affect behavioral and cognitive development (Oski, 1993).

## 1. PHARMACOLOGY

Oral iron preparations are the treatment of choice for correction of iron deficiency anemia. Parenteral iron formulations are generally considered in individuals with normal renal function only when gastrointestinal (GI) absorption is known to be impaired (Van Wyck, 1999).

The usual treatment dose for iron deficiency anemia in adults is 60 mg of elemental iron three to four times a day. For children with mild to moderate anemia, a dose of 3 mg/kg of elemental iron

From: *Nutrition and Health: Iron Deficiency and Overload*
Edited by: S. Yehuda and D.I. Mostofsky, DOI 10.1007/978-1-59745-462-9_5

given once daily or divided into two doses is recommended. Severe iron deficiency anemia in children is treated with 4–6 mg/kg/day of elemental iron and is usually given in three divided doses (Iron-containing products, 2008).

GI absorption of iron occurs primarily in the duodenum and jejunum (Walker, Paton, Cowan, & Manuel, 1989). In order for iron to be absorbed, it must be in the ferrous state ($Fe^{2+}$). The majority of dietary iron is non-heme or ferric iron ($Fe^{3+}$). Absorption is facilitated by brush border ferrireductases in the GI tract, which reduces ferric iron ($Fe^{3+}$) to ferrous iron ($Fe^{2+}$) (Andrews & Schmidt, 2007; Umbreit, 2005).

Parenteral iron formulations for the most part are available as iron complexed to a carbohydrate moiety. Following intravenous (IV) administration, the iron–carbohydrate complex is gradually removed from plasma by the reticuloendothelial system. The reticuloendothelial cells separate the iron from the iron–carbohydrate complex (Silverstein & Rodgers, 2004).

After IV administration or absorption of an oral dose, iron may be either incorporated into the body's total iron stores or can rapidly combine with transferrin. Transferrin transports the iron to the liver, spleen, and bone marrow. Hemoglobin synthesis takes place when iron binds at bone marrow receptor sites (Silverstein & Rodgers, 2004).

## 2. ORAL IRON PREPARATIONS

### *2.1. Bioavailability*

Bioavailability of oral iron can be affected by several factors. Under normal circumstances, approximately 10–35% of an oral dose of ferrous sulfate is absorbed; however, in the face of iron deficiency, the percentage of iron absorbed by the GI tract increases to 80–95% (Harju, 1989). The presence of food and the degree of GI acidity also affects absorption. Ideally, oral iron supplements should be taken on an empty stomach; however, this may not be possible due to GI distress that occurs in some individuals with this therapy. Enteric-coated preparations, which delay dissolution of iron until it reaches the intestinal tract, may have lower bioavailability compared to film-coated preparations and oral solutions. As a result, these formulations should not be used interchangeably (Walker et al., 1989).

The presence of reducing substances such as ascorbic acid facilitates the conversion of ferric iron ($Fe^{3+}$) to the readily absorbable ferrous ($Fe^{2+}$) state (Teucher, Olivares, & Cori, 2004). Administration of 50 mg of ascorbic acid may increase absorption by two- to threefold (Harju, 1989).

Oral iron supplementation is available in various salt forms. Ferrous salts are the drugs of choice due to the fact that they are most readily absorbed and absorption from the GI tract is not affected by pH (Umbreit, 2005). While variability in percentages of elemental iron exists between different salt forms (Table 1), absorption occurs at relatively the same extent for all iron salts (Crosby, 1984).

### *2.2. Adverse Drug Events with Oral Iron Preparations*

The most common adverse event reported with oral iron preparations is GI distress. Fifteen to twenty percent of patients taking oral iron preparations report some form of GI distress that may present as abdominal pain, epigastric pain, nausea, vomiting,

Table 1
**Elemental Iron Content of Iron Salts**

| *Salt Form* | *Elemental Iron Content (%)* |
|---|---|
| Ferric pyrophosphate | 12 |
| Apo-ferrous gluconate | 12 |
| Apo-ferrous sulfate | 20 |
| Ferrous aspartate | 16 |
| Ferrous carbonate, anhydrous | 48 |
| Ferrous fumarate | 33 |
| Ferrous gluconate | 12 |
| Ferrous succinate | 30 |
| Ferrous sulfate | 20 |
| Ferrous sulfate exsiccated (dried) | 32 |
| Polysaccharide–iron complex | 100 |
| Carbonyl iron | 100 |

constipation, or diarrhea. GI intolerance commonly results in non-adherence to therapy. These side effects can be avoided by taking oral iron preparations with meals. However, the disadvantage to taking these supplements with meals is that it reduces the extent to which iron is absorbed. Additionally, GI effects are likely due to the total amount of elemental iron consumed per dose (Harju, 1989). Pharmacotherapeutic approaches to reduce gastritis include administering smaller doses of iron more frequently or using carbonyl iron, iron polysaccharides, or delayed release formulations (Umbreit, 2005; Van Wyck, 1999). While these steps reduce the GI effects somewhat, GI distress remains a significant barrier to effective treatment of many patients.

### 2.3. *Drug Interactions*

Concurrent administration of oral iron preparations with a number of different medications can result in decreased efficacy of one or both drugs. Oftentimes, iron chelates with the co-administered drug leading to impaired absorption. Administration of these medications should be separated by 1–2 hours from the iron dose. See Table 2 for a detailed list of drug interactions with iron therapy.

## 3. PARENTERAL IRON PREPARATIONS

### 3.1. *Iron Dextran*

Iron dextran injection is a solution of ferric hydroxide complexed with polymerized dextran. It is the only commercially available parenteral iron product that can be given intramuscularly (IM) (Watson Pharma, 2006b). It should be administered via a z-track method into the upper quadrant of the buttock. Though iron dextran can be given IM, this is not a desirable mode of drug delivery. Administration is often associated with pain at the injection site and staining of the skin, and drug

Table 2
**Drug Interactions with Oral Iron Therapy**

| *Drug* | *Effect* |
|---|---|
| Acetohydroxamic acid | Decreased iron absorption |
| Antacids | Decreased iron absorption |
| Ascorbic acid | Concurrent administration of ≥200 mg ascorbic acid per 30 mg of elemental iron increases GI absorption of oral iron |
| Calcium | Decreased GI absorption of iron |
| Captopril | Decreased blood levels of unconjugated (active) captopril |
| Cefdinir | Decrease cefdinir absorption |
| Chloramphenicol | Response to oral iron therapy may be delayed |
| Cholestyramine | Decreased iron effectiveness |
| Gossypol | Reduced iron absorption |
| H2 receptor blockers | Hypochlorhydria may decrease iron bioavailability |
| Iron | Concurrent administration of oral and parenteral iron may result in reduced absorption of oral iron |
| Levodopa | Decreased GI absorption of levodopa |
| Levothyroxine | Variable reductions in levothyroxine efficacy |
| Methyldopa | Decreased GI absorption of methyldopa |
| Mycophenolate mofetil | Potential for decreased iron absorption; however, recent studies suggest that there may not be a drug interaction |
| Penicillamine | Decreased GI absorption of penicillamine |
| Proton pump inhibitors | Hypochlorhydria may decrease iron bioavailability |
| Quinolones | Decreased GI absorption of quinolones due to formation of an insoluble quinolone–ferric ion complex |
| Sodium bicarbonate | Decreased GI absorption of iron |
| Tetracyclines | Decreased GI absorption of both iron and tetracyclines |
| Trientine | Decreased GI absorption of both drugs |
| Vanadium | Decreased iron absorption |
| Zinc | Decreased zinc and/or iron absorption |

delivery and absorption are unpredictable (Silverstein & Rodgers, 2004). IV infusion is the preferable method of administration. Caution should be taken to maintain a rate of administration below 50 mg/min. Dosage calculation for IV infusion in iron-deficient patients is described below (Watson Pharma, 2006b).

*Calculation of iron dextran dose for adults and children over* 15 kg

$$\text{Dose (ml)} = 0.442\ [\text{Desired Hemoglobin (g/dl)} - \text{Observed Hemoglobin(g/dl)}] \times \text{LBW} + (0.26 \times \text{LBW})$$

LBW = lean body weight expressed in kg
LBW (males) = 50 kg + 2.3 kg for each inch of a patient's height over 5 feet
LBW (females) = 45.5 kg + 2.3 kg for each inch of a patient's height over 5 feet

*Calculation of iron dextran dose for children* 5–15 kg

$$\text{Dose (ml)} = 0.0442\,[\text{Desired Hemoglobin (g/dl)} - \text{ObservedHemoglobin(g/dl)}] \times W + (0.26 \times W)$$

$W$ = weight in kg

$$Weight\ in\ kg = \frac{Weight\ (lbs)}{2.2}$$

The occurrence of anaphylactic reactions is well known with iron dextran therapy. All patients should receive a 25 mg IV test dose prior to their first infusion of iron dextran. Although hypersensitivity reactions usually occur within a few minutes of exposure, it is best to wait at least an hour or longer to give the treatment dose (Watson Pharma, 2006b).

### 3.2. *Iron Sucrose (Iron Saccharate)*

Iron sucrose injection is an aqueous complex of iron hydroxide in sucrose. It can be given undiluted via slow IV push or as an IV infusion. The recommended adult dose is 100 mg of elemental iron one to three times a week to a total of 1,000 mg in 10 treatment sessions (American Regent, Inc., 2003). The safety and efficacy of iron sucrose use in children have not been established.

While hypersensitivity reactions can be problem with all parenteral iron, iron sucrose appears to have a better safety profile compared to iron dextran. Patients who previously developed sensitivity to iron dextran have successfully been treated with iron sucrose without a test dose (Van Wyck et al., 2000).

### 3.3. *Ferric Gluconate*

Ferric gluconate injection is a sodium ferric gluconate complex in sucrose. It can be given undiluted via slow IV push or as an IV infusion. The usual adult dose is 125 mg of elemental iron given with each hemodialysis session. The majority of patients will require a minimum of 1,000 mg over eight sessions for treatment of iron deficiency in hemodialysis. The recommended pediatric regimen is 1.5 mg/kg of elemental iron at each dialysis session for a total of eight doses (Watson Pharma, 2006a). Similar to iron sucrose, hypersensitivity reactions with sodium ferric gluconate are rare (Sunder-Plassmann & Hörl, 1999).

### 3.4. *Adverse Drug Events with Parenteral Iron Preparations*

Hypotension is one of the most common side effects with injectable iron therapy. This often correlates with rate of administration and total dose of iron delivered. Administering the drug slowly can reduce the incidence of infusion-related side effects.

Systemic effects can occur in single-dose as well as multiple-dose therapy. The most common problems that may present after single-dose therapy include hypotension, hypertension, dizziness, headache, cramps, chest pain, lower back pain, diarrhea, nausea, and vomiting. Frequently occurring side effects from multiple-dose therapy include hypotension, hypertension, tachycardia, fatigue, fever, abnormal erythrocytes, dizziness, headache, cramps, chest pain, abdominal pain, diarrhea, nausea, and vomiting. Dysgeusia has also been reported in post-marketing surveillance.

## 4. TOXICITY

Any drug, while effective and safe at therapeutic doses, can have detrimental effects when administered or accumulated in excess. Typically, toxicity of a drug or substance is classified as acute or chronic and treatment of these toxicities varies depending on the method of ingestion.

### *4.1. Acute Toxicity*

Most acute ingestions of iron are accidental and are seen in children, who may mistake iron tablets for candy. Prenatal vitamins contain a significant amount of iron and have been implicated in a published report of fatalities in toddlers in the Los Angeles area in 1992 (Weiss, Alkon, & Weindlar, 1993). Acute toxic effects may occur at doses of 10–20 mg/kg of elemental iron in adults with significant gastrointestinal symptoms, including nausea and diarrhea (Burkhart, Kulig, & Hammond, 1991; Ling, Hornfeldt, & Winter, 1991). Ingestion of 20–60 mg/kg of elemental iron is considered potentially toxic (Iron, n.d.). Acute toxicity can also occur after parenteral administration, such as with iron dextran, in patients being treated for anemia.

### *4.2. Clinical Effects*

There are five clinical stages of iron toxicity based on pathophysiology (Banner & Tong, 1986; Jacobs, Greene, & Gendel, 1965; Proudfoot, Simpson, & Dyson, 1986). The first stage describes a cluster of gastrointestinal effects, characterized by nausea, vomiting, abdominal pain, and diarrhea, and will always occur within 6 hours following a significant overdose. In addition, the patient may also develop intestinal ulcers, edema, and in more serious cases, small-bowel necrosis and obstruction (Tenenbein, Littman, & Stimpson, 1990).

Within the second clinical stage, typically 6–24 hours after the gastrointestinal symptoms resolve, the patient may seem to have recovered, but will have ongoing cellular organ toxicity. Patients in this "latent" stage will exhibit lethargy, tachycardia, or metabolic acidosis. Not all patients who have a resolution of gastrointestinal symptoms will have progressed into the second stage: patients with normal acid–base balance and stable vital signs will have an uneventful course (Perrone, 2006).

Profound toxicity will manifest in the third clinical stage and can be seen within the first few hours after an extreme ingestion to up to 12–24 hours after a moderate ingestion. These patients will have an ongoing metabolic acidosis and may exhibit signs of shock from hypovolemia, vasodilation, and decreased cardiac output (Vernon, Banner, & Dean, 1989). Central nervous system effects, such as lethargy, seizure, and coma, as well as iron-induced coagulopathy may also be seen (Tenenbein & Israels, 1988).

Hepatic failure is the hallmark of the fourth clinical stage and is a result of oxidative damage to the reticuloendothelial system in the liver secondary to iron update (Witzleben & Chaffey, 1966). This stage may occur from 2–3 days after ingestion (Gleason, de Mello, & de Castro, 1979).

The fifth stage of iron toxicity can develop 2–8 weeks after ingestion and involves gastrointestinal strictures and scarring from the initial injury (Tenenbein et al., 1990). This stage is rare if treatment is appropriate and timely.

### *4.3. Range of Toxicity*

Serum iron concentrations can be useful during the treatment for acute iron toxicity to monitor the efficacy of treatment and to help quantify toxicity. It is important to remember, though, that iron toxicity is based on clinical signs and symptoms. Depending on the iron product ingested, peak iron concentrations occur between 2 and 6 hours following an oral overdose (Burkhart et al., 1991; Ling et al., 1991). Significant gastrointestinal toxicity and moderate systemic toxicity typically correlate with serum iron concentrations between 300 and 500 μg/dL. Significant systemic toxicity and shock are associated with concentrations between 500 and 1,000 μg/dL, and concentrations greater than 1,000 μg/dL correlate with significant morbidity and mortality (Westlin, 1971). It is difficult, however, to predict and measure the peak serum concentration, and the value of the concentration should be kept in context and assessed with the clinical signs of the patient (Gervitz & Wasserman, 1966; Helfer & Rodgerson, 1966).

Total iron-binding capacity (TIBC) is not a useful measure of toxicity in acute overdoses. Clinical toxicity has been seen even when the TIBC level was greater than the serum iron concentration (Siff, Meldon, & Tomassoni, 1999).

### *4.4. Treatment*

Initial treatment of acute iron ingestion involves stabilizing the patient, which may include supplemental oxygen and intravenous fluids. Patients who are lethargic or unconscious will need establishment of their airway, with possible ventilation. Following stabilization and assessment, primary treatment involves limiting absorption of the ingested iron preparation, typically via gastrointestinal decontamination. Inducing emesis is not recommended (Manoguerra, Erdman, & Booze, 2005). Routine use of activated charcoal is also not recommended because iron is not well absorbed to the product (Yonker, Banner, & Picchioni, 1980). Gastric lavage is recommended in children ingesting more than 40 mg/kg of elemental iron and in all severe or persistently symptomatic patients (Iron, n.d.). However, clinical assessment and history of the ingestion should be evaluated before the decision to perform gastric lavage is made; because of morbidity with lavage, it should not be performed routinely in all patients (Vale, 1997). Complications of gastric lavage include fluid and electrolyte imbalance, mechanical injury to the throat or stomach, aspiration pneumonia, hypoxia, and hypercapnea. Following lavage, an abdominal x-ray may be helpful to determine if tablets remain in the gut; however, since dissolved tablets may not be radiopaque, a negative x-ray does not rule out the presence of potential toxicity (Jaeger, De Castro, & Barry, 1981; Ng, Perry, & Martin, 1979).

Whole bowel irrigation with a polyethylene glycol balanced electrolyte solution may be useful if the patient still has documented tablets in the gut after lavage or there are tablets seen past the pylorus (Schauben, Augenstein, & Cox, 1990). Adverse effects may include nausea, vomiting, abdominal cramping, and bloating. This method is contraindicated in patients who are seizing, or who are rapidly deteriorating, until they are intubated. Patients with bowel obstruction, perforation, gastric bleeding, or who are unstable are not candidates for whole bowel irrigation (Tenenbein, 1997).

Use of an iron chelator is indicated if the patient is symptomatic and a serum iron concentration cannot be obtained, if there is presence of free serum iron, or if the peak serum iron concentration is greater than 350 μg/dL (Iron, n.d.). Deferoxamine, a parenteral iron chelator, has been most studied in acute iron toxicity and can be administered as a continuous infusion intravenously up to 15 mg/kg/h (Iron, n.d.). The total daily dose given intravenously or intramuscularly should generally not exceed 6 g (Novartis, 2007a). The length of the infusion should be dictated by the patient's condition; with moderate toxicity the infusion is typically over 8–12 hours, while in severe cases infusions have been given over 24 hours (Tenenbein, Kowalski, & Sienko, 1992). Serum iron concentrations may be falsely low in the presence of deferoxamine (Wythe, Osterloh, & Becker, 1986). Serum iron concentration and electrolytes should be measured after the infusion is discontinued. Some patients receiving deferoxamine will exhibit a characteristic pink to orange-red color change in their urine during treatment, indicating the excretion of chelated iron (ferrioxamine), although this does not always occur (Harchelroad & Rice, 1992) and is not a very reliable indicator of serum iron concentrations (Villalobos, 1992). Pulmonary toxicity has been seen in patients receiving deferoxamine infusions over several days and is associated with high doses (10–25 mg/kg/h) (Benson & Cheney, 1992). Patients may develop hypoxemia, fever, severe tachypnea, eosinophilia, and pulmonary infiltrates, and these symptoms usually occur 3–9 days after starting therapy (Anderson & Rivers, 1992). The etiology is unknown, but hypersensitivity seems unlikely (Howland, 1996) and is thought to be related to high daily doses given over several days.

Exchange transfusion has been used in patients with an initial serum iron concentration of greater than 1,000 μg/dL who continue to deteriorate despite chelation and supportive care (Iron, n.d.).

### *4.5. Chronic Toxicity*

Chronic iron overload, also known as hemochromatosis, is the result of an excessive buildup of iron in the body tissues over time, and leads to progressive and often irreversible organ damage. Because the body does not have an efficient method for removal of excess iron, accumulation occurs in the liver, pancreas, heart, and joints. Hemochromatosis can be classified as primary or secondary. Primary hemochromatosis results from an autosomal recessive disorder from mutations on the hemochromatosis gene on chromosome 6, which causes hyperabsorption of dietary iron. This disorder affects 1 in every 200 individuals of Western European heritage (Cook, 2000). Secondary hemochromatosis typically occurs in patients who have received multiple blood transfusions, such as those with congenital anemias (sickle cell anemia or thalassemia) or myelodysplastic syndromes. A standard unit of packed red blood cells typically contains between 200 and 250 mg of iron, or approximately 1 mg of iron per mL of packed red blood cells (Schafer & Bunn, 2001). Accumulation of 20 g of iron is usually the point at which symptoms of iron overload will occur (Cook, 2000), after approximately 10–20 transfusions.

### *4.6. Clinical Effects*

Due to differences in iron deposition, the clinical signs and symptoms of chronic iron overload can vary from patient to patient (Felitti & Beutler, 1999). The major organ systems affected include the heart, endocrine system, liver, musculoskeletal system, and skin. Typically, the eyes, lungs, and urinary system are less affected. Primary hemochromatosis patients may present with a triad of diabetes, liver cirrhosis, and hyperpigmentation of the skin (Cogswell et al., 1998). Patients with iron overload also tend to have an increased incidence of infections with *Vibrio vulnificus, Escherichia coli, Listeria monocytogenes, Yersinia enterocolitica, Klebsiella pneumoniae, and Salmonella enteritidis* (Andrews, 1999).

Excess iron can deposit in the mycocardium and may lead to myocardial disease, including heart failure, cardiomegaly, or arrhythmias (Felitti & Beutler, 1999; Jensen et al., 2001). Extensive cardiac deposits of iron were seen at autopsy in patients who had received greater than 100 units of blood, while those with fewer transfusions only showed cardiac deposits if they also had evidence of hepatic fibrosis (Buja & Roberts, 1971). The clinical signs of myocardial iron overload manifest as left ventricular dysfunction and arrhythmias (Ehlers et al., 1980).

Patients with hemochromatosis are at higher risk for development of diabetes, hypothyroidism, and hypogonadism (Felitti & Beutler, 1999; Andrews, 1999). Up to half of these patients may have diabetes (Powell, 2002). Iron loading in the anterior pituitary may lead to hypopituitarism and gonadal dysfunction (Anderson, 2007).

The hepatic complications secondary to iron overload include cirrhosis, fibrosis, and elevated aminotransferases (Andrews, 1999). Hepatomegaly is seen in up to 95% of symptomatic patients, and those with cirrhosis can develop splenomegaly and portal hypertension (Felitti & Beutler, 1999; Powell, 2002). Hepatocellular carcinoma is more common in patients with hepatic damage from chronic iron overload (Powell, 2002).

Arthritis is common in patients with chronic iron overload (Anderson, 2007), as well as arthralgias, subarticular cysts at iron deposition sites, and chrondrocalcinosis (Felitti & Beutler, 1999).

Late in the course of chronic iron overload, the skin may start to change to a gray or bronze coloration, secondary to iron and melanin deposition in the tissues (Felitti & Beutler, 1999). Hair loss and skin hyperpigmentation may also be seen.

### *4.7. Range of Toxicity*

Patients with primary hemochromatosis may not develop clinical symptoms of iron overload until age 30–50 years (Powell, George, McDonnell, & Kowdley, 1998). This is in contrast to those receiving chronic transfusions, who may start to develop symptoms within 1 year of starting therapy (Wood, 2007). Because of the nature of iron toxicity over time, it is difficult to predict when and where manifestations will first appear. In chronic transfusion therapy, patients will need to be started on iron chelation relatively quickly in their treatment, typically after 10 transfusions.

The difficulty comes in a reliable measure of iron toxicity. Direct measurement of body iron status is done via liver biopsy and phlebotomy, which are quantitative and specific but invasive and not practical in all patients (Hristova & Henry, 2001). Liver biopsy has been considered the standard for measuring body iron levels, but is only reliable in patients who do not have cirrhosis. Additionally, adequate tissue for analysis must be available, typically greater than 1 mg dry weight (Pakbaz, Fischer, & Treadwell, 2005). Indirect measures include serum iron, ferritin, and transferrin, but these are not specific and/or sensitive (Olivieri, DeSilva, & Premawardena, 2000; Hristova & Henry, 2001). Serum iron represents the $Fe3^{+}$ bound to transferrin, but does not include iron in the serum as free hemoglobin (Hristova & Henry, 2001). In clinical practice, serum ferritin is the most commonly used indirect estimate of body iron stores; but while increased serum ferritin may indicate increased iron stores, it is also elevated in other conditions, such as infection, vitamin C deficiency, hemolysis, and chronic inflammation, and is not considered very sensitive in quantifying iron overload conditions (Porter, 2005; deVirgiliis, Sanna, & Cornacchia, 1980). It is a poor predictor of liver iron content, especially in iron-overloaded patients (Pakbaz et al., 2005).

Non-invasive methods for measuring iron status include magnetic resonance imaging (MRI) and biomagnetic susceptometry (Beutler, Hoffbrand, & Cook, 2003). MRI can be used to image tissue iron and document deposition of iron in the liver and other tissues, but its ability to detect organ damage is limited (Ooi, Khong, & Chan, 2004; Voskaridou, Douskou, & Terpos, 2004; Kushner, Porter, & Olivieri, 2001). Biomagnetic susceptometry uses superconducting quantum interference devices (SQUIDS) to produce an automated magnetic "biopsy" of liver ferritin and hemosiderin iron (Brittenham & Badman, 2003). It is non-invasive, reliable, and sensitive, but measures only liver and spleen iron content and it has limited availability (Neilsen, Engelhardt, Dullmann, & Fischer, 2002; Wood, 2007).

### *4.8. Treatment*

Phlebotomy and the use of chelation therapy are the only means of eliminating excess iron from the body. Phlebotomy is the gold standard for treating iron overload in patients with primary hemochromatosis (Heeney & Andrews, 2004), but is usually not practical in patients with iron overload from chronic transfusions. Phlebotomy produces an anemia, which induces iron mobilization from liver stores to allow for hemoglobin production in reticulocytes (Kontoghiorghes, Eracleous, Economides, & Kolnagou, 2005), and is recommended with ferritin levels greater than 200 ng/mL in women and 300 mg/mL in men (Barton, McDonnell, & Adams, 1998). In a phlebotomy session, approximately 500 mL of blood is removed once or twice weekly and is continued until ferritin levels are less than 20 mg/mL (Felitti & Beutler, 1999; Porter, 2001; Schilsky & Fink, 2006; Tung & Kowdley, 1998). Once the patient has reached this goal, maintenance therapy with phlebotomy several times per year is continued over the lifetime of the patient, with target ferritin levels less than 50 ng/mL (Powell, 2002; Adams, 2006; Tung & Kowdley, 1998).

The treatment of choice for iron overload associated with chronic transfusion therapy is iron chelation. The chelating agents form complexes with non-transferrin-bound iron, promoting its excretion from the body. Hepatic iron content of 2–7 mg/g dry weight (dw) liver is a goal of chelation therapy (Porter, 2005; Olivieri et al., 2000). Levels above 15 mg/g dw are linked to complications, including cardiac dysfunction (Olivieri, 1999). There are three available iron chelators, deferoxamine, deferiprone, and deferasirox.

Deferoxamine, a hexadentate chelator, has been the standard of care for iron chelation for over 30 years. It is indicated for treatment of both acute iron toxicity and chronic iron overload secondary to transfusion therapy. Because of its large molecular weight, it must be administered parenterally but may be given subcutaneously or intravenously. Because of its relatively short half-life (20 min), frequent dosing via infusion is necessary. It forms a 1:1 iron:chelator complex, and excretion of iron occurs primarily via urine, with a small amount via feces (Novartis, 2007a). Due to its urinary excretion, patients with severe renal impairment should not receive deferoxamine. Dosing is similar for all parenteral routes: 20–60 mg/kg over an 8–12 hour infusion (Novartis, 2007a), three to seven times weekly (Kushner et al., 2001; Cappellini, 2005). Because of adverse reactions such as urticaria, hypotension, and shock related to infusion rate, deferoxamine should be administered slowly. Other adverse effects tend to occur when iron stores are low secondary to therapy and include ocular and auditory disturbances. Most of these effects were reversible when treatment was discontinued. Because administration of deferoxamine is inconvenient, time-consuming, and can be painful, non-compliance with therapy is common (Kontoghiorghes et al., 2005).

Deferiprone is a bidentate chelating agent with good oral bioavailability and is available in over 50 countries, but is not licensed in the United States (Franchini, 2005). It forms a 1:3 iron:chelator complex and its excretion is via urine (Hoffbrand, 2005). Because of rapid absorption from the gut, and half-life of approximately 1.5 hours, deferiprone is administered orally three times daily (Hoffbrand, 2005). The typical standard daily dose in most patients of 75 mg/kg/day can promote negative iron balance (Franchini, 2005; Porter, 2001). Deferiprone provides better protection against heart conditions secondary to iron overload compared to monotherapy with deferoxamine (Tam et al., 2003). It has been used in combination with deferoxamine to increase iron excretion over that of either drug used alone, with better compliance and less potential toxicity (Hoffbrand, 2005). Adverse effects of deferiprone include nausea, arthropathies, agranulocytosis, neutropenia, and increased liver function tests (Kowdley & Kaplan, 1998; Cohen, Galanello, & Piga, 2000).

Deferasirox is a tridentate chelating agent with good oral bioavailability, which forms a 1:2 iron:chelator complex (Novartis, 2007b). Deferasirox tablets are to be dispersed in a liquid such as water, apple juice, or orange juice and should not be swallowed, chewed, or crushed. Half-life of deferasirox is long (8–16 hours), compared to deferiprone, and enables the dose to be administered once daily. Excretion is predominately via feces, and the daily dose varies depending on the need to decrease iron load or maintain iron load. Typical initial dose is 20–30 mg/kg/day and doses should not exceed 40 mg/kg/day (Novartis, 2007b). Adverse effects include dizziness, fever, abdominal pain, skin rash, headache, nausea, vomiting, high-frequency hearing loss, increased intraocular pressure, cough, elevation of serum creatinine or liver transaminase levels, and infections (Van Orden & Hagemann, 2006; Stumpf, 2007).

## 5. CONCLUSION

While absorption of oral iron may be slow, it remains an effective therapy for treatment of iron-deficiency anemia. Concurrent administration of oral iron and certain drugs should be avoided due to drug–drug interactions that may impair absorption of one or both drugs. Injectable iron therapy is generally reserved for cases when oral therapy has failed. Hypersensitivity reactions can occur with all injectable iron preparations; however, it is more pronounced with iron dextran. Iron toxicity can be detrimental in both acute and chronic situations. Care should be taken to monitor for iron overload in patients with predisposing conditions.

## REFERENCES


Adams, P. C. (2006). Review article: The modern diagnosis and management of haemochromatosis. *Alimentary Pharmacology and Therapeutics*, *23*, 1681–1691.

Adamson, J. W. (1999, August). Normal iron physiology. *Seminars in Dialysis*, *12*(4), 219–223.

American Regent, Inc. (2003, June). Venofer (package insert). Shirley, NY.

Anderson, G. J. (2007). Mechanisms of iron loading and toxicity. *American Journal of Hematology*, *82*, 1128–1131.

Anderson, K. J., & Rivers, R. P. A. (1992). Desferrioxamine in acute iron poisoning. *Lancet*, *339*, 1601–1602.

Andrews, N. C. (1999). Disorders of iron metabolism. *New England Journal of Medicine*, *341*(26), 1986–1995.

Andrews, N. C., & Schmidt, P. J. (2007). Iron homeostasis. *Annual Review of Physiology*, *69*, 69–85.

Banner, W., & Tong, T. G. (1986). Iron poisoning. *Pediatric Clinics of North America*, *33*, 393–409.

Barton, J. C., McDonnell, S. M., & Adams, P. C. (1998). Management of hemochromatosis. *Annals of Internal Medicine*, *129*(11S), 932–939.

Beard, J. L. (2001). Iron biology in immune function, muscle metabolism and neuronal functioning. *The Journal of Nutrition*, *131*(2), 568S–580S.

Benson, B., & Cheney, K. (1992). Survival after a severe iron poisoning treated with high dose deferoxamine (DFO) therapy. *Veterinary and Human Toxicology*, *34*, 329.

Beutler, E., Hoffbrand, A. V., & Cook, J. D. (2003). Iron deficiency and overload. *Hematology – American Society of Hematology Educational Program*, Washington, DC, pp. 40–61.

Brittenham, G. M., & Badman, D. G. (2003). Noninvasive measurement of iron: Report of an NIDDK workshop. *Blood*, *101*, 15–19.

Buja, L. M., & Roberts, W. C. (1971). Iron in the heart. Etiology and clinical significance. *American Journal of Medicine*, *51*(2), 209–221.

Burkhart, K. K., Kulig, K. W., & Hammond, K. B. (1991). The rise in the total iron-binding capacity after iron overdose. *Annals of Emergency Medicine*, *20*, 532–535.

Campbell, N., Paddock, V., & Sundaram, R. (1988, April). Alteration of methyldopa absorption, metabolism, and blood pressure control caused by ferrous sulfate and ferrous gluconate. *Clinical Pharmacology and Therapeutics*, *43*(4), 381–386.

Campbell, N. R., & Hasinoff, B. (1989, March). Ferrous sulfate reduces levodopa bioavailability: Chelation as a possible mechanism. *Clinical Pharmacology and Therapeutics*, *45*(3), 220–225.

Campbell, N. R., Hasinoff, B. B., Stalts, H., Rao, B., & Wong, N. C. (1992, December 15). Ferrous sulfate reduces thyroxine efficacy in patients with hypothyroidism. *Annals of Internal Medicine*, *117*(12), 1010–1013.

Cappellini, M. D. (2005). Iron-chelating therapy with the new oral agent ICL670 (Exjade). *Best Practices and Research in Clinical Hematology*, *18*(2), 289–298.

Cogswell, M. E., McDonnell, S. M., Khoury, M. J., Franks, A. L., Burke, W., & Brittenham, G. (1998). Iron overload, public health, and genetics: Evaluating the evidence for hemochromatosis screening. *Annals of Internal Medicine*, *129*(11), 971–979.

Cohen, A. R., Galanello, R., & Piga, A. (2000). Safety profile of the oral iron chelator deferiprone: A multicentre study. *British Journal of Haematology*, *108*, 305–312.

Carbonyl iron. (2008). *Drug facts and comparisons 4.0*. Retrieved February 12, 2008, from http://online.factsandcomparisons.com. Indy, IN: Wolters Kluwer Health, Inc.

Cook, J. D., Dassenko, S. A., & Whittaker, P. (1991, January). Calcium supplementation: Effect on iron absorption. *American Journal of Clinical Nutrition*, *53*(1), 106–111.

Cook, J. D. (2000). Hemochromatosis. In R. E. Rakel (Ed.), *Conn's current therapy* (pp. 404–406). Philadelphia: WB Saunders.

Crosby, J. D. (1984, March). The rationale for treating iron deficiency anemia. *Archives of Internal Medicine*, *144*(3), 471–472.

Deppermann, K. M., & Lode, H. (1993). Fluoroquinolones: Interaction profile during enteral absorption. *Drugs*, *45*(Suppl. 3), 65–72.

deVirgiliis, S., Sanna, G., & Cornacchia, G. (1980). Serum ferritin, liver iron stores, and liver histology in children with thalassemia. *Archives of Diseases in Childhood*, *55*, 43–45.

Ehlers, K. H., Levin, A. R., Markenson, A. L., Marcus, J. R., Klein, A. A., Hilgartner, M. W., et al. (1980). Longitudinal study of cardiac function in thalassemia major. *Annals of the New York Academy of Sciences*, *344*, 397–404.

Felitti, V. J., & Beutler, E. (1999). New developments in hereditary hemochromatosis. *American Journal of Medical Science*, *318*(4), 257–268.

Ferrous aspartate. (2008). *Drug facts and comparisons 4.0*. Retrieved February 12, 2008, from http://online.factsandcomparisons.com. Indy, IN: Wolters Kluwer Health, Inc.

Ferrous fumarate. (2008). *Drug facts and comparisons 4.0*. Retrieved February 12, 2008, from http://online.factsandcomparisons.com. Indy, IN: Wolters Kluwer Health, Inc.

Ferrous gluconate. (2008). *Drug facts and comparisons 4.0*. Retrieved February 12, 2008, from http://online.factsandcomparisons.com. Indy, IN: Wolters Kluwer Health, Inc.

Ferrous sulfate. (2008). *Drug facts and comparisons 4.0*. Retrieved February 12, 2008, from http://online.factsandcomparisons.com. Indy, IN: Wolters Kluwer Health, Inc.

Franchini, M. (2005). Recent acquisitions in the management of iron overload. *Annals of Hematology*, *84*, 640–645.

Gelone, D. K., Park, J. M., & Lake, K. D. (2007, September). Lack of an effect of oral iron administration on mycophenolic acid pharmacokinetics in stable renal transplant recipients. *Pharmacotherapy*, *27*(9), 1272–1278.

Gervitz, N. R., & Wasserman, L. R. (1966). The measurement of iron and iron-binding capacity in plasma containing deferoxamine. *Journal of Pediatrics*, *68*, 802–804.

Gleason, W. A., de Mello, D. E., & de Castro, F. J. (1979). Acute hepatic failure in severe iron poisoning. *Journal of Pediatrics*, *95*, 138–140.

Golubov, J., Flanagan, P., & Adams, P. (1991, April). Inhibition of iron absorption by omeprazole in rat model. *Digestive Diseases and Sciences*, *36*(4), 405–408.

Greene, R. J., Hall, A. D., & Hider, R. C. (1990, July). The interaction of orally administered iron with levodopa and methyldopa therapy. *The Journal of Pharmacy and Pharmacology*, *42*(7), 502–504.

Harchelroad, F., & Rice, S. (1992). Iron dextran: Treatment or overdose? *Veterinary and Human Toxicology*, *34*, 329.

Harju, E. (1989, August). Clinical pharmacokinetics of iron preparations. *Clinical Pharmacokinetics*, *17*(2), 69–89.

Heeney, M. M., & Andrews, N. C. (2004). Iron homeostasis and inherited iron overload disorders: An overview. *Hematology – Oncology Clinics of North America*, *18*(6), 1379–1403.

Helfer, R. E., & Rodgerson, D. O. (1966). The effect of deferoxamine on the determination of serum iron and iron-binding capacity. *Journal of Pediatrics*, *68*, 804–806.

Hoffbrand, A. V. (2005). Deferiprone therapy for transfusional iron overload. *Best Practice and Research in Clinical Hematology*, *18*(2), 299–317.

Howland, M. A. (1996). Risks of parenteral deferoxamine for acute iron poisoning. *Clinical Toxicology*, *34*, 491–497.

Hristova, E. N., & Henry, J. B. (2001). Metabolic intermediates, inorganic ions and biochemical markers of bone metabolism. In J. B. Henry (Ed.), *Clinical diagnosis and management of laboratory methods* (pp. 180–191). Philadelphia: WB Saunders.

Iron (management treatment protocol). (n.d.). *POISINDEX®* Retrieved January 2, 2008, from http://www.thomsonhc.com. Greenwood Village, CO: Thomson Healthcare.

Iron-containing products (2008). *Drug facts and comparisons 4.0*. Retrieved February 12, 2008, from http://online.factsandcomparisons.com. Indy, IN: Wolters Kluwer Health, Inc.

Jacobs, J., Greene, H., & Gendel, B. R. (1965). Acute iron intoxication. *New England Journal of Medicine*, *273*, 1124–1127.

Jaeger, R. W., De Castro, F. J., & Barry, R. C. (1981). Radiopacity of drugs and plants in vitro – Limited usefulness. *Veterinary and Human Toxicology*, *23*, 2–4.

Jensen, P. D., Jensen F. T., Christensen, T., Heickendorff, L., Jensen, L. G., & Ellegaard, J. (2001). Indirect evidence for the potential ability of magnetic resonance imaging to evaluate the myocardial iron content in patients with transfusional iron overload. *Magnetic Resonance Materials in Physics, Biology and Medicine*, *12*, 153–166.

Kontoghiorghes, G. J., Eracleous, E., Economides, C., & Kolnagou, A. (2005). Advances in iron overload therapies: Prospects for effective use of deferiprone (L1), deferoxamine, the new experimental chelators ICL670, GT56-252, LINAII and their combinations. *Current Medicinal Chemistry*, *12*, 2663–2681.

Kowdley, K. V., & Kaplan, M. M. (1998). Iron-chelation therapy with oral deferiprone – Toxicity or lack of efficacy. *New England Journal of Medicine*, *339*, 468–469.

Kushner, J. P., Porter, J. P., & Olivieri, N. F. (2001). Secondary iron overload. *Hematology*, 47–61.

Lehto, P., Kivisto, K. T., & Neuvonen, P. J. (1994, January). The effect of ferrous sulphate on the absorption of norfloxacin, ciprofloxacin and ofloxacin. *British Journal of Clinical Pharmacology*, *37*(1), 82–85.

Leyden, J. J. (1985, February). Absorption of minocycline hydrochloride and tetracycline hydrochloride. Effect of food, milk, and iron. *Journal of the American Academy of Dermatology*, *12*, 308–312.

Ling, L. J., Hornfeldt, C. S., & Winter, J. P. (1991). Absorption of iron after experimental overdose of chewable vitamins. *American Journal of Emergency Medicine*, *9*, 24–26.

Lorenz, M., Wolzt, M., Weigel, G., Puttinger, H., Horl, W. H., Fodinger, M., et al. (2004, June). Ferrous sulfate does not affect mycophenolic acid pharmacokinetics in kidney transplant patients. *American Journal of Kidney Diseases*, *43*(6), 1098–1103.

Manoguerra, A. S., Erdman, A. R., & Booze, L. L. (2005). Iron ingestion: An evidence based consensus guideline for out-of-hospital management. *Clinical Toxicology*, *43*(6), 553–570.

Neilsen, P., Engelhardt, R., Dullmann, J., & Fischer, R. (2002). Non-invasive liver iron quantification by SQUID-biosusceptometry and serum ferritin iron as new diagnostic parameters in hereditary hemochromatosis. *Blood Cells, Molecules and Diseases*, *29*, 451–458.

Neuvonen, P. J. (1976). Interactions with the absorption of tetracyclines. *Drugs*, *11*(1), 45–54.

Ng, R. C. W., Perry, K., & Martin, D. J. (1979). Iron poisoning: Assessment of radiography in diagnosis and management. *Clinical Pediatrics*, *18*, 614–616.

Novartis. (2007a, November). Desferal (package insert). East Hanover, NJ.

Novartis. (2007b, December). Exjade (package insert). East Hanover, NJ.

Olivares, M., Pizarro, F., & Ruz, M. (2007, April). New insights about iron bioavailability inhibition by zinc. *Nutrition*, *23*(4), 292–295.

Olivieri, N. F. (1999). The beta-thalassemias. *New England Journal of Medicine*, *341*, 99–109.

Olivieri, N. F., DeSilva, S., & Premawardena, A. (2000). Iron overload and iron-chelating therapy in hemoglobin E-β Thalassemia. *Journal of Pediatric Hematology Oncology*, *22*, 593–597.

O'Neil-Cutting, M. A., & Crosby, W. H. (1986, March 21). The effect of antacids on the absorption of simultaneously ingested iron. *The Journal of the American Medical Association*, *255*(11), 1468–1470.

Ooi, G. C., Khong, P. L., & Chan, G. C. F. (2004). Magnetic resonance screening of iron status in transfusion-dependent β-thalassemia patients. *British Journal of Haematology*, *124*, 385–390.

Oral Iron Preparations (n.d.), *Lexicomp online*. Retrieved February 12, 2008, from http://www.crlonline.com. Hudson, OH: Lexicomp, Inc.

Oski, F. A. (1993, July 15). Iron deficiency in infancy and childhood. *New England Journal of Medicine*, *329*(3), 190–193.

Osman, M. A., Patel, R. B., Schuna, A., Sundstrom, W. R., & Welling, P. G. (1983, April). Reduction in oral penicillamine absorption by food, antacid, and ferrous sulfate. *Clinical Pharmacology and Therapeutics*, *33*(4), 465–470.

Pakbaz, Z., Fischer, R., & Treadwell, M. (2005). A simple model to assess and improve adherence to iron-chelation therapy with deferoxamine in patients with thalassemia. *Annals of the New York Academy of Science*, *1054*, 486–491.

Perrone, J. (2006). Iron. In L. R. Goldfrank (Ed.), *Goldfrank's toxicologic emergencies* (pp. 548–562). New York: McGraw Hill.

Polysaccharide iron complex. (2008). *Drug facts and comparisons 4.0*. Retrieved February 12, 2008, from http://online.factsandcomparisons.com. Indy, IN: Wolters Kluwer Health, Inc.

Porter, J. B. (2001). Practical management of iron overload. *British Journal of Haematology*, *115*, 239–252.

Porter, J. B. (2005). Monitoring and treatment of iron overload: State of the art and new approaches. *Seminars in Hematology*, *42*, S14–S18.

Powell, L. W., George, D. K., McDonnell, S. M., & Kowdley, K. V. (1998). Diagnosis of hemochromatosis. *Annals of Internal Medicine*, *129*(11), 925–931.

Powell, L. W. (2002). Hereditary hemochromatosis and iron overload diseases. *Journal of Gastroenterology and Hepatology*, *7*, S191–S195.

Proudfoot, A. T., Simpson, D., & Dyson, E. H. (1986). Management of acute iron poisoning. *Medical Toxicology*, *1*, 83–100.

Schaefer, J. P., Tam, Y., Hasinoff, B. B., Tawfik, S., Peng, Y., Reimche, L., et al. (1998, October). Ferrous sulphate interacts with captopril. *British Journal of Clinical Pharmacology*, *46*(4), 377–381.

Schafer, A. I., & Bunn, H. F. (2001). Iron-deficiency and iron-loading anemias. In R. G. Petersdorf, J. B. Martin, & Braunwald, E. (Eds.), *Harrison's principles of internal medicine* (pp. 1848–1853). New York: McGraw-Hill.

Schauben, J. L., Augenstein, W. L., & Cox, J. (1990). Iron poisoning: Report of three cases and a review of therapeutic intervention. *Journal of Emergency Medicine*, *8*, 309–319.

Schilsky, M. L., & Fink, S. (2006). Inherited metabolic liver disease. *Current Opinions in Gastroenterology*, *22*, 215–222.

Siff, J. E., Meldon, S. W., & Tomassoni, A. J. (1999). Usefulness of the total iron binding capacity in the evaluation and treatment of acute iron overdose. *Annals of Emergency Medicine*, *33*, 73–76.

Silverstein, S. B., & Rodgers, G. M. (2004, May). Parenteral iron therapy options. *American Journal of Hematology*, *76*(1), 74–78.

Sunder-Plassmann, G., & Hörl, W. H. (1999, August). Comparative look at intravenous iron agents: Pharmacology, efficacy, and safety of iron dextran, iron saccharate, and ferric gluconate. *Seminars in Dialysis*, *12*(4), 243–248.

Stumpf, J. L. (2007). Deferasirox. *American Journal of Health-Systems Pharmacists*, *64*, 606–616.

Tam, T. F., Leung-Toung, R., Li, W., Wang, Y., Khashayer, K., & Spino, M. (2003). Iron chelator research: Past, present and future. *Current Medicinal Chemistry*, *10*, 983–995.

Tenenbein, M., & Israels, S. J. (1988). Early coagulopathy in severe iron poisoning. *Journal of Pediatrics*, *113*, 695–697.

Tenenbein, M., Littman, C., & Stimpson, R. E. (1990). Gastrointestinal pathology in adult iron overdose. *Journal of Toxicology and Clinical Toxicology*, *28*, 311–320.

Tenenbein, M., Kowalski, S., & Sienko, A. (1992). Pulmonary toxic effects of continuous desferrioxamine administration in acute iron poisoning. *Lancet*, 339, 669–701.

Tenenbein, M. (1997). Position statement: Whole bowel irrigation. American academy of clinical toxicology; European association of poisons centres and clinical toxicologists. *Journal of Toxicology and Clinical Toxicology*, *35*, 753–762.

Teucher, B., Olivares, M., & Cori, H. (2004, November). Enhancers of iron absorption: Ascorbic acid and other organic acids. *International Journal for Vitamin and Nutrition Research*, *74*(6), 404–419.

Tung, B. Y., & Kowdley, K. V. (1998). Clinical management of iron overload. *Gastroenterology Clinics*, *27*(3), 637–654.

Ueno, K., Tanaka, K., Tsujimura, K., Morishima, Y., Iwashige, H., Yamazaki, K., et al. (1993, November). Impairment of cefdinir absorption by iron ion. *Clinical Pharmacology and Therapeutics*, *54*(5), 473–475.

Umbreit, J. (2005, March). Iron deficiency: A concise review. *American Journal of Hematology*, *78*, 225–231.

Vale, J. A. (1997). Position statement: Gastric lavage. American academy of clinical toxicology: European association of poisons centres and clinical toxicologists. *Journal of Toxicology and Clinical Toxicology*, *35*, 711–719.

Van Orden, H. E., & Hagemann, T. M. (2006). Deferasirox-An oral agent for chronic iron overload. *Annals of Pharmacotherapy*, *40*, 1110–1117.

Van Wyck, D. B. (1999, August). Efficacy and adverse effects of oral iron supplements. *Seminars in Dialysis*, *12*(4), 235–236.

Van Wyck, D. B., Cavallo, G., Spinowitz, B. S., Adhikarla, R., Gagnon, S., Charytan, C., et al. (2000, July). Safety and efficacy of iron sucrose in patients sensitive to iron dextran: North American clinical trial. *American Journal of Kidney Diseases*, *36*(1), 88–97.

Vernon, D. D., Banner, W., & Dean, J. M. (1989). Hemodynamic effects of experimental iron poisoning. *Annals of Emergency Medicine*, *18*, 863–866.

Villalobos, D. (1992). Reliability of urine color changes after deferoxamine challenge. *Veterinary and Human Toxicology*, *34*, 330.

Voskaridou, E., Douskou, M., & Terpos, E. (2004). Magnetic resonance imaging in the evaluation of iron overload in patients with beta-thalassemia and sickle cell disease. *British Journal of Haematology*, *126*, 736–742.

Walker, S. E., Paton, T. W., Cowan, D. H., & Manuel, M. A. (1989, September 15). Bioavailability of iron in oral ferrous sulfate preparations in healthy volunteers. *Canadian Medical Association Journal*, *141*, 543–547.

Watson Pharma. (2006a, September). Ferrlecit (package insert). Corona, CA.

Watson Pharma. (2006b, March). Infed (package insert). Morristown, NJ.

Weiss, B., Alkon, E., & Weindlar, F. (1993). Toddler deaths resulting from ingestion of iron supplements – Los Angeles, 1992–1993. *Morbidity and Mortality Weekly Report*, *42*, 111–113.

Westlin, W. F. (1971). Deferoxamine as a chelating agent. *Clinical Toxicology*, *4*, 597–602.

Whittaker, P. (1998, August). Iron and zinc interactions in humans. *American Journal of Clinical Nutrition*, *68*(Suppl. 2), 442S–446S.

Witzleben, C. L., & Chaffey, N. J. (1966). Acute ferrous sulphate poisoning: A histochemical study of its effects on the liver. *Archives of Pathology and Laboratory Medicine*, *82*, 454–460.

Wood, J. C. (2007). Diagnosis and management of transfusion iron overload: The role of imaging. *American Journal of Hematology*, *82*, 1132–1135.

Wythe, E. T., Osterloh, J. D., & Becker, C. E. (1986). The reliability of serum iron levels after deferoxamine treatment: An in vitro study. *Veterinary and Human Toxicology*, *28*, 478.

Yonker, J., Banner, W., & Picchioni, A. (1980). Absorption characteristics of iron and deferoxamine onto charcoal. *Veterinary and Human Toxicology*, *22*(S2), 75.

# II

# Iron Overload and Deficiency Pathologies

# 6 Iron Deficiency and Excess in the Brain: Implications for Cognitive Impairment and Neurodegeneration

*Moussa B.H. Youdim, Manfred Gerlach, and Peder Riederer*

**Summary**

- Iron is a two-way sword. Either its brain iron deficiency (ID) or excess profoundly affects brain function.
- ID can result in reduction of brain iron by roughly 35% as contrast to a 90% depletion in the liver. Thus it is tightly controlled. It is associated with impairment of cognition and learning processes which may result from alteration in dopaminergic, at the level of its receptor subsensitivity, and increased opiate neurotransmission. Other aminergic systems are not profoundly affected.
- The effect of ID on brain function is age dependent, and it is more severe in newborn rats than adults and is irreversible in newborn even after long-term supplementation with iron.
- The exact mechanisms by which dopamine receptors are affected by ID and their effects cognition are not well understood, but may involve dopamine interaction with the endogenous opiates, enkephalin, and dynorphins, involving the hippocampus and striatum.
- One of the major findings on brain iron metabolism is its accumulation at neuronal sites which degenerate and give rise to neurodegenerative disorders such as Parkinson's disease, Alzheimer's disease, Huntington's diseases. Some are familial disorders, with mutation of genes involved in iron metabolism, such as Freidreich's ataxia, PANK2, aceruloplasminemia.
- The role of iron and its accumulation in substantia nigra pars compacta of parkinsonian brains, where melanized dopamine neuron selectively degenerates, has indicated that iron participates in the Fenton reaction to induce oxidative stress-dependent damage to the neurons.
- Confirmation for participation of iron in Parkinson's disease has come from its 6-hydroxydopmaine, MPTP (*N*-methy-4-phenyl-1,2,3,6-tetrahydropyridine), and lactacystin neurotoxin models, where similar iron accumulation occurs in substantia nigra pars compacta and pretreatment with iron chelators are neuroprotective. Several iron chelators have been developed as neuroprotective agents for Parkinson's disease and other neurodegenerative disorders.
- It is apparent that iron accumulation may have a pivotal role in the degeneration of dopamine neurons in Parkinson's disease. Future studies must illuminate why the process of neurodegeneration results in iron deposition and from where it is transported when it has limited access across the blood–brain barrier.

**Key Words:** Nutritional iron deficiency; iron accumulation; dopamine; enkephalins; cognition; neurodegeneration

From: *Nutrition and Health: Iron Deficiency and Overload*
Edited by: S. Yehuda and D.I. Mostofsky, DOI 10.1007/978-1-59745-462-9_6

## 1. NUTRITIONAL IRON DEFICIENCY AND ITS NEUROCHEMICAL ASPECT

It is well recognized that nutritional iron deficiency (NID) is the most prevalent nutritional deficiency in the world. It can affect more than 400 million individuals (WHO) and is indeed most prevalent in infants and young children. The importance of iron in systemic cellular biochemistry, where it is utilized in the synthesis of DNA and proteins and is involved as cofactor for numerous enzymes, structural protein and physiological responses, is well recognized. The vast literature that has been published on its various functions and dysfunctions in systemic organs, as a consequence of its deficiency, is too numerous to be summarized in this short chapter. However, what is not known and not readily recognized is that early iron deficiency can have a profound long-term effect on brain function, with possible irreversible brain damage at cellular and neuronal level. Even so until 1974, little or no attention was paid to brain iron metabolism and brain function. Since then there has been an active interest in brain iron metabolism, not only as a consequence of its deficiency with an effect on learning and cognitive processes but also on the role of excess brain iron accumulation and its involvement in neurodegeneration and progressive neurodegenerative diseases (Parkinson's disease, Alzheimer's disease, Huntington's chorea, Hallervorden-Spatz disease, etc.) (Dobbing, 1990a; Youdim, 1990; Youdim & Reiderer, 1999; Youdim & Riederer, 1997). To appreciate the effect of NID on brain one must consider its distribution.

The first studies of iron in human brain were those of Spatz (1922) and Hallgren and Sourander (1958) who showed that adult brain iron was unevenly distributed and some brain regions, namely the extrapyramidal regions (globus pallidus, substantia nigra, thalamus, venteral thalamus, red nucleus, intrapeduncular nucleus, dentate gyrus, cingula nucleus), had the highest concentrations and in some cases there was more iron per gram weight wet in these regions than in the liver. Ferritin (FER) is similarly distributed. These data have consistently been confirmed for human, monkey, dog, and rat brains.

However, there is no correlation between the distributions of iron–ferritin concentration and those of transferrin–transferrin receptors. Yet, the highest concentration of the latter is found in the hippocampal and cortical regions, which have relatively low iron and ferritin contents (Hill, 1988; Riederer et al., 1989; Dwork, Schon, & Herbert, 1988; Connor et al., 1987). By contrast, at birth in rat brain most of the iron is found in cortical and hippocampal areas. Studies involving brain $^{95}$Fe uptake in newborn rats with limited blood–brain barrier (BBB) have shown two crucial aspects of brain iron metabolism: (1) The major portion of $^{59}$Fe is found in the globus pallidus, substantia nigra, intrapeduncular nucleus, dentate gyrus, etc. (2) More than 90% of the iron ($^{59}$Fe) was present in newborn rats brain 24 hour after its injection is still in the brain of adult animal. This clearly indicates that iron is highly conserved in the brain and has a very slow turnover (Dwork, Lawler, Zybert, & Durkin, 1990; Ben-Shachar, Ashkenazi, & Youdim, 1986). Although iron transport into the brain is via transferrin receptors residing in capillary endothelial cells, the mechanism(s) by which iron is transported from one brain site to another is not known. The most puzzling question, which cannot be discussed at length in this chapter (due to lack of space), is why should such brain regions as globus pallidus, substantia nigra, dentate gyrus, caudate nucleus, etc. accumulate the highest concentration of iron in the brain. More recent studies point to iron-induced oxidative stress in the neurodegenerative processes in these regions, and the consequences of it are some of the most devastating neurodegenerative diseases (Parkinson's disease, Alzheimer's Disease, Huntington's chorea, Hallervorden-Spatz disease). There have been several reviews dealing with brain iron metabolism and brain function in iron deficiency (Dobbing, 1990a, 1990b; Pollitt & Leibel, 1982; Pollitt, Haas, & Levitsky, 1989) and iron in neurodegenerative diseases (Youdim & Riederer, 1999; Youdim & Riederer, 1997). This chapter will concentrate in updating the newer aspect of iron deficiency on brain function.

## 2. THE IMPACT OF NUTRITIONAL IRON DEFICIENCY ON BRAIN IRON

The first studies that dealt with the effects of NID on the brain were those of Werkman, Shifman, and Shelly (1964), Webb and Oski (1973), Dallman, Siimes, and Manies (1975), and Dallman and Spirito (1977). These investigators reported respectively that NID in children induced behavioral abnormalities that included reduction of learning abilities (cognitive impairments) and that NID in rats fed an iron-deficient diet results in the reduction of brain iron, albeit not as much that in the liver. These reports together with the earlier studies of Spatz (1922) and Hallgren and Sourander (1958) on the uneven distribution of iron in human brain prompted us to investigate the brain biochemical, pharmacological, physiological, and behavioral effects of NID in rats as a model for the human condition (see Youdim & Green, 1977; Youdim, Ben-Shachar, & Yehuda, 1989). Our original hypothesis was based on the notion that the behavioral changes noted in iron-deficient children by Webb and Oski (1973) were related to changes in the metabolism of CNS aminergic neurotransmitters, dopamine, serotonin, and noradrenaline. Abnormality in the metabolism and function of these neurotransmitters were implicated in behavior and learning processes and several neuropsychiatric diseases. There was good reason for this since the rate-limiting enzymes for the synthesis (tyrosine and tryptophan hydroxylases) and catabolizing (monoamine oxidase) the aminergic neurotransmitters were shown to be dependent on iron for their full enzymatic activity. Thus, any changes in the activities of these enzymes may alter the brain level of these neurotransmitters at specific sites (hypothalamus, striatum, raphe nucleus, frontal cortex, and hippocampus) in the brain and alter the physiology of their respective neurons as a consequence of over- or under-production of the neurotransmitters. Indeed, we demonstrated that while NID in rats, as induced by feeding them a diet low in iron (5 pp million), results in the reduction of iron-dependent enzymes (monoamine oxidase, phenylalanine hydroxylase, succinic dehydrogenase, cytochrome oxidase to mention a few) in peripheral tissues, by contrast none of the brain enzymes containing iron as a cofactor (including tyrosine hydroxylase, tryptophan hydroxylase, and monoamine oxidase) were changed (Youdim & Green, 1977; Youdim et al., 1989, Table 1). This was in spite of the fact that rat brain iron was reduced by 30–40% in adult (48 days old) in the striatum, hippocampus, cortex, and raphe nucleus. The effect is region dependent. It is now apparent that the effect of NID on tissue (brain and liver) iron is also dependent on the age of the animal and time on the nutritionally iron-deficient diet. While rat

**Table 1**
**Effect of ID on Brain Enzymes***

| | |
|---|---|
| Phenylalanine hydroxylase | Unchanged |
| Tyrosine hydroxylase | Unchanged |
| Tryptophan hydroxylase | Unchanged |
| Monoamine oxidase | Unchanged |
| Aldehyde dehydrogenase | Unchanged |
| Cytochrome oxidase C | Unchanged |
| Succinic dehydrogenase | Unchanged |
| Aminobutyric acid transaminase | Decreased |
| Glutamate decarboxylase | Decreased |

*Adult (aged 48 days) male rats were made nutritionally iron-deficient by feeding them a semisynthetic diet deficient in iron. Control animals received the same diet, to which iron sulfate had been added. In both groups the animals were pair-fed to maintain similar weight. Decrease in liver, heart, and adrenal glands.

(47 days old) liver iron and ferritin stores can be reduced relatively fast (within 2 weeks by 80–90%), brain iron is hardly changed until 3–5 weeks on the ID diet. Indeed, newborn pups (10 days old) are more readily made ID than young (21 days old) animals (Ben-Shachar et al., 1986; Dallman & Siimes, 1975; Dallman & Spirito, 1977; Youdim & Green, 1977; Youdim et al., 1989).

The unchanged activities of the brain neurotransmitter enzymes in ID rats are complimented with unaltered brain (striatum, caudate nucleus, and raphe nucleus) levels and turnover of dopamine, noradrenaline, and serotonin (Table 2). Nevertheless, our animal behavioral studies with functional activities of neurotransmitters dopamine and serotonin indicated a highly significant degree of deficit, which for the first time complimented the "behavioral" deficits reported by Webb and Oski (1973) in children with NID. The neurochemical explanation for the behavioral deficits was not easily forthcoming, and we suggested that brain ID may result in alteration in receptor number and function for any of these neurotransmitters (Youdim & Green, 1977). However, the abilities to measure various brain neurotransmitter receptor $B_{max}$ (receptor number) and $K_a$, employing radioligands, did not become available until 1976. As shown in Table 3,

Table 2
**Striatal Neurotransmitters and Their Precursor Levels in Brains of ID Rats**

| | *Concentration* | *Turnover* |
|---|---|---|
| Serotonin | Decreased | Unchanged |
| Dopamine | Unchanged | Increased |
| Noradrenaline | Unchanged | Unchanged |
| Tryptophan | Unchanged | – |
| Tyrosine | Unchanged | – |
| 5-Hydroxyindole acetic acid | Decreased | – |
| Met-enkephalin | Increased | |
| Dynorphin B | Increased | |

Table 3
**Effect of ID on Brain Neurotransmitter Receptors as Identified by Specific Radioligands**

| *Receptors* | $K_a$* | $B_{max}$ |
|---|---|---|
| γ-Adrenoceptor ($^3$H-WBA101) | Unchanged | Unchanged |
| β-Adrenoceptor ($^3$H-DHA) | Unchanged | Unchanged |
| Muscrinic-cholinergic receptor ($^3$H-ONB) | Unchanged | Unchanged |
| Dopamine $D_2$ receptor ($^3$H-spiperone) | Unchanged | Decreased |
| Dopamine $D_1$ receptor | Decreased | Unchanged |
| 5-$HT_2$ receptor ($^3$H-serotonin) | Unchanged | Unchanged |
| GABA receptor ($^3$H-musimol) | Unchanged | Increased |
| Benzodiazepine | ? | ? |

* Affinity constant for the receptor.

the only neurotransmitter receptors that were affected were those of dopamine (Youdim et al., 1989). Indeed, employing radioligand analysis of dopamine D1 and D2 receptors, we observed an increase in $K_a$ of dopamine D1 and a decrease of dopamine D2 $B_{max}$ in the striatum of NID rats, which complimented the significant diminution of dopamine-dependent behaviors as elicited by the treatments of rats with the dopamine agonist, apomorphine. This was the first time that a neurochemical change could be associated with the behavioral effects observed in NID. Indeed, our numerous behavioral and neurochemical investigations related to reduction of dopamine D2 receptor $B_{max}$ clearly indicate a subsensitivity of this receptor via the initiation of NID (see Table 4). There was direct parallelism between time-dependent reduction of brain (striatum) iron, dopamine D2 receptor $B_{max}$, and apomorphine-elicited dopamine-dependent behavior (Ben-Shachar et al., 1986; Youdim et al., 1989). This effect is related to iron deficiency and not the anemia resulting from it, since hemolytic anemia induced by chronic treatment of rats with phenylhydrazine does not alter brain dopamine D2 receptor number nor their behavioral responses (Ben-Shachar et al., 1986). Furthermore, supplementation of ID rats with iron plus diet (control) can result in restoration of brain iron dopamine receptor $B_{max}$ and behavioral responses. Again, this is an age-dependent phenomenon and has clear clinical implications in children with NID. One obvious but extremely important finding in our studies was the handling of iron by brain versus liver during iron supplementation. While rat liver iron could be restored within 1–2 weeks, brain iron increased very gradually, reaching its pre iron deficiency level within 3–4 weeks. Continuing iron supplementation for some 6 months resulted in liver iron being increased by some 20folds whereas brain iron remained constant. This discrepancy between iron handling of liver and brain indicates that iron transport in the brain is handled differently and may be related to BBB since in adult rats serum iron has no access to the brain. Furthermore, the turnover of brain iron is significantly much slower than the liver and almost all the iron that is present in the brain is conserved throughout life.

**Table 4**
**Biochemical and Behavioral Consequences of Reduced Dopamine $D_2$ Receptor in the Brains of ID Rats***

| | *Response* |
|---|---|
| 1. Monoamine oxidase inhibitor plus tryptophan (serotonin behavioural syndrome) | Decreased |
| 2. Monoamine oxidase inhibitor plus L-dopa (dopamine behavioural syndrome) | Decreased |
| 3. Monoamine oxidase inhibitor plus 5-hydroxy-tryptophan (serotonin behavioral syndrome) | Decreased |
| 4. 5-methoxy-*N,N*-dimethyltryptamine (behavioral syndrome) | Decreased |
| 5. D-amphetamine (dopamine release-induced stereotypy) | Decreased |
| 6. Apomorphine (dopamine receptor agonism stereotypy) | Decreased |
| 7. Learning processes | Decreased |
| 8. Thyrotropin-releasing hormone (TRH) and its analogue | Unchanged |
| 9. Phenobarbitone sleeping time | Increased |
| 10. Serum prolactin | Increased |
| 11. Serum testosterone | Increased |
| 12. Liver prolactin receptor | Increased |
| 13. Antinociceptive response to β-endorphin and enkephalins | Increased |
| 14. Dynorphin and met- and leu-enkephalins concentrations in globus pallidus, substantia nigra, caudate nucleus, and central gray and antinociception increased | Increased |
| 15. Response to neurotoxin (kainite, 6-hydroxydoapmine) induced neurodegeneration | Decreased |

Examination of BBB in NID rats indicated selective alteration and we suggested this could be at the level of gap or tight junctions of capillary endothelial cells that constitute the BBB (Ben-Shachar, Yehuda, Finberg, Spanier, & Youdim, 1988). However, Taylor and coworkers (Taylor, Crowe, & Morgan, 1991) have also provided evidence for upregulation of transferrin and transferrin receptors during NID and their downregulation when brain iron is restored. It is possible that both mechanisms are involved, and clearly more work needs to be done to clarify the differences between liver and brain handling of iron. Certainly, the roles of the recently described iron-regulatory proteins IRP1 and IRP2 during iron deficiency and repletion in the brain need clarification (Eisenstein & Blemings, 1998; Haile, 1999).

## 3. EARLY IRON DEFICIENCY AND ITS CONSEQUENCE ON BRAIN FUNCTION AND BEHAVIOR

It is in the first decade of child's life (first 4 years) that the bulk of iron deficiency is seen (Pollitt & Leibel, 1982). This is apparently the most crucial period of brain development, where DNA and protein synthesis, neuronal growth and differentiation take place and maturation of enzymes occurs. In this period myelination of neurons is at it fastest period and there is an essential role for iron in myelin deposition by oligodendrocytes (Erikson, Pinero, Connor, & Beard, 1997). Indeed, iron deficiency significantly interferes with myelination of the neurons (Connor & Menzies, 1996). Numerous studies on rat brain development confirm this. The obvious question would be what are the long-term consequences of iron deficiency in this period on brain development and function. Dallman (1973, 1975) reported persistent deficiency of brain iron during short-term deprivation in young rats followed by iron supplementation. He has attributed this to the very slow turnover of iron in the brain as compared to the liver.

We re-examined this in rats of different ages (newborn, young, and adult) made nutritionally iron deficient. Not only did we confirm Dallamn's findings in newborn rats but we also showed this feature to be age dependent (Ben-Shachar et al., 1986). While young and adult rats could recover their brain iron, newborn could not alter iron repletion. Furthermore, newborn rats had unrecoverable behavioral deficit, which was related to the deficiency of striatal dopamine D2 receptor and this and brain iron could not be restored even after 6 months of iron therapy, in spite of the normalization of their hematological indices. These findings point to long-term irreversible consequences of early iron deficiency on brain function. They may go some way to support what Lozzof and co-workers and others (Lozoff, 1988; Lozoff & Brittenham, 1986; Parks & Wharton, 1990; Felt & Lozoff, 1996) have consistently reported in iron-deficient infants and young children with impaired attentional problems where long-term iron therapy was ineffective. Whether our animal models reflect the human condition may be a matter of debate and all animal models do have their drawbacks. Nevertheless, early iron deficiency does impair brain biochemistry and function and its consequences need to be appreciated, considering the susceptibility of human brain to undernourishment in the first decade of life (Guesry, 1998; Rao et al., 1999), when the major portion (80%) of iron found in the adult brain is deposited and interaction of iron with other metals may be crucial (Rao et al., 1999; Georgieff, Petry, Wobken, & Oyer, 1996; Chua & Morgan, 1996; Adhami, Husain, Husain, & Seth, 1996). Although our original behavioral studies were related to dopamine neurotransmission deficit in iron deficiency, we have extended our work to closely investigate learning parameters in Morris Water Maze. Indeed, iron-deficient young rats were poorer performers (longer time and more trials) in finding the platform in the Morris maze and had lower activity (Yehuda, Youdim, & Mostofsky, 1986; Yehuda & Youdim, 1989; Yehuda, 1990), and 4 weeks of iron therapy (repletion) did not alter the learning performance of these rats. Confirmation of this result has recently come from Felt and Lozzoff (1996). These results raise the concern that iron deficiency during the course of early brain development, prenatally and postnatally, is damaging. Thus it is crucial to maintain normal brain iron concentration (Guesry, 1998; Rao et al., 1999; Georgieff et al., 1996; Chua & Morgan, 1996; Adhami et al., 1996) where neuronal iron uptake is age dependent and susceptible to iron deficiency as a consequence of its dependence on transferrin receptor (Moos, Oates, & Morgan, 1998). The one puzzling factor in comparing the effects of NID on newborn and adult rat brain iron is that adult rat brain recovers its iron but not the newborn. This would suggest some other underlying irreversible cause, which we have not identified as yet.

## 4. BRAIN IRON DEFICIENCY AND DOPAMINE–ENDOGENOUS OPIATE INTERACTION AND FUNCTION

The role of dopamine in learning and cognitive processes has been discussed at length by Yehuda and Youdim (1989) and Yehuda (1990). Nevertheless, consideration has to be given also to other mechanisms and changes that occur in the brain during ID, as a consequence of reduction in dopamine neurotransmission or other processes. For example, we showed that iron deficiency alters several brain proteins as identified by two-dimensional electrophoresis, and among them a protein with a molecular weight identical to that of dopamine D2 receptor decreased while other proteins are increased (Youdim, Sills, Neydron, Creed, & Jacobowitz, 1986). We were not able to identify many of the protein changes. However, consideration has to be given to the alterations in these proteins. What roles they have in brain function clearly need thorough investigation.

The brain areas known to have the highest concentration of iron (globus pallidus, substantia nigra, dentate gyrus, caudate nucleus, thalamus, putamen, ventral tegmentum) are innervated with the densest population of opiate-peptides (enkephalins, endorphins, and dynorphin B). The importance of endogenous opiate-peptides alone and their interaction with dopamine in learning process has been investigated, and it is now evident that they are closely involved in learning and cognition processes. On several occasions it has been reported that administration of the opiate antagonists (e.g., naloxone, MIF) improves learning (Pablo Huidobro-Toro & Leong Way, 1983, 1985) and this may be dependent on dopamine transmission functional activity and learning processes; as a consequence of dopamine D2 receptor subsensitivity, we investigated the function of central opiates in these animals. Indeed, ID rats showed a highly significant antinociception, which was further exaggerated when treated intraperitoneally with the opiates, morphine, met-enkephalin, leu-enkephalin, or endorphin. Naloxone and melanocyte-inducing factor (MIF) (44–46) could block these effects. Normal rats do not show antinociception to opiate-peptides, since these peptides do not cross the BBB and are rapidly metabolized by zinc-dependent metalopeptidase in the systemic organs. Thus, in Newborn the metabolism of opiate-peptides and their brain transport are affected. BBB studies in iron deficiency have clearly shown uptake of opiate-peptide, β-endorphin in ID rats but not control rats (Ben-Shachar et al., 1988). The latter results may indicate the reason why ID but not control rats exhibit antinociception in response to opiate-peptide (met-enkephalin and dynorphin B) as measured in globus pallidus, caudate nucleus, substantia nigra, midbrain tegmentum, and central gray (Pablo Huidobro-Toro & Leong Way, 1983, 1985; Yehuda & Youdim, 1984; Yehuda, Youdim, & Zamir, 2000; Youdim, Zamir, & Yehuda, 2000). The mechanism whereby NID brings about increased brain levels of opiate peptides is not well understood. It is well established that dopamine is inhibitory to opiates (Pablo Huidobro-Toro & Leong Way, 1983, 1985; Tang, Costa, & Schartz, 1983), and antagonism of dopamine receptors with dopamine D2 receptor antagonists (haloperidol, chlorpromazine) results in brain elevation of opiate-peptides similar to those as shown by us in ID rats (47–50). The explanation for this may be found in studies where it has been demonstrated that dopamine D2 receptor antagonists induces the pro-enkephalin mRNA (Tang et al., 1983; Durham, Johnson, Moore, & Lookingland, 1996; Angulo, 1992; Morris, Höllt, & Herz, 1988). Whether NID brings about the same changes in opiate mRNAs and opiate antagonists can reverse the diminished learning processes remains to be investigated.

## 5. IRON AND ZINC INTERACTION IN THE HIPPOCAMPUS

The involvement of hippocampus in cognition has prompted our investigation into distribution and development of the iron-storage protein ferritin (FER) in rat hippocampus (Shoham & Youdim, 2002). (a) In normal rats, FER-positive cells appeared first in lateral CA3 of hippocampus and hilus of dentate gyrus and then spread over the entire mossy fiber (MF) system. No such spread was observed in hippocampal CA1 field. (b) NID retarded development of FER in the MF system. No change in FER was observed in CA1 field. (c) Zinc distribution can be altered by iron deficiency. Thus, the effect of zinc added to iron supplementation was tested in iron-deficient rats. Significant FER recovery was observed only in hippocampal MF of rats receiving both zinc and iron. It is apparent that for accelerating recovery of hippocampal function in iron deficiency, both zinc and iron are required.

The background for our study (Shoham & Youdim, 2002) was the cognitive impairment and resistance to nutritional iron therapy in young iron-deficient (ID) children (52–55) (Lozoff, Jimenez, & Wolf, 1991; Lozoff, Wolf, & Jimenez, 1996; Parks & Wharton, 1989; Walter, De Andraca, Chadud, & Perales, 1989) and their confirmation in our animal studies (Ben-shachar et al., 1986; Youdim & Green, 1977; Youdim et al., 1989; Yehuda & Youdim, 1989). The main objectives of the study were (a) to chart the normal development of ferritin distribution in the hippocampus, (b) examine the effects of ID on FER immunohistochemical distribution, and (c) study the consequences of nutritional therapy with iron alone compared to zinc alone and compared to zinc added to iron therapy (Shoham & Youdim, 2002).

### *5.1. The Normal Development of Ferritin Distribution in the Hippocampus*

The study revealed a spatial pattern of FER distribution in the hippocampal MF system and a spatiotemporal order in the development of FER cells in this hippocampal system. It should be noted that the sensitivity of the immunohistochemical methods used in the present study depend on the quality and affinity of the antibody. Thus, some cells that appeared to lack ferritin, in the present study, might have actually contained some ferritin. In other words, lack of FER cells in a given region of the hippocampus should not be taken to mean absence of ferritin. Nevertheless, assuming that the threshold for detection of ferritin was the same for all groups compared in the study, we have been able to detect a spatiotemporal trend in the development of FER cells in the hippocampal MF system. Several previous studies have touched the subject of iron and ferritin in the hippocampus (Dwork et al., 1990; Connor, Pavlick, Karli, Menzies, & Palmer, 1995; Dwork, 1995). However, an association of FER distribution with the hippocampal MF system has not been noted in previous studies. Noting this association is important, since it provides a potential clue to the effects of brain iron deficiency on cognitive function.

### *5.2. Effects of Iron Deficiency on Distribution of Ferritin in the Hippocampus*

Previous studies on the impact of iron deficiency on the hippocampus have not reported any effect specific to the hippocampal MF system (Taylor et al., 1991; Shoham & Youdim, 2002;

De Los Monteros et al., 2000; Han, Day, Thomson, Connor, & Beard, 2000; Shoham & Youdim, 2000, 2002; Hansen, Nielsen, Bernth, & Moos, 1999; Pinero, Li, Connor, & Beard, 2000). Furthermore, in these studies 2 weeks of iron supplementation to iron-deficient rats was sufficient to restore iron and ferritin to the hippocampus as measured in a homogenate of the dissected hippocampus. Since the MF terminal zone comprises only a small fraction of hippocampal tissue, it is not surprising that only with the resolution power of immunohistochemistry as employed in the present study it was possible to discover that ID had a specific effect on the hippocampal MF system, and that 2 weeks of iron supplementation did not restore ferritin distribution to this anatomical system.

It is also important to note that despite the impact of ID, no change in MF neuro-anatomy was detected by the sulfide/silver stain, or by immunohistochemical staining with markers of hippocampal innervation such as the potassium channel Kv1.4 or calbindin D28k. This suggests that the retarded development of ferritin distribution was not secondary to an effect of iron deprivation on MF development. On the other hand, the fact that ferritin distribution could be retarded without a gross change in MF development led to the search for subtle effects of ID on hippocampal MF composition and one candidate aspect was zinc. Although zinc accumulates in the hippocampus, MF zinc comprises only 8% of hippocampal zinc (Frederickson, Klitenick, Manton, & Kirkpatrick, 1983; Howell, Welch, & Frederickson, 1984). Nevertheless, MF zinc appears to have an important role in signal transduction in the MF system (Frederickson et al., 1983; Howell et al., 1984). Thus, we examined the potential impact of zinc added to iron therapy in iron-deficient rats.

### 5.3. *Effects of Zinc Alone and Zinc Added to Iron Therapy*

The diet employed in the study was not zinc-deficient and there was no reason to consider the iron-deprived rats were zinc-deprived. However, based on previous studies, alterations in zinc levels can occur in some tissues secondary to iron deficiency (Yokoi, Kimura, & Itokawa, 1991; Shukla, Agrawal, & Shukla, 1989). Thus, a subtle change in MF zinc under iron deficiency was considered as a potential contributing factor in resistance of learning ability to iron therapy. In the present study, zinc supplementation alone failed to increase the number of FER cells in the MF system of ID rats. But addition of zinc to iron therapy significantly increased the number of FER cells in the hippocampal MF. The mechanisms underlying this effect remain to be investigated. One possible line of investigation may be interactions of iron and zinc with endogenous opioid-peptide neurotransmission. There is evidence suggesting that zinc modulates enkephalinergic neurotransmission (Stengaard-Pedersen, Fredens, & Larson, 1981). Met-enkephalin and dynorphin B levels were increased in several brain regions in ID rats including the striatum, substantia nigra, ventreal tegmentum, and pallidum (Yehuda et al., 1986; Youdim et al., 2000), and these animals exhibit highly significant antinociception, which could be blocked by naloxane and MIF (Youdim et al., 2000). Normally, rats do not exhibit antinociception to systemic administration of enkepalins. However, iron-deficient rats do so to Met- and Leu-enkephalins (Youdim et al., 2000) because they are metabolized rapidly by zinc-dependent metalopeptidases (Gulya, Kovacs, & Kasa, 1991). This may be the result of the fact that in normal circumstances enkephalin-peptides are metabolized by zinc-dependent metaloproteases. Since iron deficiency affects zinc metabolism, it is most likely that metabolism of the enkephalins by zinc-metaloproteases is reduced and they would have access to the brain. Intracerebral administration of enkephalin analogs causes partial depletion of zinc in several brain regions including hippocampus (Gulya et al., 1991). Thus, brain zinc may be affected in ID through effects on enkephalinergic neurotransmission. In the hippocampal MF system there are opioid neurotransmitters. Both enkephalin and dynorphin are released from glutamatergic nerve terminals of the hippocampal MF system and modulate hippocampal pyramidal cell excit-Iron zinc and ferritin in hippocampus of iron-deficient rats (Morris & Johnston, 1995). The present study may provide clues to further investigation of the alterations in opioid neurotransmission in the hippocampal MF in iron-deficiency. Another domain in which zinc may interact with opioid-peptides in the phenomenology of iron deficiency may be the regulation of food intake and body weight. Iron deficiency is associated with reduction in spontaneous food intake and reduction in body weight (Dhur, Galan, & Hercberg, 1990). Zinc deficiency is also associated with reduced food intake and body weight (Essatara, Levine, Morley, & McClain, 1984). However, the present study is the first, to the best of our knowledge, to show that zinc supplementation to iron-deficient rats is sufficient to restore food intake and body weight. This finding suggests that the anorexia of iron deficiency may be mediated by a secondary deficiency in zinc in some brain regions. Given the interaction of zinc with enkephalin (Stengaard-Pedersen et al., 1981), it is possible that ID indirectly affects zinc and hence enkephalinergic modulation of food intake (Gosnell, Levine, & Morley, 1986).

The neurobiological significance of the present findings on ferritin distribution remains to be elucidated. In the present study, the developmental spread of FER cells in the rat hippocampus follows the pattern of developmental synaptic plasticity in this region (Bayer, 1985). Thus, in the present study, FER cells were mostly localized in the vicinity of the stems of apical dendrites of pyramidal cells in CA3. These apical dendrites receive multiple afferents, which arrive in the course of development with a temporal order (Bayer, 1985). In the hippocampal dentate gyrus (DG), cell division continues into adult life (Bayer, 1985). Thus, according to the present findings, the formation of new MF synaptic contacts appears to be accompanied by the increase in ferritin, possibly reflecting increased accumulation of iron. Possibly, iron in glial cells, localized along the MF system, has a role in the support of developmental synaptic plasticity. In the present study and in previous studies by others (Connor, Boeshore, Benkovic, & Menzies, 1994; Kaneko, Kitamoto, Tateishi, & Yamaguchi, 1989; Kaur & Ling, 1995), ferritin immunohistochemistry revealed cells with microglial morphology in the hippocampus. Iron has been detected in amoeboid microglia in early development (Kaur & Ling, 1995). Possibly, iron is important in some microglial "macrophagic" functions in the hippocampal MF system. With normal development, synaptic reorganization in the MF system requires removal of old synaptic structures as well as formation of new structures. Microglia are involved in the removal of synaptic structures in various paradigms of synaptic plasticity (Nakajima & Kohsaka, 1993). Possibly, iron stored in microglia participates in this "macrophagic function" of microglia. Indeed, there is evidence for release of iron from ferritin stored in microglia (Yoshida, Tanaka, Sotomatsu, & Hirai, 1995). In iron deficiency, lower availability of iron to microglia may slow down developmental plasticity in the MF system, which may be manifested in cognitive deficits.

More research is required to understand how the addition of zinc to iron therapy may accelerate the recovery of iron storage in glial cells along the MF system and how this may affect cognitive deficits in ID. In another study, our finding that zinc added to iron therapy potentiates kainate neurotoxicity in ID (Shoham & Youdim, 2000) suggests that zinc added to iron therapy enhances glutamatergic neurotransmission in the hippocampus. Glutamatergic neurotransmission in hippocampus is important for learning processes (Bliss & Collingridge, 1993). Since microglia are sensitive to glutamate via *N*-methyl-D-aspartate receptors (Tikka & Koistinaho, 2001), it is possible that the addition of zinc modulates the functional states of microglia via zinc modulation of NMDA receptor function (Xie & Smart, 1994). Furthermore, there is evidence that microglia secrete factors that enhance neuronal excitability in the hippocampus (Hegg &

Thayer, 1999). It remains to be further explored whether this function is modulated by iron in microglia and whether this process is subject to modulation by zinc levels. Furthermore, studies are now under way to assess the impact of zinc added to iron therapy on learning ability in ID rats.

## 6. BRAIN IRON AND PARKINSON'S DISEASE

### *6.1. Transition Metals in Parkinson's Disease*

The participation of iron in Parkinson's disease and other neurodegenerative disorders have been investigated and recently reviewed by Zecca, Youdim, Riederer, Connor, and Crichton (2004). Occupational and dietary metal exposure is thought to be associated with the occurrence of Parkinson's disease (PD) (Lai, Marion, Teschke, & Tsui, 2002; Powers et al., 2003). Gorell et al. (1997, 1999) reported significant associations of PD with copper and iron in workers with more than 20 years of occupational contact and an increased risk for patients with family history (Rybicki, Johnson, Peterson, Kortsha, & Gorell, 1999). A combination of manganese, iron, aluminum, and mercury might favor the development of PD after 30 years of exposure (Zayed et al., 1990; Ngim & Devathasan, 1989; Seidler et al., 1996). In contrast to Logroscino et al. (1998), Powers et al. (2003) reported a moderate association between iron intake from foods and PD and an apparent joint effect of iron and manganese. These epidemiological findings might point to a role of transition metals in PD but cannot explain most of cases of idiopathic parkinsonism. Thus, transition metal alterations described in the brain of parkinsonian patients and of other neurodegenerative diseases might result from endogenous dysregulation of iron uptake, transport, distribution, and storage (Table 5), which has been reviewed (Youdim & Green, 1977; Youdim, 1985; Youdim et al., 1989; Youdim, Ben-Shachar, & Riederer, 1993; Hirsch, 1994; Jellinger, 1999; Jellinger, 2003; Berg et al., 2001; Berg et al., 2002; Double, Zecca, Costi, Gerlach, & Riederer, 2000; Double, Ben-Shachar, Youdim, & Riederer, 2002; Gerlach et al., 2004; Gerlach, Double, Ben-Shachar, Youdim, & Riederer, 2003; Perry et al., 2002; Sipe, Lee, & Beutler, 2002; Wolozin & Golts, 2002; Friedman & Galazka-Friedman, 2001; Zecca et al., 2004).

**Table 5**
**Increased Localized Brain Ferritin and Iron Deposits in Neurodegenerative Diseases**

| |
|---|
| Aceruloplasminemia |
| Alzheimer's disease |
| Amyotropic lateral sclerosis |
| Acquired immune deficiency syndrome |
| Friedreich's ataxia |
| Hallervorden Syndrome |
| Huntington's chorea |
| Juvenile Parkinson's disease |
| Multiple sclerosis |
| Parkinson's disease |
| Prion diseases |

Adapted from Youdim and Riederer (2003) with kind permission from Elsevier Amsterdam.

## 7. IRON IN PARKINSONIAN BRAIN

Iron is the most abundant transition metal in the body and has a unique distribution in the brain. A quantitative regional distribution of non-hemin iron in the normal brain was presented in 1958 by Hallgren and Sourander (1958) and confirmed by Riederer et al. (1989). Accordingly, iron levels range from 1.4 mg to 100 g fresh weight in the medulla oblongata up to 21.3 mg/100 g fresh weight in the globus pallidus in individuals older than 29 years. The substantia nigra (SN), one of the most vulnerable brain regions in PD, contains 18.5 mg/100 g fresh weight. These values were confirmed when analyzed with extended X-ray absorption fine structure (Griffiths, Dobson, Jones, & Clarke, 1999). Iron concentrations in the SN and the globus pallidus are higher than those of the liver. Other brain regions where iron is found in high concentrations are the dentate gyrus, interpeduncular nucleus, thalamus, ventral pallidus, nucleus basalis, and red nucleus.

Increased levels of iron in the brain of parkinsonian patients were demonstrated first by Lhermitte, Kraus, and McAlpine (1924), Earle (1968), Riederer, Sofic, and Rausch (1985), and Dexter et al. (1987). The increase in non-hemin chelatable ironIII (Riederer et al., 1989; Sofic, Riederer, Heinsen, Riederer, & Youidim, 1988) was not seen in patients with mild neuropathological changes in the SN. However, total iron content, determined following reduction of ironIII to ironII by using the ironII chelator ferrozine and granulated ascorbic acid as a reductant for ironIII, increased only in the SN in more severe cases of PD, but not in incidental Lewy body disease (Dexter et al., 1995; Owen, Schapira, & Jenner, 1997). Spectrophotometry studies showed increased total iron and ironIII contents in the SN pars compacta from parkinsonian but not from Alzheimer subjects (Sofic, Paulus, Jellinger, Riederer, & Youdim, 1991). Histochemical iron staining of paraffin sections using Perl's stain of ironIII after pretreatment with ferrocyanide (Gomori, 1993) revealed ironIII in astrocytes, microglia, the walls of arterioles and veins in putamen and pallidum but only rarely in neurons. In the SN pars compacta ironIII was localized in microglia, in astrocytes often localized next to neurons, and in single non-pigmented neurons. The selective increase in total iron in the parkinsonian SN pars compacta dopamine neurons was detected as well with inductively coupled plasma spectroscopy (ICP) and energy-dispersive X-ray microanalysis (EDX) (Table 5) (Dexter et al., 1987; Dexter, Wells, Lees, Marsden, & Jenner, 1989; Dexter et al., 1991; Jellinger, Kienzl, Rumpelmair, Riederer, & Youdim, 1992; Jellinger, Kienzl, Rumpelmair, Riederer, & Youdim, 1993; Hirsch, Brandel, Galle, Agid, & Agid, 1991). Several other studies could not find significant changes in total iron content in the SN of parkinsonian patients using ICP, atomic absorption and emission (AAS), or Mössbauer spectroscopy (MS) (Table 5) (Uitti et al., 1989; Mann, Cooper, & Daniel, 1994; Galazka-Friedman et al., 1996). Explanations for the divergent findings of different groups may be based on the usage of brain tissue at different stages of neurodegeneration at the time of death as well as different dissection and tissue handling protocols. Moreover, sensitivities of methods vary considerably. For example, Mössbauer spectroscopy only measures $^{57}Fe$, which is a low-abundance isotope in brain tissue (Gerlach, Trautwein, Zecca, Riererer, & Youdim, 1995; Gerlach, Double, Riederer, & Youdim, 1997). Other methods do not give total levels of iron, but detailed microstructural informations such as EDX and laser microprobe mass analysis (LAMMA). Using EDX on an electron microscope working in the scanning transmission mode, neuromelanin-bound iron could be detected only in pigmented neurons of the SN pars compacta of parkinsonian patients (Jellinger et al., 1993) and confirmed using the sensitive LAMMA technique to be associated with neuromelanin granules (Good, Olanow, & Perl, 1992; Iancu, Perl, Sternlieb, & Olanow, 1996). Probe sites directed to nonmelanized portions of cytoplasm of these cells or to the adjacent neurophil revealed lower concentrations of both metals with EDX and LAMMA. Further, the use of X-ray absorption fine structure (EXAFS) and cryo-electron transmission microscopy confirmed the increased iron in parkinsonian nigra and the lateral globus pallidus and revealed that ferritin was more heavily loaded with iron in PD when compared with age-matched controls (Griffiths et al., 1999). When iron levels are correlated with dopamine concentrations, the highly significant negative association was found between dopamine and ironIII in the putamen and not in the SN in severe PD (Gerlach, Ben-Shachar, Riederer, & Youdim, 1994). However, in putamen total iron levels are not significantly different from controls (Table 1). In the globus pallidus there is a subregional alteration of iron levels in the lateral versus the medial part (Table 6) (Griffiths et al., 1999; Dexter et al., 1989, 1991). These findings may be indicative of retrograde degeneration

**Table 6**
**Alterations in Levels of Iron and of Parameters Proposed to Reflect Iron Content (e.g., $T_2$ Relaxation Time in MRI or Echogenicity in TCS) Determined by Different Histochemical, Biochemical, and Physicochemical Methods in Parkinson's Disease**

| | *SN* | *Putamen* | *Globus Pallidus* |
|---|---|---|---|
| Semiquantitative Estimations | | | |
| Lhermitte (1924) (H) | Normal | – | Increase |
| Earle (1967) (XF) | General but nonspecific increase in PD | | |
| Jellinger et al. (1990) (H) | Increase (S) | (NS) | (NS) |
| Jellinger et al. (1992) (EDX) | Increase (S) | – | – |
| Gorell et al. (1997, 1999) (MRI) | Increase (S) | – | – |
| Ryvlin et al. (1995) (MRI) | Increase (S) | Decrease (S) | Decrease (S) |
| Becker et al. (1995) (TCS) | | Basal ganglia increase (S) | |
| Ye et al. (1996) (MRI) | | Basal ganglia increase (S) | |
| Quantitative Determinations | | | |
| Riederer et al. (195) (SP) | 1.22 (a) | 1.17 (a) | 0.87 (a) |
| Dexter et al. (1997) (ICP) | 1.35 (S) | – | – |
| Sofić et al. (1988) (SP) | 1.89 (S) | 0.81 (NS) | 1.20 (NS) |
| Riederer et al. (1989) (SP) | 1.77 (S) | 0.81 (NS) | 1.20 (NS) |
| Uitti et al. (1989) (AAS) | 1.07 (NS) | – | – |
| Dexter et al. (1989) | 1.34 (S) (t) | 1.04 (NS)(l) | 0.71 (S)(l) |
| Dexter et al. (1991) (ICP) | 1.30 (S) (pc) | 0.83 (NS)(m) | 0.71 (S)(m) |
| Sofic et al. (1991) (SP) | 1.50 (S) | – | – |
| Hirsch et al. (1991) (XMA) | 3.40 (S) (b) | – | – |
| Good et al. (1992) (LAMMA) | 1.45 (S) (c) | – | – |
| Mann et al. (1994) (ICP) | 1.56 (S) | – | – |
| Galazka- Friedman et al. (1996) (MS) | 0.98 (NS) | – | – |
| Loeffler et al. (1995) (Col) | 0.82 (NS) | 0.64 (NS) | 1.8 (NS) |
| Griffiths et al. (1999) (EXAFS) | 2.01 (S) | 1.23 (NS) | 1.43 (S) (l) |

Values express fold change of arithmetic mean values compared to control means. (S) statistically significant, (NS) statistically not significant, (a) no statistics calculated, (b) on zones lacking neuromelanin, (c) on neuromelanin granules, – not determined; (pc) substantia nigra pars compacta, (l) lateral, (m) medial, (t) total, (AAS) atomic absorption spectroscopy, (Col) colorimetry, (EDX) energy dispersive x-ray analysis, (EXAFS) extended X-ray absorption fine structure, (H) histological staining, (ICP) inductively coupled plasma spectroscopy, (LAMMA) laser microprobe mass analysis, (MRI) magnetic resonance imaging, (MS) Mössbauer spectroscopy, (SP) spectrophotometry, (TCS) transcranial ultrasound, (XF) X-ray fluorescence spectroscopy, (XMA) X-ray microprobe analysis.

of catecholaminergic neurons in PD. However, unlike the presence of oxidative stress and neurochemical changes reported for SN pars compacta, where iron is increased, the striatum is relatively unaltered biochemically.

The nigral increase in iron level was also identified in patients as assessed by magnetic resonance imaging (MRI) (Gorell et al., 1995; Ryvlin et al., 1995; Ye, Allen, & Martin, 1996; Bartzokis et al., 1999). The prominent contrast changes seen by MRI on $T_2$-weighted images correlate with sites of ferric iron that dephase the excited proton spins and thus lead to decreased $T_2$ relaxation times in MRI experiments. $T_2$-weighted images demonstrate prominent low-signal areas in the red nucleus, and the SN pars reticulata may be indicative of high ferric iron content since iron concentrations in the adult are much higher than those of paramagnetic manganese or copper (Martin, 2001).

Transcranial ultrasound (TCS) may reflect alterations in brain metal constituents since PD patients exhibit a substantially increased echogenicity in the SN (Becker, Seufert, Bogdahn Reichmann, & Reiners, 1995). In more than 90% of PD patients, the SN is superimposed by extended white signals, reflecting increased echogenicity, which predominate contralateral to the clinically more affected body side (Berg, Becker, & Zeiler, 1999; Berg et al., 2001, 2002; Walter, Wittstock, Benecke, & Dressler, 2002; Zecca et al., 2008). A recent postmortem study using brains from normal subjects at different ages suggests an association of SN echogenicity with higher levels of iron, L-ferritin, and H-ferritin, and reduced neuromelanin concentration (Zecca et al., 2003). This molecular constellation of different iron species may describe a noxious cellular milieu promoting the generation of oxyradicals and cell damage. This may explain the increased susceptibility of subjects with SN hyperechogenicity for nigral injury as demonstrated by positron emission tomography (PET) studies.

## 8. SOURCES OF IRON AND ITS INTERACTION WITH NEUROMELANIN

Transferrin-mediated iron transport can result in highest levels of iron being bound to ferritin and neuromelanin in the brain. Ferritin is a 450-kDa protein with 24 subunits forming a cavity which can store up to 4,500 atoms of ferric iron. It is expressed in oligodendrocytes, astrocytes, and microglia, but hardly in neurons (Connor, Menzies, St. Martin, & Mufson, 1990; Zecca et al., 2001a and b). In PD the number of ferritin-immunoreactive microglial cells in the SN increases with many reactive microglial cells located in close proximity to melanin-containing or degenerating neurons (Jellinger, Paulus, Grundke-Iqbal, Riederer, & Youdim, 1990; Jellinger et al., 1992; Riederer, Rausch, Schmidt, & Gerlach, 1988). Ferritin cores in the SN of PD patients are reported to be denser and contain more iron than those in the SN of healthy subjects (Griffiths et al., 1999). As long as iron is bound to ferritin, cytotoxic reactions are not expected. However, iron can be released from ferritin by various exogenous (Monteiro, Ville, & Winterbourn, 1989; Lapenna, Degioia, & Ciofani, 1995; Linert et al., 1996; Double, Maywald, Schmittel, & Riederer, 1997) and endogenous substances via reductive mechanisms (Monteiro & Winterbourn, 1988; Boyer, Grabill, & Petrovich, 1988). If released from ferritin, low-molecular ironII complexes can undergo redox reactions resulting in cytotoxic damage of proteins, DNA, or lipids (Halliwell & Gutteridge, 1986; Götz, Künig, Riederer, & Youdim, 1994). In vitro experiments revealed that *ortho*-dyhydroxyphenyl compounds such as the endogenous neurotransmitter dopamine potently release ironII from ferritin (Double et al., 1997; Double, Riederer, & Gerlach, 1998). Since ferritin is predominantly located in glial cells, oxidative stress from glial cells might be a secondary event following high dopamine turnover, neuronal cell dysfunction, and death.

An interesting intraneuronal iron source or iron deposit is neuromelanin. Ben-Shachar et al. (1991) demonstrated for the first time that synthetic dopamine derived melanin has a capacity to bind highly significant amount of iron at two sites, and this has recently been confirmed by the studies of Ben-Shachar et al. (1991) and more recently confirmed by Double et al. (2003). Neuromelanin contains considerable amounts of iron in the SN of patients with PD (Jellinger et al., 1992, 1993), a dark pigment produced in catecholaminergic neurons of the human SN and locus coeruleus, and is generally regarded as the result of the reaction of oxidized catechols with a variety of nucleophiles including thiols from glutathione and proteins. The involvement of enzymes in neuromelanin synthesis is still under debate (Zecca et al., 2001a and b). This pigment may be different in some respects as compared to epidermal melanocytes and synthetic dopamine melanins (Double, Gerlach, Youdim, & Riederer, 2000). It appears that iron is bound to catecholic groups. EPR studies showed that in the SN the ferric iron is bound to neuromelanin as a high spin complex with an octahedral configuration (Zecca & Swartz, 1993; Zecca, Shima, & Stroppolo, 1996; Shima, Sarna, Stroppolo, Gerbasi, & Zecca, 1997; Zecca et al., 2008). Mössbauer spectroscopy demonstrates that ferric iron is bound to ferritin-like oxyhydroxide clusters (Friedman & Galazka-Friedman, 2001; Galazka-Friedman et al., 1996; Gerlach et al., 1995). In the SN, neuromelanin is only about 50% saturated with ironIII. The remaining binding capacity can be used for further metal binding or binding of other cationic compounds such as paraquat and methyl-phenylpyridinium ($MPP^+$) as well as of dopamine oxidation products. Thus, neuromelanin may have a cytoprotective role as long as transition metals are bound to it, or it may trigger cytotoxicity if iron is released within neurons depending on the reducing cellular environment and probably other yet unknown factors.

The number of pigmented and non-pigmented neurons is constant in normal aging while in PD there is a preferential loss of pigmented neurons (Hirsch, Graybiel, & Agid, 1988). Precise analysis of the dopaminergic neurons in the midbrain demonstrates that the loss of dopaminergic neurons in the mesencephalon is not uniform. Some dopaminergic cell groups are more vulnerable than others. The degree of cell loss is severe in the SN pars compacta, intermediate in the ventral tegmental area and cell group A8, but nonexistent in the central gray substance. This heterogeneity provides a good paradigm for analyzing the factors implicated in the differential vulnerability of dopaminergic neurons. So far, the neurons that degenerate have been shown to contain neuromelanin, high amounts of iron, no calbindin 28 K, and are poorly protected against oxidative stress. By contrast, the neurons that survive in PD are free of neuromelanin, calbindinD28-positive, contain low amounts of iron, and are better protected against oxidative stress (Hirsch, 1994).

The absolute concentration of nigral neuromelanin is less than 50% in PD with respect to age-matched controls (Zecca, Fariello, & Riederer, 2002). This may lead to the conclusion that neuromelanin might be somehow involved in neurotoxicity in PD. On the other hand, it is discussed that in PD either not enough neuromelanin is produced or the structure of neuromelanin is changed. Hence, the ability to bind cytotoxic components is reduced and thus neuromelanin would be rather a neuroprotectant than a neurotoxicant in PD brains. This view is supported by neuropathological investigations that show that pigmented cells in PD contain less neuromelanin compared with those in control brains (Kastner et al., 1992). Furthermore, it was reported (Gibb, 1992) that the more vulnerable nigral ventral tier cells contain less neuromelanin than the more heavily pigmented cells in the dorsal tier, suggesting that neuromelanin may confer an advantage upon the cells in which it is found. Further support for the hypothesis that neuromelanin can act as a protective substance comes from in vitro studies. Human neuromelanin can significantly reduce both basal and iron-stimulated lipid peroxidation in rat cortical homogenates (Ben-Shachar et al., 1991; Double, Riederer, & Gerlach, 1999; Double et al., 2003). Thus, neuromelanin may attenuate oxidative damage by directly interacting with, and inactivating, free radical species. The ability of neuromelanin to bind potentially damaging species such as transition metals may represent another mechanism by which it is neuroprotective. However, if high-affinity binding capacity is overcome, low-affinity binding may result in iron overload prone to leak back iron into the cytosol (Ben-Shachar et al., 1991; Double et al., 1999). Alternatively, it is possible that iron bound to neuromelanin may remain redox-active. Although ferrous iron bound to synthetic melanin is reported to be not very efficient for decomposing hydrogen peroxide in vitro (Pilas, Sarna, Kalyanaraman, & Swartz, 1988), redox-active iron has recently been reported on neuromelanin granules in both the normal and the parkinsonian brain (Castellani, Siedlak, Perry, & Smith, 2000). It is suggested from structural analysis using nuclear magnetic resonance spectroscopy and electron paramagnetic resonance spectroscopy that neuromelanin isolated from parkinsonian brain may have decreased ability to bind iron (Aime et al., 2000; Lopiano et al., 2000). Consequently, a reduction in iron-binding ability of neuromelanin would render catecholaminergic neurons more vulnerable due to increased redox-capable iron levels (Double et al., 2002). In fact, Faucheux, Martin, Beaumont, and Hirsch (2003) investigated the redox activity of neuromelanin aggregates in a group of parkinsonian patients, who presented a statistically significant reduction (–70%) in the number of melanized neurons and an increased non-heme ironIII content as compared with a group of matched control subjects. The level of redox activity detected in neuromelanin aggregates was significantly increased (+69%) in parkinsonian patients and was highest in patients with the most severe neuronal loss. This change was not observed in tissue in the immediate vicinity of melanized neurons. These results strongly support the hypothesis that neuromelanin–iron interactions are involved in neurodegeneration in PD. However, whether neuromelanin acts as a toxifying or detoxifying component in PD depends on the human SN intracellular environment and, most probably, the stage of the disease.

Important further clues to the understanding of elevated cerebral iron are provided by the findings of mutated genes relevant for iron metabolism in other neurodegenerative disorders (Table 7) such as HFE, the gene most commonly mutated in patients with hereditary hemochromatosis, and of TFR2, a mutated transferrin receptor, which is important in non-HFE-associated iron-overload disorders. How these mutated genes operate and interact to induce abnormal brain iron metabolism, transport, and accumulation in the CNS and how iron in turn interacts with proteins (e.g., α-synuclein) causing them to aggregate into toxic inclusions are under current investigation as emphasized below.

Table 7
**Disorders of Iron Metabolism and Their Expressed Mutated Genes**

| | *Defect in Ferritin Accumulation (Relevance in PD)* |
|---|---|
| DCYTB | Mutated iron transporter |
| Ferroportin1 | Iron exporter across membrane |
| FTL | Ferritin light polypeptide (abnormal ferritin accumulation) |
| HFE | Hemochromatosis protein (iron metabolism, relevance in PD) |
| Ireg1 | Iron-regulated transporter gene |
| IRP2 | Iron-regulated protein 2 (degeneration, ataxia, bradykinesia) |
| MTP1 | Mouse transition protein 1 |

(*Continued*)

Table 7
**(Continued)**

| | *Defect in Ferritin Accumulation (Relevance in PD)* |
|---|---|
| NRAMP1 | Iron transporter (relevance in Multiple sclerosis) |
| Nramp2 | Iron importer |
| P53 | Mutations in Wilson's disease, PD and hemochromatosis |
| PANK2 | Pantothenate kinase defect (PD and Hallervorden Syndrome) |
| Sfxn1 | Mutated transmembrane protein (important for iron utilization) |
| SLC11A3 | Ferroprotein gene |
| Tfc2 | Mutated transferrin receptor (relevance in Alzheimer's disease) |
| TFR2 | Mutated transferrin receptor (linked to neurodegeneration) |
| YFH1 | Friedreich's ataxia (mitochondrial iron accumulation, neurodegeneration) |

Adapted from Youdim (2003) with kind permission from Springer Wien, New York, as well as from Youdim and Riederer (2003) with kind permission from Elsevier Amsterdam.

## 9. CONSEQUENCES OF IRON OVERLOAD IN THE PARKINSONIAN SUBSTANTIA NIGRA

There are suggestive findings that iron is triggering protein aggregation in Lewy bodies, the major neuropathological hallmark of PD. Lewy bodies contain many lipids and proteins, including ubiquitin, tyrosine hydroxylase, nitrosylated iron regulatory protein 2 (IRP2), and α-synuclein. The association of mutations in α-synuclein and familial PD (Polymeropoulos, Lavedan, & Leroy, 1997; Krüger et al., 1998; Mizuno, Hattori, & Kitada, 2001) and the accumulation of α-synuclein in Lewy bodies (178–180) (Spillantini, Schmidt, & Lee, 1997; Markopoulou, Wszolek, & Pfeiffer, 1999) suggest that α-synuclein may be part of the pathogenetic mechanism at least in familial PD. α-Synuclein associated with the presynaptic vesicles tends to self-aggregation, but as long as it is associated with the presynaptic membrane, it is not toxic (Spillantini et al., 1998). Recent studies showed that it forms stable aggregates in the presence of iron or calcium (181–183) (Ostrerova-Golts et al., 2000; Turnbull et al., 2001; Nielsen, Vorum, Lindersson, & Joseph, 2001). Iron-catalyzed oxidative reactions convert α-helical α-synuclein conformation into β-pleated sheet conformation, which is the form of synuclein found in Lewy bodies and glial cytoplasmic inclusions (Hashimoto, Rockenstein, & Masliah, 2003; Hashimoto et al., 1999; Paik, Shin, & Lee, 1999; Paik, Lee, Cho, Lee, & Chang, 2003). Furthermore, it has been shown in vitro that α-synuclein promotes the production of hydroxyl radicals as detected with spin trapping agents by electron spin resonance spectroscopy in the presence of ironII (Turnbull et al., 2001; Tabner, Turnbull, El-Agnaf, & Allsop, 2002). Crosslinking of α-synuclein may in addition be promoted by advanced glycation end products (Münch et al., 2000). Interestingly, the formation of advanced glycation end products is accelerated by iron since the reaction products formed (Amadori products) from reducing sugars with primary or secondary amino groups are further oxidized. These advanced glycation end products may be involved in protein crosslinking in various neurodegenerative diseases (Münch, Gasic-Milenkovic, & Arendt, 2003).

Very interestingly, catecholamines stabilize oligomers by covalent ligation (Conway, Rochet, Bieganski, & Lansbury, 2001). Thus, iron-catalyzed oxidation of catechols may lead to α-synuclein protofibrils. Protofibrils of α-synuclein interact with membranes of vesicles and mitochondria, leading to transient permeabilization and leakage of transmitters or mitochondrial factors triggering cell death (Tabrizi et al., 2001; Hsu, Sagarra, & Arroyo, 2001; Saha, Ninkina, & Hanger, 2001). In addition, α-synuclein may bind iron leading to aggregation of α-synuclein (Wolozin & Olts, 2002; Kim, Choi, & Kwon, 2002; Youdim, Eshel, & Ben-Shachar, 2003). In this process mainly, the oligomers, not the mature aggregates of α-synuclein, appear to be selectively toxic to dopaminergic neurons (197–201) (Forloni, Bertani, & Calella, 2001; Lo Bianco, Ridet, Schneider, Deglon, & Aebischer, 2002; Volles et al., 2001; Volles & Lansbury, 2002; Volles & Lansbury, 2003).

One of the most significant features of 6-hydroxydopamine and MPTP-induced dopaminergic neurotoxicity is that both these neurotoxins induce a selective increase of iron in SN pars compacta of rats, mice, and monkeys (Youdim, Eshel, & Ben-Shachar, 2003; Youdim et al., 2004; Youdim, 2003; Youdim & Riederer, 2003; Oestreicher, Sengstock, Riederer, & Olanow, 1994; Sengstock, Zawia, Olanow, Dunn, & Arendash, 1997; Ben-Shachar et al., 1991; Ben-Shachar, Kahana, Kampel, Warshawsky, & Youdim, 2004; Ben-Shachar & Youdim, 1991). While iron deficiency is not perceived as a life-threatening disorder, it is the most prevalent nutritional abnormality in the world, and a better understanding of modes and sites of action can help devise better treatment programs for those who suffer from it. Nowhere this is more important than in young infants and children that make up the bulk iron deficiency in the society. Although the effects of iron deficiency have been extensively studied in systemic organs, until very recently little attention was paid to its effects on brain function. The studies of Oski at Johns Hopkin Medical School in 1974 demonstrating the impairment of learning in young school children with iron deficiency prompted us to study its relevance to brain biochemistry and function in animal model of iron deficiency. Indeed, rats made iron-deficient have lowered brain iron and impaired behavioral and learning. This can become irreversible, specially in newborn animals, even after long-term iron supplementation. We have shown that in this condition it is the brain striatal dopaminergic-opiate system which becomes defective, resulting in alterations in circadian behaviors, cognitive impairment, and neurochemical changes closely associated with them. More recently, we have extended these studies and have established the cognitive impairment may be closely associated with neuroanatomical damage and zinc metabolism in the hippocampus due to iron deficiency and which may result from abnormal cholinergic function. The hippocampus is the focus of many studies today, since this brain structure has high zinc concentration and is highly involved in many forms of cognitive deficits as a consequence of cholinergic deficiency and has achieved prominence in dementia in ageing and Alzheimer's disease. Thus, it is now apparent that cognitive impairment may not be attributed to a single neurotransmitter, but rather alterations and interactions of several in different brain regions. In animal model of iron deficiency, it is apparent that dopaminergic interaction with the opiate system and cholinergic neurotransmission may be defective. The levels of iron in postmortem brains from patients with Parkinson's disease as compared to those from individuals not suffering from neurological disorders are increased with the severity of neuropathological changes in Parkinson's disease substantia nigra pars compacta (SNpc), presumably due to increased transport through the BBB in late stages of parkinsonism. Glial iron is mainly stored as ferric iron in ferritin, whilst neuronal iron is predominantly bound to neuromelanin. Iron overload may induce progressive degeneration of nigro-striatal neurons by facilitating oxidative stress and the formation or reactive biological intermediates including reactive oxygen species (ROS) and the formation of cytotoxic protein aggregates. There are indications that iron-mediated neuronal death in Parkinson's disease proceeds retrogradely. These results are also discussed with respect to their relevance for disease progression in relation to cytotoxic α-synuclein protofibril formation and relation to the MPTP (*N*-methyl-4-phenyl-1,2,3,6-tetrahydropyridine) and 6-hydroxydoapmine models of PD, where similar increases in iron are seen in SNpc and iron chelators are neuroprotective in these models. Desferal and VK-28 and multifunctional iron chelator M30 (Ben-Shachar et al., 2004; Zheng, Weiner, et al., 2005; Zheng, Gal, et al., 2005; Gal, Zheng, Fridkin, & Youdim, 2005; Zhu et al., 2007) pretreatment are neuroprotective against these neurotoxins (Ben-Shachar et al., 1991, 2004; Ben-Shachar & Youdim, 1991) and prevent the appearance of iron, IRP2 (iron-responsive protein 2), and α-synuclein in SN pars compacta. These results might encourage clinical studies in the future with the aim to slow down disease progression in PD and possibly other neurodegenerative diseases as well (Zecca et al., 2004).

## 10. CONCLUSION

The effect of iron deficiency on brain function is relatively a new subject. Never the less, it is clear from animal studies that ID can profoundly affect the CNS structural components, neurons, its neurotransmitter metabolism and function. The most obvious systems that are affected are the dopaminergic and enkephalinergic systems which interact with each other. This may not be unexpected since iron plays a crucial role in many physiological processes. Furthermore, iron metabolism is one of the most tightly regulated events within the cells, since both its deficiency and its excess can effect many enzymatic and structural proteins. Thus, iron homeostasis is crucial for the brain function. What is obvious is that the abnormality of iron in brain metabolism and function has not received as much attention as in the studies in systemic organs; this may be related to the notion that brain was impervious to such changes. For example, it is now well recognized that there are a number of very important neurodegenerative diseases (Freidriech ataxia, Parkinson's disease, Alzheimer's disease, Hallervorden-Spatz disease, Wilson's disease) where iron has access to the brain by accumulating in specific neurons and may be involved in the neurodegenerative processes in these diseases.

This short chapter has dealt with the effects of ID on the dopamine–opiate system in the striatum and its interaction with hippocampal zinc metabolism and function, mainly because little attention has been paid to other brain neurotransmitter systems (e.g., GABA, glutamate, nitric oxide), which could also be affected (Li, 1998). Because dopamine–opiate interaction plays such a crucial central role in the brain neurotransmission and effects other neuronal systems, it is most likely that the effects of nutritional ID on brain are more complex than so far studied (Youdim & Yehuda, 2000).

Finally, more recent work from our own laboratory has indicated that brain iron deficiency is a two-edged sword. Although throughout this chapter we have demonstrated that deficiency of iron can profoundly affect brain biochemistry and function, we now have evidence that in certain circumstances iron deficiency can be protective to the adult brain. Thus, rats made iron-deficient, where brain iron fall by about 30%, are less susceptible to brain neurodegeneration in response to neurotoxins (such as kainate and 6-hydroxydopamine), which are used as tools for animal models of epilepsy and Parkinson's disease (Li, 1998; Shoham, Glinka, Tanne, & Youdim, 1996). These neurotoxins induce neurodegeneration by a mechanism that initiates oxidative stress and proliferation of reactive microglia that generate the reactive oxygen species. The mechanism of neurotoxin-dependent neurodegeneration has been attributed to the ability of these neurotoxins to release ferritin-dependent chelatable iron and the participation of the metal in redox generation of oxygen radical species, with the consequential onset of oxidative stress, which includes activation and proliferation of reactive microglia. Under the condition of reduced brain iron, these neurotoxins do not induce proliferation of reactive microglia. Thus it is suspected that generation of reactive oxygen species is limited. There might be interactions of several pathogenetic pathways being active on the background of normal human brain aging and aggravated by individual susceptibility that lead to the histopathological changes in PD because complete pathology cannot be mimicked so far in mice that solely overexpressed α-synuclein (Matsuoka et al., 2001; Dong, Ferger, Feldon, & Bueler, 2002), or following intranigral iron injections to rats (Youdim et al., 2003, 2004; Youdim, 2003; Youdim & Riederer, 2003; Oestreicher et al., 1994; Sengstock et al., 1997; Ben-Shachar et al., 1991, 2004; Ben-Shachar & Youdim, 1991). Iron chelators desferal and VK-28 and multifunctional iron chelator M30 (Zheng, Weiner, et al., 2005; Zheng, Gal, et al., 2005; Gal et al., 2005; Zhu et al., 2007) have neuroproctive and neurorestorative activity in animal models of Parkinson's disease. Future research using viral vectors to increase cerebral overexpression of putatively pathogenetic proteins in rodents may elucidate the complex interactions between iron, oxidative stress, and protein aggregation in neurodegeneration and hopefully pave the way for the development of novel therapeutic strategies to combat neurodegeneration.

## REFERENCES


Adhami, V. M., Husain, R., Husain, R., & Seth, P. K. (1996). Influence of iron deficiency and lead treatment on behavior and cerebellar and hippocampal polyamine levels in neonatal rats. *Neurochemical Research, 21*(8), 915–922.

Aime, S., Bergamasco, B., Casu, M., Digilio, G., Fasano, M., Giraudo, S., et al. (2000). Isolation and 13C-NMR characterization of an insoluble proteinaceous fraction from substantia nigra of patients with Parkinson's disease. *Movement Disorder, 15*(5), 977–981.

Angulo, J. A. (1992). Involvement of dopamine D1 and D2 receptors in the regulation of proenkephalin mRNA abundance in the striatum and accumbens of the rat brain. *Journal of Neurochemistry, 58*(3), 1104–1109.

Bartzokis, G., Cummings, J. L., Markham, C. H., Marmarelis, P. Z., Treciokas, L. J., Tishler, T. A., et al. (1999, February). MRI evaluation of brain iron in earlier- and later-onset Parkinson's disease and normal subjects. *Magn Reson Imaging, 17*(2), 213–222.

Bayer, S. A. (1985). Hippocampal region. In G. Paxinos (Ed.), *The rat nervous system* (pp. 335–352). Australia: Academic Press.

Becker, G. J., Seufert, U., Bogdahn Reichmann, H., & Reiners, K. (1995). Degeneration of substantia nigra in chronic Parkinson's disease visualized by transcranial color-coded real-time sonography. *Neurology, 45*, 182–184.

Ben-Shachar, D., Ashkenazi, R., & Youdim, M. B. H. (1986). Long term consequences of early iron-deficiency on dopaminergic neurotransmission. *International Journal of Developmental Neuroscience, 4*, 81–88.

Ben-Shachar, D., Yehuda, S., Finberg, J. P. M., Spanier, I., & Youdim, M. B. H. (1988). Selective alteration in blood brain barrier and insulin transport in iron-deficient rat. *Journal of Neurochemistry, 50*, 1434–1437.

Ben-Shachar, D., & Youdim, M. B. H. (1991). Intranigral iron injection induces behavioural and biochemical "parkinsonism" in rats. *Journal of Neurochemistry, 57*, 2133–2135.

Ben-Shachar, D., Eshel, G., Finberg, J. P., & Youdim, M. B. H. (1991). The iron chelator desferrioxamine (Desferal) retards 6-hydroxydopamine-induced degeneration of nigrostriatal dopamine neurons. *Journal of Neurochemistry, 56*, 1441–1444.

Ben-Shachar, D., Riederer, P., & Youdim, M. B. H. (1991). Iron-melanin interaction and lipid peroxidation: Implications for Parkinson's disease. *Journal of Neurochemistry, 57*, 1609–1614.

Ben-Shachar, D., Kahana, N., Kampel, V., Warshawsky, A., & Youdim, M. B. H. (2004). Neuroprotection by a novel brain permeable iron chelator, VK-28, against 6-hydroxydopamine lesion in rats. *Neuropharmacology, 46*, 254–263.

Berg, D., Becker, G., & Zeiler, B. (1999). Vulnerability of the nigrostriatal system as detected by transcranial ultrasound. *Neurology, 53*, 1026–1031.

Berg, D., Gerlach, M., Youdim, M. B. H., & Riederer, P. (2001). Brain iron pathways and their relevance to Parkinson's disease. *Journal of Neurochemistry, 79*, 225–236.

Berg, D., Roggendorf, W., Schröder, U., Klein, R., Tatschner, T., Benz, P., et al. (2002). Echogenicity of the substantia nigra: Association with increased iron content and marker for susceptibility to nigrostriatal injury. *Archive of Neurology, 599*, 999–1005.

Berg, D., Siefker, C., Ruprecht-Dörfler, P., & Becker, G. (2001). Echo pattern of substantia nigra and its relevance for motor function and motility in elderly subjects. *Neurology, 56*, 13–17.

Björklund, A., & Kirik, D. (2003). Modeling CNS neurodegeneration by overexpression of disease-causing proteins using viral vectors. *TINS*, *26*, 386–392.

Bliss, T. V., & Collingridge, G. L. (1993). A synaptic model of memory: Long-term potentiation in the hippocampus. *Nature*, *361*(6407), 31–39.

Boyer, R., Grabill, Y., & Petrovich, R. (1988). Reactive release of ferritin iron: A kinetic assay. *Analytical Biochemistry*, *174*, 17–22.

Castellani, R., Siedlak, S., Perry, G., & Smith, A. (2000). Sequestration of iron by Lewy bodies in Parkinson's disease. *Acta Neuropathology*, *100*, 111–114.

Chua, A. C., & Morgan, E. H. (1996). Effect of iron deficiency and iron overload on manganese uptake and deposition in the brain and other organs of the rat. *Biological Trace Element Research*, *55*(1–2), 39–54.

Connor, J. R., Boeshore, K. L., Benkovic, S. A., & Menzies, S. L. (1994). Isoforms of ferritin have aspecific cellular distribution in the brain. *Journal of Neuroscience Research*, *37*, 461–465.

Connor, J., Menzies, S., St. Martin, S., & Mufson, G. L. (1990). The cellular distribution of transferrin, ferritin and iron in the human brain. *Journal of Neuroscience Research*, *27*, 595–611.

Connor, J. R., & Menzies, S. L. (1996). Relationship of iron to oligodendrocytes and myelination. *GLIA*, *17*(2), 83–93.

Connor, J. R., Pavlick, G., Karli, D., Menzies, S. L., & Palmer, C. (1995). A histochemical study of iron-positive cells in the developing rat brain. *Journal of Comparative Neurology*, *355*, 111–123.

Connor, J. R., Pillips, T. M., Lakshman, M. R., Baron, K. D., Fine, R. E. & Csiza, C. K. (1987). Regional variation in the levels of transferrin in the CNS of normal and myelin-deficient rats. *Journal of Neurochemistry*, *49*(5), 1523–1529.

Conway, K. A., Rochet, J. C., Bieganski, R. M., & Lansbury, P. T., Jr. (2001). Kinetic stabilization of the alpha-synuclein protofibril by a dopamine alpha-synuclein adduct. *Science*, *294*, 1346–1349.

Dallman, P. R., Siimes, M. A., & Manies, E. C. (1975). Brain iron: Persistent deficiency following short-term iron deprivation in the young rat. *British Journal of Haematology*, *31*(3), 209–215.

Dallman, P. R., & Spirito, R. A. (1977). Brain iron in the rat: Extremely slow turnover in normal rats may explain the long-lasting effects of early iron deficiency. *Journal of Nutrition*, *107*, 1075–1081.

De los Monteros, A. E., Korsak, R. A., Tran, T., Vu, D., de Vellis, J., & Edmond, J. (2000). Dietary iron and the integrity of the developing rat brain: A study with the artificially-reared rat pup. *Cellular Molecular Biology (Noisy-le-grand)*, *46*, 501–515.

Dexter, D., Florence, A., Aouad, F., Hider, R., Jenner, P., & Crichton, R. R. (1995). Brain iron in the ferrocene-loaded rat: Its chelation and influence on dopamine metabolism. *Biochemical Pharmacology*, *49*(12), 1821–6.

Dexter, D. T., Carayon, A., Javoy-Agid, F., Agid, Y., Marsden, D., & Jenner, P. (1991). Alterations in the levels of iron, ferritin and other trace metals in Parkinson's disease and other neurodegenerative diseases affecting the basal ganglia. *Brain*, *114*, 1953–1975.

Dexter, D. T., Sian, J., Rose, S., Marsden, D., & Jenner, P. (1994). Indices of oxidative stress and mitochondrial function in individuals with incidental Lewy body disease. *Annals of Neurology*, *35*, 38–44.

Dexter, D. T., Wells, F. R., Agid, J., Agid, Y., Marsden, D., & Jenner, P. (1987). Increased nigral iron content in post-mortem parkinsonian brain. *Lancet*, *341*, 1219–1220.

Dexter, D. T., Wells, F. R., Lees, A. J., Marsden, D., & Jenner, P. (1989). Increased nigral iron content and alterations in other metal ions occurring in brain in Parkinson's disease. *Journal of Neurochemistry*, *52*, 1830–1836.

Dexter, D. T., Brooks, D. J., Harding, A. E., Burn, D. J., Muller, D. P., Goss-Sampson, M. A., Jenner, P. G., & Marsden, C. D. (1994). Nigrostriatal function in vitamin E deficiency: clinical, experimental, and positron emission tomographic studies. *Annals of Neurology*, *35*(3), 298–303.

Dhur, A., Galan, P., & Hercberg, S. (1990). Effect of decreased food consumption during iron deficiency upon growth rate and iron status indicators in the rat. *Annals of Nutrition and Metabolism*, *34*, 280–287.

Dobbing, J. (1990a). Vulnerable periods in developing brain. In J. Dobbing (Ed.), *Brain behavior and iron in the infant diet* (pp. 1–26). New York: Springer-Verlag.

Dobbing, J. (Ed.). (1990b). *Brain behavior and iron in the infant diet*. Berlin: Springer-Verlag.

Dong, Z., Ferger, B., Feldon, J., & Bueler, H. (2002). Overexpression of Parkinson's disease associated alpha-synuclein A53T by recombinant adeno-associated virus in mice does not increase the vulnerability of dopaminergic neurons to MPTP. *Journal of Neurochemistry and Neurobiology*, *53*, 1–10.

Double, K. L., Ben-Shachar, D., Youdim, M. B. H., & Riederer, P. (2002). Influence of neuromelanin on oxidative pathways within the human substantia nigra. *Neurotoxicology and Teratology*, *24*, 621–628.

Double, K. L., Gerlach, M., Schünemann, V., Ben Shachar, D., Youdim, M. B. H., & Riederer, P. (2003). Iron-binding characteristics of neuromelanin of the human substantia nigra. *Biochemical Pharmacology*, *66*, 489–494.

Double, K. L., Gerlach, M., Youdim, M. B. H., & Riederer, P. (2000). Impaired iron homeostasis in Parkinson's disease. *Journal of Neural Transmission*, *60*(Suppl.), 37–58.

Double, K. L., Maywald, M., Schmittel, M., & Riederer, P. (1997). In vitro studies of ferritin iron release and neurotoxicity. *Journal of Neurochemistry*, *70*, 2492–2499.

Double, K. L., Riederer, P., & Gerlach, M. (1998). The role of iron in 6-hydroxydopamine neurotoxicity. *Advances in Neurology*, *80*, 287–296.

Double, K. L., Riederer, P., & Gerlach, M. (1999). The significance of neuromelanin in Parkinson's disease. *Drug News Development*, *12*, 333–340.

Double, K. L., Zecca, L., Costi, P., Gerlach, M., & Riederer, P. (2000). Structural characteristics of human substantia nigra neuromelanin and synthetic dopamine melanins. *Journal of Neurochemistry*, *75*, 2583–2589.

Durham, R. A., Johnson, J. D., Moore, K. E., & Lookingland, K. J. (1996, September 2). Evidence that D2 receptor-mediated activation of hypothalamic tuberoinfundibular dopaminergic neurons in the male rat occurs via inhibition of tonically active afferent dynorphinergic neurons. *Brain Research*, *732*(1–2), 113–120.

Dwork, A. J. (1995). Effects of diet and development upon the uptake and distribution of cerebral iron. *Journal of Neurological Sciences*, *134*(Suppl.), 45–51.

Dwork, A. J., Lawler, G., Zybert, P. A., & Durkin, M. (1990, June 4). An autoradiographic study of the uptake and distribution of iron by the brain of the young rat. *Brain Research*, *518*(1–2), 31–39.

Dwork, A. J., Schon, E. A., & Herbert, J. (1988). Non-identical distribution of transferrin and ferric iron in human brain. *Neuroscience*, *27*, 333–345.

Earle, K. M. (1968). Studies in Parkinson's disease including x-ray fluorescent spectroscopy of formalin-fixed tissues. *Journal of Neuropathology and Experimental Neurology*, *27*, 1–14.

Eisenstein, R. S., & Blemings, K. P. (1998). Iron regulatory proteins, iron responsive elements and iron homeostasis. *Journal of Nutrition*, *128*(12), 2295–2298.

Erikson, K. M., Pinero, D. J., Connor, J. R., & Beard, J. L. (1997). Regional brain iron, ferritin and transferrin concentrations during iron deficiency and iron repletion in developing rats. *Journal of Nutrition*, *127*(10), 2030–2038.

Essatara, M. B., Levine, A. S., Morley, J. E., & McClain, C. J. (1984). Zinc deficiency and anorexia in rats: Normal feeding patterns and stress induced feeding. *Physiology and Behavior*, *32*, 469–474.

Faucheux, B. A., Martin, M. E., Beaumont, C., & Hirsch, E. (2003). Neuromelanin associated redox-active iron is increased in the substantia nigra of patients with Parkinson's disease. *Journal of Neurochemistry*, *86*, 1142–1148.

Felt, B. T., & Lozoff, B. (1996). Brain iron and behavior of rats are not normalized by treatment of iron deficiency anemia during early development. *Journal of Nutrition*, *126*(3), 693–701.

Forloni, G., Bertani, I., & Calella, A. M. (2001). α-Synuclein and Parkinson's disease: Selective neurodegenerative effect of α-synuclein fragment on dopaminergic neurons in vitro and in vivo. *Annnals of Neurology*, *47*, 632–640.

Frederickson, C. J., Klitenick, M. A., Manton, W. I., & Kirkpatrick, J. B. (1983). Cytoarchitectonic distribution of zinc in the hippocampus of man and the rat. *Brain Research*, *273*, 335–339.

Friedman, A., & Galazka-Friedman, J. (2001). The current state of free radicals in Parkinson's disease. Nigral iron as a trigger of oxidative stress. In D. Calne & S. Calne (Eds.), *Parkinson's disease: Advances in neurology* (Vol. 86, pp. 137–142). Philadelphia, PA: Lippincott Williams & Wilkins.

Gal, S., Zheng, H., Fridkin, M., & Youdim, M. B. H. (2005). Novel multifunctional neuroprotective iron chelator-monoamine oxidase inhibitor drugs for neurodegenerative diseases. In vivo selective brain monoamine oxidase inhibition and prevention of MPTP-induced striatal dopamine depletion. *Journal of Neurochemistry*, *95*(1), 79–88.

Galazka-Friedman, J., Bauminger, E. R., Friedman, A., Barcikowska, M., Hechel, D., & Nowik, I. (1996). Iron in parkinsonian and control substantia nigra, a Mössbauer spectroscopy study. *Movement Disorder*, *11*, 8–16.

Georgieff, M. K., Petry, C. D., Wobken, J. D., & Oyer, C. E. (1996). Liver and brain iron deficiency in newborn infants with bilateral renal agenesis (Potter's syndrome). *Pediatric Pathology and Laboratory Medicine*, *16*(3), 509–519.

Gerlach, M., Ben-Shachar, D., Riederer, P., & Youdim, M. B. (1994). Altered brain metabolism of iron as a cause of neurodegenerative diseases. *Journal of Neurochemistry*, *63*(3), 793–807.

Gerlach, M., Double, K., Riederer, P., & Youdim, M. B. H. (1997). Iron in the parkinsonian substantia nigra. *Movement Disorder*, *12*, 258–260.

Gerlach, M., Double, K. L., Ben-Shachar, D., Youdim, M. B. H., & Riederer, P. (2003). Neuromelanin and its interaction with iron as a potential risk factor for dopaminergic neurodegeneration underlying Parkinson's disease. *Neurotoxicity Research*, *5*, 35–44.

Gerlach, M., Trautwein, A. X., Zecca, L., Riererer, P., & Youdim, M. B. H. (1995). Mössbauer spectroscopic studies of human neuromelanin isolated from the substantia nigra. *Journal of Neurochemistry*, *65*, 923–926.

Gibb, W. (1992). Melanin, tyrosine hydroxylase, calbindin and substance P in the human midbrain and substantia nigra in relation to nigrostriatal projections and differential neuron susceptibility in Parkinson's disease. *Brain Research, 581*, 283–291.

Gomori, G. (1993). Microtechnical demonstration of iron. *American Journal of Pathology, 12*, 655–663.

Good, P. F., Olanow, C. W., & Perl, D. P. (1992). Neuromelanin-containing neurons of the substantia nigra accumulate iron and aluminum in Parkinson's disease. A LAMMA study. *Brain Research, 593*, 343–346.

Gorell, J. M., Johnson, C. C., Rybicki, B. A., Peterson, E. L., Kortsha, G. X., Brown, G. G., et al. (1997). Occupational exposures to metals as risk factors for Parkinson's disease. *Neurology, 48*, 650–658.

Gorell, J. M., Johnson, C. C., Rybicki, B., Peterson, E. L., Kortsha, G. X., Brown, G. G., et al. (1999). Occupational exposure to manganese, copper, lead, iron, mercury, and zinc and the risk of Parkinson's disease. *Neurotoxicology, 20*, 239–247.

Gorell, J. M., Ordidge, R. J., Brown, G. G., Deniau, J. C., Buderer, N. M., & Helpern, J. A. (1995). Increased iron-related MRI contrast in the substantia nigra in Parkinson's disease. *Neurology, 45*, 1138–1143.

Gosnell, B. A., Levine, A. S., & Morley, J. E. (1986). The stimulation of food intake by selective agonists of mu, kappa and delta opioid receptors. *Life Sciences, 38*(12), 1081–1088.

Götz, M. E., Künig, G., Riederer, P., & Youdim, M. B. H. (1994). Oxidative stress: Free radical production in neural degeneration. *Pharmacology and Therapeutics, 63*, 37–122.

Griffiths, P. D., & Crossman, A. R. (1993). Distribution of iron in the basal ganglia and neocortex in postmortem tissue in Parkinson's disease and Alzheimer's disease. *Dementia, 4*(2), 61–65.

Griffiths, P. D., Dobson, B. R., Jones, G. R., & Clarke, D. T. (1999). Iron in the basal ganglia in Parkinson's disease. An in vitro study using extended X-ray absorption fine structure and cryo-electron microscopy. *Brain, 122*, 667–673.

Guesry, P. (1998). The role of nutrition in brain development. *Prevention Medicine, 27*(2), 189–194.

Gulya, K., Kovacs, G. L., & Kasa, P. (1991). Partial depletion of endogenous zinc level by (DPen2, D-Pen5) enkephalin in the rat brain. *Life Sciences, 48*(12), PL57–PL62.

Haile, D. J. (1999). Regulation of genes of iron metabolism by the iron-response proteins. *American Journal of Medical Sciences, 318*(4), 230–240.

Hallgren, B., & Sourander, P. (1958). The effect of age on the non-haemin iron in the human brain. *Journal of Neurochemistry, 3*, 41–51.

Halliwell, B., & Gutteridge, J. (1986). Iron and free radical reactions: Two aspects of antioxidant protection. *Trends in Biological Sciences, 11*, 1372–1375.

Han, J., Day, J. R., Thomson, K., Connor, J. R., & Beard, J. L. (2000). Iron deficiency alters H- and L-ferritin expression in rat brain. *Cellular Molecular Biology (Noisy-le-grand), 46*, 517–528.

Hansen, T. M., Nielsen, H., Bernth, N., & Moos, T. (1999). Expression of ferritin protein and subunit mRNAs in normal and iron deficient rat brain. *Molecular Brain Research, 65*, 186–197.

Hashimoto, M., Hsu, L. J., Xia, Y., Takeda, A., Sisk, A., Sundsmo, M., et al. (1999). Oxidative stress induces amyloid-like aggregate formation of NACP/α-synuclein in vitro. *Neuroreport, 10*, 717–721.

Hashimoto, M., Rockenstein, E., & Masliah, E. (2003). Transgenic models of α-synuclein pathology. *Annals of New York Academy of Sciences, 991*, 171–188.

Hegg, C. C., & Thayer, S. A. (1999). Monocytic cells secrete factors that evoke excitatory synaptic activity in rat hippocampal cultures. *European Journal of Pharmacology, 385*(2–3), 231–237.

Hill, J. M. (1988). The distribution of iron in the brain. In M. B. H. Youdim (Ed.), *Brain iron: neurochemistry and behavioural aspects* (pp. 1–24). London: Taylor and Francis.

Hirsch, E. C. (1994). Biochemistry of Parkinson's disease with special reference to the dopaminergic systems. *Molecular Neurobiology, 9*, 135–142.

Hirsch, E. C., Brandel, J.-P., Galle, P., Agid, Y. A., & Agid, J. (1991). Iron and aluminum increase in the substantia nigra of patients with Parkinson's disease: An x-ray microanalysis. *Journal of Neurochemistry, 56*, 446–451.

Hirsch, E. C., Graybiel, A. M., & Agid, Y. A. (1988). Melanized dopaminergic neurons are differentially susceptible to degeneration in Parkinson's disease. *Nature, 334*, 345–348.

Howell, G. A., Welch, M. G., & Frederickson, C. J. (1984). Stimulation-induced uptake and release of zinc in hippocampal slices. *Nature (London), 308*, 736–738.

Hsu, L. J., Sagarra, Y., & Arroyo, A. (2001). α-Synuclein promotes mitochondrial deficit and oxidative stress. *American Journal of Pathology, 157*, 401–410.

Iancu, T. C., Perl, D. P., Sternlieb, I., & Olanow, W. (1996). The application of laser microprobe mass analysis to the study of biological material. *Biometals, 9*, 57–65.

Jellinger, K. A. (1999). The role of iron in neurodegeneration: Prospects for pharmacotherapy of Parkinson's disease. *Drugs Aging*, *14*, 115–140.

Jellinger, K. A. (2003). General aspects of neurodegeneration. *Journal of Neural Transmission*, *65*(Suppl.), 101–144.

Jellinger, K., Kienzl, E., Rumpelmair, G., Riederer, P., & Youdim, M. B. H. (1992). Iron-melanin complex in substantia nigra of parkinsonian brains: An x-ray microanalysis. *Journal of Neurochemistry*, *59*, 1168–1171.

Jellinger, K., Kienzl, E., Rumpelmair, G., Riederer, P., & Youdim, M. B. H. (1993). Iron and ferritin in substantia nigra in Parkinson's disease. In H. Narabayashi, T. Nagatsu, N. Yanagisawa, & Y. Mizuno (Eds.), *Parkinson's disease: Advances in neurology* (Vol. 60, pp. 267–272). New York: Raven Press Ltd.

Jellinger, K., Paulus, W., Grundke-Iqbal, I., Riederer, P., & Youdim, M. B. H. (1990). Brain iron and ferritin in Parkinson's and Alzheimer's disease. *Journal of Neural Transmission*, *2*, 327–340.

Kaneko, Y., Kitamoto, T., Tateishi, J., & Yamaguchi, K. (1989). Ferritin immunohistochemistry as a marker for microglia. *Acta Neuropathology (Berl)*, *79*(2), 129–136.

Kastner, A., Hirsch, E., Lejeune, O., Javoy-Agid, F., Rascol, O., & Agid, Y. (1992). Is the vulnerability of neurons in the substantia nigra of patients with Parkinson's disease related to their neuromelanin content? *Journal of Neurochemistry*, *59*, 1080–1089.

Kaur, C., & Ling, E. A. (1995). Transient expression of transferrin receptors and localisation of iron in amoeboid microglia in postnatal rats. *Journal of Anatomy*, *186*(Pt. 1), 165–173.

Kim, K. S., Choi, S. Y., & Kwon, H. Y. (2002). Aggregation of α-synuclein induced by the Cu,Zn-superoxide dismutase and hydrogen peroxide system. *Free Radicals in Biology and Medicine*, *32*, 544–550.

Krüger, R., Kuhn, W., Müller, T., Woitalla, D., Graeber, M., Kösel, S., et al. (1998). Ala30Pro mutation in the gene encoding α-synuclein in Parkinson's disease. *Nature Genetic*, *18*, 106–108.

Lai, B. C. L., Marion, S. A., Teschke, K., & Tsui, A. J. (2002). Occupational and environmental risk factors for Parkinson's disease. *Parkinsonism and Related Disorders*, *8*, 297–309.

Lapenna, D., Degioia, S., & Ciofani, G. (1995). Captopril induces iron release from ferritin and oxidative stress. *Journal of Pharmacy and Pharmacology*, *47*, 1–11.

Lhermitte, J., Kraus, W. M., & McAlpine, D. (1924). On the occurrence of abnormal deposits of iron in the brain in Parkinsonism with special reference to its localisation. *Journal of Neurology and Psychopathology*, *5*, 195–208.

Li, D. (1998). Effect of iron deficiency on iron distribution and gamma-aminobutyric acid (GABA) metabolism in young rat brain tissues. Hokkaido Igaku Zasshi – Hokkaido. *Journal of Medical Sciences*, *73*(3), 215–225.

Linert, W., Herlinger, E., Jameson, R. F., Kienzl, E., Jellinger, K., & Youdim, M. B. H. (1996). Dopamine, 6-hydroxydopamine, iron, and dioxygen, their mutual interactions and possible implication in the development of Parkinson's disease. *Biochimica et Biophysica Acta*, *1316*, 160–168.

Lo Bianco, C., Ridet, J. L., Schneider, B. L., Deglon, N., & Aebischer, P. (2002). α-Synucleinopathy and selective dopaminergic loss in a rat lentiviral-based model of Parkinson's disease. *Proceeding of National Academy of Sciences, USA*, *99*, 10813–10818.

Loeffler, D. A., Connor, J. R., Juncau, P. L., Snyder, B. S., Kanaley, L., DeMaggio, A. J., et al. (1995). Transferrin and iron in normal, Alzheimer's disease, and Parkinson's disease brain regions. *Journal of Neurochemistry*, *65*, 710–716.

Logroscino, G., Marder, K., Graziano, J., Freyer, G., Slavkovich, V., Lojacono, N., et al. (1998). Dietary iron, animal fats, and risk of Parkinson's disease. *Movement Disorder*, *13*(Suppl. 1), 13–16.

Lopiano, L., Chiesa, M., Digilio, D., Giraudo, S., Bergamasco, B., Torre, E., et al. (2000). Q-band EPR investigations of neuromelanin in control and Parkinson's disease patients. *Biochimica et Biophysica Acta*, *1500*, 306–312.

Lozoff, B., & Brittenham, G. M. (1986). Behavioral aspects of iron deficiency. *Progress in Hematology*, *14*, 23–53.

Lozoff, B. (1988). Behavioral alteration in iron deficiency. *Advances in Pediatrics*, *6*, 331–359.

Lozoff, B., Jimenez, E., & Wolf, A. W. (1991). Long-term developmental outcome of infants with iron deficiency. *New England Journal of Medicine*, *325*, 687–694.

Lozoff, B., Wolf, A. W., & Jimenez, E. (1996). Iron-deficiency anemia and infant development: Effects of extended oral iron therapy. *Journal of Pediatric*, *129*, 382–389.

Mann, V. M., Cooper, J. M., & Daniel, S. E. (1994). Complex, I., iron, and ferritin in Parkinson's disease substantia nigra. *Annals of Neurology*, *36*, 876–881.

Markopoulou, K., Wszolek, Z., & Pfeiffer, R. (1999). Reduced expression of the G209A α-synuclein allele in familial parkinsonism. *Annals of Neurology*, *46*, 374–381.

Martin, W. R. W. (2001). Magnetic resonance imaging and spectroscopy in Parkinson's disease. In D. Calne & S. Calne (Eds.), *Parkinson's disease: Advances in neurology* (Vol. 86, pp. 197–203). Philadelphia, PA: Lippincott Williams & Wilkins.

Matsuoka, Y., Vila, M., Lincoln, S., McCormack, A., Picciano, M., LaFrancois, J., et al. (2001). Lack of nigral pathology in transgenic mice expressing human α-synuclein driven by the tyrosine hydroxylase promoter. *Neurobiology of Disease*, *8*, 535–539.

Mizuno, Y., Hattori, N., & Kitada, T. (2001). Familial Parkinson's disease, α-synuclein and parkin. In D. Calne & S. Calne (Eds.), *Parkinson's disease: Advances in neurology* (Vol. 86, pp. 13–21). Philadelphia: Lippincott Williams & Wilkins.

Monteiro, H., & Winterbourn, C. (1988). The superoxide-dependent transfer of iron from ferritin to transferrin and lactoferrin. *The Biochemical Journal*, *256*, 923–928.

Monteiro, H., Ville, G., & Winterbourn, C. (1989). Release of iron from ferritin by semiquinone, anthracycline, bipyridyl and nitroaromatic radicals. *Free Radicals in Biology and Medicine*, *6*, 587–591.

Moos, T., Oates, P. S., & Morgan, E. H. (1998). Expression of the neuronal transferrin receptor is age dependent and susceptible to iron deficiency. *Journal of Comparative Neurology*, *398*(3), 420–430.

Morris, B. J., & Johnston, H. M. (1995). A role for hippocampal opioids in long-term functional plasticity. *Trends in Neuroscience*, *18*, 350–355.

Morris, B. J., Höllt, V., & Herz, A. (1988). Dopaminergic regulation of striatal proenkephalin mRNA and prodynorphin mRNA contrasting effects of D1 and D2 antagonists. *Neuroscience*, *25*(2), 525–532.

Münch, G., Gasic-Milenkovic, J., & Arendt, T. (2003). Effect of advanced glycation endproducts on cell cycle and their relevance for Alzheimer's disease. *Journal of Neural Transmission*, *65*(Suppl.), 63–71.

Münch, G., Lüth, H. J., Wong, A., Arendt, T., Hirsch, E., Ravid, R., et al. (2000). Crosslinking of α-synuclein by advanced glycation endproducts – An early pathophysiological step in Lewy body formation? *Journal of Chemical Neuroanatomy 20*, 253–257.

Nakajima, K., & Kohsaka, S. (1993). Functional roles of microglia in the brain. *Neuroscience Research*, *17*, 187–203.

Ngim, C. H., & Devathasan, G. (1989). Epidemiologic study on the association between body burden mercury level and idiopathic Parkinson's disease. *Neuroepidemiology*, *8*, 128–141.

Nielsen, M. S., Vorum, H., Lindersson, E., & Joseph, P. H. (2001). $Ca2^+$ binding to α-synuclein regulate ligand binding and oligomerization. *Journal of Biological Chemistry*, *276*, 22680–22684.

Oestreicher, E., Sengstock, G. J., Riederer, P., & Olanow, W. (1994). Degeneration of nigrostriatal dopaminergic neurons increases iron within the substantia nigra: A histochemical and neurochemical study. *Brain Research*, *660*, 8–18.

Ostrerova-Golts, N., Petrucelli, L., Hardy, J., Lee, J. M., Farer, M., & Wolozin, B. (2000). The A53T α-synuclein mutation increases iron-dependent aggregation and toxicity. *Journal of Neuroscience*, *20*, 6048–6054.

Owen, A. D., Schapira, A. H. V., & Jenner, P. (1997). Indices of oxidative stress in Parkinson's disease, Alzheimer's disease and dementia with Lewy bodies. *Journal of Neural Transmission*, *51*(Suppl.), 167–173.

Pablo Huidobro-Toro, J., & Leong Way, E. (1983). Opiates. In D. G. Grahame-Smith & P. J. Cowen (Eds.), *Part 1, Preclinical psychopharmacology* (pp. 300–343). Amsterdam: Excerpta Medica.

Pablo Huidobro-Toro, J., & Leong Way, E. (1985). Opiates. In D. G. Grahame-Smith & P. J. Cowen (Eds.), *Part 1. Preclinical psychopharmacology* (pp. 283–343). Amsterdam: Elsevier.

Paik, S. R., Lee, D. Y., Cho, H. J., Lee, E. N., & Chang, C. S. (2003). Oxidized glutathione stimulated the amyloid formation of α-synuclein. *FEBS Letters*, *537*, 63–67.

Paik, S. R., Shin, H., & Lee, J. (1999). Copper(II)-induced self oligomerization of α-synuclein. *The Biochemical Journal*, *340*, 821–828.

Parks, Y. A., & Wharton, B. A. (1989). Iron deficiency and the brain. *Acta Paediatrica Scanddinavia*, *361*, 71–77.

Parks, Y. A., & Wharton, B. (1990). Iron-deficiency and the brain clinical significance of behavioral changes. In J. Dobbing (Ed.), *Brain, behavior and iron in the infant diet* (pp. 157–176). Berlin: Springer-Verlag.

Perry, G., Sayre, L. M., Atwood, C. S., Castellani, R. J., Cash, A. D., Rottkamp, C. A., et al. (2002). The role of iron and copper in the aetiology of neurodegenerative disorders, therapeutic implications. *CNS Drugs*, *16*, 339–352.

Pilas, B., Sarna, T., Kalyanaraman, B., & Swartz, H. M. (1988). The effect of melanin on iron associated decomposition of hydrogen peroxide. *Free Radicals in Biology and Medicine*, *4*, 285–293.

Pinero, D. J., Li, N. Q., Connor, J. R., & Beard, J. L. (2000). Variations in dietary iron alter brain iron metabolism in developing rats. *Journal of Nutrition*, *130*(2), 254–263.

Pollitt, E., Haas, J., & Levitsky, D. A. (Eds.). (1989). International conference of iron deficiency and behavioural development. *American Journal of Clinical Nutrition*, *50*, 565–705.

Pollitt, E., & Leibel, R. L. (Eds.). (1982). Iron-deficiency, brain biochemistry and behavior. New York: Raven Press.

Polymeropoulos, M., Lavedan, C., & Leroy, E. (1997). Mutation in the α-synuclein gene identified in families with Parkinson's disease. *Science*, *276*, 2045–2047.

Powers, K. M., Smith-Weller, T., Franklin, G., Longstreth, W. T. Jr., Swanson, P. D., & Checkoway, H. (2003). Parkinson's disease risks associated with dietary iron, manganese, and other nutrient intakes. *Neurology*, *60*, 1761–1766.

Rao, R., de Ungria, M., Sullivan, D., Wu, P., Wobken, J. D., Nelson, C. A., et al. (1999). Perinatal brain iron deficiency increases the vulnerability of rat hippocampus to hypoxic ischemic insult. *Journal of Nutrition*, *129*(1), 199–206.

Riederer, P., Sofic;E., Rausch, W. D., Birkmyer, W., Riederer, P., & Youdim, M. B. H. (1989). Transition metals, ferritin, glutathione, and ascorbic acid in parkinsonian brains. *Journal of Neurochemistry*, *52*, 515–520.

Riederer, P., Rausch, W. D., Schmidt, B., & Gerlach, M. (1988). Biochemical fundamentals in Parkinson's disease. *Mount Sinai Journal of Medicine*, *55*, 21–28.

Riederer, P., Sofic, E., Rausch, W. D., & Youdim, M. B. H. (1989). Transition metal, ferritin, glutathime and ascorbic acid in Parkinsonian brains. *Journal of Neurochemistry*, *52*, 515–521.

Riederer, P., Sofic, E., & Rausch, W. D. (1985). Dopaminforschung heute und morgen – L-Dopa in der Zunkunft. In P. Riederer & H. Umek (Eds.), *L-Dopa Substitution der Parkinson-Krankheit, Geschichte-Gegenwart-Zukunft* (pp. 127–144). New York: Springer Wien.

Rybicki, B. A., Johnson, C. C., Peterson, E. L., Kortsha, G. X., & Gorell, J. M. (1999). A family history of Parkinson's disease and its effect on other PD risk factors. *Neuroepidemiology*, *18*, 270–278.

Ryvlin, P., Broussolle, E., Piollet, H., Viallet, F., Khalfallah, Y., & Chazot, G. (1995). Magnetic resonance imaging evidence of decreased putamenal iron content in idiopathic Parkinson's disease. *Archives of Neurology*, *52*, 583–588.

Saha, A. R., Ninkina, N. N., & Hanger, D. P. (2001). Induction of neuronal death by α-synuclein. *European Journal of Neuroscience*, *12*, 3073–3077.

Seidler, A., Hellenbrand, W., Robra, B. P., Vieregge, P., Nischan, P., Joerg, J., et al. (1996). Possible environmental, occupational, and other etiologic factors for Parkinson's disease: A case control study in Germany. *Neurology*, *46*, 1275–1284.

Sengstock, G. J., Zawia, N. H., Olanow, C. W., Dunn, A. J., & Arendash, G. W. (1997). Intranigral iron infusion in the rat. Acute elevations in nigral lipid peroxidation and striatal dopaminergic markers with ensuing nigral degeneration. *Biology of Trace Element Research*, *58*, 177–195.

Shima, T., Sarna, T., Stroppolo, A., Gerbasi, R., & Zecca, L. (1997). Binding of iron to neuromelanin of human substantia nigra and synthetic melanin: An electron paramagnetic resonance spectroscopy study. *Free Radicals in Biology and Medicine*, *23*, 110–119.

Shoham, S., Glinka, Y., Tanne, Z., & Youdim, M. B. H. (1996). Brain iron: Function and dysfunction in relation to cognitive processes. In L. Hallberg & N. G. Asp (Eds.), *Iron nutrition in health and disease* (pp. 205–218). London: John Libbey & Co.

Shoham, S., & Youdim, M. B. H. (2000). Iron involvement in neural damage and microgliosis in models of neurodegenerative diseases. *Cellular and Molecular Biology (Noisy-le-grand)*, *46*, 743–760.

Shoham, S., & Youdim, M. B. (2002). The effects of iron deficiency and iron and zinc supplementation on rat hippocampus ferritin. *Journal of Neural Transmission*, *109*(10), 1241–1256.

Shukla, A., Agrawal, K. N., & Shukla, G. S. (1989). Effect of latent iron deficiency on metal levels of rat brain regions. *Biology of Trace Element Research*, *22*, 141–152.

Sipe, J. C., Lee, P., & Beutler, E. (2002). Brain iron metabolism and neurodegenerative disorders. *Developmental Neuroscience*, *24*, 188–196.

Sofić, E., Paulus, W., Jellinger, K., Riederer, P., & Youdim, M. B. H. (1991). Selective increase of iron in substantia nigra zona compacta of parkinsonian brains. *Journal of Neurochemistry*, *56*, 978–982.

Sofić, E., Riederer, P., Heinsen, H., Riederer, P., & Youidim, M. B. H. (1988). Increased iron(III) and total iron content in post-mortem substantia nigra of parkinsonian brain. *Journal of Neural Transmission*, *74*, 199–205.

Spatz, H. (1922). Uber des eisennachewis in gehrin besonders in zentren des extra-pyramidal motorrischen systems. *Neural Psychiatry*, *77*, 261–390.

Spillantini, M. G., Crowther, R. A., Jakes, R., Hasegawa, M., & Goedert, M. (1998). α-Synuclein in filamentous inclusions of Lewy bodies from Parkinson's disease and dementia with Lewy bodies. *Proceedings of National Academy of Sciences USA*, *95*, 6469–6473.

Spillantini, M. G., Schmidt, M. L., & Lee, V. M. (1997). α-Synuclein in Lewy bodies. *Nature*, *388*, 839–840.

Stengaard-Pedersen, K., Fredens, K., & Larson, L. I. (1981). Enkephalin and zinc in the mossy fiber system. *Brain Research*, *212*, 230–233.

Tabner, B. J., Turnbull, S. O., El-Agnaf, O. M. A., & Allsop, D. (2002). Formation of hydrogen peroxide and hydroxyl radicals from Aβ and α-synuclein as a possible mechanism of cell death in Alzheimer's disease and Parkinson's disease. *Free Radicals in Biology and Medicine*, *32*, 1076–1083.

Tabrizi, S. J., Orth, M., Wilkinson, J. M., Taanman, J. W., Warner, T. T., Cooper, J. M., et al. (2001). Expression of mutant α-synuclein causes increased susceptibility to dopamine toxicity. *Human Molecular Genetics*, *9*, 2683–2689.

Tang, F. E., Costa, E., & Schartz, J. P. (1983). Increase of proenkephalin mRNA and enkephalin content of rat striatum after daily injection of haloperidol for 2 to 3 weeks. *Proceedings of National Academy of Sciences USA*, *80*, 3841–3846.

Taylor, E. M., Crowe, A., & Morgan, E. H. (1991). Transferrin and iron uptake by the brain: Effects of altered iron status. *Journal of Neurochemistry*, *57*(5), 1584–1592.

Tikka, T. M., & Koistinaho, J. E. (2001). Minocycline provides neuroprotection against N-methyl-D-aspartate neurotoxicity by inhibiting microglia. *Journal of Immunology*, *166*(12), 7527–7533.

Turnbull, S., Tabner, B. J., El-Agnaf, O. M. A., Moore, S., Davies, Y., & Allsop, D. (2001). α-Synuclein implicated in Parkinson's disease catalyses the formation of hydrogen peroxide in vitro. *Free Radicals in Biology and Medicine*, *30*, 1163–1170.

Uitti, R. J., Rajput, A. H., Rozdilsky, B., Bickis, M., Wollin, T., & Yuen, W. K. (1989). Regional metal concentrations in Parkinson's disease, other chronic neurological diseases, and control brains. *Canadian Journal of Neurology Sciences*, *16*, 310–314.

Volles, M. J., & Lansbury, P. T., Jr. (2002). Vesicle permeabilization by protofibrillar α-synuclein is sensitive to Parkinson's disease-linked mutations and occurs by a pore-like mechanism. *Biochemistry*, *41*, 4595–4602.

Volles, M. J., & Lansbury, P. T., Jr. (2003). Zeroing in on the pathogenic form of alpha-synuclein and its mechanism of neurotoxicity in Parkinson's disease. *Biochemistry*, *42*, 7871–7878.

Volles, M. J., Lee, S. J., Rochet J-C, Shtilerman, M. D., Ding, T. T., Kessler, J. C., & Lansbury, P. T., Jr. (2001). Vesicle permeabilization by protofibrillar α-synuclein: Implications for the pathogenesis and treatment of Parkinson's disease. *Biochemistry*, *40*, 7812–7819.

Walter, T., De Andraca, I., Chadud, P., & Perales, C. G. (1989). Iron deficiency anemia: Adverse effects on infant psychomotor development. *Pediatrics*, *84*, 7–17.

Walter, U., Wittstock, M., Benecke, R., & Dressler, D. (2002). Substantia nigra echogenicity is normal in non-extrapyramidal cerebral disorders but increased in Parkinson's disease. *Journal of Neural Transmission*, *109*, 191–196.

Webb, T. F., & Oski, F. A. (1973). Iron deficiency anemia and scholastic achievements: Behavioral stability and perceptual sensitivity to adolescents. *Journal of Pediatrics*, *82*, 827–830.

Werkman, S., Shifman, L., & Shelly, T. (1964). Psychosocial correlates of iron deficiency in early childhood. *Psychosomatic Medicine*, *26*, 125–134.

Wolozin, B., & Golts, N. (2002). Iron and Parkinson's disease. *Neuroscientist*, *8*, 22–32.

Xie, X., & Smart, T. G. (1994). Modulation of long-term potentiation in rat hippocampal pyramidal neurons by zinc. *Pflugers Archives*, *427*, 481–486.

Ye, F. Q., Allen, P. S., & Martin, W. R. W. (1996). Basal ganglia iron content in Parkinson's disease measured with magnetic resonance. *Movement Disorder*, *11*, 243–249.

Yehuda, S., & Youdim, M. B. H. (1984). The increased opiate action of β-endorphin in iron-deficient rats: The possible involvement of dopamine. *European Journal of Pharmacology*, *105*, 245–251.

Yehuda, S., & Youdim, M. B. H. (1989). Brain iron: A lesson from animal models. *American Journal of Clinical Nutrition*, *50*(Suppl), 618–625.

Yehuda, S. (1990). Neurochemical bases of behavioral effects o brain iron-deficiency in animals. In J. Dobbing (Ed.), *Brain, behavior and iron in the infant diet* (pp. 63–82). Berlin: Springer-Verlag.

Yehuda, S., Youdim, M. B. H., & Mostofsky, M. (1986). Brain iron deficiency causes reduced learning capacity in rats. *Pharmacology Biochemistry and Behavior*, *25*, 141–145.

Yehuda, S., Youdim, M. B. H., & Zamir, N. (2000). Iron-deficiency induces increased brain met-enkaphalin and pain threshold in response to opiate peptides. *Nutri Neurosci. 1*, 78–85.

Yokoi, K., Kimura, M., & Itokawa, Y. (1991). Effect of dietary iron deficiency on mineral levels in tissues of rats. *Biology of Trace Element Research*, *29*, 257–265.

Yoshida, T., Tanaka, M., Sotomatsu, A., & Hirai, S. (1995). Activated microglia cause superoxide- mediated release of iron from ferritin. *Neuroscience Letters*, *190*(1), 21–24.

Youdim, M. B. H. (1985). Brain iron metabolism. Biochemical and behavioural aspects of iron in relation to dopaminergic neurotransmission. In A. Lajtha (Ed.), *Handbook of neurochemistry* (Vol. 10, pp. 731–756). New York: Plenum Press.

Youdim, M. B. H. (1990). Neuropharmacological and neurochemical aspects of iron deficiency. In J. Dobbing (Ed.), *Brain behavior and iron in the infant diet* (pp. 83–106). Berlin: Springer-Verlag.

Youdim, M. B. H. (2003). What have we learnt from cDNA microarray gene expression studies about the role of iron in MPTP-induced neurodegeneration and Parkinson's disease. *Journal of Neural Transmission, 65*(Suppl.), 73–88.

Youdim, M. B., Ben-Shachar, D., & Riederer, P. (1989). Is Parkinson's disease a progressive siderosis of substantia nigra resulting in iron and melanin induced neurodegeneration? *Acta Neurologica Scandinavia Supplementum, 126*, 47–54.

Youdim, M. B., Ben-Shachar, D., & Riederer, P. (1993). The possible role of iron in the etiopathology of Parkinson's disease. *Movement Disorder, 8*, 1–12.

Youdim, M. B. H., Ben-Shachar, D., & Yehuda, S. (1989). Putative biological mechanisms of the effect of iron-deficiency on brain biochemistry and behavior American. *Journal of Clinical Nutrition, 50*, 607–617.

Youdim, M. B. H., Eshel, G., & Ben-Shachar, D. (2003). Ironing iron out in Parkinson's disease and other neurodegenerative diseases with iron chelators; a lesson from 6-hydroxydopamine and iron chelators desferal and VK-28. *Annals of New York Academy of Sciences*. New York. 1012, 306–325.

Youdim, M. B., & Green, A. R. (1977). Biogenic monoamine metabolism and functional activity in iron-deficient rats: Behavioural correlates. *Ciba Foundation Symposium, 51*, 201–225.

Youdim, M. B. H., & Riederer, P. (1997). Understanding Parkinson's disease. *Scientific American, 257*, 59–64.

Youdim, M. B. H., & Riederer, P. (1999). Iron in the brain, normal and pathological. In G. Adelman & B. H. Smith (Eds.), *Encyclopedia of neuroscience* (pp. 983–987). Amsterdam: Elsevier.

Youdim, M. B. H., & Riederer, P. (2003, in press). Iron in normal and pathological brain diseases. In B. Smith & G. Adleman (Eds.), *Encyclopedia of neuroscience*. Amsterdam: Elsevier.

Youdim. M. B., Stephenson, G., & Ben Shachar, D. (2004). Ironing iron out in Parkinson's disease and other neurodegenerative diseases with iron chelators: A lesson from 6-hydroxydopamine and iron chelators, desferal and VK-28. *Annals of New York Academy of science, 1012*, 306–25.

Youdim, M. B. H., Sills, M. A., Neydron, W. E., Creed, G. J., & Jacobowitz, D. H. (1986). Iron deficiency alters discrete proteins in rat caudate nucleus and nucleus accumbens. *Journal of Neurochemistry, 47*, 794–799.

Youdim, M. B. H., & Yehuda, S. (2000). The neurochemical basis of cognitive deficits induced by brain iron deficiency: Involvement of dopamine-opiate system. *Cellular Molecular Biology, 46*, 491–500.

Youdim, M. B. H., Zamir, N., & Yehuda, S. (2000). Antinociception in iron-deficient rats related to subsensitivity of dopamine D2 receptor induced increase of opiate peptides. *Nutrition Neuroscience, 3*, 357–365.

Zayed, J., Ducic, S., Campanella, G., Panisset, J. C., André, P., Masson, H., et al. (1990). Facteurs environnementaux dans l'étiologie de la maladie de Parkinson. *Canadian Journal of Neurological Sciences, 17*, 286–291.

Zecca, L., Berg, D., & Arzberger, T., et al. (2008). The in vivo detection of iron and neuromelanin by transcranial sonography: A new approach for early detection of substantia nigra damage. *Brain* (submitted).

Zecca, L., Gallorini, M., & Schünemann, V., et al. (2001a). Iron, neuromelanin and ferritin content in the substantia nigra of normal subjects at different ages: Consequences for iron storage and neurodegenerative processes. *Journal of Neurochemistry, 76*, 1766–1773.

Zecca, L., Tampellini, D., & Gerlach, M., et al. (2001b). Substantia nigra neuromelanin: Structure, synthesis, and molecular behaviour. *Molecular Pathology, 54*, 414–418.

Zecca, L., Fariello, R., & Riederer, P. (2002). The absolute concentration of nigral neuromelanin, assayed by a new sensitive method, increases throughout the life and is dramatically decreased in Parkinson's disease. *FEBS Letters, 510*, 216–220.

Zecca, L., Shima, T., & Stroppolo, A. (1996). Interaction of neuromelanin and iron in substantia nigra and other areas of human brain. *Neuroscience, 73*, 407–415.

Zecca, L., & Swartz, H. M. (1993). Total and paramagnetic metals in human substantia nigra and its neuromelanin. *Journal of Neural Transmission Parkinson's Disease and Dementias Section, 5*, 203–213.

Zecca, L., Youdim, M. B., Riederer, P., Connor, J. R., & Crichton, R. R. (2004). Iron, brain ageing and neurodegenerative disorders. *Nature Reviews. Neuroscience, 5*(11), 863–873.

Zecca, L., Zucca, F. A., Wilms, H., & Sulzer, D. (2003). Neuromelanin of the substantia nigra: A neuronal black hole with protective and toxic characteristics. *Trends in Neuroscience, 26*(11) 578–80.

Zheng, H., Gal, S., Weiner, L. M., Bar-Am, O., Warshawsky, A., Fridkin, M., & Youdim, M. B. (2005). Novel multifunctional neuroprotective iron chelator-monoamine oxidase inhibitor drugs for neurodegenerative diseases: In vitro studies on antioxidant activity, prevention of lipid peroxide formation and monoamine oxidase inhibition. *Journal of Neurochemistry, 95*(1), 68–78.

Zheng, H., Weiner, L. M., Bar-Am, O., Epsztejn, S., Cabantchik, Z. I., Warshawsky, A., et al. (2005). Design, synthesis, and evaluation of novel bifunctional iron-chelators as potential agents for neuroprotection in Alzheimer's, Parkinson's, and other neurodegenerative diseases. *Bioorganic Medical Chemistry*, *13*(3), 773–783.

Zhu, W., Xie, W., Pan, T., Xu, P., Fridkin, M., Zheng, H., et al. (2007, December). Prevention and restoration of lactacystin-induced nigrostriatal dopamine neuron degeneration by novel brain-permeable iron chelators. *FASEB Journal*, *21*(14), 3835–3844.

# 7 Brain Iron Deposition in Aging and Disease: Role of HO-1

*Hyman M. Schipper*

**Summary**

- Mechanisms responsible for the pathological deposition of redox-active iron in the aging and degenerating human brain remain incompletely understood.
- Heme oxygenase-1 (HO-1) is a 32-kDa stress protein that degrades heme to biliverdin, free iron, and carbon monoxide.
- Brain HO-1 expression increases with advancing age, and the enzyme is further induced in CNS tissues affected by Alzheimer's disease, Parkinson's disease, and other neurodegenerative and neuroinflammatory conditions.
- Upregulation of HO-1 in astrocytes exacerbates intracellular oxidative stress and promotes sequestration of non-transferrin-derived iron by the mitochondrial compartment.
- The glial mitochondrial iron catalyzes the bio-activation of protoxins (e.g., catechols, MPTP) to potent neurotoxins (*o*-semiquinones, MPP+) and may further facilitate neural injury by attenuating glutathione biosynthesis and other ATP-dependent processes.
- Suppression of glial HO-1 induction or activity may constitute a rational therapeutic approach to curtail pathological iron deposition and mitochondrial insufficiency in disorders of the aging human CNS.

**Key Words:** Aging; Alzheimer's disease; astrocyte; heme oxygenase-1; iron; mitochondria; neurodegeneration; oxidative stress; Parkinson's disease

## 7.1. INTRODUCTION

Iron is essential for normal neural development and participates in a wide range of cellular functions including electron transport, antioxidant enzyme activity, biogenic amine metabolism, cell cycle traverse, and myelination. To enable these vital functions, iron homeostasis in neural and peripheral tissues is tightly regulated by diverse proteins controlling its absorption, extracellular transport, valence configuration, cellular flux, chemical signaling activities, and intracellular storage (Ponka, 2004). Despite this elaborate control, iron accumulates in the aging mammalian CNS, and a fraction of the iron pool in cerebrospinal fluid (CSF) and brain substance is maintained in a redox-active state. The latter may contribute to neural damage in diverse neuropathological conditions (Table 1) by (i) mediating the reduction of hydrogen peroxide to

From: *Nutrition and Health: Iron Deficiency and Overload*
Edited by: S. Yehuda and D.I. Mostofsky, DOI 10.1007/978-1-59745-462-9_7

Table 1
**Acquired Human Nervous System Conditions Implicating Pathological Iron Deposition in Their Etiopathogenesis. PANK-2, Pantothenate Kinase-Type 2. Modified after H. M. Schipper (2004) with permission**

- CNS senescence
- Cerebral hemorrhage
- Alzheimer's disease
- Parkinson's disease
- Amyotrophic lateral sclerosis
- Progressive supranuclear palsy
- Corticobasal ganglionic degeneration
- Multiple sclerosis
- Superficial siderosis
- Restless legs syndrome
- HIV-1 encephalitis

highly reactive hydroxyl radicals (Fenton catalysis), (ii) behaving as a non-enzymatic peroxidase activity capable of converting endogenous catechols (e.g., dopamine, 2-hydroxyestradiol) to neurotoxic semiquinone intermediates, and (iii) facilitating the bioactivation of pro-toxins (e.g. MPTP) to potent neurotoxins (MPP+) (DiMonte, Schipper, Hetts, & Langston, 1995; H. M. Schipper, Kotake, & Janzen, 1991). The advent of effective therapeutic interventions to offset this metal-dependent neural injury presupposes a thorough understanding of the biological pathways subserving iron sequestration in aging and degenerating neural tissues.

## 7.2. IRON DEPOSITION IN THE AGING AND DEGENERATING CNS

### 7.2.1. *Aging*

Oxidative stress, aberrant iron mobilization, and mitochondrial insufficiency have been amply documented in the aging mammalian CNS (H. M. Schipper, 2004a). Within the aging brain, there appears to be selective regional susceptibility to the development of this pathological triad and considerable topographical overlap of these changes within affected areas (M. Beal, 1995). In the senescent human brain, markers of free radical injury, excessive iron accumulation, and mitochondrial DNA deletions are particularly robust in the basal ganglia, hippocampus, and certain cerebellar nuclei and less so in the cerebral cortices and other regions (Soong, Hinton, Cortopassi, & Arnheim, 1992). It is noteworthy that those brain loci prone to iron sequestration in the course of normal aging tend to accumulate the metal to a significantly greater extent in numerous degenerative hereditary and acquired disorders of cognition and movement. Little is currently known concerning the cellular mechanisms imposing regional predilections on iron deposition in the aging and diseased CNS. Nor is it clear whether primary derangements in iron homeostasis predispose to mitochondrial injury or, conversely, whether iron mismanagement occurs downstream of oxidative stress accruing from electron transport infidelity within senescent and diseased mitochondrial membranes. On the basis of evidence garnered from human neuropathological studies, animal models of aging-related neurodegeneration, and cell culture experiments, we posited that augmented iron deposition, oxidative stress, and bioenergetic failure (mitochondrial insufficiency) are features of a single, fairly ubiquitous, and self-reinforcing "lesion" that constitutes a vital link between normal brain aging and associated neurodegenerative disorders (H. M. Schipper, 2004a). As discussed below, upregulation of the heme-degrading enzyme, heme oxygenase-1 (HO-1), may be instrumental in binding the components of this tri-partite lesion.

### 7.2.2. *Alzheimer's Disease*

Alzheimer's disease (AD) is a dementing illness featuring progressive neuronal degeneration, gliosis, and the accumulation of extracellular deposits of amyloid (senile plaques) and intracellular inclusions (neurofibrillary tangles) in basal forebrain, hippocampus, and association cortices (Selkoe, 1991). Excessive iron deposition, oxidative stress, and mitochondrial deficits have been consistently implicated in the pathogenesis of this condition (M. Beal, 1995; Corral-Debrinski et al., 1994; Gibson, Sheu, & Blass, 1998; Mattson, 2002; Reichmann & Riederer, 1994; H. M. Schipper, 2004a; Tanno, Okuizumi, & Tsuji, 1998) (Bonilla et al., 1999; Fukuyama et al., 1994; Minoshima et al., 1997). Potential sources of oxidative stress in the AD brain include baseline ROS generation by senescent mitochondria, accelerated β-amyloid deposition (Butterfield, 2002), production of pro-inflammatory cytokines (TNFα, IL-1β) and nitric oxide (NO) by activated microglia (McGeer & McGeer, 1995), and excessive deposition of redox-active iron in association cortices and basal forebrain (Sayre, Smith, & Perry, 2001; H. M. Schipper, 1998). In both the AD and the Parkinson brain, increased expression of tissue ferritin, the major intracellular iron storage protein, parallels the distribution of the excess iron and largely implicates non-neuronal (glial, endothelial) cellular compartments (H. M. Schipper, 1998). In both conditions, regional concentrations of transferrin-binding sites remain unchanged or vary inversely with the increased iron stores. The latter observations suggest that the transferrin pathway of iron mobilization contributes little to the pathological accumulation of brain iron in these aging-related neurodegenerative conditions, despite the importance of this route for normal iron delivery to most peripheral tissues (H. M. Schipper, 1999). This realization has led several laboratories to consider alternate pathways for deranged iron compartmentalization in the aging and degenerating CNS. The potential role(s) of lactoferrin, melanotransferrin (p97), and their receptors in pathological brain iron mobilization are discussed elsewhere (Jefferies et al., 1996; H. M. Schipper, 1998, 1999), and the putative involvement of heme oxygenase-1 (HO-1) in these processes is reviewed in Section 7.3.

### 7.2.3. *Parkinson's Disease*

Idiopathic PD is a late-onset movement disorder of uncertain etiology characterized pathologically by progressive degeneration of dopaminergic neurons in the substantia nigra pars compacta, formation of intraneuronal fibrillar inclusions (Lewy bodies) in this cell population, and variable depletion of noradrenaline and serotonin in other brain stem nuclei. As in the case of AD, there is abundant evidence of transferrin-independent iron sequestration, oxidative substrate damage, and bioenergetic failure in PD-affected brain tissues and in animal models of the disease (H. M. Schipper, 1998, 1999, 2004a; Storm et al., 2002; Bowen et al., 1995). The pathological iron deposits, electron transport chain (ETC) abnormalities, ROS derived from accelerated dopamine turnover ($H_2O_2$, *o*-semiquinones), Th1 cytokines, NO, and MPTP-like xenobiotics may predispose to oxidative injury in the PD basal ganglia (Jenner, 2003).

### 7.2.4. *Other Neurological Disorders*

In addition to AD and PD, disturbances in iron homeostasis, oxidative stress, and mitochondrial lesions have been described in other aging-related human neurodegenerative conditions, including Huntington's disease, amyotrophic lateral sclerosis, progressive supranuclear palsy, corticobasal degeneration, and aceruloplasminemia (Calne, 1994; Connor, 1997; Miyajima, Kono, Takahashi, & Sugimoto, 2002; H. M. Schipper, 2004b). This pathological triad may also compromise neural tissues affected by various ischemic (cerebral infarction), hemorrhagic (cerebral hematoma), traumatic (CNS contusion), immunologic (multiple sclerosis), and infectious (HIV-1 encephalitis) disorders (H. M. Schipper, 2004b).

### 7.2.5. *Glial Senescence and Iron Sequestration*

In rodents, humans, and other vertebrates, a subpopulation of astrocytes residing within subcortical brain regions progressively accumulates discrete, iron-laden cytoplasmic granules as a function of advancing age (Mydlarski, Brawer, & Schipper, 1998; H. M. Schipper, 1996). In the rat substantia nigra, for example, these gliosomes increase in abundance by a factor of four between the ages of 4 and 14 months (H. M. Schipper, Vininsky, Brull, Small, & Brawer, 1998). Also, at 3 and 14 months of age, the density of these inclusions within periventricular astrocytes is considerably greater in senescence-accelerated (SAMP10) mice relative to age-matched control values (Lee & Lee, 2001). The inclusions exhibit intense, iron-mediated (non-enzymatic) peroxidase activity capable of oxidizing neutral catechols to potentially neurotoxic semiquinone radicals (H. M. Schipper et al., 1991) and the pro-toxin MPTP to the dopaminergic neurotoxin MPP+ (DiMonte et al., 1995). Thus, the progressive accretion of these glial granules may predispose senescent neural tissues to oxidative and toxicant injury.

#### 7.2.5.1. The Cysteamine Model

In young adult rats, subcutaneous injections of the aminothiol compound, 2-mercaptoethylamine or cysteamine (CSH; 150–300 mg/kg twice weekly for 3 weeks) induced two- to threefold increases in numbers of peroxidase-positive astrocyte granules in the basal ganglia, hippocampus, and other subcortical brain regions (H. M. Schipper, Mydlarski, & Wang, 1993). Similar results were obtained following direct intracerebroventricular instillation of CSH by mini-pump (1.0 mg/day × 3 weeks) (St-Jacques, Chapman, Lacaille, Mohr, & Schipper, 1999). In both models, astrocyte hypertrophy (gliosis) accompanied granule accumulation, whereas a panel of histochemical stains failed to disclose any neuronal or white matter pathology. In dissociated fetal or neonatal rat brain cell cultures, CSH administration (880 μM with each culture feed from in vitro days 6–18) stimulates the appearance of peroxidase-positive astrocytic inclusions that are structurally and histochemically identical to those which spontaneously accumulate in subcortical astroglia of the intact aging brain (H. Schipper, Scarborough, Lechan, & Reichlin, 1990; H. M. Schipper, 1996). As in situ elemental iron was detected in the inclusions by electron microprobe analysis, and the presence and concentration of the metal correlated closely with the presence and intensity of diaminobenzidine (peroxidase) staining (McLaren, Brawer, & Schipper, 1992).

#### 7.2.5.2. Mitochondrial Precursors of Senescent Glial Granules

In the CSH-treated astroglia, the earliest morphological changes appeared restricted to the mitochondrial compartment. Within 24–72 hours of CSH exposure, many astroglial mitochondria exhibited swelling, rearrangement or dissolution of their cristae, iron sequestration and fusion with lysosomes and occasional strands of endoplasmic reticulum (ER) (Brawer, Reichard, Small, & Schipper, 1994). As in the case of the CSH-treated cultures, DAB-positive glial granules in the intact rat and human brain invariably exhibit mitochondrial epitopes in immunohistochemical preparations (Brawer, Stein, Small, Cisse, & Schipper, 1994; Cissé & Schipper, 1995; H. M. Schipper & Cissé, 1995). Our observations indicate that (a) the iron-laden astrocyte granules are derived from abnormal mitochondria engaged in a complex autophagic process and (b) CSH accelerates the appearance of a senescent phenotype in these cells. Several lines of evidence suggested further that intracellular oxidative stress is a "final common pathway" responsible for the transformation of normal astrocyte mitochondria to iron-laden inclusions in vitro and in situ.

#### 7.2.5.3. Non-Transferrin Iron Sequestration in "Stressed" Astroglial Mitochondria

We showed that CSH attenuates the incorporation of the heme precursors, $\delta$-amino[$^{14}$C]-levulinic acid and [$^{14}$C]glycine into porphyrin and heme in astroglial cultures before and during the time when augmented iron concentrations are detectable in distended astrocyte mitochondria by microprobe analysis (Brawer, Reichard et al., 1994; H. M. Schipper, Small, Wang, & Brawer, 2002; Wang, Manganaro, & Schipper, 1995). Thus, an accumulation of heme iron is not responsible for the peroxidase activity in these cells. Following inhibition of porphyrin-heme biosynthesis, CSH significantly increased the uptake of $^{59}$Fe (or $^{55}$Fe) into astroglial mitochondria without affecting disposition of the metal in whole-cell and lysosomal compartments. Mitochondrial iron sequestration following CSH challenge only occurred when low-molecular-weight $^{59}FeCl_3$, but not $^{59}$Fe-diferric transferrin, served as the metal donor (Wang et al., 1995). These in vitro data are commensurate with the fact that (a) pathological iron accumulation in the AD and PD brain appears to be a transferrin-independent event and (b) mitochondrial insufficiency is characteristic of AD, PD, and other neural tissues experiencing iron overload (Section 7.2).

## 7.3. HEME OXYGENASE-1 AND BRAIN IRON HOMEOSTASIS

### 7.3.1. *Heme Oxygenase*

Heme oxygenases (E.C. 1:14:99:3; heme-hydrogen donor:oxygen oxidoreductase) are ER enzymes that function in concert with NADPH cytochrome P450 reductase to oxidize heme to biliverdin, free ferrous iron, and carbon monoxide (CO; Fig. 1). Biliverdin is metabolized further to bilirubin by the action of biliverdin reductase (Ryter & Tyrrell, 2000). Mammalian cells express at least two isoforms of heme oxygenase, HO-1 (a.k.a. HSP32) and HO-2. Whereas HO-2 protein is distributed widely within the rodent neuraxis (Verma, Hirsch, Glatt, Ronnett, & Snyder, 1993), basal HO-1 expression in the normal brain is limited to small groups of scattered neurons and neuroglia (Baranano & Snyder, 2001). The mammalian *ho-1* promoter contains a panoply of response elements that render the gene highly inducible by numerous pro-oxidant and inflammatory stimuli, including heme, transition metals, $H_2O_2$, UV light, Th1 cytokines, prostaglandins, lipopolysaccharide, β-amyloid, and dopamine (Dennery, 2000; H. M. Schipper, 2000). In various tissues, oxidative stress may transiently increase the intracellular 'free heme pool' by impelling the conformational modification and accelerated proteolysis of vulnerable hemoproteins (Ryter & Tyrrell, 2000). Upregulation of HO-1 may confer protection in these stressed cells by enhancing the degradation of pro-oxidant heme to the radical-scavenging bile pigments, biliverdin and bilirubin (Baranano & Snyder, 2001; Dore et al., 1999; Llesuy & Tomaro, 1994; Nakagami, Toyomura, Kinoshita, & Morisawa, 1993; Stocker, Yamamoto, McDonagh, Glazer, & Ames, 1987). In many instances, co-stimulation of apoferritin synthesis, a major iron storage pathway, obviates potential toxicity resulting from the intracellular liberation of heme-derived ferrous iron (Dennery, 2000; Ryter & Tyrrell, 2000). Under certain circumstances, iron and CO originating from heme may *exacerbate* intracellular oxidative damage by stimulating free radical generation within the mitochondrial and other subcellular compartments (Frankel, Mehindate, & Schipper, 2000; Ryter & Tyrrell, 2000; Zhang & Piantadosi, 1992). Evidence supporting both protective and endangering aspects of HO-1 activity in neural and systemic tissues is reviewed elsewhere (Dennery, 2000; Mawal, Berlin, Kravitz, & Schipper, 2002; Ryter & Tyrrell, 2000).

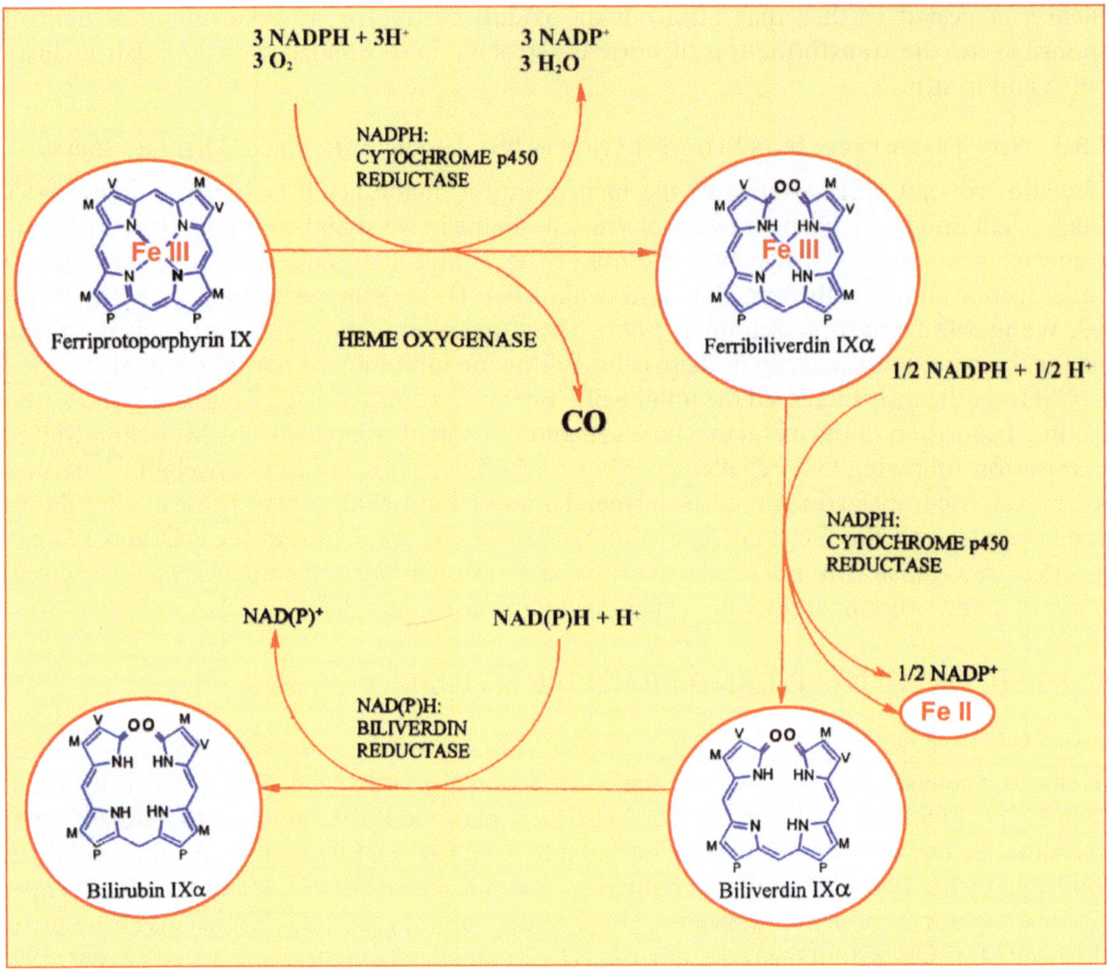


**Fig. 1.** The heme catabolic pathway. M = methyl; V = vinyl; P = propionate. Modified after Ryter & Tyrrell (2000) with permission.

### *7.3.2. HO-1 and Astroglial Iron*

The role of HO-1 in glial iron homeostasis has been intensively investigated using the astroglial culture model described in Section 7.2.5. In these cultures, CSH (880 μM), β-amyloid $_{40/42}$ (3–15 μM), dopamine (1 μM), TNFα (20 ng/mL), and IL-1β (20 ng/mL) upregulated HO-1 mRNA, protein, and/or activity levels within 3–12 hours of treatment. Within 3–6 days, uptake of non-transferrin-derived $^{59/55}$Fe (but not diferric transferrin-derived iron) by the mitochondrial compartment was significantly augmented in the treated cells relative to untreated control cultures (Ham & Schipper, 2000; Mehindate et al., 2001; H. M. Schipper, 1999; H. M. Schipper, Bernier, Mehindate, & Frankel, 1999; Wang et al., 1995). Oxidative stress is a likely common mechanism mediating glial *ho-1* gene induction under these experimental conditions because (i) the effects of these stimuli on HO-1 expression and mitochondrial iron sequestration were recapitulated by hydrogen peroxide (300–500 μM) or menadione (100 μM) treatment and (ii) co-administration of potent antioxidants (ascorbate, melatonin, or *trans*-resveratrol) suppressed the HO-1 response to CSH, DA, and the pro-inflammatory cytokines in these cells (Mehindate et al., 2001; H. M. Schipper et al., 1999). Importantly, co-incubation with tin mesoporphyrin

(SnMP; 1 μM), a competitive inhibitor of heme oxygenase activity, or dexamethasone (DEX; 50 μg/ml), a transcriptional suppressor of the *ho-1* gene, significantly attenuated mitochondrial iron trapping in cultured astrocytes exposed to DA (H. M. Schipper et al., 1999), TNFα, or IL-1β (Mehindate et al., 2001). Along similar lines, the administration of SnMP or DEX obviated the pathological accumulation of mitochondrial $^{55}$Fe in rat astroglia transiently transfected with the human (h) *ho-1* gene (H. M. Schipper et al., 1999). These observations indicated that upregulation of HO-1 is a pivotal event in the cascade leading to excessive mitochondrial iron deposition in oxidatively challenged astroglia.

*How does heme-derived iron find its way into mitochondria?* Treatment with SnMP or antioxidants (ascorbate, melatonin, or resveratrol) blocked the late, presumably compensatory, induction of the MnSOD gene in astrocytes challenged with dopamine or transiently transfected with hHO-1 cDNA (Frankel et al., 2000). Furthermore, the levels of protein carbonyls (protein oxidation), 8-epiPGF2α (lipid peroxidation), and 8-OHdG (nucleic acid oxidation) in glial mitochondrial fractions were significantly increased after 4 days of hHO-1 transfection relative to sham-transfected controls and HO-1-transfected cells receiving SnMP (W. Song, Su, Song, Paudel, & Schipper, 2006). HO-1 transfection also stimulated oxidation of the synthetic reporter molecules, linoleoyl-tyrosine, and linoleoyl-tyrosine-deoxyguanosyl ester to hydroperoxides and 8-oxo-guanosine in glial whole-cell and mitochondrial compartments (Vaya, Song, Khatib, Geng, & Schipper, 2007). These convergent data clearly indicate that HO-1 over-expression in astroglia exacerbates intracellular oxidative stress that targets the mitochondrial compartment. Treatment with cyclosporin A or trifluoperazine, potent inhibitors of the mitochondrial permeability transition pore, also curtailed mitochondrial iron trapping in hHO-1 transfected glia and cells exposed to DA (Fig. 2), TNFα, or IL-1β (Mehindate et al., 2001; H. M. Schipper et al., 1999).

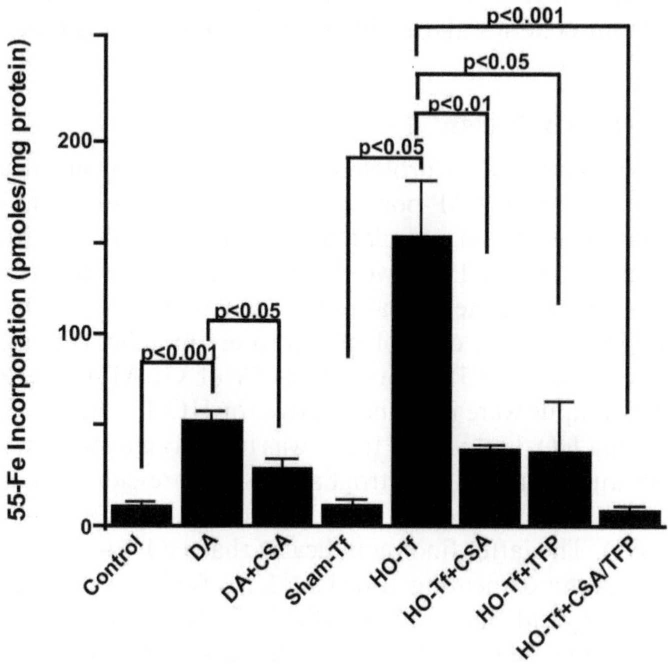


**Fig. 2.** Effects of DA (1 μM) stimulation and hHO-1 transfection (HO-Tf) on mitochondrial sequestration of $^{55}FeCl_3$-derived iron in the presence and absence of the mitochondrial permeability transition pore inhibitors, cyclosporin A (CSA; 0.5 μM) and/or trifluoperazine (TFP; 30 μM). $n = 4$/group. Pore inhibitors attenuate mitochondrial iron deposition in DA-exposed and hHO-1-transfected astroglia. From H. M. Schipper et al. (1999) with permission.

Conceivably, intracellular oxidative stress accruing from HO-1 activity promotes pore opening (Broekemeier & Pfeiffer, 1995; Petronilli, Cola, Massari, Colonna, & Bernardi, 1993) and influx of cytosolic iron into the mitochondrial matrix. CO stimulates mitochondrial transition pore opening in liver cells (Piantadosi, Carraway, & Suliman, 2006) and may similarly engage the pore in astroglia. Additional or alternative modes of iron delivery to the mitochondrial compartment may be envisioned here. Ultrastructural studies of the biogenesis of iron-laden astroglial inclusions have revealed occasional close apposition and possibly membrane fusion of ER strands with osmiophilic cytoplasmic granules derived from damaged mitochondria (Brawer & Sonnenschein, 1975). Thus, in stressed astroglia, putative organellar fusions or transient 'kiss-and-run' relationships of the ER with mitochondria may facilitate "delivery" of HO-1 enzyme, and hence heme-derived iron, to mitochondrial matrices. Another intriguing possibility is that HO-1 enzyme *native* to the mitochondrial compartment may contribute to the sequestration of heme-derived iron in this organelle. HO-1 protein has been detected in *mitochondria* of rat pulmonary endothelial cells (Kim, Wang, Galbiati, Ryter, & Choi, 2004) and liver cells (Converso et al., 2006) where it appears to modulate heme content and metabolism. It is not yet known whether some fraction of HO-1 protein in astrocytes similarly localizes to the mitochondrial compartment.

### *7.3.3. HO-1 and Human Brain Aging*

HO-1 expression in human brain has not been rigorously mapped or quantified. However, one report indicated that numbers of human neuroglia immunoreactive for HO-1 increase with advancing aging (Hirose, Ikematsu, & Tsuda, 2003). In accord with the data reviewed in Section 7.3.2 and the tenets of Free Radical-Mitochondrial theory of aging (H. M. Schipper, 2004), progressive induction of glial HO-1, provoked by gradually intensifying ambient oxidative stress, may contribute to mitochondrial iron deposition and worsening bioenergetic failure in the senescent human CNS.

### *7.3.4. HO-1 and Alzheimer's Disease*

In AD-affected neural tissues, HO-1 protein co-localizes to neurons, neurofibrillary tangles, senile plaques, corpora amylacea, GFAP-positive astrocytes, choroid plexus epithelial cells, ependymocytes, and some endothelial and vascular smooth muscle cells (H. M. Schipper, Cissé, & Stopa, 1995; Smith et al., 1994). In 1995, we reported that Western blots of protein extracts derived from AD hippocampus and temporal cortex exhibited strong HO-1 bands, whereas the latter were faint or undetectable in control preparations matched for age and post-mortem interval (H. M. Schipper et al., 1995). Moreover, 86% of GFAP-positive astrocytes residing within the the AD hippocampus were immunoreactive for HO-1, whereas the fraction of hippocampal astroglia expressing HO-1 in normal tissue was in the range of only 6–7%. Similarly, in a recent study, significant augmentation of astroglial HO-1 expression was noted in post-mortem brain specimens procured from individuals with MCI (mild cognitive impairment), a frequent harbinger of incipient AD. The latter finding indicates that HO-1 induction is a relatively early event in the pathogenesis of this dementing disorder (H. M. Schipper et al., 2006). Oxidative stress resulting from excessive amyloid burden (Butterfield, Castegna, Lauderback, & Drake, 2002; Ham & Schipper, 2000) or the secretion of pro-inflammatory cytokines (Mehindate et al., 2001) may be responsible for the elaboration of HO-1 in the Alzheimer-diseased cerebral cortex and hippocampus. Dysregulation of iron homeostasis and the mitochondriopathy observed in AD brain (Section 7.2.2) may, in turn, represent distal effects of sustained HO-1 over-production in the diseased tissues. Jofre-Monseny et al. recently reported greater basal and lipopolysaccharide-stimulated HO-1 expression in an apolipoprotein E4-transfected murine macrophage line (RAW

264.7 cells) than apoE3-transfected cells (Jofre-Monseny et al., 2007). It remains to be determined whether HO-1 expression is similarly enhanced in the brains of E4 allele carriers relative to E3 and E2 carriers. If so, and in light of the above considerations, augmented HO-1 elaboration and attendant brain iron dysregulation may be an additional mechanism whereby the E4 genotype confers risk for the development of AD (Saunders et al., 1993).

In contradistinction to the augmented HO-1 expression in AD brain parenchyma, HO-1 protein or mRNA levels are *suppressed* in AD CSF, choroid plexus epithelial cells, plasma, and blood mononuclear cells relative to control values (Anthony et al., 2003; H. M. Schipper et al., 2000). The diminished CSF HO-1 concentrations in this condition may reflect decreased synthesis and release of the protein by the choroid plexus or, alternatively, curtailed delivery (transudation) from the systemic circulation (*vide infra*). Using a glial bioassay developed in our laboratory, a *heme oxygenase-1 suppressor (HOS) factor* was detected in AD plasma that could not be accounted for by disproportionate antioxidant exposure, increased plasma total antioxidant capacity, hypercortisolemia, apolipoprotein E ε4 carrier status (Maes et al., 2006), or over-representation of specific *ho-1* promoter polymorphisms (Kimpara et al., 1997). Biochemical analyses indicated that the plasma HOS factor is a 50–100 kDa heat-labile, heparin-binding glycoprotein (Maes et al., 2006). In a related proteomic study, the acute-phase reactant, α1-antitrypsin, was found to be over-abundant in HOS-positive AD plasma fractions relative to normal elderly control (NEC) values (Yu, Chertkow, Bergman, & Schipper, 2003). Moreover, exogenous α1-antitrypsin recapitulated HOS activity in the glial bioassay and immunodepletion of α1-antitrypsin attenuated HOS activity of AD plasma (Maes et al., 2006). α1-Antitrypsin immunoreactivity is augmented in AD brain and co-distributes with HO-1 (ibid.). Thus, HOS activity of α1-antitrypsin may curtail HO-1-dependent derangement of cerebral iron homeostasis and account for diminished HO-1 expression in AD peripheral tissues. We conjecture that net HO-1 mRNA and protein levels remain elevated in AD brain because the HOS activity of α1-antitrypsin is overwhelmed by the pro-oxidant effects of β-amyloid, Th1 cytokines, and other endogenous inducers of the *ho-1* gene (Fig. 3).

### 7.3.5. HO-1 and Parkinson's Disease

Moderate HO-1 immunoreactivity was observed in dopaminergic neurons of the substantia nigra in both normal and PD human brain (H. M. Schipper, Liberman, & Stopa, 1998). In the PD sections, cytoplasmic Lewy bodies within affected dopaminergic neurons were prominently decorated with HO-1 staining (Castellani, Smith, Richey, & Perry, 1996; H. M. Schipper, Liberman, et al., 1998). The proportion of GFAP-positive astroglia expressing HO-1 in the PD nigra was significantly increased (77.1%) relative to age-matched control subjects (18.7%). Percentages of GFAP-positive astroglia co-expressing HO-1 in other subcortical nuclei, such as the caudate, putamen, and globus pallidus, were relatively low in both the PD and the control specimens (H. M. Schipper, Liberman, et al., 1998). Dopamine-derived pro-oxidant intermediates, MPTP-like neurotoxins generated endogenously or stemming from the environment, and TH1 cytokines are plausible inducers of astroglial *ho-1* gene expression in the PD nigra (Mehindate et al., 2001; H. M. Schipper, 1999). Enhanced glial HO-1 activity may, in turn, promote the transferrin receptor-independent accumulation of iron and mitochondrial electron transport (Complex I) deficits consistently reported in the basal ganglia of PD subjects (M. F. Beal, 1996; H. M. Schipper, 2001).

HO-1-dependent iron sequestration by astroglial mitochondria may have important consequences for the viability of nearby neuronal constituents. With reference to PD, glial mitochondrial iron (augmented by CSH pre-treatment) was shown using paramagnetic resonance spectroscopy to promote the oxidation of dopamine to neurotoxic *o*-semiquinone radicals (H. M. Schipper, 2001;

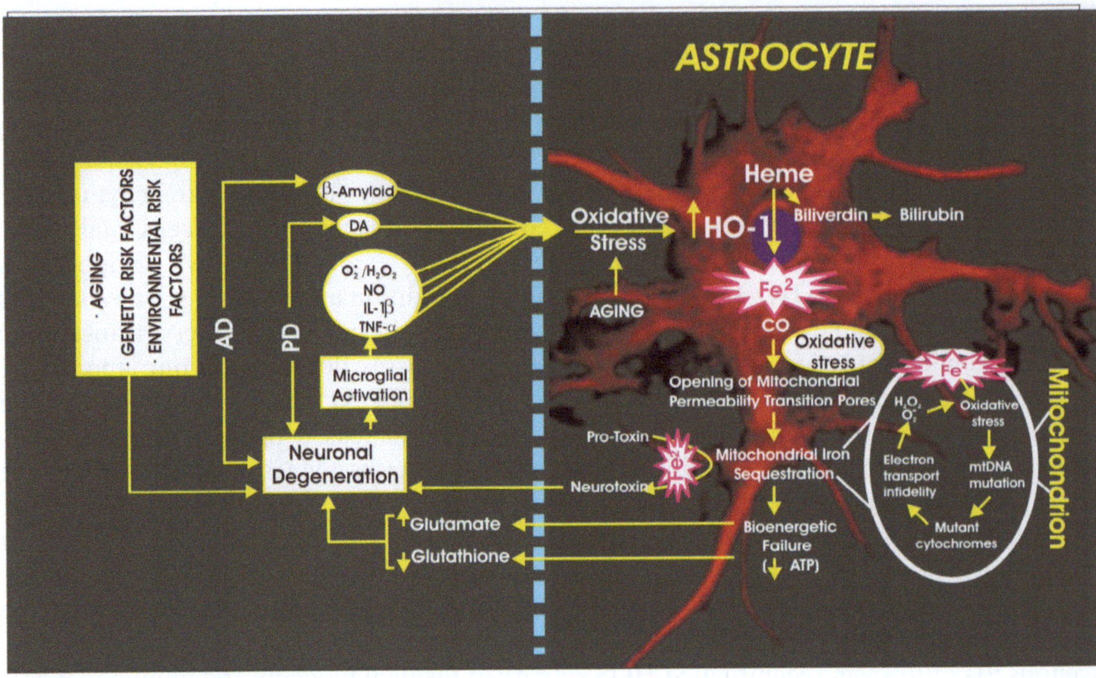


**Fig. 3.** A model for pathological brain iron deposition in aging and disease. Intrinsic aging processes and extracellular pro-oxidant stressors induce HO-1 in astrocytes, generating heme-derived free ferrous iron and carbon monoxide. The latter promote intracellular oxidative stress that triggers opening of mitochondrial permeability transition pores and ingress of iron to the mitochondrial matrix. The redox-active iron exacerbates oxidative injury to the electron transport chain machinery (mtDNA, cytochromes), resulting in a vicious spiral of mitochondrial ROS production in accord with the prevailing Free Radical–Mitochondrial theory of aging. The mitochondrial iron catalyzes the bio-activation of protoxins (e.g., catechols, MPTP) to potent neurotoxins (*o*-semiquinones, MPP+). The latter may egress to the extracellular milieu and exert direct dystrophic effects on vulnerable neuronal targets. Diminished ATP levels accruing from glial bioenergetic failure may further predispose to neuronal degeneration by augmenting extracellular glutamate concentrations (excitotoxicity), curtailing GSH delivery to the neuronal compartment and limiting the degradation of potentially toxic protein aggregates by the ubiquitin–proteosome system. Neuronal degeneration activates indigent microglia, resulting in the release of NO, ROS, and proinflammatory cytokines. The latter further induce the *ho-1* gene in astroglia, completing a self-sustaining loop of pathological cellular interactions that perpetuates oxidative damage and mitochondrial insufficiency within senescent and degenerating neural tissues. Environmental and genetic risk factors may confer disease specificity by superimposing unique pathological signatures on this core lesion. In the case of PD and AD, for example, DA release from dying nigrostriatal projections and β-amyloid deposition in the hippocampus and association cortices, respectively, feed into the pathological cascade by stimulating HO-1 activity in regional astroglia. Progressive perturbation of astroglial iron mobilization and mitochondrial insufficiency would then drive the primary neurodegenerative process regardless of its etiology. AD, Alzheimer's disease; CO, carbon monoxide; DA, dopamine; $Fe^2$, ferrous iron; GSH, glutathione; $H_2O_2$, hydrogen peroxide; HO-1, heme oxygenase-1; IL-1β, interleukin-1β; mtDNA, mitochondrial DNA; NO, nitric oxide; PD, Parkinson's disease; ROS, reactive oxygen species; TNF-α, tumor necrosis factor-α. Modified after H. M. Schipper (2004a) with permission.

H. M. Schipper et al., 1991). Moreover, catecholaminergic PC12 cells grown on a substratum of astrocytes replete with mitochondrial iron induced by CSH pre-treatment (Frankel & Schipper, 1999) or *hho-1* cDNA transfection (L. Song, Song, & Schipper, 2007) were determined to be far more vulnerable to dopamine/$H_2O_2$-related killing than PC12 cells co-cultured with control, "iron-poor" astroglia. In the experimental co-cultures, dopamine/$H_2O_2$-mediated PC12 cell death was significantly attenuated by co-administration of SnMP, ascorbate, or iron chelators (deferoxamine, phenanthroline), attesting to the biological potency of HO-1 and the role of glia-dependent oxidative stress in this paradigm (L. Song et al., 2007). Of further relevance to PD, the glial mitochondrial iron may also mediate bioactivation of MPTP to the dopaminergic neurotoxin, MPP+, in the face of monoamine oxidase (MAO) blockade (DiMonte et al., 1995). These observations raise the possibility that PD patients treated with MAO inhibitors for the purpose of arresting the conversion of endogenous dopamine or putative MPTP-like environmental pro-toxins to dopaminergic neurotoxins may still experience chronic, low-level exposure to the latter upon their synthesis in glia via iron-mediated reactions (DiMonte et al., 1995; H. M. Schipper, 2001).

### *7.3.6. HO-1 and Other Human CNS Disorders*

Oxidative stress and mitochondrial iron deposition have been implicated in the pathogenesis of multiple sclerosis (MS), an autoimmune demyelinating disorder of central white matter (LeVine, 1997; Mehindate et al., 2001). In a neuropathological survey (Mehindate et al., 2001), the proportion of GFAP-positive astrocytes expressing HO-1 in spinal cord plaques derived from MS patients (57.3%) was noted to be significantly higher than that recorded in the spinal white matter of normal subjects (15.4%). Glial HO-1 over-expression in MS may be secondary to the enhanced release of IL-1β, TNFα (Section 7.3.2), or myelin basic protein (Businaro et al., 2002) within the affected tissues. Upregulation of HO-1 may amplify intracellular oxidative stress and give rise to the mitochondrial iron deposits reported in this condition. Robust HO-1 induction has also been documented in the brains of patients with Pick's disease, corticobasal ganglionic degeneration, progressive supranuclear palsy, ischemic and hemorrhagic stroke, and cerebral malaria. The pathological triad of oxidative molecular damage, aberrant iron mobilization, and bioenergetic failure occurs in many, if not all, of these conditions and may represent an obligatory response to HO-1 over-expression in "stressed" astroglia (H. M. Schipper, 2004a).

## 7.4. CONCLUSIONS

Induction of the heme-degrading enzyme HO-1 in astrocytes stressed by aging or disease promotes the sequestration of non-transferrin iron by the mitochondrial compartment. The mitochondrial iron behaves as a non-enzymatic (pseudo-) peroxidase activity capable of catalyzing the conversion of various pro-toxins to potent neurotoxins. As such, the progressive accumulation of mitochondrial iron within senescent astroglia may contribute to the enhanced susceptibility of the aging CNS to a host of degenerative, inflammatory, and ischemic conditions (Fig. 3).

As a potent transducer of mitochondrial iron deposition under oxidative stress, curtailment of glial HO-1 activity by pharmacological or other means should be further explored, perhaps using appropriate transgenic mouse models, as a potential therapeutic strategy for the management of AD, PD, and other CNS disorders characterized by sustained over-activity of this critical enzyme.

**Acknowledgments** The author thanks Adrienne Liberman for assistance with the preparation of this manuscript. Contributions by the Schipper laboratory were enabled by grants from the Canadian Institutes of Health Research, the Fonds de la Recherche en Santé du Québec, the Alzheimer's Association (US), and the Parkinson Foundation of Canada.

## REFERENCES


Anthony, S. G., Schipper, H. M., Tavares, R., Hovanesian, V., Cortez, S. C., Stopa, E. G., et al. (2003). Stress protein expression in the Alzheimer-diseased choroid plexus. *Journal of Alzheimer's Disease, 5*(3), 171–177.

Baranano, D. E., & Snyder, S. H. (2001). Neural roles for heme oxygenase: contrasts to nitric oxide synthase. *Proceedings of the National Academy of Sciences, USA, 98*(20), 10996–11002.

Beal, M. (1995). *Mitochondrial dysfunction and oxidative damage in neurodegenerative diseases.* Austin, TX: R.G. Landes Co.

Beal, M. F. (1996). Mitochondria, free radicals, and neurodegeneration. *Current Opinion in Neurobiology, 6*(5), 661–666.

Bonilla, E., Tanji, K., Hirano, M., Vu, T. H., DiMauro, S., & Schon, E. A. (1999). Mitochondrial involvement in Alzheimer's disease. *Biochimica et Biophysica Acta, 1410*(2), 171–182.

Bowen, B. C., Block, R. E., Sanchez-Ramos, J., Pattany, P. M., Lampman, D. A., Murdoch, J. B., et al. (1995). Proton MR spectroscopy of the brain in 14 patients with Parkinson disease. *AJNR American Journal of Neuroradiology, 16*(1), 61–68.

Brawer, J. R., Reichard, G., Small, L., & Schipper, H. M. (1994). The origin and composition of peroxidase-positive granules in cysteamine-treated astrocytes in culture. *Brain Research, 633*(1–2), 9–20.

Brawer, J. R., & Sonnenschein, C. (1975). Cytopathological effects of estradiol on the arcuate nucleus of the female rat. A possible mechanism for pituitary tumorigenesis. *American Journal of Anatomy, 144*(1), 57–88.

Brawer, J. R., Stein, R., Small, L., Cisse, S., & Schipper, H. M. (1994). Composition of Gomori-positive inclusions in astrocytes of the hypothalamic arcuate nucleus. *Anatomical Record, 240*(3), 407–415.

Broekemeier, K. M., & Pfeiffer, D. R. (1995). Inhibition of the mitochondrial permeability transition by cyclosporin A during long time frame experiments: relationship between pore opening and the activity of mitochondrial phospholipases. *Biochemistry, 34*(50), 16440–16449.

Businaro, R., Fabrizi, C., Caronti, B., Calderaro, C., Fumagalli, L., & Lauro, G. M. (2002). Myelin basic protein induces heme oxygenase-1 in human astroglial cells. *Glia, 37*(1), 83–88.

Butterfield, D. A. (2002). Amyloid beta-peptide (1–42)-induced oxidative stress and neurotoxicity: Implications for neurodegeneration in Alzheimer's disease brain. A review. *Free Radical Research, 36*(12), 1307–1313.

Butterfield, D. A., Castegna, A., Lauderback, C. M., & Drake, J. (2002). Evidence that amyloid beta-peptide-induced lipid peroxidation and its sequelae in Alzheimer's disease brain contribute to neuronal death. *Neurobiology of Aging, 23*(5), 655–664.

Calne, D. B. (1994). *Neurodegenerative diseases.* Philadelphia: W.B. Saunders Co.

Castellani, R., Smith, M. A., Richey, P. L., & Perry, G. (1996). Glycoxidation and oxidative stress in Parkinson disease and diffuse Lewy body disease. *Brain Research, 737*(1–2), 195–200.

Cissé, S., & Schipper, H. M. (1995). Experimental induction of corpora amylacea-like inclusions in rat astroglia. *Neuropathology and Applied Neurobiology, 21*(5), 423–431.

Connor, J. R. (1997). *Metals and oxidative damage in neurological disorders.* New York: Plenum Press.

Converso, D. P., Taille, C., Carreras, M. C., Jaitovich, A., Poderoso, J. J., & Boczkowski, J. (2006). HO-1 is located in liver mitochondria and modulates mitochondrial heme content and metabolism. *The Federation of American Societies for Experimental Biology Journal, 20*(8), 1236–1238.

Corral-Debrinski, M., Horton, T., Lott, M. T., Shoffner, J. M., McKee, A. C., Beal, M. F., et al. (1994). Marked changes in mitochondrial DNA deletion levels in Alzheimer brains. *Genomics, 23*(2), 471–476.

Dennery, P. A. (2000). Regulation and role of heme oxygenase in oxidative injury. *Current Topics in Cellular Regulation, 36*, 181–199.

DiMonte, D., Schipper, H., Hetts, S., & Langston, J. (1995). Iron-mediated bioactivation of 1-methl-4-phenyl-1,2,3,6-tetrahydropyridine (MPTP) in glial cultures. *Glia, 15*, 203–206.

Dore, S., Takahashi, M., Ferris, C. D., Zakhary, R., Hester, L. D., Guastella, D., et al. (1999). Bilirubin, formed by activation of heme oxygenase-2, protects neurons against oxidative stress injury. *Proceedings of the National Academy of Sciences, USA, 96*(5), 2445–2450.

Frankel, D., Mehindate, K., & Schipper, H. M. (2000). Role of heme oxygenase-1 in the regulation of manganese superoxide dismutase gene expression in oxidatively-challenged astroglia. *Journal of Cellular Physiology, 185*(1), 80–86.

Frankel, D., & Schipper, H. M. (1999). Cysteamine pretreatment of the astroglial substratum (mitochondrial iron sequestration) enhances PC12 cell vulnerability to oxidative injury. *Experimental Neurology, 160*(2), 376–385.

Fukuyama, H., Ogawa, M., Yamauchi, H., Yamaguchi, S., Kimura, J., Yonekura, Y., et al. (1994). Altered cerebral energy metabolism in Alzheimer's disease: A PET study. *Journal of Nuclear Medicine, 35*(1), 1–6.

Gibson, G. E., Sheu, K. F., & Blass, J. P. (1998). Abnormalities of mitochondrial enzymes in Alzheimer disease. *Journal of Neural Transmission, 105*(8–9), 855–870.

Ham, D., & Schipper, H. M. (2000). Heme oxygenase-1 induction and mitochondrial iron sequestration in astroglia exposed to amyloid peptides. *Cellular and Molecular Biology (Noisy-le-grand), 46*(3), 587–596.

Hirose, W., Ikematsu, K., & Tsuda, R. (2003). Age-associated increases in heme oxygenase-1 and ferritin immunoreactivity in the autopsied brain. *Legal Medicine (Tokyo), 5*(Suppl.), S360–S366.

Jefferies, W. A., Food, M. R., Gabathuler, R., Rothenberger, S., Yamada, T., Yasuhara, O., et al. (1996). Reactive microglia specifically associated with amyloid plaques in Alzheimer's disease brain tissue express melanotransferrin. *Brain Research, 712*(1), 122–126.

Jenner, P. (2003). Oxidative stress in Parkinson's disease. *Annals of Neurology, 53*(Suppl. 3), S26–S36; discussion S36–S28.

Jofre-Monseny, L., Loboda, A., Wagner, A. E., Huebbe, P., Boesch-Saadatmandi, C., Jozkowicz, A., et al. (2007). Effects of apoE genotype on macrophage inflammation and heme oxygenase-1 expression. *Biochemical and Biophysical Research Communications, 357*(1), 319–324.

Kim, H. P., Wang, X., Galbiati, F., Ryter, S. W., & Choi, A. M. (2004). Caveolae compartmentalization of heme oxygenase-1 in endothelial cells. *The Federation of American Societies for Experimental Biology Journal, 18*(10), 1080–1089.

Kimpara, T., Takeda, A., Watanabe, K., Itoyama, Y., Ikawa, S., Watanabe, M., et al. (1997). Microsatellite polymorphism in the human heme oxygenase-1 gene promoter and its application in association studies with Alzheimer and Parkinson disease. *Human Genetics, 100*(1), 145–147.

Lee, E. Y., & Lee, K. L. (2001). Accumulation of peroxidase-positive granules with ageing in SAMP and 10 SAMR1 mouse brains. *Korean Journal of Anatomy, 34*, 645–651.

LeVine, S. M. (1997). Iron deposits in multiple sclerosis and Alzheimer's disease brains. *Brain Research, 760*(1–2), 298–303.

Llesuy, S. F., & Tomaro, M. L. (1994). Heme oxygenase and oxidative stress. Evidence of involvement of bilirubin as physiological protector against oxidative damage. *Biochimica et Biophysica Acta, 1223*(1), 9–14.

Maes, O. C., Kravitz, S., Mawal, Y., Su, H., Liberman, A., Mehindate, K., et al. (2006). Characterization of alpha(1)-antitrypsin as a heme oxygenase-1 suppressor in Alzheimer plasma. *Neurobiology of Disease, 24*, 89–100.

Mattson, M. P. (2002). Contributions of mitochondrial alterations, resulting from bad genes and a hostile environment, to the pathogenesis of Alzheimer's disease. *International Review of Neurobiology, 53*, 387–409.

Mawal, Y., Berlin, D., Kravitz, S., & Schipper, H. (2002). Heme oxygenase-1 and Alzheimer disease. In N. G. Abraham, J. Alam, & K. A. Nath (Ed.), *Heme oxygenase in biology and medicine* (pp. 145–155). New York: Kluwer Academic/Plenum Publishers.

McGeer, P. L., & McGeer, E. G. (1995). The inflammatory response system of brain: implications for therapy of Alzheimer and other neurodegenerative diseases. *Brain Research Brain Research Reviews, 21*(2), 195–218.

McLaren, J., Brawer, J. R., & Schipper, H. M. (1992). Iron content correlates with peroxidase activity in cysteamine-induced astroglial organelles. *Journal of Histochemistry and Cytochemistry, 40*(12), 1887–1897.

Mehindate, K., Sahlas, D. J., Frankel, D., Mawal, Y., Liberman, A., Corcos, J., et al. (2001). Proinflammatory cytokines promote glial heme oxygenase-1 expression and mitochondrial iron deposition: implications for multiple sclerosis. *Journal of Neurochemistry, 77*(5), 1386–1395.

Minoshima, S., Giordani, B., Berent, S., Frey, K. A., Foster, N. L., & Kuhl, D. E. (1997). Metabolic reduction in the posterior cingulate cortex in very early Alzheimer's disease. *Annals of Neurology, 42*(1), 85–94.

Miyajima, H., Kono, S., Takahashi, Y., & Sugimoto, M. (2002). Increased lipid peroxidation and mitochondrial dysfunction in aceruloplasminemia brains. *Blood Cells Molecules and Diseases, 29*(3), 433–438.

Mydlarski, M. B., Brawer, J. R., & Schipper, H. M. (1998). The peroxidase-positive subcortical glial system. In H. M. Schipper (Ed.), *Astrocytes in brain aging and neurodegeneration* (pp. 191–206). Austin: R.G. Landes Co.

Nakagami, T., Toyomura, K., Kinoshita, T., & Morisawa, S. (1993). A beneficial role of bile pigments as an endogenous tissue protector: Anti-complement effects of biliverdin and conjugated bilirubin. *Biochimica et Biophysica Acta, 1158*(2), 189–193.

Petronilli, V., Cola, C., Massari, S., Colonna, R., & Bernardi, P. (1993). Physiological effectors modify voltage sensing by the cyclosporin A-sensitive permeability transition pore of mitochondria. *Journal of Biological Chemistry, 268*(29), 21939–21945.

Piantadosi, C. A., Carraway, M. S., & Suliman, H. B. (2006). Carbon monoxide, oxidative stress, and mitochondrial permeability pore transition. *Free Radical Biology and Medicine, 40*(8), 1332–1339.

Ponka, P. (2004). Hereditary causes of disturbed iron homeostasis in the central nervous system. *Annals of the New York Academy of Sciences, 1012*, 267–281.

Reichmann, H., & Riederer, P. (1994). *Mitochondrial disturbances in neurodegeneration*. Philadelphia: Saunders.

Ryter, S. W., & Tyrrell, R. M. (2000). The heme synthesis and degradation pathways: Role in oxidant sensitivity. Heme oxygenase has both pro- and anti-oxidant properties. *Free Radical Biology and Medicine, 28*(2), 289–309.

Saunders, A. M., Strittmatter, W. J., Schmechel, D., George-Hyslop, P. H., Pericak-Vance, M. A., Joo, S. H., et al. (1993). Association of apolipoprotein E allele epsilon 4 with late-onset familial and sporadic Alzheimer's disease. *Neurology, 43*(8), 1467–1472.

Sayre, L. M., Smith, M. A., & Perry, G. (2001). Chemistry and biochemistry of oxidative stress in neurodegenerative disease. *Current Medical Chemistry, 8*(7), 721–738.

Schipper, H., Scarborough, D., Lechan, R., & Reichlin, S. (1990). Gomori-positive astrocytes in primary culture: Effects of in vitro age and cysteamine exposure. *Developmental Brain Research, 54*, 71.

Schipper, H. M. (1996). Astrocytes, brain aging, and neurodegeneration. *Neurobiology of Aging, 17*(3), 467–480.

Schipper, H. M. (1998). Glial iron sequestration and neurodegeneration. In H. M. Schipper (Ed.), *Astrocytes in brain aging and neurodegeneration* (pp. 235–251). Austin: R.G. Landes Co.

Schipper, H. M. (1999). Glial HO-1 expression, iron deposition and oxidative stress in neurodegenerative diseases. *Neurotoxicity Research, 1*(1), 57–70.

Schipper, H. M. (2000). Heme oxygenase-1: Role in brain aging and neurodegeneration. *Experimental Gerontology, 35*(6–7), 821–830.

Schipper, H. M. (2001). Mitochondrial iron deposition in aging astroglia: Mechanisms and disease implications. In M. Ebadi, J. Marwah, & R. K. Chopra (Eds.), *Mitochondrial ubiquinone (Coenzyme Q): Biochemical, functional, medical, and therapeutic aspects in human health and disease* (pp. 267–280). Scottsdale, AZ: Prominent Press.

Schipper, H. M. (2004a). Brain iron deposition and the free radical-mitochondrial theory of ageing. *Ageing Research Reviews, 3*, 265–301.

Schipper, H. M. (2004b). Heme oxygenase-1: Transducer of pathological brain iron sequestration under oxidative stress. In S. LeVine, J. R. Connor, & H. M. Schipper (Eds.), *Redox-active metals in neurological disorders* (Vol. 1012, pp. 84–93). New York: Annals of the New York Academy of Sciences.

Schipper, H. M., Bennett, D. A., Liberman, A., Bienias, J. L., Schneider, J. A., Kelly, J., et al. (2006). Glial heme oxygenase-1 expression in Alzheimer disease and mild cognitive impairment. *Neurobiology of Aging, 27*(2), 252–261.

Schipper, H. M., Bernier, L., Mehindate, K., & Frankel, D. (1999). Mitochondrial iron sequestration in dopamine-challenged astroglia: role of heme oxygenase-1 and the permeability transition pore. *Journal of Neurochemistry, 72*(5), 1802–1811.

Schipper, H. M., Chertkow, H., Mehindate, K., Frankel, D., Melmed, C., & Bergman, H. (2000). Evaluation of heme oxygenase-1 as a systemic biological marker of sporadic AD. *Neurology, 54*(6), 1297–1304.

Schipper, H. M., & Cissé, S. (1995). Mitochondrial constituents of corpora amylacea and autofluorescent astrocytic inclusions in senescent human brain. *Glia, 14*(1), 55–64.

Schipper, H. M., Cissé, S., & Stopa, E. G. (1995). Expression of heme oxygenase-1 in the senescent and Alzheimer-diseased brain. *Annals of Neurology, 37*(6), 758–768.

Schipper, H. M., Kotake, Y., & Janzen, E. G. (1991). Catechol oxidation by peroxidase-positive astrocytes in primary culture: An electron spin resonance study. *Journal of Neuroscience, 11*(7), 2170–2176.

Schipper, H. M., Liberman, A., & Stopa, E. G. (1998). Neural heme oxygenase-1 expression in idiopathic Parkinson's disease. *Experimental Neurology, 150*(1), 60–68.

Schipper, H. M., Mydlarski, M. B., & Wang, X. (1993). Cysteamine gliopathy in situ: A cellular stress model for the biogenesis of astrocytic inclusions. *Journal of Neuropathology and Experimental Neurology, 52*(4), 399–410.

Schipper, H. M., Small, L., Wang, X., & Brawer, J. R. (2002). Role of porphyrin sequestration in the biogenesis of iron-laden astrocytic inclusions in primary culture. *Developmental Neuroscience, 24*(2–3), 169–176.

Schipper, H. M., Vininsky, R., Brull, R., Small, L., & Brawer, J. R. (1998). Astrocyte mitochondria: A substrate for iron deposition in the aging rat substantia nigra. *Experimental Neurology, 152*(2), 188–196.

Selkoe, D. J. (1991). The molecular pathology of Alzheimer's disease. *Neuron, 6*(4), 487–498.

Smith, M. A., Kutty, R. K., Richey, P. L., Yan, S. D., Stern, D., Chader, G. J., et al. (1994). Heme oxygenase-1 is associated with the neurofibrillary pathology of Alzheimer's disease. *American Journal of Pathology, 145*(1), 42–47.

Song, L., Song, W., & Schipper, H. M. (2007). Astroglia overexpressing heme oxygenase-1 predispose co-cultured PC12 cells to oxidative injury. *Journal of Neuroscience Research, 85*(10), 2186–2195.

Song, W., Su, H., Song, S., Paudel, H. K., & Schipper, H. M. (2006). Over-expression of heme oxygenase-1 promotes oxidative mitochondrial damage in rat astroglia. *Journal of Cellular Physiology, 206*(3), 655–663.

Soong, N. W., Hinton, D. R., Cortopassi, G., & Arnheim, N. (1992). Mosaicism for a specific somatic mitochondrial DNA mutation in adult human brain. *Nature Genetics, 2*(4), 318–323.

St-Jacques, R., Chapman, A., Lacaille, J. C., Mohr, G., & Schipper, H. M. (1999). Acceleration of ageing-related gliopathic changes and hippocampal dysfunction following intracerebroventricular infusion of cysteamine in adult rats. *Neuroscience, 90*(3), 1103–1113.

Stocker, R., Yamamoto, Y., McDonagh, A. F., Glazer, A. N., & Ames, B. N. (1987). Bilirubin is an antioxidant of possible physiological importance. *Science, 235*(4792), 1043–1046.

Storm, T., Rath, S., Mohamed, S. A., Bruse, P., Kowald, A., Oehmichen, M., et al. (2002). Mitotic brain cells are just as prone to mitochondrial deletions as neurons: A large-scale single-cell PCR study of the human caudate nucleus. *Experimental Gerontology, 37*(12), 1389–1400.

Tanno, Y., Okuizumi, K., & Tsuji, S. (1998). mtDNA polymorphisms in Japanese sporadic Alzheimer's disease. *Neurobiology of Aging, 19*(Suppl. 1), S47–51.

Vaya, J., Song, W., Khatib, S., Geng, G., & Schipper, H. M. (2007). Effects of heme oxygenase-1 expression on sterol homeostasis in rat astroglia. *Free Radical Biology and Medicine, 42*(6), 864–871.

Verma, A., Hirsch, D. J., Glatt, C. E., Ronnett, G. V., & Snyder, S. H. (1993). Carbon monoxide: a putative neural messenger. *Science, 259*(5093), 381–384.

Wang, X., Manganaro, F., & Schipper, H. M. (1995). A cellular stress model for the sequestration of redox-active glial iron in the aging and degenerating nervous system. *Journal of Neurochemistry, 64*(4), 1868–1877.

Yu, H.-L., Chertkow, H. M., Bergman, H., & Schipper, H. M. (2003). Aberrant profiles of native and oxidized glycoproteins in Alzheimer plasma. *Proteomics, 3*, 2240–2248.

Zhang, J., & Piantadosi, C. A. (1992). Mitochondrial oxidative stress after carbon monoxide hypoxia in the rat brain. *Journal of Clinical Investigation, 90*(4), 1193–1199.

# 8 Iron Deficiency and Neuropharmacology

*Laura Bianco, Erica Unger, and John Beard*

**Summary**

- Iron deficiency alters functioning of the dopaminergic system with effects on both receptors and transporters.
- Early developmental iron deficiency may produce persistent alterations in neural functioning.
- The metabolism of a number of drugs whose target of action is reuptake of monoamines may be dramatically altered by existing brain iron deficiency.
- The expansion of the list of neurotransmitters altered by iron deficiency is likely to grow as new investigations explore adenosine, glutamate, and GABA metabolism.

**Key Words:** Iron deficiency; brain iron; striatum; neurotransmitters; dopamine

## 1. INTRODUCTION

Iron is essential for many peripheral and central biological processes including electron transfer, cell growth, and oxygen transport, and there is considerable evidence that iron is also an important nutrient in neurological functioning and development (Yehdua, 1990; Roncagliolo, Garrido, Walter, Peirano, & Lozoff, 1998; Youdim, 2000; Beard & Connor, 2003; Lozoff et al., 2006). Iron deficiency during infancy causes impaired social interactions, learning deficits, and increased fearfulness (Lozoff, 1989; Lozoff, Jimenez, Hagen, Mollen, & Wolf, 2000; Walker et al., 2007). These effects may be transient or they may persist into adolescence and adulthood depending on the timing of iron deficiency in development. The biological basis of the behavioral and cognitive deficits observed in iron-deficient infants and adults is not completely understood, but likely involves changes in neurotransmitter metabolism (Ben-Shachar, Finberg, & Youdim, 1985; Yehdua, 1990; Erikson, Jones, & Beard, 2000), decreased myelin formation (Yu, Steinkirchner, Rao, & Larkin, 1986; Beard, Wiesinger, & Connor, 2003; Ward et al., 2007), and alterations in energy metabolism (Ill, Mitchell, Neely, & Connor, 2006; Ward et al., 2007). Rodent studies have shown that the synthesis and metabolism of several neurotransmitters, including dopamine (Ben-Shachar et al., 1985; Yehdua, 1990; Erikson et al., 2000), norepinephrine (Burhans et al., 2005; Beard, Wiesinger, & Jones, 2006), serotonin (Kaladhar & Narasinga Rao, 1982), and GABA/glutamate (Rao, Tkac, Townsend, Gruetter, & Georgieff, 2003), are influenced by iron deficiency. Moreover, transport and receptor expression within these

From: *Nutrition and Health: Iron Deficiency and Overload*
Edited by: S. Yehuda and D.I. Mostofsky, DOI 10.1007/978-1-59745-462-9_8

neurotransmitter systems are also affected. These changes in monoaminergic systems modulate behavior and the pharmacological responses to drugs of abuse (Erikson et al., 2000; Kwik-Uribe, Golub, & Keen, 2000; Dancheck et al., 2005).

## 2. MONOAMINES

Intra-neuronal iron metabolism involves the incorporation of iron into the binding sites of enzymes involved in electron transport, synthesis, packaging of neurotransmitters, and uptake and degradation of the neurotransmitters. In addition, secondary effects on peroxide reduction, amino acid metabolism, and fatty acid elongation and desaturation have implications for the potential mechanisms of action of iron on neuronal functioning. There are conflicting reports regarding the effects of dietary iron deficiency on energy metabolism of the brain. Mackler and colleagues (Mackler, Person, Miller, & Finch, 1979) demonstrated that mitochondrial cytochrome concentrations and rates of oxidative phosphorylation were normal in brains of iron-deficient rats. In addition, tyrosine hydroxylase, tryptophan hydroxylase, monoamine oxidase, succinate hydroxylase, and cytochrome *c* activities are reportedly normal in the brains of iron-deficient animals (Ashkenazi, Ben-Shachar, & Youdim, 1982). However, more recent studies noted a diminution of cytochrome *c* oxidase levels in the hippocampus (Siddappa et al., 2002). Bioenergetic evaluations of brain functioning using $^1$H-NMR showed dramatic changes in energy substrates in both the hippocampus and the striatum of rodents during early life iron deficiency (Ward et al., 2007). These more recent in vivo data indicate that nearly all processes that are energy-dependent in the brain are likely affected by regional brain iron deficiency. Unfortunately, the extent of these alterations in bioenergetics across neural systems is relatively unexplored and a dose–response relationship between severity of iron deficiency and magnitude of change in energy metabolism is lacking.

### *2.1. Dopamine*

#### 2.1.1. Dopaminergic Brain Regions and Consequences of ID

The two most well-studied dopamine pathways in the brain are the nigrostriatal system, linking the substantia nigra to the striatum, and the mesolimbic system, connecting the ventral tegmentum to the nucleus accumbens (Fig. 1). These dopaminergic tracts appear to be consistently sensitive to regional brain iron deficiency (Ben-Shachar et al., 1985; Pinero, Li, Connor, & Beard, 2000). Dopamine deficits in these regions inhibit the ability to process environmental information, leading to altered perception and motivation as well as impaired movement and bradykinesia (Cooper, Bloom, & Roth, 2003b). Although DA neurons can be found widely distributed in the brain, particularly high concentrations are found in the terminal fields of the striatum and nucleus accumbens.

#### 2.1.2. Synthesis

The conversion of tyrosine to L-dihydroxyphenylalanine (L-DOPA) by tyrosine hydroxylase (TH) is the initial and rate-limiting step in the catecholamine synthesis pathway (Fig. 2). TH activity is dependent on the presence of tetrabiopterin and oxygen (Cooper et al., 2003b), and is regulated by substrate availability, feedback inhibition, and phosphorylation status (Dunkley, Bobrovskaya, Graham, von Nagy-Felsobuki, & Dickson, 2004). Because TH is an iron-containing enzyme, the redox state of iron is also important in determining enzymatic activity. In the rat, TH exists in four forms, two forms containing ferrous iron (phosphorylated and not phosphorylated) and two forms containing ferric iron also existing in a phosphorylated and non-phosphorylated form (Dunkley

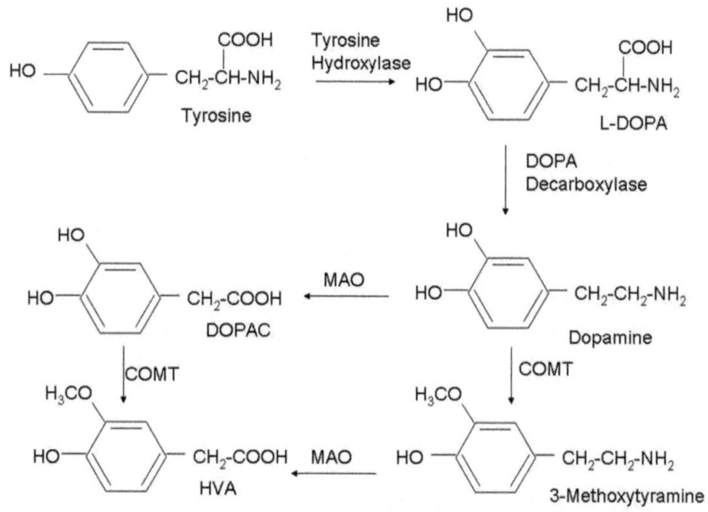


**Fig. 1.** Synthesis of dopamine: Tyrosine hydroxylase is the rate-limiting step in this pathway. This is followed by decarboxylation with dopa decarboxylase. Monoamine oxidase (MAO) and catechol-*O*-methyl-transferase (COMT) are the primary catabolic enzymes.

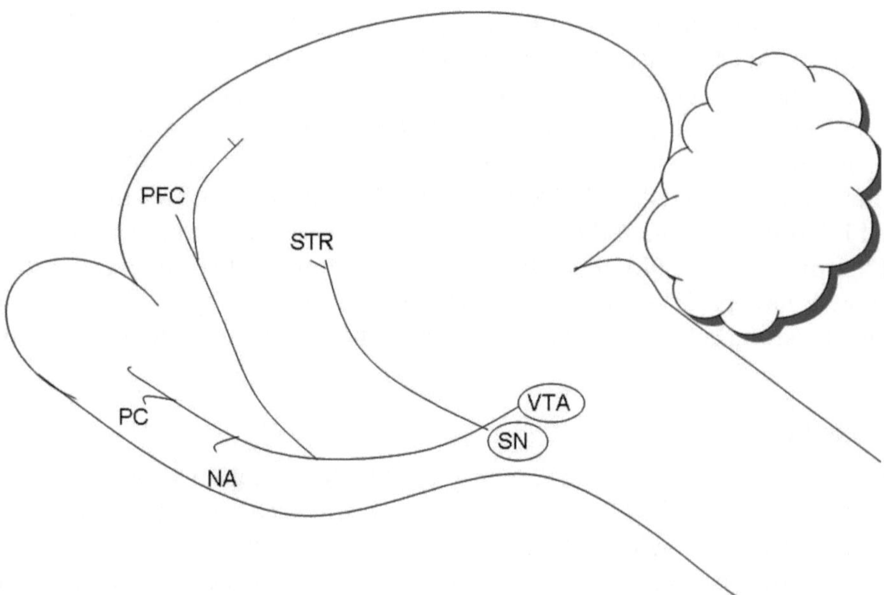


**Fig. 2.** Dopaminergic innervation of the rodent brain. STR – striatum, VTA – ventral tegmental area, PC – perirhinal cortex, PFC – prefrontal cortex, SN – substantia nigra, NA – nucleus accumbens.

et al., 2004). The ferric forms of TH are inactive and form complexes with catecholamines (Ramsey & Fitzpatrick, 1998) while the ferrous forms are enzymatically active with the phosphorylated form being the most active. Iron can also play an indirect role in TH activity through protein phosphatase 2A (PP2A). This enzyme dephosphorylates TH and it too may be an iron-sensitive protein (Yu, 1998).

Because TH plays a critical role in dopamine synthesis and iron is vital for its functioning, it would seem that iron deficiency would result in decreased activities of this enzyme. However, evidence of this is mixed. Initial studies by Youdim et al. found that post-weaning ID in rats reduces brain iron by 40% without affecting TH activity levels in whole brain (Youdim & Green, 1978; Youdim, Ben-Shachar, & Yehuda, 1989). However, Beard et al. reported decreased TH activity in striatum but not pons of iron-deficient 63-day-old rats when dietary treatment began on day 21. Earlier initiation of ID at P4 had no effect on TH in 21-day-old animals (Beard, Wiesinger et al., 2003), while initiating treatment at gestation day 15 resulted in increased TH levels in ID animals at postnatal day 15 but not postnatal day 9 or 21 compared to CN rats (Unger et al., 2007). The aggregate of these data point to a potential developmental window where iron deficiency may have particular effects on the dopamine systems that are not observed at other times in the life span.

### 2.1.3. Catabolism

The catabolism of DA requires activity of both intracellular and extracellular enzymes in order to produce the two principal catabolites, DOPAC and HVA (Fig. 2) (Cooper et al., 2003b). Intracellular DA is converted to DOPAC by monoamine oxidase B (MAO-B). The activity of this enzyme is reduced by iron deficiency in both brain and platelets, resulting in decreased levels of DOPAC (Patiroglu & Dogan, 1991; Hu, Wei, & Ding, 1996). Catechol-*O*-methyltransferase (COMT) converts extracellular DA to 3-methoxy tyramine, 3-MT (Sharman, 1973; Dedek, Baumes, Tien-Duc, Gomeni, & Korf, 1979), where it is further converted to HVA by aldehyde dehydrogenase or MAO-B. Often DOPAC and HVA levels are used as an index for DA production or turnover. The ratio of DOPAC + HVA/DA can provide insight into the metabolic rate of DA catabolism (Beard, Chen, Connor, & Jones, 1994). For example, an elevated HVA/DA ratio in CSF or dialysate could be attributed to both elevated extracellular DA, due to reduced DA transporter functioning, and reduced MAO activity. These shifts would result in reduced DOPAC and increased HVA production in the steady state. This was exactly what was observed in one in vivo study (Nelson, Erikson, Pinero, & Beard, 1997), but not in two others (Beard et al., 1994; Chen, Beard, & Jones, 1995). It is feasible that these changes are highly sensitive to dopamine activation, but these earlier studies did not specifically probe the system with pharmacologic agents.

### 2.1.4. Dopamine Receptors

The physiologic actions of dopamine are mediated by five receptor subtypes that are grouped into $D_1$-like ($D_1$ and $D_5$) and the $D_2$-like receptor ($D_2$, $D_3$, and $D_4$) subtypes. The $D_1$ receptors are located postsynaptically and, when activated, these receptors couple to the stimulatory G protein ($G_s$) and activate adenylyl cyclase, which serves to increase intracellular cAMP. Postsynaptic $D_2$-like receptors inhibit adenylyl cyclase and activate $K^+$ channels (Cooper et al., 2003b). In the striatum, postsynaptic dopamine receptors regulate the activity of neuronal feedback pathways by which striatal neurons can communicate with dopamine cell bodies in the substantia nigra. This enables dopamine-innervated cells in the striatum to modulate the physiological activity of the nigrostriatal dopamine neurons. In general, increased postsynaptic activity translates to decreased nigrostriatal dopamine activity.

$D_2$ receptors are also located presynaptically, where they regulate dopamine synthesis and release (Jones et al., 1999). Autoreceptors in the somatodendritic region slow the firing rate of dopamine neurons while the stimulation of autoreceptors on the nerve terminal inhibits dopamine synthesis and release. Thus, autoreceptors work in concert with somatodendritical terminals to control dopamine activity. Numerous studies exploring the effects of ID on $D_1$-and $D_2$-receptor densities have been performed (Youdim, Ben-Shachar, Yehuda, & Ashkenazi, 1983; Beard et al., 1994; Nelson et al., 1997; Erikson et al., 2000; Erikson, Jones, Hess, Zhang, & Beard, 2001), and these studies consistently show that $D_2R$ protein levels are reduced in the iron-deficient striatum. The mechanism of the effect of neuronal iron deficiency on DR gene expression or metabolism is not entirely understood. In 1998, Yajima et al. reported that the $D_2R$ gene is transcribed from a TATA-less promoter that has an initiator-like sequence and several putative Sp1/Sp3 and Ap1 transcriptional binding sites (Yajima, Lee, Minowa, & Mouradian, 1998). Iron chelation was found to alter the levels of these transcription factors without influencing mRNA levels (Kramer-Stickland, Edmonds, Bair, & Bowden, 1999; Ruiz et al., 2000). Microarray analysis of DFO-treated PC12 cells also failed to reveal any effect of iron chelation on other possible transcription factors (unpublished data). However, regulation of $D_2R$ functionality occurs due to the regulation of trafficking by DR multiplex proteins (Kabbani & Levenson, 2007). Clardy and colleagues recently showed that a number of these DR-associated proteins are altered by iron deficiency in early life (Clardy et al., 2006). These findings suggest a potential mechanism through which $D_2R$ regulation is altered by iron deficiency.

#### 2.1.5. DA Transport

The ability of neurons to process environmental information is dependent upon appropriate rates of dopamine clearance from the interstitial space. Thus, alterations in dopamine metabolism in the mesolimbic and nigrostriatal tracts could easily be related to altered perception and motivation (Cooper et al., 2003b). The dopamine transporter (DAT) is the primary method of clearance of DA from the synaptic cleft and is estimated to remove between 80% and 90% of DA from the extracellular space. DAT is located on the extrasynaptic region of the axonal terminal and is believed to be responsible for the inactivation of dopamine that diffuses away from the synapse (Ciliax et al., 1995). Pharmacologic inhibition of the transporter by GBR 12909 or cocaine results in an increase in extracellular DA (Smith & Justice, 1994). DAT density is diminished by iron deficiency in striatum and nucleus accumbens, both terminal fields of neurons originating in the substantia nigra and ventral tegmentum (Lipschitz, Cook, & Finch, 1974; Erikson et al., 2000). The first studies to report this finding focused on a post-weaning rat model, as this is developmentally similar to when most human infants are experiencing an iron-deficient environment (Ben-Shachar, Ashkenazi, & Youdim, 1986; Yehuda & Youdim, 1989; Beard et al., 1994). In support of these data, in vivo microdialysis studies using a similar post-weaning model found that dietary iron deficiency increased extracellular dopamine in striatum while tissue levels were reduced by 20% (Chen, Beard, et al., 1995; Kwik-Uribe et al., 2000; Beard et al., 2007). Pharmacologic studies with cocaine using the same post-weaning model demonstrated a $\sim$50% reduction in the sensitivity of striatal synaptosomes in ID animals, implying changes in both transporter density and functioning (Chen, Connor, & Beard, 1995; Erikson et al., 2000). These observations suggest that drug efficacy for those compounds which target DAT are likely to be adversely affected by iron deficiency. There is a sparse amount of documentation regarding the impact of iron deficiency in human populations on consumption of drugs like cocaine or methylphenidate. One study by Semba noted an increased use of "speedball" by iron-deficient drug users in Baltimore compared to non-anemic drug users (Dancheck et al., 2005). Dietary iron repletion of rodents restores striatal DAT to normal levels (Bianco, Wiesinger, Earley, Jones, & Beard, 2008). This is consistent with recent human studies showing that decreased reliance of iron-deficient ADHD children on methylphenadate after iron supplementation corrected their iron status.

### 2.1.6. $D_2$R-DAT Link

Several animal studies provide evidence that there is a relationship between $D_2$R activity and DAT movement on and off the plasma membrane (Meiergerd, Patterson, & Schenk, 1993; Cass & Gerhardt, 1994; Dickinson et al., 1999). In 1993, it was found that the application of the $D_2$R agonist quinpirole resulted in increased DA transport velocity in striatal synaptosomes (Meiergerd et al., 1993). Later studies showed that activation of the $D_2$R enhances DAT function by increasing the number of cell surface transporters through $G_{i/o}$-dependant mechanisms (Mayfield & Zahniser, 2001). Knockout mice provided further evidence for this connection, with $D_2$R knockout mice exhibiting a loss in DAT functioning in all dopaminergic fields without a change in gene expression (Dickinson et al., 1999). Furthermore, DAT knockout mice show decreased $D_2$R densities in dopaminergic neurons (Jones et al., 1999).

Since $D_2$R and DAT are both affected by iron deficiency, it has been suggested that the linkage between them may be compromised by iron deficiency (Unger et al., 2007). In 2007, a study of developmental iron deficiency reported alterations in $D_2$R levels that preceded the alterations in DAT and in tissue DA concentrations. This indicated a site of major influence on monoamine metabolism and a sequence of sensitivity to regional iron deprivation (Unger et al., 2007). Additionally, there are also two lines of evidence that suggest that the PKC/PKA pathways and the ERK1/2 pathway alter the $D_2$R regulation of DAT. First, cell culture experiments showed that cell surface DAT and DAT uptake are decreased as a result of iron chelation and that changes in protein kinase C (PKC) and protein kinase A (PKA) expression and function may mediate this effect (Wiesinger et al., 2007). Although it has not been explored in relation to iron deficiency, Bolan et al. demonstrated that $D_2$ autoreceptors regulate DAT expression via the extracellular signal-regulated kinases 1 and 2 (ERK1/2) (Bolan et al., 2007). Thus, PKC and ERK 1/2 are potential targets through which iron deficiency could disrupt $D_2$R–DAT communication.

### 2.1.7. Iron Deficiency During Development

In rodents, the effects of post-weaning iron deficiency are largely reversible with iron therapy. This finding, however, does not appear to translate to human infants. This is believed to be due to the dramatically different timing of neurological development in rodents and humans (Clancy, Darlington, & Finlay, 2001). When iron deficiency was started in rodents at mid-lactation, P10, or P14 and extended to P21 (Pinero et al., 2000; Pinero, Jones, & Beard, 2001), there was a very severe reduction in brain iron and changes in behaviors that were not corrected with several weeks of iron therapy begun at weaning (Beard, 2003; Beard, Erikson, & Jones, 2003). The findings from these studies pointed to at least one critical period in the second half of lactation at which iron deficiency permanently altered the course of neurological development. Moving the window of iron deficiency to P4 followed by iron repletion at P21 produced essentially the same result (Erikson et al., 2000; Beard, Felt, et al., 2006). When iron deprivation started in mid-gestation but stopped early in lactation and prior to the period of rapid striatal dopamine receptor differentiation and development, dams became mildly anemic by parturition and thus the pups were only mildly iron-deficient. The nearly complete lack of change in brain monoamines, iron, and behavioral measures in these rats shows that a period of iron deficiency before the period of maximal neurogenesis and differentiation in the rodent had no lasting effects.

These studies indicate that brain iron repletion is possible in many regions, and that iron-repleted rats had higher levels of brain iron than CN rats. This excessive accumulation of iron may have long-term deleterious consequences (McArdle, Andersen, Jones, & Gambling, 2006). Two brain regions, ventral midbrain and frontal cortex, showed an over-compensation in brain iron concentration in adult rats that had been iron deficient from G15-P4 but then iron sufficient into adulthood (Pinero et al., 2000). Aggressive iron therapy following fetal iron deficiency in C57BL/6 mice was recently claimed to be related to development of Parkinson-like neurodegeneration (Kaur et al., 2006). The fetal programming of the set-point for brain iron concentrations has not been carefully explored, but the previous work and the current observations suggest that resetting of the set-point for iron homeostasis may occur when iron deficiency commences in early life. Iron deficiency may involve prioritization and even redistribution of iron across tissues, an effect that may be related to the stage of particular organ differentiation (Georgieff, Mills, Gordon, & Wobken, 1995; Kretchmer, Beard, & Carlson, 1996; Guiang, Georgieff, Lambert, Schmidt, & Widness, 1997; Siddappa et al., 2004; McArdle et al., 2006).

## 2.2. *Norepinephrine*

Norepinephrine in the central nervous system affects alertness and arousal and influences the reward system (Cooper, Bloom, & Roth, 2003c). The major noradrenergic tracts in the brain project from the locus cerelus to the medial forebrain bundle, cortices, hippocampus, cerebellum, and spinal cord (Fig. 3).

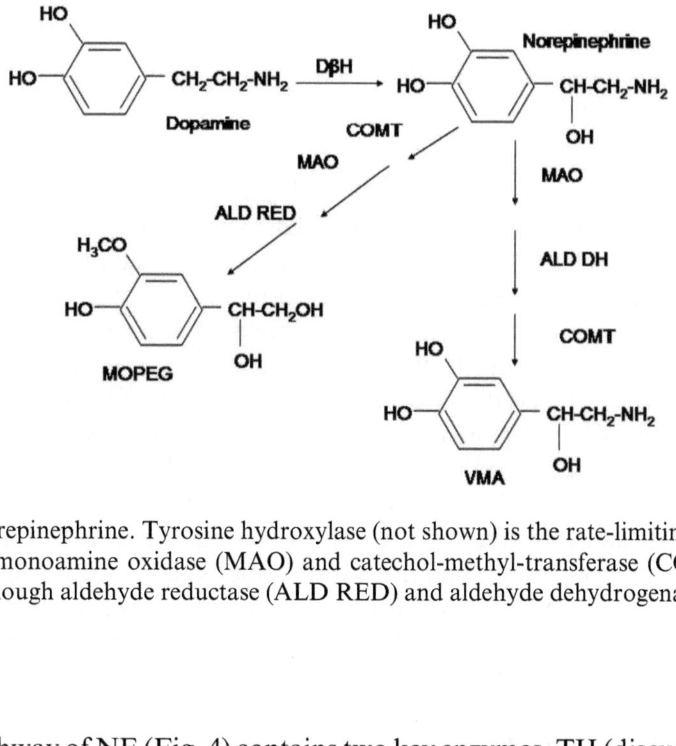


**Fig. 3.** Synthesis of norepinephrine. Tyrosine hydroxylase (not shown) is the rate-limiting step in this pathway. Similar to dopamine, monoamine oxidase (MAO) and catechol-methyl-transferase (COMT) are the primary catabolic enzymes, although aldehyde reductase (ALD RED) and aldehyde dehydrogenase (ALD DH) are also important.

### 2.2.1. Synthesis

The synthetic pathway of NE (Fig. 4) contains two key enzymes, TH (discussed previously) and Dopamine-β-hydroxylase (DβH). DβH is a copper, not iron, containing enzyme localized within vesicles that store catecholamines (Axelrod, 1972). Most DβH is bound to the inner vesicle membrane, but some is free within the vesicle and is released into the extracellular space with NE by reverse pinocytosis (Weinshilboum, Thoa, Johnson, Kopin, & Axelrod, 1971). In situations where NE tissue levels are reduced (α-methyl-paratyrosine or reserpine treatment), DβH activity and thus NE are increased (Molinoff, Brimijoin, & Axelrod, 1972), suggesting that DβH activity can be regulated by NE concentration. In post-weaning ID rats both DβH activity and extracellular NE levels in striatum were increased.

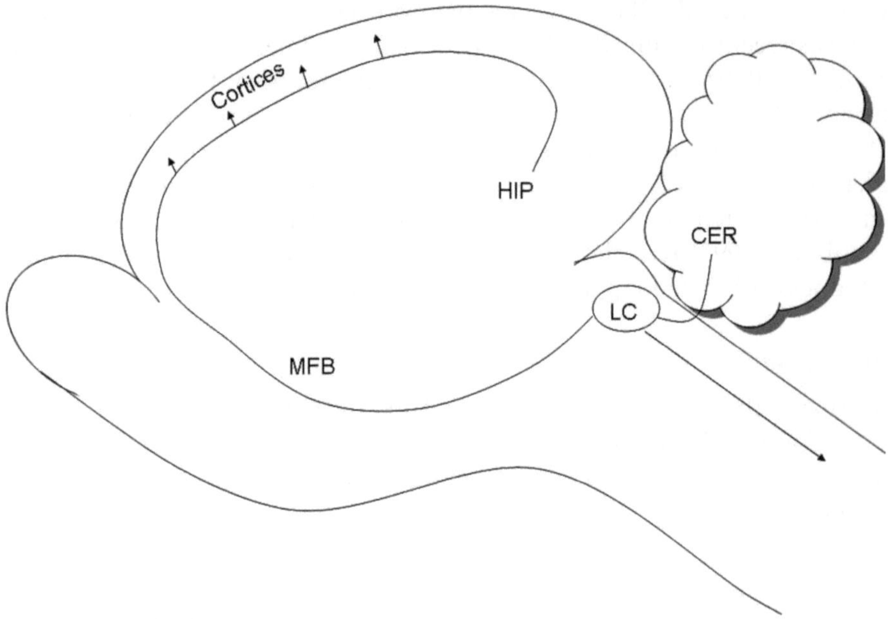


**Fig. 4** Noradrenergic innervation of the rodent brain. LC – locus ceruleus, CER – cerebellum, MFB – medial forebrain bundle, HIP – hippocampus.

Norepinephrine signaling is mediated by α and β receptors (Jhanwar-Uniyal, Roland, & Leibowitz, 1986). The α adrenergic receptors inhibit adenylyl cyclase activity (Bylund, 1992), while β adrenergic receptors stimulate synthesis of cAMP, resulting in activation of PKA (Minneman, Dibner, Wolfe, & Molinoff, 1979). In 1982, Ashkenazi reported that post-weaning iron deficiency did not affect the density of either class of adrenergic receptors in the brain (Ashkenazi et al., 1982).

One of the first studies of neuronal effects of ID in humans was performed by Oski and colleagues in ID anemic infants. They observed increased urinary NE in these ID infants, which returned to normal with iron therapy (Voorhess, Stuart, Stockman, & Oski, 1975). Studies in ID women showed that levels of plasma NE are increased when cold-stressed (Borel, Smith, Brigham, & Beard, 1991). Other studies with rodent models demonstrated that NE turnover is increased in post-ganglionic noradrenergic terminals and elevated levels of NE in plasma during IDA (Smith & Beard, 1989; Tobin & Beard, 1990). Cell culture experiments also demonstrated a dose–response effect of iron chelators on NET levels and NE uptake (Burhans et al., 2005; Beard, Wiesinger, et al., 2006), indicating that NET is responsive to available iron in the cell. Whether the effect of iron deficiency on NET works through a mechanism similar to that of DAT is likely, but for now unproven.

#### 2.2.2. Degradation and Transport

COMT and MAO-A are the two main enzymes involved in the degradation of NE (Cooper et al., 2003c). There is no evidence to indicate that either of these enzymes is altered by iron deficiency. However, reuptake of NE into the cell by the NET may be affected. Burhans et al. reported that NET density was reduced in the ID rodent brain in the thalamic nuclei and locus cerelus (Burhans et al., 2005). Follow-up cell culture experiments demonstrated a dose-dependent loss of NET protein levels on the cell membrane and reduced NET mRNA within 24 hours of iron chelation (Beard, Wiesinger, et al., 2006). Levels of NET protein in thalamus and locus cerelus tissue, evaluated by western blotting, were also reduced by iron deficiency.

## *2.3. Serotonin*

The serotonin neurotransmitter system is well known for its involvement in the modulation of mood (Merens, Willem Van der Does, & Spinhoven, 2007). Serotonin cell bodies lie in the raphe nuclei and the upper brain stem. Projections from these cell bodies extend to many regions of the brain, including striatum, thalamus, hippocampus, and cerebral cortices (Cooper, Bloom, & Roth, 2003a) (Fig. 5).

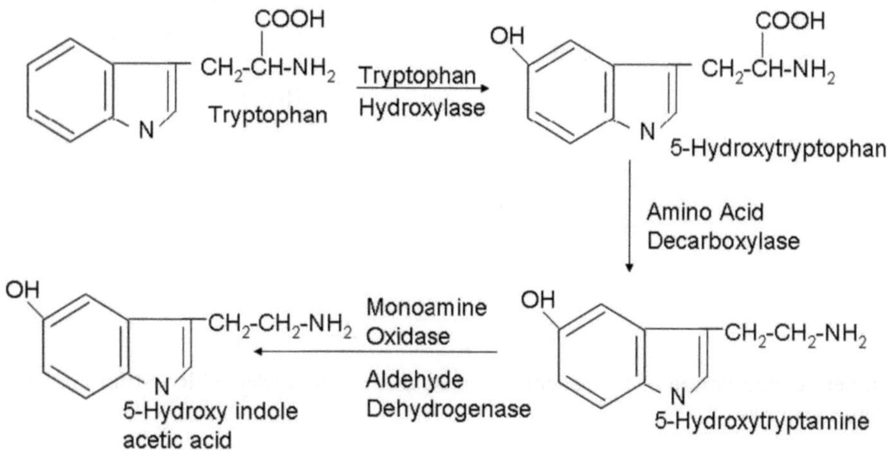


**Fig. 5.** Synthesis of serotonin: Tryptophan hydroxylase is the rate-limiting step. This is followed by decarboxylation with amino acid decarboxylase. Finally, serotonin is degraded by monoamine oxidase and aldehyde dehydrogenase.

### 2.3.1. Synthesis

Serotonin (5-HT) is found throughout the body, but it cannot cross the blood–brain barrier and thus must be synthesized in the brain from the amino acid tryptophan (Fig. 6). Tryptophan hydroxylase contains an iron-binding site and is regulated by phosphorylation with PKA (Johansen, Jennings, Cotton, & Kuhn, 1996). The question of whether iron deficiency affects this enzyme in vivo is under debate. Initial reports indicate that tryptophan hydroxylase, along with several other brain enzymes, remains unchanged during conditions of iron deficiency (Green & Youdim, 1977; Youdim et al., 1989). However, other work in cell culture demonstrated that iron chelation inhibits tryptophan hydroxylase activity (Kuhn, Ruskin, & Lovenberg, 1980; Hasegawa, Oguro, Naito, & Ichiyama, 1999).

### 2.3.2. Transport

Similar to the catecholamine systems, 5-HT is transported across the cell membrane by the serotonin transporter (5-HTT). This protein is the main site of pharmacologic action for a number of classes of psychoactive drugs including tricyclic antidepressants, such as imipramine and amitriptyline, and the serotonin reuptake inhibitors (Fuller, Perry, & Molloy, 1975; Blakely, De Felice, & Hartzell, 1994; Keller, 1999). Previous work from several laboratories indicate that pre- and post-weaning iron deficiency alter 5-HTT protein expression in the rat brain (Burhans et al., 2005, 2006; Beard et al., 2007), and that 5-HT uptake in synaptic vesicles is reduced by moderate and severe iron deficiency in rats (Kaladhar & Narasinga Rao, 1982). A decrease in

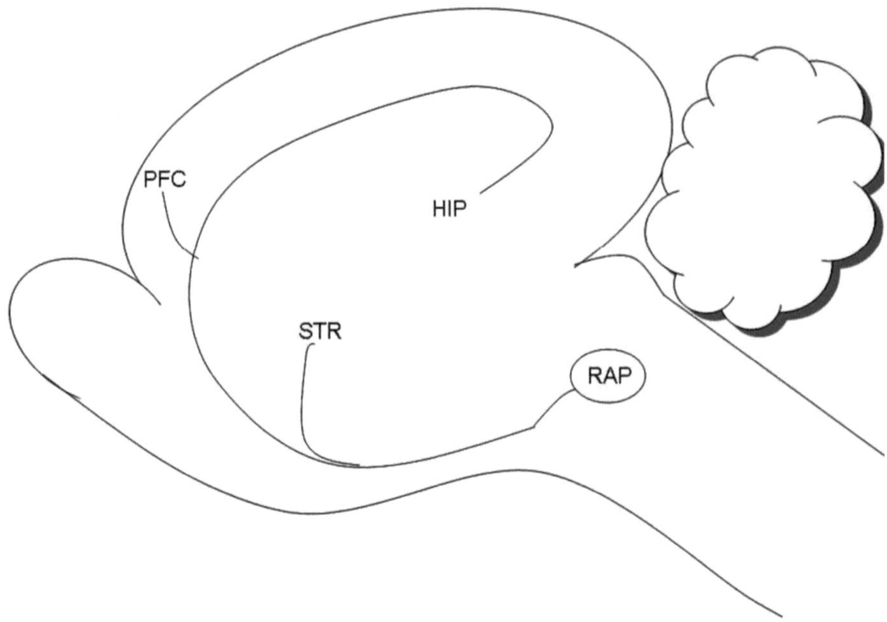


**Fig. 6.** Serotoninergic innervation of the rodent brain. RAP – raphe nuclei, STR – striatum, PFC – prefrontal cortex, HIP – hippocampus.

uptake generally results in a depletion of intracellular tissue 5-HT which has been reported in prefrontal cortex, striatum, and ventral midbrain (Shukla, Agarwal, Chansuria, & Taneja, 1989; Beard et al., 2007). Most likely, decreases in transport are also accompanied by increased extracellular 5-HT; however, this has not been explored to date.

#### 2.3.3. Receptors

5-HT levels are regulated by at least 14 different 5-HT receptor subtypes, most of which have been linked to anxiety and/or depression (Parks, Robinson, Sibille, Shenk, & Toth, 1998; Ramboz et al., 1998). Despite the potential relationships between 5-HT and many of the behavioral responses to iron deficiency in humans and animal models, 5-HT receptor expression and sensitivity have not been addressed within the context of iron deficiency.

#### 2.3.4. Catabolism

Serotonin is catabolized to 5-hydroxyindolacetic acid (5-HIAA) by deamination with MAO-A. There are reports of decreased 5-HIAA levels in tissue (Shukla et al., 1989; Beard et al., 2007). In a lactation iron-deficiency model, 5-HIAA levels were reduced; however, this coincided with decreased 5-HT levels. Because the ratio of 5-HIAA/5-HT was not altered, changes in the concentration of 5-HIAA likely result from decreased 5-HT and not altered catabolism. To date, there is no evidence that MAO-A function is directly affected by iron deficiency.

### *2.4. GABA/Glutamate*

Gamma amino butyric acid (GABA) and glutamate are the major inhibitory and excitatory neurotransmitters in the mammalian central nervous system. These neurotransmitters have been implicated in neurological and psychiatric disorders in humans, and pharmacological manipulation of GABAergic transmission is effective in the treatment of anxiety (Humphrey et al., 1995).

The work on iron deficiency and GABA and glutamate is far less extensive than that of iron deficiency and monoamines. Most of the recent studies have had a focus on interactions with Mn toxicity when dietary iron deficiency is imposed (Erikson, Shihabi, J. L. Aschner, & M. Aschner, 2002; Anderson, Cooney, & Erikson, 2007).

### 2.4.1. Synthesis

GABA and glutamate are formed by the GABA shunt (Fig. 7). This closed loop process begins with the transamination of α-ketoglutarate into glutamate by gamma-aminobutyric acid transaminase (GABA-T). Glutamate is converted to glutamic acid and then to GABA by glutamic acid decarboxylase (GAD). Iron deficiency in utero and post-weaning causes a downregulation of the GABAergic system, including decreases in glutamate decarboxylase, glutamate dehydrogenase, and GABA transaminase activities (Taneja, Mishra, & Agarwal, 1986; Li, 1998). Concentrations of GABA were also found to be decreased in the hippocampus, striatum, and globus pallidus of iron-deficient rodents (Erikson et al., 2002) most likely due to decreased GABA transport (Anderson et al., 2007) or synthesis. Another study examined the relationship between iron deficiency and the glutaminergic system and observed that the ratio of glutamate to glutamine was increased in the striatum (Ward et al., 2007). Glutaminergic input into the striatum is important in regulating dopaminergic systems. Alterations to the glutaminergic as well as the GABAergic tone of the system may increase the likelihood that dopaminergic neurons will fire (Lisman & Grace, 2005). This is a potential explanation for the efficacy of gabapentin, a $Ca^{++}$ channel blocker that alters the GABA system in RLS patients (Winkelman, Allen, Tenzer, & Hening, 2007). Alterations in GABAergic regulation of DA release could accomplish the same efficacy as DA agonist or L-DOPA treatment of these patients with a deficit in brain iron content. This provides a secondary route through which iron deficiency could modulate the dopaminergic system and associated behaviors.

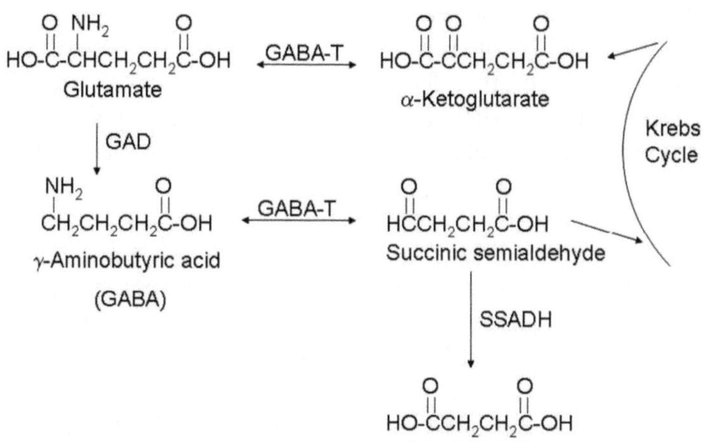


**Fig. 7.** Synthesis of GABA: Transamination of α-ketoglutarate into glutamate by gamma-aminobutyric acid transaminase (GABA-T). Glutamate is then converted to glutamic acid, which is decarboxylated to GABA by glutamic acid decarboxylase (GAD). Succinic semialdehyde is converted to succinic acid by succinic semialdehyde dehydrogenase.

### 2.4.2. Receptors

The GABAergic system has two major receptors, $GABA_A$ and $GABA_B$. $GABA_A$ is the major inhibitory neurotransmitter receptor and the site of many psychoactive drugs, while $GABA_B$ serves as an autoreceptor and regulates release (Ben-Ari, Khazipov, Leinekugel, Caillard, & Gaiarsa, 1997). Glutamate is regulated by a complex series of receptors including the *N*-methyl-D-aspartate (NMDA), kainate, and α-amino-3-hydroxy-5-methylisoxazole-4-propionic acid (AMPA) receptors (Ben-Ari et al., 1997). The effect of iron deficiency on these receptors has not been well studied. However, one study employing the $GABA_A$ agonist, muscimol, found increased muscimol and decreased glutamate binding in synaptosomes prepared from iron-deficient rats (Agarwal, 2001). GABA and glutamate play such a crucial role in excitatory and inhibitory pathways of the central nervous system that the influence of ID on alterations in AMPA or NMDA receptor binding could indicate a "ripple" influence of ID on other neurotransmitter systems in the brain.

### 2.4.3. Iron Deficiency and Drugs of Abuse

Changes in monoaminergic systems caused by iron deficiency can modulate behavior and change drug efficacy. Iron deficiency decreases the sensitivity of rats to the locomotor-activating effect of cocaine, and it causes a right shift in the $IC_{50}$ for cocaine, indicating that more cocaine is required to inhibit DAT (Erikson et al., 2000; Jones, Wheeler, Beard, & Grigson, 2002). This first finding is not surprising considering that iron deficiency reduces DAT and alters dopamine receptor expression. However, the second finding shows that the functioning of DAT is also altered in iron deficiency independent of DAT expression.

Impairment of dopamine systems has wide-ranging effects on behavior from psychotic and psychoaffective problems to propensity for drug abuse, attention-deficit hyperactivity disorder, and perhaps conduct disorders among others (Dancheck et al., 2005; Konofal et al., 2008; Oner, Alkar, & Oner, 2008). In 2005, Dancheck et al. reported an association between iron deficiency and injection drug usage among HIV-positive and HIV-negative women in Baltimore (Dancheck et al., 2005). The authors could not conclude from this study whether there was a causal association; however, they theorized two possible explanations for their results. First, they hypothesized that drug injection could lead to iron deficiency through high prevalence of skin abscesses or endocarditis caused by the injection itself. Second, it is possible that iron deficiency increases the risk of addiction through a decrease in drug sensitivity at the DAT. Approximately 80% of injection drug use in this study involved cocaine mixed with heroin, making it quite plausible that a causal relationship between iron status and drug usage may exist among these women.

### 2.4.4. ADHD

Attention-deficit hyperactivity disorder (ADHD) affects between 5% and 10% of school-age children (Biederman, 2005). This disease manifests itself as a persistent pattern of inattention and/or hyperactivity/impulsivity (American Psychiatric Association, 1994). The pathophysiology is not well understood; however, generally it is thought that an imbalance of norepinephrine and dopamine are responsible for the behavioral effects exhibited by patients (Biederman, 2005). Because iron deficiency is known to severely impact the catecholaminergic systems, the iron status of these individuals is being explored as an underlying cause. There have been several reports that support a relationship between lower serum ferritin levels and higher hyperactivity scores (Oner & Oner, 2007; Oner et al., 2008). Iron treatment with oral ferrous iron supplementation can greatly improve scores on the ADHD rating scale in patients with low (<30 ng/mL) serum ferritin levels

(Konofal et al., 2008). Similarly, iron repletion studies in rats have found that DAT and extracellular DA return to nearly normal levels in a short period of time (Nelson et al., 1997; Bianco et al., 2008). Thus, it appears that iron supplementation either in conjunction with or instead of traditional drug treatments may be an effective avenue in some cases. Traditional treatment of ADHD with methylphenidate and atomoxetine target the DAT/NET and NET, respectively. Decreases in both of these transporters occur in iron deficiency, providing a possible mechanism through which iron may modulate ADHD symptoms and treatment (Erikson et al., 2000; Burhans et al., 2005).

### 2.5. *Endorphins*

Endorphins are the "feel good" molecules in the brain (Goldstein & Lowery, 1975). They are released from the hypothalamus and pituitary gland and act as natural painkillers which resemble opiates in their ability to produce analgesia and a sense of well-being. Studies discussing the effects of iron deficiency on endorphins are rare. However, one study performed by Yehuda and Youdim measured pain threshold and circadian rhythm (Yehuda & Youdim, 1984). They found that peripherally administered beta-endorphin elevated pain threshold while administration of naloxene abolished these effects in ID rats only and that pain threshold in ID animals was different depending on when in the diurnal cycle it was measured. Furthermore, neuroleptics increased the pain threshold in CN and ID rats implicating the dopamine system in this response. These results suggest that the rate of opiate degradation in the brain is diminished and/or the uptake of opiates across the blood–brain barrier is enhanced by iron deficiency (Ben-Shachar, Yehuda, Finberg, Spanier, & Youdim, 1988).

### 2.6. *Estrogen*

Several studies indicate that male and female rodents respond differently to iron deficiency (Erikson et al., 2000, 2001), yet most studies are primarily performed in male rats. Female rats are known to exhibit an estrous cycle-dependent variation in basal extracellular concentration of striatal DA, amphetamine-stimulated DA release, and striatal DA-mediated behaviors (Becker, 1990a, 1990b; Becker, Jamieson, & Brown, 1993). These differences are believed to be due to estrogen modification of $D_2$ receptors and DAT densities resulting in increased sensitivity to pharmacological stimulus (Levesque & Di Paolo, 1990; Le Saux & Di Paolo, 2006). Although previously documented in ID female rats, a mechanism by which ID may modulate estrogen metabolism has not been explored. While the effects of estrogen regulation on the iron-uptake proteins transferrin and lactoferrin have been documented (Lee, McKnight, & Palmiter, 1978; Teng, 1995), the effect of iron deficiency on these interactions is unknown

## 3. CONCLUSIONS

Brain iron deficiency can have lasting effects on neurotransmitter systems in the brain resulting in sensorimotor deficits, decreased cognitive abilities, and increased emotional behaviors. In some cases, depending on the timing of onset of iron deficiency these alterations can be reversed. However, further studies should be performed to elucidate the critical time points during which iron supplementation can be executed without risk of damage. In particular, relatively little information is known about the influence of gestational and lactational iron deficiency on the serotonin, GABA, and glutamate systems. What aspects of these systems are altered, and can the adverse effects be reversed with iron supplementation? Once these questions are answered, we can better define the mechanisms through which these neurotransmitter systems are related as it pertains to iron deficiency. Iron deficiency has been linked to several disorders including drug abuse and ADHD. Further work focusing on iron supplementation in individuals that are afflicted with these disorders can help to elucidate the role of iron status in disease states.

## REFERENCES

Agarwal, K. N. (2001). Iron and the brain: Neurotransmitter receptors and magnetic resonance spectroscopy. *British Journal of Nutrition, 85*(Suppl. 2), S147–S150.

American Psychiatric Association. (1994). *Diagnostic criteria from DSM-IV*. Washington, DC: The Association.

Anderson, J. G., Cooney, P. T., & Erikson, K. M. (2007). Brain manganese accumulation is inversely related to gamma-amino butyric acid uptake in male and female rats. *Toxicological Sciences, 95*, 188–195.

Ashkenazi, R., Ben-Shachar, D., & Youdim, M. B. (1982). Nutritional iron and dopamine binding sites in the rat brain. *Pharmacology Biochemistry and Behavior, 17*(Suppl. 1), 43–47.

Axelrod, J. (1972). Dopamine-P-hydroxylase: Regulation of its synthesis and release from nerve terminals. *Pharmacological Reviews, 24*, 233–243.

Beard, J. (2003). Iron deficiency alters brain development and functioning. *Journal of Nutrition, 133*, 1468S–1472S.

Beard, J., Erikson, K. M., & Jones, B. C. (2003). Neonatal iron deficiency results in irreversible changes in dopamine function in rats. *Journal of Nutrition, 133*, 1174–1179.

Beard, J. L., Chen, Q., Connor, J., & Jones, B. C. (1994). Altered monamine metabolism in caudate-putamen of iron-deficient rats. *Pharmacology Biochemistry and Behavior, 48*, 621–624.

Beard, J. L., & Connor, J. R. (2003). Iron status and neural functioning. *Annual Review of Nutrition, 23*, 41–58.

Beard, J. L., Felt, B., Schallert, T., Burhans, M., Connor, J. R., Georgieff, M. K. (2006). Moderate iron deficiency in infancy: biology and behavior in young rats. *Behavioral Brain Research, 170*, 224–232.

Beard, J. L., Unger, E. L., Bianco, L. E., Paul, T., Rundle, S. E., Jones, B. C. (2007). Early postnatal iron repletion overcomes lasting effects of gestational iron deficiency in rats. *Journal of Nutrition, 137*, 1176–1182.

Beard, J. L., Wiesinger, J. A., & Connor, J. R. (2003). Pre- and post-weaning iron deficiency alters myelination in Sprague-Dawley rats. *Developmental Neuroscience, 25*, 308–315.

Beard, J. L., Wiesinger, J. A., & Jones, B. C. (2006). Cellular iron concentrations directly affect the expression levels of norepinephrine transporter in PC12 cells and rat brain tissue. *Brain Research, 1092(1)*, 47–58.

Becker, J. B. (1990a). Direct effect of 17 beta-estradiol on striatum: Sex differences in dopamine release. *Synapse, 5*, 157–164.

Becker, J. B. (1990b). Estrogen rapidly potentiates amphetamine-induced striatal dopamine releasc and rotational behavior during microdialysis. *Neuroscience Letters, 118*, 169–171.

Becker, P. M., Jamieson, A. O., & Brown, W. D. (1993). Dopaminergic agents in restless legs syndrome and periodic limb movements of sleep: Response and complications of extended treatment in 49 cases. *Sleep 16*, 713–716.

Ben-Ari, Y., Khazipov, R., Leinekugel, X., Caillard, O., & Gaiarsa, J. L. (1997). GABAA, NMDA and AMPA receptors: A developmentally regulated 'menage a trois'. *Trends in Neuroscience, 20*, 523–529.

Ben-Shachar, D., Ashkenazi, R., & Youdim, M. B. (1986). Long-term consequence of early iron-deficiency on dopaminergic neurotransmission in rats. *International Journal of Developmental Neuroscience, 4*, 81–88.

Ben-Shachar, D., Finberg, J. P., & Youdim, M. B. (1985). Effect of iron chelators on dopamine D2 receptors. *Journal of Neurochemistry, 45*, 999–1005.

Ben-Shachar, D., Yehuda, S., Finberg, J. P., Spanier, I., & Youdim, M. B. (1988). Selective alteration in blood-brain barrier and insulin transport in iron-deficient rats. *Journal of Neurochemistry, 50*, 1434–1437.

Bianco, L. E., Wiesinger, J. A., Earley, C. J., Jones, B. C., & Beard, J. (2008, in press). Iron deficiency alters dopamine uptake and response to L-DOPA injection in Sprague Dawley rats. *Journal of Neurochemistry, 106(1)*, 205–15.

Biederman, J. (2005). Attention-deficit/hyperactivity disorder: A selective overview. *Biological Psychiatry, 57*, 1215–1220.

Blakely, R. D., De Felice, L. J., & Hartzell, H. C. (1994). Molecular physiology of norepinephrine and serotonin transporters. *Journal of Experimental Biology, 196*, 263–281.

Bolan, E. A., Kivell, B., Jaligam, V., Oz, M., Jayanthi, L. D., Han, Y., et al. (2007). D2 receptors regulate dopamine transporter function via an extracellular signal-regulated kinases 1 and 2-dependent and phosphoinositide 3 kinase-independent mechanism. *Molecular Pharmacology, 71*, 1222–1232.

Borel, M. J., Smith, S. H., Brigham, D. E., & Beard, J. L. (1991). The impact of varying degrees of iron nutriture on several functional consequences of iron deficiency in rats. *Journal of Nutrition, 121*, 729–736.

Burhans, M. S., Dailey, C., Beard, Z., Wiesinger, J., Murray-Kolb, L., Jones, B. C., et al. (2005). Iron deficiency: Differential effects on monoamine transporters. *Nutritional Neuroscience, 8*, 31–38.

Burhans, M. S., Dailey, C., Wiesinger, J., Murray-Kolb, L. E., Jones, B. C., & Beard, J. L. (2006). Iron deficiency affects acoustic startle response and latency, but not prepulse inhibition in young adult rats. *Physiology and Behavior, 87*, 917–924.

Bylund, D. B. (1992). Subtypes of alpha 1- and alpha 2-adrenergic receptors. *FASEB Journal, 6*, 832–839.

Cass, W. A., & Gerhardt, G. A. (1994). Direct in vivo evidence that D2 dopamine receptors can modulate dopamine uptake. *Neuroscience Letters, 176*, 259–263.

Chen, Q., Beard, J., & Jones, B. (1995). Abnormal rat brain monoamine metabolism in iron deficiency anemia. *Nutritional Biochemistry, 6*, 486–493.

Chen, Q., Connor, J. R., & Beard, J. L. (1995). Brain iron, transferrin and ferritin concentrations are altered in developing iron-deficient rats. *Journal of Nutrition 125*, 1529–1535.

Ciliax, B. J., Heilman, C., Demchyshyn, L. L., Pristupa, Z. B., Ince, E., Hersch, S. M., et al. (1995). The dopamine transporter: Immunochemical characterization and localization in brain. *Journal of Neuroscience 15*, 1714–1723.

Clancy, B., Darlington, R. B., & Finlay, B. L. (2001). Translating developmental time across mammalian species. *Neuroscience, 105*, 7–17.

Clardy, S. L., Wang, X., Zhal, W., Liu, W., Chase, G. A., Beard, J. L., et al. (2006). Acute and chronic effects of developmental iron deficiency on mRNA expression patterns in the brain. *Journal of Neural Transmission Supplementation, 71*, 173–196.

Cooper, J. R., Bloom, F. E., & Roth, R. H. (Eds.). (2003a). Serotonin, histamine, and adenosine. In *The biochemical basis of neuropharmacology* (pp. 271–320). Oxford: Oxford Press.

Cooper, J. R., Bloom, F. E., & Roth, R. H. (Eds.). (2003b). Dopamine. In *The biochemical basis of neuropharmacology* (pp. 225–270). Oxford: Oxford Press.

Cooper, J. R., Bloom, F. E., & Roth, R. H. (Eds.). (2003c). Norepinephrine and Epinephrine. In *The biochemical basis of neuropharmacology* (pp. 181–224). Oxford: Oxford Press.

Dancheck, B., Tang, A. M., Thomas, A. M., Smit, E., Vlahov, D., & Semba, R. D. (2005). Injection drug use is an independent risk factor for iron deficiency and iron deficiency anemia among HIV-seropositive and HIV-seronegative women. *Journal of Acquired Immune Deficiency Syndrome, 40*, 198–201.

Dedek, J., Baumes, R., Tien-Duc, N., Gomeni, R., & Korf, J. (1979). Turnover of free and conjugated (sulphonyloxy) dihydroxyphenylacetic acid and homovanillic acid in rat striatum. *Journal of Neurochemistry, 33*, 687–695.

Dickinson, S. D., Sabeti, J., Larson, G. A., Giardina, K., Rubinstein, M., Kelly, M. A., et al. (1999). Dopamine D2 receptor-deficient mice exhibit decreased dopamine transporter function but no changes in dopamine release in dorsal striatum. *Journal of Neurochemistry, 72*, 148–156.

Dunkley, P. R., Bobrovskaya, L., Graham, M. E., von Nagy-Felsobuki, E. I., & Dickson, P. W. (2004). Tyrosine hydroxylase phosphorylation: Regulation and consequences. *Journal of Neurochemistry, 91*, 1025–1043.

Erikson, K. M., Jones, B. C., & Beard, J. L. (2000). Iron deficiency alters dopamine transporter functioning in rat striatum. *Journal of Nutrition, 130*, 2831–2837.

Erikson, K. M., Jones, B. C., Hess, E. J., Zhang, Q., & Beard, J. L. (2001). Iron deficiency decreases dopamine D1 and D2 receptors in rat brain. *Pharmacology Biochemistry and Behavior, 69*, 409–418.

Erikson, K. M., Shihabi, Z. K., Aschner, J. L., & Aschner, M. (2002). Manganese accumulates in iron-deficient rat brain regions in a heterogeneous fashion and is associated with neurochemical alterations. *Biological Trace Element Research, 87*, 143–156.

Fuller, R. W., Perry, K. W., & Molloy, B. B. (1975). Effect of 3-(p-trifluoromethylphenoxy). N. N. methyl-3-phenylpropylamine on the depletion of brain serotonin by 4-chloroamphetamine. *Journal of Pharmacology and Experimental Therapeutics, 193*, 793–803.

Georgieff, M. K., Mills, M. M., Gordon, K., & Wobken, J. D. (1995). Reduced neonatal liver iron concentrations after uteroplacental insufficiency. *Journal of Pediatrics, 127*, 308–304.

Goldstein, A., & Lowery, P. J. (1975). Effect of the opiate antagonist naloxone on body temperature in rats. *Life Science, 17*, 927–931.

Green, A. R., & Youdim, M. B. (1977). The effect of iron deficiency on brain monoamine metabolism and the behavioural responses to increased brain 5-hydroxytryptamine and dopamine synthesis [proceedings]. *British Journal of Pharmacology, 59*, 470P–471P.

Guiang, S. F., III, Georgieff, M. K., Lambert, D. J., Schmidt, R. L., & Widness, J. A. (1997). Intravenous iron supplementation effect on tissue iron and hemoproteins in chronically phlebotomized lambs. *American Journal of Physiology, 273*, R2124–R2131.

Hasegawa, H., Oguro, K., Naito, Y., & Ichiyama, A. (1999). Iron dependence of tryptophan hydroxylase activity in RBL2H3 cells and its manipulation by chelators. *European Journal of Biochemistry, 261*, 734–739.

Hu, R., Wei, M., & Ding, X. (1996). Changes in brain monoamine neurotransmitter in iron deficiency nonanemic rats. *Zhonghua Yu Fang Yi Xue Za Zhi (Article in Chinese), 30*, 351–353.

Humphrey, P. P., Buell, G., Kennedy, I., Khakh, B. S., Michel, A. D., Surprenant, A., et al. (1995). New insights on P2X purinoceptors. *Naunyn-Schmiedeberg's Archive of Pharmacology, 352*, 585–596.

Ill, A. M., Mitchell, T. R., Neely, E. B., & Connor, J. R. (2006). Metabolic analysis of mouse brains that have compromised iron storage. *Metabolic Brain Disease, 21*, 77–87.

Jhanwar-Uniyal, M., Roland, C. R., & Leibowitz, S. F. (1986). Diurnal rhythm of alpha 2-noradrenergic receptors in the paraventricular nucleus and other brain areas: Relation to circulating corticosterone and feeding behavior. *Life Science, 38*, 473–482.

Johansen, P. A., Jennings, I., Cotton, R. G., & Kuhn, D. M. (1996). Phosphorylation and activation of tryptophan hydroxylase by exogenous protein kinase A. *Journal of Neurochemistry, 66*, 817–823.

Jones, B. C., Wheeler, D. S., Beard, J. L., & Grigson, P. S. (2002). Iron deficiency in rats decreases acquisition of and suppresses responding for cocaine. *Pharmacology Biochemistry and Behavior, 73*, 813–819.

Jones, S. R., Gainetdinov, R. R., Hu, X. T., Cooper, D. C., Wightman, R. M., White, F. J., et al. (1999). Loss of autoreceptor functions in mice lacking the dopamine transporter. *Nature Neuroscience, 2*, 649–655.

Kabbani, N., & Levenson, R. (2007). A proteomic approach to receptor signaling: Molecular mechanisms and therapeutic implications derived from discovery of the dopamine D2 receptor signalplex. *European Journal of Pharmacology, 572*, 83–93.

Kaladhar, M., & Narasinga Rao, B. S. (1982). Effects of iron deficiency on serotonin uptake in vitro by rat brain synaptic vesicles. *Journal of Neurochemistry, 38*, 1576–1581.

Kaur, D., Peng, J., Chinta, S. J., Rajagopalan, S., Di Monte, D. A., Cherny, R. A., et al. (2006). Increased murine neonatal iron intake results in Parkinson-like neurodegeneration with age. *Neurobiology of Aging, 106(1)*, 205–15.

Keller, M. B. (1999). The long-term treatment of depression. *Journal of Clinical Psychiatry, 60*(Suppl. 17), 41–45; discussion 46–48.

Konofal, E., Lecendreux, M., Deron, J., Marchand, M., Cortese, S., Zaim, M., et al. (2008). Effects of iron supplementation on attention deficit hyperactivity disorder in children. *Pediatric Neurology, 38*, 20–26.

Kramer-Stickland, K., Edmonds, A., Bair, W. B., III, & Bowden, G. T. (1999). Inhibitory effects of deferoxamine on UVB-induced AP-1 transactivation. *Carcinogenesis, 20*, 2137–2142.

Kretchmer, N., Beard, J. L., & Carlson, S. (1996). The role of nutrition in the development of normal cognition. *American Journal of Clinical Nutrition, 63*, 997S–1001S.

Kuhn, D. M., Ruskin, B., & Lovenberg, W. (1980). Tryptophan hydroxylase. The role of oxygen, iron, and sulfydryl groups as determinants of stability and catalytic activity. *Journal of Biological Chemistry, 255*, 4137–4143.

Kwik-Uribe, C. L., Golub, M. S., & Keen, C. L. (2000). Chronic marginal iron intakes during early development in mice alter brain iron concentrations and behavior despite postnatal iron supplementation. *Journal of Nutrition, 130*, 2040–2048.

Le Saux, M., & Di Paolo, T. (2006). Influence of oestrogenic compounds on monoamine transporters in rat striatum. *Journal of Neuroendocrinology, 18*, 25–32.

Lee, D. C., McKnight, G. S., & Palmiter, R. D. (1978). The action of estrogen and progesterone on the expression of the transferrin gene. A comparison of the response in chick liver and oviduct. *Journal of Biological Chemistry, 253*, 3494–3503.

Levesque, D., & Di Paolo, T. (1990). Effect of the rat estrous cycle at ovariectomy on striatal D-1 dopamine receptors. *Brain Research Bulletin, 24*, 281–284.

Li, D. (1998). Effects of iron deficiency on iron distribution and gamma-aminobutyric acid (GABA) metabolism in young rat brain tissues. *Hokkaido Igaku Zasshi, 73*, 215–225.

Lipschitz, D. A., Cook, J. D., & Finch, C. A. (1974). A clinical evaluation of serum ferritin as an index of iron stores. *New England Journal of Medicine, 290*, 1213–1216.

Lisman, J. E., & Grace, A. A. (2005). The hippocampal-VTA loop: Controlling the entry of information into long-term memory. *Neuron, 46*, 703–713.

Lozoff, B. (1989). Iron and learning potential in childhood. *Bulletin of the New York Academy of Medicine, 65*, 1050–1066; discussion 1085–1058.

Lozoff, B., Beard, J., Connor, J., Barbara, F., Georgieff, M., & Schallert, T. (2006). Long-lasting neural and behavioral effects of iron deficiency in infancy. *Nutritional Reviews, 64*, S34–S43; discussion S72–S91.

Lozoff, B., Jimenez, E., Hagen, J., Mollen, E., & Wolf, A. W. (2000). Poorer behavioral and developmental outcome more than 10 years after treatment for iron deficiency in infancy. *Pediatrics, 105*, E51.

Mackler, B., Person, R., Miller, L. R., & Finch, C. A. (1979). Iron deficiency in the rat: Effects on phenylalanine metabolism. *Pediatric Research, 13*, 1010–1011.

Mayfield, R. D., & Zahniser, N. R. (2001). Dopamine D2 receptor regulation of the dopamine transporter expressed in *Xenopus laevis* oocytes is voltage-independent. *Molecular Pharmacology, 59*, 113–121.

McArdle, H. J., Andersen, H. S., Jones, H., & Gambling, L. (2006). Fetal programming: Causes and consequences as revealed by studies of dietary manipulation in rats – A review. *Placenta, 27*(Suppl. A), S56–S60.

Meiergerd, S. M., Patterson, T. A., & Schenk, J. O. (1993). D2 receptors may modulate the function of the striatal transporter for dopamine: Kinetic evidence from studies in vitro and in vivo. *Journal of Neurochemistry, 61*, 764–767.

Merens, W., Willem Van der Does, A. J., & Spinhoven, P. (2007). The effects of serotonin manipulations on emotional information processing and mood. *Journal of Affective Disorders, 103*, 43–62.

Minneman, K. P., Dibner, M. D., Wolfe, B. B., & Molinoff, P. B. (1979). beta1- and beta2-Adrenergic receptors in rat cerebral cortex are independently regulated. *Science, 204*, 866–868.

Molinoff, P. B., Brimijoin, S., & Axelrod, J. (1972). Induction of dopamine hydroxylase and tyrosine hydroxylase in rat hearts and sympathetic ganglia. *Journal of Pharmacology and Experimental Therapeutics, 182*, 116–129.

Nelson, C., Erikson, K., Pinero, D. J., & Beard, J. L. (1997). In vivo dopamine metabolism is altered in iron-deficient anemic rats. *Journal of Nutrition, 127*, 2282–2288.

Oner, O., Alkar, O. Y., & Oner, P. (2008). Relation of ferritin levels with symptom ratings and cognitive performance in children with attention deficit-hyperactivity disorder. *Pediatrics International, 50*, 40–44.

Oner, P., & Oner, O. (2007). Relationship of ferritin to symptom ratings children with attention deficit hyperactivity disorder: Effect of comorbidity. *Child Psychiatry and Human Development, 39(3)*, 323–330.

Parks, C. L., Robinson, P. S., Sibille, E., Shenk, T., & Toth, M. (1998). Increased anxiety of mice lacking the serotonin1A receptor. *Proceedings of the National Academy of Science USA, 95*, 10734–10739.

Patiroglu, T., & Dogan, P. (1991). Iron deficiency anemia and catecholamine metabolism. *Indian Pediatrics, 28*, 51–56.

Pinero, D., Jones, B., & Beard, J. (2001). Variations in dietary iron alter behavior in developing rats. *Journal of Nutrition, 131*, 311–318.

Pinero, D. J., Li, N. Q., Connor, J. R., & Beard, J. L. (2000). Variations in dietary iron alter brain iron metabolism in developing rats. *Journal of Nutrition, 130*, 254–263.

Ramboz, S., Oosting, R., Amara, D. A., Kung, H. F., Blier, P., Mendelsohn, M., et al. (1998). Serotonin receptor 1A knockout: An animal model of anxiety-related disorder. *Proceedings of the National Academy of Sciences USA, 95*, 14476–14481.

Ramsey, A. J., & Fitzpatrick, P. F. (1998). Effects of phosphorylation of serine 40 of tyrosine hydroxylase on binding of catecholamines: Evidence for a novel regulatory mechanism. *Biochemistry, 37*, 8980–8986.

Rao, R., Tkac, I., Townsend, E. L., Gruetter, R., & Georgieff, M. K. (2003). Perinatal iron deficiency alters the neurochemical profile of the developing rat hippocampus. *Journal of Nutrition, 133*, 3215–3221.

Roncagliolo, M., Garrido, M., Walter, T., Peirano, P., & Lozoff, B. (1998). Evidence of altered central nervous system development in infants with iron deficiency anemia at 6 mo: Delayed maturation of auditory brainstem responses. *American Journal of Clinical Nutrition, 68*, 683–690.

Ruiz, I. G., de la Torre, P., Diaz, T., Esteban, E., Morillas, J. D., Munoz-Yague, T., et al. (2000). Sp family of transcription factors is involved in iron-induced collagen alpha1(I) gene expression. *DNA and Cell Biology, 19*, 167–178.

Sharman, D. F. (1973). The catabolism of catecholamines. Recent studies. *British Medical Bulletin, 29*, 110–115.

Shukla, A., Agarwal, K. N., Chansuria, J. P., & Taneja, V. (1989). Effect of latent iron deficiency on 5-hydroxytryptamine metabolism in rat brain. *Journal of Neurochemistry, 52*, 730–735.

Siddappa, A. J., Rao, R. B., Wobken, J. D., Leibold, E. A., Connor, J. R., & Georgieff, M. K. (2002). Developmental changes in the expression of iron regulatory proteins and iron transport proteins in the perinatal rat brain. *Journal of Neuroscience Research, 68*, 761–775.

Siddappa, A. M., Georgieff, M. K., Wewerka, S., Worwa, C., Nelson, C. A., & Deregnier, R. A. (2004). Iron deficiency alters auditory recognition memory in newborn infants of diabetic mothers. *Pediatric Research, 55*, 1034–1041.

Smith, A. D., & Justice, J. B. (1994). The effect of inhibition of synthesis, release, metabolism and uptake on the microdialysis extraction fraction of dopamine. *Journal of Neuroscience Methods, 54*, 75–82.

Smith, S. M., & Beard, J. L. (1989). Norepinephrine turnover in iron deficiency: Effect of two semi-purified diets. *Life Science, 45*, 341–347.

Taneja, V., Mishra, K., & Agarwal, K. N. (1986). Effect of early iron deficiency in rat on the gamma-aminobutyric acid shunt in brain. *Journal of Neurochemistry, 46*, 1670–1674.

Teng, C. (1995). Mouse lactoferrin gene: A marker for estrogen and epidermal growth factor. *Environmental Health Perspectives, 103*(Suppl. 7), 17–20.

Tobin, B. W., & Beard, J. L. (1990). Interactions of iron deficiency and exercise training relative to tissue norepinephrine turnover, triiodothyronine production and metabolic rate in rats. *Journal of Nutrition, 120*, 900–908.

Unger, E. L., Paul, T., Murray-Kolb, L. E., Felt, B., Jones, B. C., & Beard, J. L. (2007). Early iron deficiency alters sensorimotor development and brain monoamines in rats. *Journal of Nutrition, 137*, 118–124.

Voorhess, M. L., Stuart, M. J., Stockman, J. A., & Oski, F. A. (1975). Iron deficiency anemia and increased urinary norepinephrine excretion. *Journal of Pediatrics, 86*, 542–547.

Walker, S. P., Wachs, T. D., Gardner, J. M., Lozoff, B., Wasserman, G. A., Pollitt, E., et al. (2007). Child development: risk factors for adverse outcomes in developing countries. *Lancet, 369*, 145–157.

Ward, K. L., Tkac, I., Jing, Y., Felt, B., Beard, J., Connor, J., et al. (2007). Gestational and lactational iron deficiency alters the developing striatal metabolome and associated behaviors in young rats. *Journal of Nutrition, 137*, 1043–1049.

Weinshilboum, R. M., Thoa, N. B., Johnson, D. G., Kopin, I. J., & Axelrod, J. (1971). Proportional release of norepinephrine and dopamine- -hydroxylase from sympathetic nerves. *Science, 174*, 1349–1351.

Wiesinger, J. A., Buwen, J. P., Cifelli, C. J., Unger, E. L., Jones, B. C., & Beard, J. L. (2007). Down-regulation of dopamine transporter by iron chelation in vitro is mediated by altered trafficking, not synthesis. *Journal of Neurochemistry, 100*, 167–179.

Winkelman, J. W., Allen, R. P., Tenzer, P., & Hening, W. (2007). Restless legs syndrome: Nonpharmacologic and pharmacologic treatments. *Geriatrics, 62*, 13–16.

Yajima, S., Lee, S. H., Minowa, T., & Mouradian, M. M. (1998). Sp family transcription factors regulate expression of rat D2 dopamine receptor gene. *DNA and Cell Biology, 17*, 471–479.

Yehdua, S. (1990). Neurochemical basis of behavioral effects of brain iron deficiency in animals. In J. Dobbing (Ed.), *Brain, behavior, and iron in the infant diet* (pp. 83–106). London: Springer Verlag.

Yehuda, S., & Youdim, M. B. (1984). The increased opiate action of beta-endorphin in iron-deficient rats: the possible involvement of dopamine. *European Journal of Pharmacology, 17*, 104(3–4), 245–251.

Yehuda, S., & Youdim, M. B. (1989). Brain iron: A lesson from animal models. *American Journal of Clinical Nutrition, 50*, 618–625; discussion 625–619.

Youdim, M. B. (2000). Nutrient deprivation and brain function: Iron. *Nutrition, 16*, 504–508.

Youdim, M. B., Ben-Shachar, D., & Yehuda, S. (1989). Putative biological mechanisms of the effect of iron deficiency on brain biochemistry and behavior. *American Journal of Clinical Nutrition, 50*, 607–615; discussion 615–607.

Youdim, M. B., Ben-Shachar, D., Yehuda, S., & Ashkenazi, R. (1983). Brain iron and dopamine receptor function. In P. Mandel & F. DeFeudis (Eds.), *CNS receptors from molecular pharmacology to behavior* (pp. 309–322). New York: Raven Press.

Youdim, M. B., & Green, A. R. (1978). Iron deficiency and neurotransmitter synthesis and function. *Proceedings of the Nutrition Society, 37*, 173–179.

Yu, G. S., Steinkirchner, T. M., Rao, G. A., & Larkin, E. C. (1986). Effect of prenatal iron deficiency on myelination in rat pups. *American Journal of Pathology, 125*, 620–624.

Yu, J. S. (1998). Activation of protein phosphatase 2A by the Fe2+/ascorbate system. *Journal of Biochemistry (Tokyo), 124*, 225–230.

# 9 Peripheral Effects of Iron Deficiency

*Daniel B. Costa and Reed E. Drews*

**Summary**

- Clinical manifestations of iron deficiency were described since 1500 BC and were well known in 16th and 17th century Europe as part of the disease "chlorosis".
- The major cause of iron deficiency is blood loss, commonly from the gastro-intestinal tract in adults.
- The hematologic changes characteristic of iron deficiency include hypochromic and microcytic anemia.
- The tongue and mouth, hypopharynx and esophagus, stomach, nails, and hair are common epithelial tissues affected by iron deficiency.
- Glossitis, cheilitis, koilonychia, dysphagia, and pica are the signs and symptoms commonly associated with iron deficiency and iron deficiency anemia.

**Key Words:** Iron deficiency; anemia; glossitis; cheilitis; koilonychias

## 1. HISTORICAL ACCOUNT OF IRON DEFICIENCY AND ITS CLINICAL MANIFESTATIONS

In-depth reviews of the history of iron deficiency have been published elsewhere (Beutler, 2002; Poskitt, 2003; Lee, 1998; London, 1980). According to these accounts, descriptions of a disease in which patients had pallor, edema, and dyspnea date to 1,500 BC (Bryan, 1931; Beutler, 2006; London, 1980). Quite possibly, this ancient disease was iron deficiency anemia from chronic hookworm infestation. However, the clear association of signs and symptoms of a disorder due to iron deficiency only occurred as physicians revealed the possible pathophysiology of "chlorosis."

Derived from the Greek word for "green" (Lee, 1998), chlorosis was described by 16th and 17th century physicians (Fowler, 1936) as a disorder most prevalent in adolescent girls who had inadequate dietary intake of iron and high requirements for iron due to increased iron loss from menses (Brumberg, 1982; Lee, 1998). Characterized by greenish pallor, palpitations, breathlessness, trace ankle edema, and propensity for thrombosis (Lee, 1998), one hypothesis relates the development of this disease to tight-lacing corsets used by young women (Lee, 1998), resulting either in decreasing dietary intake (Hudson, 1977) or in aggravated reflux esophagitis with subsequent blood loss (Lee, 1998). William Shakespeare used chlorosis often in his plays (Mercer & Wangensteen, 1985). For example, a reference to the disorder appears in *Romeo and Juliet*

From: *Nutrition and Health: Iron Deficiency and Overload*
Edited by: S. Yehuda and D.I. Mostofsky, DOI 10.1007/978-1-59745-462-9_9

where Romeo says, "Her vestal livery is but sick and green," referring to Juliet's protracted virginity that subjected her to the "green-sickness." Later in the play, Capulet screams at his daughter Juliet, "Out, you greensickness carrion," referring to Juliet's refusal to marry the man he has chosen for her (Stolz et al., 2007). Dutch painters Gerard Dou (Gerrit Douw), Jan Steen, Gabriel Metsu, and Frans van Mieris depicted pale young women dressed in fur-trimmed jackets and rich gowns (indicating their wealthier status) while being examined by their 17th century physicians (Garrison, 1921). Metsu's "Doctor's Visit" and Steen's "Doctor's Visit" from 1660 AD are examples of such paintings (Fig. 1).

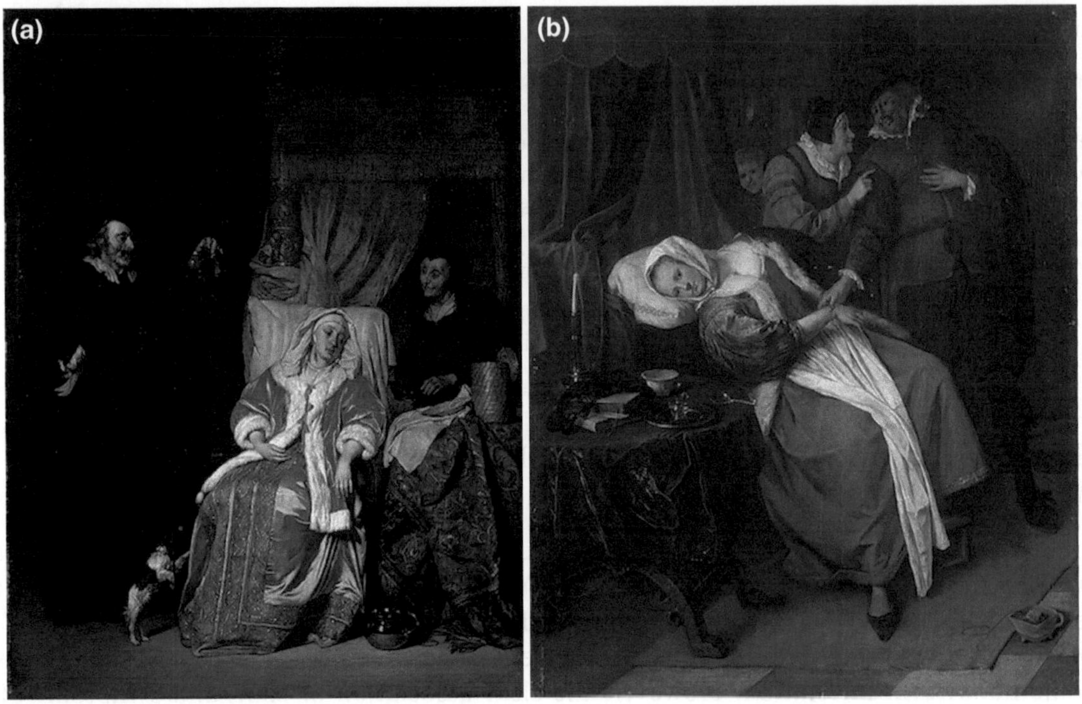


**Fig. 1.** Paintings of 17th century European artists possibly depicting young women with chlorosis: (**A**) Gabriel Metsu, Doctor's Visit 1660; (**B**) Jan Steen, Doctor's Visit circa 1660. Both courtesy of Hermitage Museum: http://www.hermitagemuseum.org

It was not until the 1800s that anemia, hypochromia, and decreased content of iron in the blood were identified in patients with chlorosis (Fowler, 1936), leading Ashwell to classify chlorosis as a disease of the blood (Ashwell, 1836). In the same era, Blaud and others described improvement of chlorosis with the use of increasing concentrations of pills containing potassium carbonate and ferrous sulfate (Haden, 1938).

By the 1920s and 1930s, the term "hypochromic anemia" was used to describe a form of anemia affecting women beyond their fourth decade of life, often with poor diets, multiple pregnancies, and menstrual irregularities (Wintrobe, 1933). Distinguished from chlorosis by its appearance in older women, hypochromic anemia was often associated with striking epithelial changes now known to be secondary to iron deficiency, including changes in the nails, tongue, and stomach (Witts, 1931). In 1932, Heath, Strauss, and Castle confirmed iron deficiency as the main etiology of hypochromic anemia (Heath, Strauss, & Castle, 1932).

## 2. PREVALENCE OF IRON DEFICIENCY AND ITS CAUSES

Iron deficiency is a common worldwide problem. By applying a multiple-indicator model to data from the United States of America 1999–2000 National Health and Nutrition Examination Survey (NHANES 1999–2000), the Centers for Disease Control and Prevention (CDC) calculated the prevalence of iron deficiency (low iron stores without anemia) and iron deficiency anemia (low iron stores with anemia) as: 7% among toddlers aged 1–2 years; 9–16% among adolescent and adult females aged 12–49 years; and 3% among adult males aged 70 years or above (Looker, Cogswell, & Gunter, 2002). While the specific causes of this negative iron balance will be discussed in detail elsewhere in this book, it is important to note that a negative iron balance in adults most commonly arises from disorders that lead to blood loss (Lee, 1998; Beutler, 2006). Table 1 lists some of the known causes of iron deficiency.

**Table 1**
**Causes of Iron Deficiency and Iron Deficiency Anemia**

I. Inadequate iron supply
- A. Poor nutritional intake in children
- B. Malabsorption
    - Celiac disease
    - Crohn's disease
    - Gastric bypass surgery
    - Other miscellaneous disorders affecting the stomach and duodenum
- C. Abnormal transferrin function
    - Congenital atransferrinemia
    - Autoantibodies to transferrin receptor
    - Transferrin polymorphisms

II. Increased iron requirements
- A. Blood loss
- A.1. Gastrointestinal Bleeding
    - Malignant neoplasms
    - Hookworm
    - Peptic ulcer disease
    - Esophageal varices
    - Hiatal hernia
    - Ulcerative colitis
    - Hemorrhoids
    - Gastritis
    - Angiodysplasia
    - *Helicobacter pylori* infection
    - Hemangioma
    - Amebiasis
    - Diverticulum
    - Polyps
    - Leiomyoma
    - Hypergastrinemia

(*Continued*)

Table 1
**(Continued)**

| |
|---|
| Milk allergy in infants |
| Schistosomiasis |
| Trichuriasis |
| A.2. Excessive Menstrual Losses or Abnormal Uterine Bleeding in Women |
| Menstrual bleeding |
| Uterine fibroids |
| Malignant neoplasms |
| A.3. Respiratory tract bleeding |
| Malignant neoplasms |
| Epistaxis |
| Infections |
| Telangiectasias |
| Idiopathic pulmonary hemosiderosis |
| Goodpasture's syndrome |
| A.4. Biliary Tract Bleeding |
| Malignant neoplasms |
| Cholelithiasis |
| Intrahepatic bleeding |
| Trauma |
| A.5. Urinary Tract Bleeding |
| Malignant neoplasms |
| Trauma |
| Urolithiasis |
| Inflammatory disorders |
| Glomerulonephritis |
| A.6. Blood Donation |
| A.7. Self-induced Bleeding (Factitious Anemia) |
| A.8. Intravascular Hemolysis |
| Paroxysmal nocturnal hemoglobinuria |
| Mechanical erythrocyte trauma (as in valvular heart disease) |
| High-performance athletic activities |
| Other hemolytic disorders |
| B. Chronic Renal Failure and Hemodialysis |
| C. Disorders of Hemostasis |
| D. Increased Physiologic Requirements |
| Infancy |
| Pregnancy |
| Lactation |
| E. Idiopathic |

Adapted from Lee (1998) and Beutler (2006).

## 3. PATHOGENESIS OF THE MANIFESTATIONS OF IRON DEFICIENCY

### 3.1. *Proteins and Enzymes*

No clear unifying mechanism can explain all symptoms and signs encountered in the clinic when confronting a patient with iron deficiency. However, it is likely that key proteins and enzymes that either depend on or use iron as a co-factor account for some, if not most, of the clinical findings of iron deficiency in humans. As iron deficiency ensues, changes in the quantities of storage iron, hemoglobin iron, transport iron, and enzyme iron may explain in part the clinical findings observed in patients (Beutler, 2006).

Depletion of iron leads to decreased levels of hemosiderin and ferritin from bone marrow and other storage sites (Beutler, 2006). Thus, serum ferritin is used as a clinical marker of iron deficiency (Lipschitz, Cook, & Finch, 1974; Beutler, 2002). It is believed that when transferrin saturation falls below 16%, the supply of iron to hematopoietic bone marrow is inappropriate to meet hemoglobin production, which leads to increased free erythrocyte protoporphyrin and decreased hemoglobin levels (Bainton & Finch, 1964). As impaired hemoglobin synthesis ensues, each individual red cell that is produced carries less hemoglobin. In animal models, transferrin iron is essential to induce the proliferation of erythroid precursors (Rich, Sawatzki, & Kubanek, 1981), and this effect may explain in part the lack of significant bone marrow hyperplasia in iron deficiency anemia (Lee, 1998).

However, radio-ferrokinetic studies performed in humans during the 1960s and 1970s showed that the amount of iron delivered to the bone marrow, even in the face of iron deficiency, is nearly normal and that marrow elements may actually use iron more efficiently during iron deficiency anemia (Finch et al., 1970; Pollycove, 1966). Since mild to moderate shortening of erythroid survival is seen in iron deficiency anemia (Loria, Sanchez-Medal, Lisker, De Rodriguez, & Labardini, 1967; Rasch, Cotton, Griggs, & Harris, 1976) as a consequence of splenic destruction (Macdougall, Judisch, & Mistry, 1970), it is possible that erythroid iron is reused in a shunt pathway (Lee, 1998; Cavill, Ricketts, Napier, & Jacobs, 1977). Mechanisms underlying the observed decreased red cell survival in iron deficiency anemia are not well understood; but investigators have postulated an increase in erythrocyte stiffness due to either oxidative damage (Yip et al., 1983) or reduced glutathione peroxidase activity (Rodvien, Gillum, & Weintraub, 1974). In iron deficiency anemia, plasma iron clearance is quiet rapid and this is inversely correlated with serum iron levels (Lee, 1998; Beutler, 2006). All these factors may indeed lead to partially ineffective erythropoiesis during iron deficiency and subsequent anemia.

In addition to decreased hemoglobin concentration, other iron-containing proteins are decreased in iron deficiency (Beutler, Larsh, & Tanzi, 1960; Beutler, 1957; Beutler & Blaisdell, 1960; Beutler & Blaisdell, 1958; Beutler, 1959a). Decreased levels or function of these non-hemoglobin proteins are responsible for many of the non-hematologic clinical manifestations of iron deficiency. The depletion of such enzymes seems to occur in parallel with the degree of anemia observed in patients (Siimes, Refino, & Dallman, 1980). For example, iron is a major component of myoglobin, cytochromes, catalase, and peroxidase. Decreased protein levels and enzymatic activities have been observed in iron deficiency for cytochrome *c* in the muscle and intestine (Hagler et al., 1981), cytochrome oxidase in the buccal mucosa and intestine (Dallman & Schwartz, 1965; Dallman, Beutler, & Finch, 1978), myoglobin and alpha-glycerophosphate oxidase in muscle (Hagler et al., 1981; Finch et al., 1979; Celsing, Ekblom, Sylven, Everett, & Astrand, 1988), and succinic dehydrogenase and aconitase in other tissues (Beutler, 2006; Lee, 1998). It is believed that these and many other iron-dependent proteins are diminished during iron deficiency.

Enzymes that do not require or contain iron can also have their activity decreased, such as some oxidative glycolysis cycle enzymes (Beutler, 2006). For example, the conversion of thyroxine to triiodothyronine is iron-dependent and therefore impaired in iron deficiency (Dillman et al., 1980). A disturbance in catecholamine metabolism, perhaps mediated by decreased tissues levels of monoamine oxidase, can also be seen in states of iron deficit (Youdim, Woods, Mitchell, Grahame-Smith, & Callender, 1975; Wagner, Fortier, Giroux, Lukes, & Snyder, 1979).

While a complete account of all protein enzymes affected in iron deficiency is beyond the scope of this chapter, suffice it to say that iron plays essential roles in a variety of physiologic and metabolic pathways, which affect many cellular compartments and manifest as the signs and symptoms encountered in clinical practice as a consequence of iron deficiency.

### 3.2. *Epithelial Cells and Skeleton*

In iron deficiency, rapidly proliferating epithelial cells of the alimentary mucosa are susceptible to many histological abnormalities (Beutler, 2006). While the exact mechanism for these histological effects are not known in most cases, reports include atrophy of the mucosa of the small intestine (Naiman, Oski, Diamond, Vawter, & Shwachman, 1964), stomach (Cheli, Dodero, Celle, & Vassalotti, 1959), esophagus (Baird, Dodge, Palmer, & Wawman, 1961), tongue (Baird et al., 1961; Scott, Valentine, St. Hill, & West, 1985), and mouth (Jacobs, 1960; Macleod, Hamilton, & Soames, 1988). These changes may account for the frequent epithelial-related clinical signs found in iron deficiency anemia (Lee, 1998). However, it is difficult to know if co-existing nutritional deficiencies also play a role in some of these epithelial changes (Jacobs & Cavill, 1968). Changes in bones of the skull have also been seen in children with iron deficiency, but their clinical significance is unclear (Shahidi & Diamond, 1960).

## 4. LABORATORY EVALUATION OF IRON DEFICIENCY

While a comprehensive review of laboratory tests currently used to diagnose iron deficiency is beyond the scope of this chapter, a concise exploration of hematological parameters and basic laboratory tests is warranted. This will help familiarize the reader to terminologies and tests that have been used in examining associations between iron deficiency and certain peripheral manifestations of this disorder. Table 2 summarizes clinically useful and emerging parameters for measuring iron status in humans. However, all mentioned tests have their limitations.

Historically, serum iron levels were used as a determinant of iron body stores (Beutler, 2006). This test is usually low in iron deficiency, but not always (Beutler, 1959b; Ellis, Jensen, & Westerman, 1964). For example, serum iron has a diurnal rhythmic variation (Hamilton, Gubler, Caertwright, & Wintrobe, 1950; Speck, 1968; Dale, Burritt, & Zinsmeister, 2002) and is affected by many processes, such as inflammation (Bainton & Finch, 1964), bleeding (Beutler, 2006; Zilva & Patston, 1966), malignancy (Banerjee & Narang, 1967), chemotherapy (Follezou & Bizon, 1986), myocardial infarction (Syrkis & Machtey, 1973), and iron-containing vitamins or preparations (Seligman & Schleicher, 1999), among others (Lee, 1998).

Total iron-binding capacity (TIBC) is the sum of the plasma iron and the unsaturated iron-binding capacity (Stojceski, Malpas, & Witts, 1965), which is calculated from the level of transferrin in blood (Beutler, 2006; Lee, 1998). Serum iron saturation is the ratio of serum iron to TIBC. In anemia of iron deficiency, TIBC is often increased and iron saturation is usually below 10% (Beutler, Robson, & Buttenwieser, 1958; Beutler, 2002).

Serum ferritin levels correlate best with total-body iron stores in most circumstances (Lipschitz, Cook, & Finch, 1974; Beutler, 2002). However, inflammatory disorders and other

**Table 2**
**Clinically Significant and Emerging Tests to Assess Iron Status**

| *Test* | *Value Compared to Normal Standards in Iron Deficiency and Iron Deficiency Anemia* |
|---|---|
| Fasting serum IRON | Decreased (or normal) |
| Total iron-binding capacity (TIBC) | Increased (or normal) |
| Serum iron saturation (percentage) | Decreased |
| Serum ferritin | Decreased* |
| Serum transferrin receptor | Increased* |
| Hepcidin | Increased |
| Red cell indices | |
| Mean corpuscular volume (MCV) | Decreased |
| Mean corpuscular hemoglobin (MCH) | Decreased |
| Mean corpuscular hemoglobin concentration (MCHC) | Decreased |
| Red cell distribution width (RDW) | Increased |
| Reticulocyte hemoglobin content (CHr) | Decreased |

* Unless confounded by inflammation (see text for details).

circumstances can increase serum ferritin levels, as in rheumatoid arthritis (Hansen & Hansen, 1986), chronic kidney disease (Dennison, 1999), malignancies (Matzner, Konijn, & Hershko, 1980), Gaucher's disease (Morgan, Hoffbrand, Laulicht, Luck, & Knowles, 1983), hepatitis (Ioannou, Tung, & Kowdley, 2002), and use of parental iron (Wheby, 1980), among others.

Serum transferrin receptor can be measured, and levels increase in iron deficiency (Ahluwalia, 1998; Junca et al., 1998). However, this test has not been completely standardized to clinical practice and variations with concomitant disorders are poorly understood (North, Dallalio, Donath, Melink, & Means, 1997; Pettersson, 1994). The ratio of serum transferrin receptor to serum ferritin may be a better assessment of body iron stores (Beutler, 2006; Cook, Flowers, & Skikne, 2003).

Red cell indices become abnormal in adults, and the red cell distribution width (RDW) can be increased when the degree of iron deficiency is already moderate to severe and anemia is present (Beutler, 1959b). In such cases, mean corpuscular volume (MCV) and mean corpuscular hemoglobin (MCH) are decreased alongside decreased serum hemoglobin levels, reflecting the microcytic and hypochromic changes seen in the peripheral blood (Lee, 1998). In one series, the average MCV and MCH of iron-deficient patients were 74 fL and 20 pg, respectively (Bainton & Finch, 1964).

Novel laboratory measurements are entering clinical practice (Wish, 2006). Among them is a measure of hemoglobin in reticulocytes called the reticulocyte hemoglobin content (CHr) (Chuang, Liu, Wei, Huang, & Tarng, 2003; Cullen et al., 1999; Mast, Blinder, Lu, Flax, & Dietzen,

2002; Mast, Blinder, & Dietzen, 2007). Another surrogate marker of iron deficiency is hepcidin, which increases in iron deficiency anemia (Dallalio, Fleury, & Means, 2003; Kemna, Tjalsma, Podust, & Swinkels, 2007; Ganz, 2006).

## 5. CLINICAL MANIFESTATIONS OF IRON DEFICIENCY AND IRON DEFICIENCY ANEMIA

### *5.1. Clinical Manifestations of Anemia*

Symptoms of anemia can accompany severe iron deficiency anemia. When blood loss resulting in iron deficiency is indolent and protracted, it may take many years until patients seek medical attention. Due to such a delay, hemoglobin concentrations can be quiet depressed, as patients acclimate to the physiologic consequences of slowly evolving anemia.

The clinical manifestations of anemia occur as a compound function of the degree of tissue hypoxia and the compensatory mechanisms activated in the presence of decreased oxygen-carrying capacity (Prchal, 2006). Hypoxia-inducible transcription factor 1 (HIF-1) is pivotal in one of the major pathways used by the human body in response to hypoxia; it regulates energy metabolism, glycolytic enzyme genes, and respiratory control, among other functions (Semenza, 2004). Other pathways are also involved in sensing hypoxia and activating compensatory mechanisms (Prchal, 2006), but a discussion of these actions is beyond the scope of this text.

In chronic anemia, overall intravascular volume is not changed; however, there is a redistribution of tissue perfusion from "non-vital" to vital organs. Cutaneous tissue is often vasoconstricted, and the characteristic pallor of anemia is a consequence of this effect (Marks & Shuster, 1970; Prchal, 2006). Examination of mucous membranes, conjunctivae, nail beds, and palmar creases (tissues lacking pigmentation) may reveal pallor (Bushnell, 1992). Interestingly, clinical judgment of pallor is often faulty and does not correlate well with measurements of hemoglobin levels in the blood (Ingram & Lewis, 2000).

Another compensatory mechanism is increased cardiac output. Increased cardiac output will not occur until the hemoglobin concentration decreases to below 7 g/dL (Prchal, 2006). Some of the signs of cardiac compensation include tachycardia, increased arterial pulsation, and "flow murmurs." In patients with underlying coronary artery disease, symptoms of angina may develop. In cases when an underlying cardiomyopathy precedes the diagnosis of anemia, the presence of increased cardiac hyperactivity may lead to pulmonary congestion and edema.

In the respiratory system, dyspnea on exertion or orthopnea is a characteristic finding of severe anemia. Increase in the respiratory rate is thought to be secondary to the demands imposed by the augmented cardiac output, and also as a by-product of the decreased oxygen affinity mediated by enhancement in the production of 2,3-biphosphoglycerate, which leads to decreased affinity of hemoglobin for oxygen and improved oxygen delivery (Brewer, 1974; Thomas, Lefrak, Irwin, Fritts, & Caldwell, 1974). This is accomplished by increasing the intracellular pH of red cells by respiratory alkalosis.

Despite the compensatory mechanisms detailed above, severe tissue hypoxia to organs can still ensue and lead to further symptoms, such as intermittent claudication (hypoxia to muscles), fatigue, and abdominal cramps. The pathophysiologic mechanisms underlying some of these changes are unknown (Prchal, 2006).

### *5.2. Effects on the Hematopoietic System*

The earliest blood cell abnormality that develops in iron deficiency anemia is anisocytosis (Bessman & Feinstein, 1979; Bessman, Gilmer, & Gardner, 1983; Fairbanks, 1971). The difference in size between red cells as measured by the RDW can help differentiate iron deficiency anemia (in which RDWs are increased) from thalassemia minor (in which RDWs are normal) (Bessman & Feinstein, 1979). Sometimes the anisocytosis is accompanied by mild ovalocytosis (Beutler, 2006).

Erythrocyte morphologies arising as a consequence of iron deficiency were evaluated in the 1960s by controlled human phlebotomies (Conrad & Crosby, 1962). As total body iron deficiency reaches its peak, the characteristic picture of hypochromia and microcytosis becomes increasingly evident in erythrocytes (Conrad & Crosby, 1962; Beutler, 2006). The decreased amount of hemoglobin in each individual red cell generates increased central pallor, which is visually seen as hypochromia (Figs. 2 and 3). In severe cases, a moderate number of poikilocytes with tailed and elongated elliptical forms can be seen (Lee, 1998). These have been called "pencil forms" (Fig. 3).

Morphologic changes in the bone marrow are variable in iron deficiency anemia and do not correlate with the degree of anemia (Lee, 1998; Beutler, 2006). Erythroid hyperplasia with small

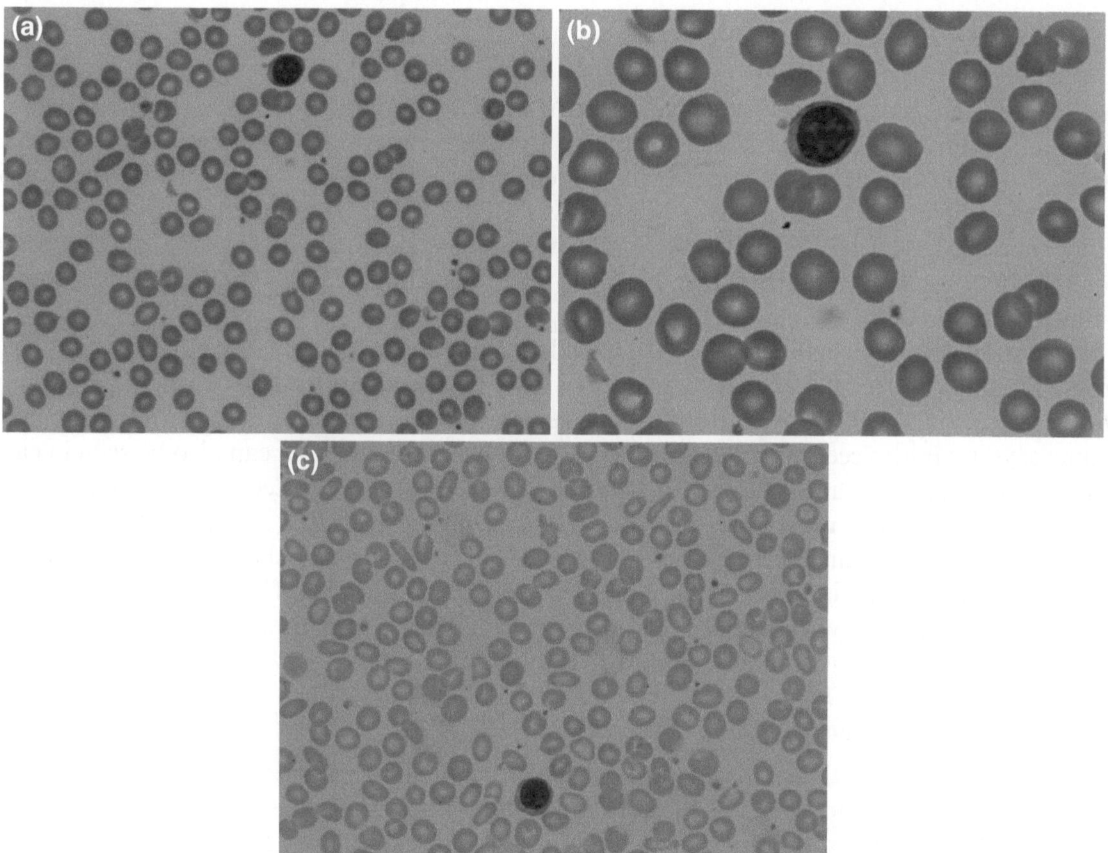


**Fig. 2.** Peripheral blood in a normal individual and a patient with iron deficiency anemia. (**A**) Wright's stain, 500X. Peripheral blood red cell morphology of a patient without iron deficiency or anemia. (**B**) 1000X. Red cells without increased central pallor. (**C**) Wright's stain, 500X. Peripheral blood of a patient with iron deficiency and anemia. The patient was a 38-year old woman with menometrorrhagia. The hemoglobin was 11 g/dL, hematocrit 38.4%, MCV 79 fL, MCH 24.3 pg/RBC, MCHC 30.8 g/dL of RBCs, iron 17 μg/dL, TIBC 451 μg/dL, and ferritin 4.7 ng/dL. Shown are red cells with the characteristic loss of central pallor and a pattern consistent with hypochromia and microcytosis.

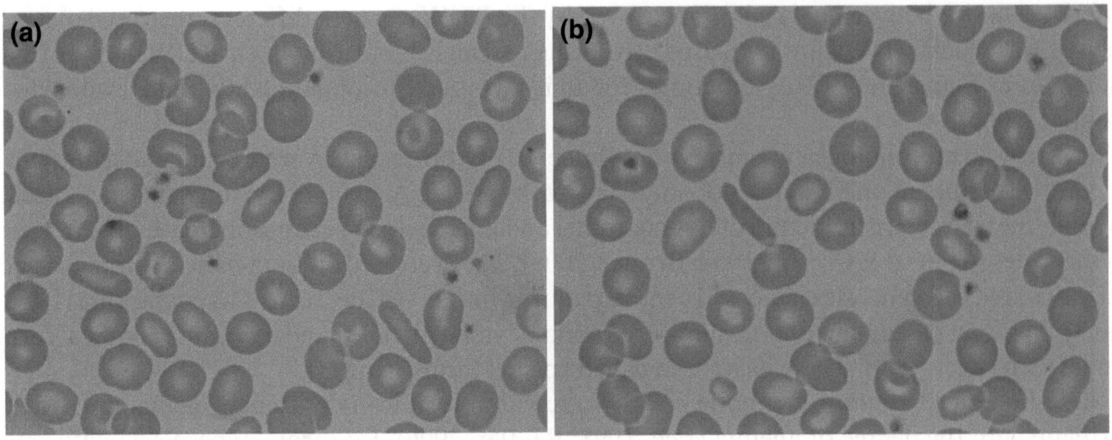


**Fig. 3.** (**A**) Detailed view of microcytic and hypochromic red cells of the patient described in Fig. 2. (**B**) Also shown are "pencil form" red cells, which are poikilocytes with tailed and elongated elliptical forms seen occasionally in iron deficiency.

erythroblasts and normoblasts that have irregular nuclear borders have been described (Beutler, Drennan, & Block, 1954). Decreased or absent iron hemosiderin in the bone marrow is characteristic of iron deficiency anemia, as measured by Prussian Blue staining to detect iron in marrow macrophages (Beutler et al., 1958; Cavill, 2003). While the reticulocyte count can be mildly increased (Kasper, Whissell, & Wallerstein, 1965; de Lima & Grotto, 2003), normal (Beutler, 2006) or decreased (Stevens, 1956) in iron deficiency anemia, the former is the most common finding.

The platelet count is usually increased in iron deficiency anemia (Lee, 1998; Kasper et al., 1965; Gross, Keefer, & Newman, 1964). Thrombocytosis may be a reflection of ongoing bleeding (Dincol & Aksoy, 1969; Beutler, 2006). However, in animal models of dietary iron deficiency, thrombocytosis is also seen (Choi & Simone, 1973). Thrombocytopenia can also be seen in cases of iron deficiency anemia (Soff & Levin, 1988; Berger & Brass, 1987; Lee, 1998). The leukocyte count is not changed in most cases of iron deficiency anemia (Kasper et al., 1965; Lee, 1998). However, there have been descriptions of neutropenia in cases of established anemia in the setting of iron deficiency anemia (Lee, 1998; Voigt, Dieterich, Brushke, & Herrmann, 1967). Other leukocytes are not usually affected. In the case of iron deficiency anemia secondary to hookworm infestation, eosinophilia is common (Bakta & Budhianto, 1994).

### 5.3. *Effects on Non-hematopoietic Systems*

Many changes in epithelial tissues have been attributed to iron deficiency. As previously described, the exact pathogenesis of these changes is not known. Tissues affected include tongue and mouth, hypopharynx, esophagus, stomach, nails, and scalp hair (Lee, 1998).

### 5.4. *Tongue and Mouth*

In patients with iron deficiency anemia, atrophy of the lingual papillae has been described as occurring in more than 5–10% of patients (Jacobs & Cavill, 1968; Beveridge, Bannerman, Evanson, & Witts, 1965; Uchida, Matsuno, Ide, & Kawachi, 1998). Some authors have speculated that some of the tongue changes may be due to concomitant pyridoxine deficiency (Jacobs & Cavill, 1968). In iron deficiency–related glossitis, the filiform papillae of the anterior third of the tongue atrophy first (Lee, 1998; Baird et al., 1961) followed by changes in the whole tongue. This involvement leads to a smooth and waxy appearance of the tongue (Fig. 4). Patients may report burning of the tongue, but this symptom is common in the general population and may not be specific to iron deficiency (Beutler, 2006). Glossitis can be reversed with adequate iron replacement therapy, and the clinical re-appearance of tongue papillae may occur within weeks of therapy (Lee, 1998).

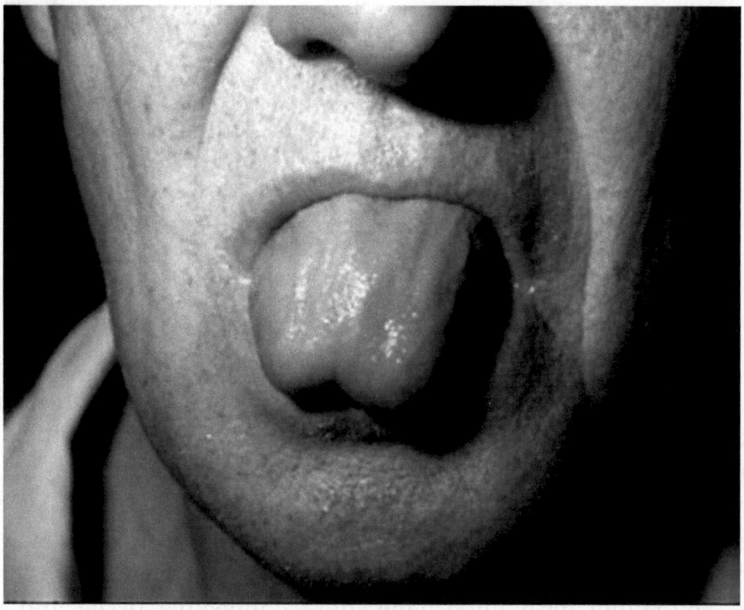

**Fig. 4.** Smooth tongue that can accompany iron deficiency in a male patient with iron deficiency anemia. The picture is courtesy of Drs. A. J. Chandrasekhar and Harry Messmore, Loyola University Medical Education; http://www.lumen.luc.edu

Angular stomatitis or cheilitis has also been attributed to iron deficiency (Fig. 5). Ulcerations or fissures of the mouth are the characteristic findings (Lu & Wu, 2004). This form of cheilitis can also been seen in other nutritional deficiencies, such as that of pyridoxine (Wray, Ferguson, Hutcheon, & Dagg, 1978; Lee, 1998) or riboflavin (Blanck et al., 2002).

### 5.5. *Hypopharynx and Esophagus*

In 1919, Paterson and Kelly described the association of dysphagia with angular cheilitis and lingual abnormalities in patients with iron deficiency anemia (Paterson, 1919; Kelly, 1919; Lee, 1998). In 1922, Vinson reported similar cases (Vinson, 1922) and referred to prior observations made by Plummer in 1912 (Plummer, 1912). This syndrome has since been called Paterson-Kelly, Plummer-Vinson (Lee, 1998), or sideropenic dysphagia (Lee, 1998). While rare, the syndrome continues to be described in the medical literature (Novacek, 2006). Most patients are Caucasian women in their fourth to seventh decade of life (Novacek, 2006). However, the syndrome has also been described in younger individuals (Crawfurd, Jacobs, Murphy, & Peters, 1965) and is not infrequent in developing countries such as India (Khosla, 1984).

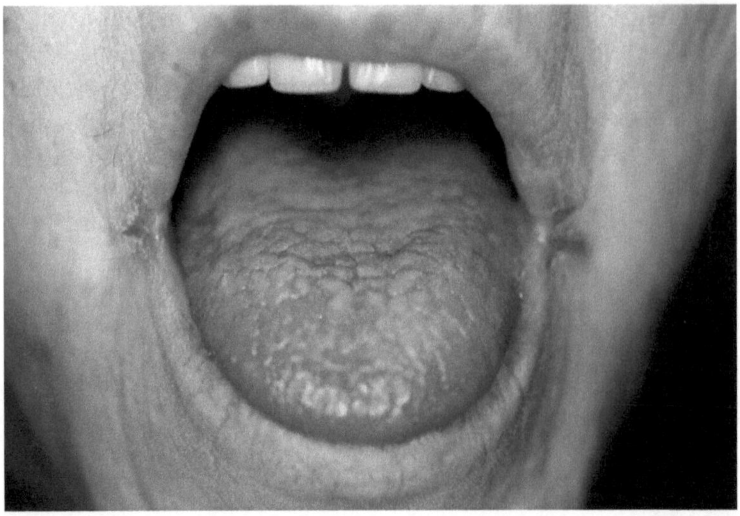

**Fig. 5.** Angular cheilitis. The picture is courtesy of Dr. Jerzy Pawlak, © Dermatlas; http://www.dermatlas.org

The dysphagia is commonly progressive and limited to solids (Novacek, 2006). The symptoms may persist for many years prior to the patient's referral to a health care professional (Lee, 1998). The characteristic symptom is post-cricoid dysphagia, and esophageal motility may be impaired (Miranda & Dantas, 2003). The most common anatomic lesion identified in such patients is a web of normal-appearing mucosa between the junction of the hypopharynx and esophagus (Hoffman & Jaffe, 1995). Upper esophageal webs can be demonstrated by contrast X-ray, videofluoroscopy, or endoscopy (Hoffman & Jaffe, 1995; Novacek, 2006). Biopsies of such webs have demonstrated normal squamous epithelium with underlying loose connective tissue and an inflammatory reaction (Entwistle & Jacobs, 1965; Baird et al., 1961). There have been reports of the association of esophageal webs with development of esophageal squamous cell carcinomas (Chisholm, 1974; Messmann, 2001; Larsson, Sandstrom, & Westling, 1975; Entwistle & Jacobs, 1965).

The exact pathogenesis of esophageal webs is unknown. Despite the clinical association with iron deficiency (Dantas, 1999), it seems that iron deficiency is neither necessary nor a sufficient cause of web formation (Novacek, 2006). Some authors dispute the hypothesis that the alimentary tract loses iron-dependent enzymes due to its high cell turnover, which then leads to mucosal degeneration and web formation (Novacek, 2006). Other authors favor etiologic factors such as inherited predisposition (Lee, 1998), malnutrition, and autoimmune processes (Rashid, Kumar, & Komar, 1999; Medrano, 2002; Jessner et al., 2003; Jacobs & Kilpatrick, 1964).

Anecdotal reports have described improvement in dysphasia in some patients receiving iron supplementation alone (Hoffman & Jaffe, 1995). However, for most patients with visible webs, mechanical dilation is required (Novacek, 2006; Hoffman & Jaffe, 1995).

### *5.6. Stomach*

Gastritis has been described in patients with iron deficiency anemia. In the 1950s, it was thought that this was a common manifestation or complication of iron deficiency (Davidson & Markson, 1955; Lee, 1998). While atrophic gastritis has been reported in iron deficiency anemia, the pattern is nonspecific and can mimic changes seen with other nutritional deficiencies and normal aging (Hershko, Patz, & Ronson, 2007). Dating back to the 1920s, it was already known that decreased acid secretion could be seen with hypochromic anemia (Wintrobe, 1933) and sometimes in a pattern similar to pernicious anemia (Hershko et al., 2007). In such cases, iron repletion therapy was sometimes sub-optimal to correct the anemia, and it was thought that lack of hydrochloric acid somehow impaired absorption of iron (Wintrobe, 1933). The concept of gastric atrophy as a cause of iron deficiency anemia was a point of doubt in the medical literature, but in more than a quarter of cases of refractory iron deficiency anemia without gastrointestinal symptoms, atrophic gastritis has been identified (Annibale et al., 2001).

The relationship between iron deficiency anemia and pernicious anemia is underscored by the observation that patients with iron deficiency anemia and non-bleeding gastrointestinal lesions may have chronic infections with *Helicobacter pylori* as the underlying mechanism that connects iron deficiency and autoimmune gastritis (Hershko et al., 2007; Hershko et al., 2005). To this effect, it has been reported that therapy with antibiotics for *H. pylori* may enhance the recovery of anemia and iron parameters in patients with iron deficiency and concomitant *H. pylori* infection (Chen & Luo, 2007; Choe et al., 1999). It is possible that antigenic mimicry between $H^+ K^+$-ATPase and *H. pylori* promotes immunity to auto-antigens that can lead to pernicious anemia in these circumstances (Rad, Schmid, & Prinz, 2006).

## 5.7. *Nails*

Nails represent another rapidly proliferating epithelial tissue that can be affected by iron deficiency (Fawcett, Linford, & Stulberg, 2004; Marks & Shuster, 1970). The characteristic lesion seen is koilonychia, defined as a concavity of the outer surface of the nail (Fig. 6). Thinning and flattening of the nail, as well as brittle nails, may precede the development of koilonychia (Marks & Shuster, 1970). The term "spoon-shaped nails" is also used to describe these changes (Kumar, Vaidyanathan, & Stead, 2007; Fawcett et al., 2004). It is unknown why iron deficiency leads to the nail changes described above, but finding koilonychia should raise a suspicion for iron deficiency (Beutler, 2006). The characteristic "spoon-shaped" appearance of nails was reported to occur in

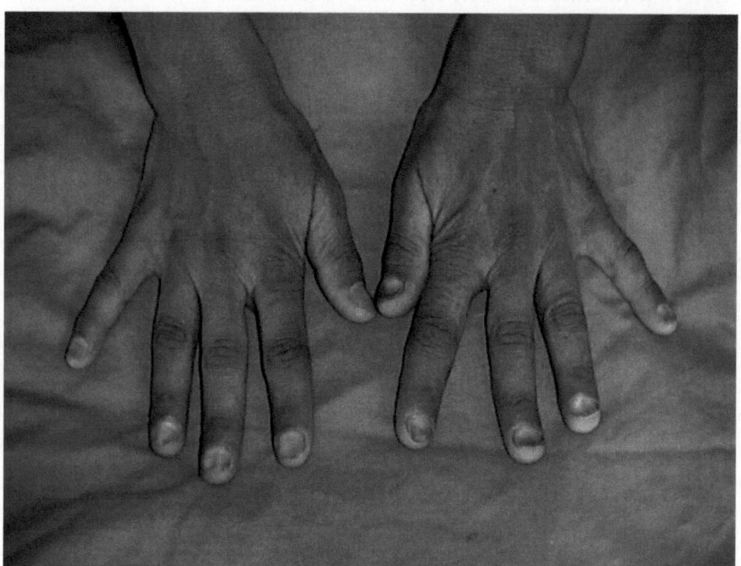

**Fig. 6.** Koilonychia. Nail changes of a 38 year-old woman who presented with symptoms of severe iron deficiency anemia due to long standing menorrhagia. The picture is courtesy of Dr. Jayalath Thilak, © Dermatlas; http://www.dermatlas.org

around 20% of iron-deficient patients diagnosed between the 1940s and the 1960s (Beveridge et al., 1965), but it seems that this finding is rare today (Beutler, 2006), possibly due to earlier detection of iron deficiency.

Koilonychia is not specific to iron deficiency anemia and can also be seen in a myriad of other systemic or genetic diseases and as a consequence of local injuries. It may result from occupational exposure of the hands to petroleum-based solvents, trauma, and other caustic agents (Lee, 1998; Samman, 1978). It has also been described in association with hemochromatosis (Barnett, Scher, & Taylor, 1991) and the autosomal dominant nail-patella syndrome (Fawcett et al., 2004). It can be seen in populations living at high altitudes, with or without concomitant iron deficiency (Sawhney, 2003; Patial, 1999). Alcoholics (Rao, 2004) and patients with chronic renal failure (Udayakumar et al., 2006) can also have koilonychia. Familial forms have been described as well (Gao, Li, Zhao, Wang, & Chen, 2001).

### *5.8. Hair*

Alopecia is not uncommon in women, and it is estimated that about one-third of all women will experience some hair loss during their lifetime (Shapiro, 2007). Iron deficiency may be associated with hair loss in women (Olsen et al., 2005). The data on this topic are limited, and cross-sectional studies of women with iron deficiency and hair loss have led to conflicting results (Sinclair, 2002; Rushton, Ramsay, James, Norris, & Gilkes, 1990; Kantor, Kessler, Brooks, & Cotsarelis, 2003; Trost, Bergfeld, & Calogeras, 2006). Telogen effluvion, or the rapid shift of hair from anagen (growing period) to telogen (resting period) phase, has been described as the mechanism underlying hair loss in women with iron deficiency (Trost et al., 2006; Shapiro, 2007). However, in one cross-sectional study, only women with androgenic alopecia or alopecia arreata had significantly lower ferritin levels than controls (Kantor et al., 2003). Iron is required as a cofactor for the activity of ribonucleotide reductase, a rate-limiting enzyme controlling DNA synthesis and required by rapidly dividing hair matrix cells (Shapiro, 2007). It is possible that in iron deficiency this enzyme is less active and may explain the hair loss seen.

Despite the controversy regarding the link between iron deficiency and hair loss in women, reviews of the topic still advise physicians to obtain ferritin levels and treat women with iron supplementation if iron deficiency co-exists (Shapiro, 2007; Trost et al., 2006; Olsen et al., 2005). However, it should be noted that iron supplementation has not been studied in well-conducted randomized trials for women with hair loss, and case series have reported lack of efficacy of this approach (Sinclair, 2002; Trost et al., 2006; Olsen et al., 2005).

### *5.9. Other Manifestations*

*Pica:* Pica is defined as an eating disorder, in which objects thought to be non-nutritional are eaten persistently. Pica originates from the Latin term for magpie, a bird that gleans all sorts of things for its nest (Woywodt & Kiss, 2002). The craving to eat non-nutritional substances such as ice, dirt, clay, starch, salt, and cardboard among other items is considered a classic manifestation of iron deficiency (Lee, 1998; Beutler, 2006; Coltman, 1969). It is interesting to note that reports of pica date back to the writings of Hippocrates (Lee, 1998; Woywodt & Kiss, 2002). A change in appetite and "perversion of appetite" were also known symptoms of chlorosis (Ashwell, 1836). Miguel de Cervantes in his1605 *Don Quixote* reported behaviors characteristic of pica, writing: "women that by caprice eat soil, plaster coal and other disgusting substances" (Larrain, 2005).

The cause of pica in iron deficiency is not well established. Pica has been described in animals with iron deficiency, and it is possible that pica is a direct effect of iron deficiency (Hyslop, 1977).

Some authors have questioned if pica serves as a compensatory response to other peripheral effects of iron deficiency. Changes in the tongue mucosa and mouth can lead to pain, and it is possible that part of the explanation for pacophagia (the ingestion of ice) is the analgesic effect of ice in the oral mucosa (Kettaneh et al., 2005; Osaki, Ueta, Arisawa, Kitamura, & Matsugi, 1999; Brown & Dyment, 1972). In the case of geophagia (the consumption of earth, soil, or clay), some authors speculate that soil may be viewed as a source of nutrients and that in the face of nutritional deficiencies, including iron deficiency, the urge of geophagia would be an atavistic response to behaviors that may have been common to early human beings (Woywodt & Kiss, 2002; Dreyer, Chaushev, & Gledhill, 2004). Rapid resolution of pica can be seen with adequate iron supplementation (Lee, 1998; Beutler, 2006; Osman, Wali, & Osman, 2005; Coltman, 1969).

The true incidence of pica in patients with iron deficiency is not clear. In the 1960s and 1970s, it was estimated that almost half of all patients with iron deficiency had some form of pica, with pacophagia being the most common pica (Reynolds, Binder, Miller, Chang, & Horan, 1968; Crosby, 1976). More recent reports from the 1990s and 2000s continue to identify a high percentage of iron-deficient patients who report pica, with estimates between 5% and 50% (Munoz et al., 1998; Simpson, Mull, Longley, & East, 2000; Kettaneh et al., 2005).

*Muscular function and exercise tolerance*: In animal models of iron deficiency, decreased exercise tolerance and increased propensity to lactic acidosis with exercise have been observed (Finch et al., 1979; Mackler, Person, & Grace, 1985). In humans, objective measurements of work performance and oxygen consumption have on occasion shown that in iron deficiency there is a decrease in work capacity (Haas & Brownlie, 2001). Other reports have demonstrated improved performance and oxygen consumption parameters with iron supplementation in patients with iron deficiency, even in the absence of anemia (Friedmann, Weller, Mairbaurl, & Bartsch, 2001; Hinton, Giordano, Brownlie, & Haas, 2000; Zhu & Haas, 1998).

*Immune system manifestations*: Iron deficiency may alter immune function by increasing the susceptibility to some forms of infection, as shown in animal models (Beard, 2001) and humans (Ahluwalia, Sun, Krause, Mastro, & Handte, 2004).

*Restless leg syndromes*: The first description of this syndrome was made in the 1940s and 1950s, and an association with iron deficiency was proposed then (Allen & Earley, 2001; Nordlander, 1953; Nordlander, 1954). Restless leg syndrome is a common neurologic disorder characterized by an irresistible urge to move the legs and is one of the major causes of sleep deprivation (Sun, Chen, Ho, Earley, & Allen, 1998; Stefansson et al., 2007; Trenkwalder, Paulus, & Walters, 2005). A common variant in an intron of *BTBD9* on chromosome 6p21.2 was recently described in affected individuals (Stefansson et al., 2007). The correlation of low ferritin levels and this syndrome is now well characterized (Stefansson et al., 2007; Trenkwalder et al., 2005).

## REFERENCES

Ahluwalia, N. (1998). Diagnostic utility of serum transferrin receptors measurement in assessing iron status. *Nutrition Reviews, 56*, 133–141.

Ahluwalia, N., Sun, J., Krause, D., Mastro, A., & Handte, G. (2004). Immune function is impaired in iron-deficient, homebound, older women. *The American Journal of Clinical Nutrition, 79*, 516–521.

Allen, R. P., & Earley, C. J. (2001). Restless legs syndrome: A review of clinical and pathophysiologic features. *Journal of Clinical Neurophysiology, 18*, 128–147.

Annibale, B., Capurso, G., Chistolini, A., D'Ambra, G., DiGiulio, E., Monarca, B., et al. (2001). Gastrointestinal causes of refractory iron deficiency anemia in patients without gastrointestinal symptoms. *The American Journal of Medicine, 111*, 439–445.

Ashwell, S. (1836). Observations on chlorosis and its complications. *Guy's Hospital Reports, 1*, 529.

Bainton, D. F., & Finch, C. A. (1964). The diagnosis of iron deficiency anemia. *The American Journal of Medicine, 37*, 62–70.

Baird, I. M., Dodge, O. G., Palmer, F. J., & Wawman, R. J. (1961). The tongue and oesophagus in iron-deficiency anaemia and the effect of iron therapy. *Journal of Clinical Pathology, 14*, 603–609.

Bakta, I. M., & Budhianto, F. X. (1994). Hookworm anemia in the adult population of Jagapati village, Bali, Indonesia. *The Southeast Asian Journal of Tropical Medicine and Public Health, 25*, 459–463.

Banerjee, R. N., & Narang, R. M. (1967). Haematological changes in malignancy. *British Journal of Haematology, 13*, 829–843.

Barnett, J. M., Scher, R. K., & Taylor, S. C. (1991). Nail cosmetics. *Dermatologic Clinics, 9*, 9–17.

Beard, J. L. (2001). Iron biology in immune function, muscle metabolism and neuronal functioning. *The Journal of Nutrition, 131*, 568S–579S.

Berger, M., & Brass, L. F. (1987). Severe thrombocytopenia in iron deficiency anemia. *American Journal of Hematology, 24*, 425–428.

Bessman, J. D., & Feinstein, D. I. (1979). Quantitative anisocytosis as a discriminant between iron deficiency and thalassemia minor. *Blood, 53*, 288–293.

Bessman, J. D., Gilmer, P. R., Jr., & Gardner, F. H. (1983). Improved classification of anemias by MCV and RDW. *American Journal of Clinical Pathology, 80*, 322–326.

Beutler, E. (1957). Iron enzymes in iron deficiency. I. Cytochrome c. *The American Journal of Medical Sciences, 234*, 517–527.

Beutler, E. (1959a). Iron enzymes in iron deficiency. IV. Cytochrome oxidase in rat kidney and heart. *Acta Haematologica, 21*, 371–377.

Beutler, E. (1959b). The red cell indices in the diagnosis of iron-deficiency anemia. *Annals of Internal Medicine, 50*, 313–322.

Beutler, E. (2002). History of iron in medicine. *Blood Cells, Molecules & Diseases, 29*, 297–308.

Beutler, E. (2006). Disorders of iron metabolism. In M. A. Lichtman, T. J. Kipps, K. Kaushansky, E. Beutler, U. Seligsohn, & J. T. Prchal (Eds.), *Williams hematology* (7th ed., pp. 511–553). New York: McGraw-Hill.

Beutler, E., & Blaisdell, R. K. (1958). Iron enzymes in iron deficiency. II. Catalase in human erythrocytes. *The Journal of Clinical Investigation, 37*, 833–835.

Beutler, E., & Blaisdell, R. K. (1960). Iron enzymes in iron deficiency. V. Succinic dehydrogenase in rat liver, kidney and heart. *Blood, 15*, 30–35.

Beutler, E., Drennan, W., & Block, M. (1954). The bone marrow and liver in iron-deficiency anemia: A histopathologic study of sections with special reference to the stainable iron content. *The Journal of Laboratory and Clinical Medicine, 43*, 427–439.

Beutler, E., Felitti, V., Ho, N. J., & Gelbart, T. (2002). Relationship of body iron stores to levels of serum ferritin, serum iron, unsaturated iron binding capacity and transferrin saturation in patients with iron storage disease. *Acta Haematologica, 107*, 145–149.

Beutler, E., Hoffbrand, A. V., & Cook, J. D. (2003). Iron deficiency and overload. *Hematology/The Education Program of the American Society of Hematology*, 40–61.

Beutler, E., Larsh, S., & Tanzi, F. (1960). Iron enzymes in iron deficiency: VII. Oxygen consumption measurements in iron-deficient subjects. *The American Journal of Medical Sciences, 239*, 759–765.

Beutler, E., Robson, M. J., & Buttenwieser, E. (1958). A comparison of the plasma iron, iron-binding capacity, sternal marrow iron and other methods in the clinical evaluation of iron, stores. *Annals of Internal Medicine, 48*, 60–82.

Beveridge, B. R., Bannerman, R. M., Evanson, J. M., & Witts, L. J. (1965). Hypochromic anaemia. A retrospective study and follow-up of 378 in-patients. *The Quarterly Journal of Medicine, 34*, 145–161.

Blanck, H. M., Bowman, B. A., Serdula, M. K., Khan, L. K., Kohn, W., & Woodruff, B. A. (2002). Angular stomatitis and riboflavin status among adolescent Bhutanese refugees living in southeastern Nepal. *The American Journal of Clinical Nutrition, 76*, 430–435.

Brewer, G. J. (1974). 2,3–DPG and erythrocyte oxygen affinity. *Annual Review of Medicine, 25*, 29–38.

Brown, W. D., & Dyment, P. G. (1972). Pagophagia and iron deficiency anemia in adolescent girls. *Pediatrics, 49*, 766–767.

Brumberg, J. J. (1982). Chlorotic girls, 1870–1920: A historical perspective on female adolescence. *Child Development, 53*, 1468–1477.

Bryan, C. P. (1931). *The Papyrus Ebers*. New York: Appleton-Century-Crofts.

Bushnell, F. K. (1992). A guide to primary care of iron-deficiency anemia. *The Nurse Practitioner, 17*, 68, 71–68, 74.

Cavill, I., Ricketts, C., Napier, J. A., & Jacobs, A. (1977). Ferrokinetics and erythropoiesis in man: Red-cell production and destruction in normal and anaemic subjects. *British Journal of Haematology, 35*, 33–40.

Cavill, I. A. (2003). Iron status indicators: Hello new, goodbye old? *Blood, 101*, 372–373.

Celsing, F., Ekblom, B., Sylven, C., Everett, J., & Astrand, P. O. (1988). Effects of chronic iron deficiency anaemia on myoglobin content, enzyme activity, and capillary density in the human skeletal muscle. *Acta Medica Scandinavica, 223*, 451–457.

Cheli, R., Dodero, M., Celle, G., & Vassalotti, M. (1959). Gastric biopsy and secretory findings in hypochromic anaemias. *Acta Haematologica, 22*, 1–11.

Chen, L. H., & Luo, H. S. (2007). Effects of H pylori therapy on erythrocytic and iron parameters in iron deficiency anemia patients with H pylori-positive chronic gastritis. *World Journal of Gastroenterology, 13*, 5380–5383.

Chisholm, M. (1974). The association between webs, iron and post-cricoid carcinoma. *Postgraduate Medical Journal, 50*, 215–219.

Choe, Y. H., Kim, S. K., Son, B. K., Lee, D. H., Hong, Y. C., & Pai, S. H. (1999). Randomized placebo-controlled trial of Helicobacter pylori eradication for iron-deficiency anemia in preadolescent children and adolescents. *Helicobacter, 4*, 135–139.

Choi, S. I., & Simone, J. V. (1973). Platelet production in experimental iron deficiency anemia. *Blood, 42*, 219–228.

Chuang, C. L., Liu, R. S., Wei, Y. H., Huang, T. P., & Tarng, D. C. (2003). Early prediction of response to intravenous iron supplementation by reticulocyte haemoglobin content and high-fluorescence reticulocyte count in haemodialysis patients. *Nephrology, Dialysis, Transplantation, 18*, 370–377.

Coltman, C. A., Jr. (1969). Pagophagia and iron lack. *Journal of the American Medical Association, 207*, 513–516.

Conrad, M. E., & Crosby, W. H. (1962). The natural history of iron deficiency induced by phlebotomy. *Blood, 20*, 173–185.

Cook, J. D., Flowers, C. H., & Skikne, B. S. (2003). The quantitative assessment of body iron. *Blood, 101*, 3359–3364.

Crawfurd, M. D., Jacobs, A., Murphy, B., & Peters, D. K. (1965). Paterson-Kelly syndrome in adolescence: A report of five cases. *British Medical Journal, 1*, 693–695.

Crosby, W. H. (1976). Pica. *Journal of the American Medical Association, 235*, 2765.

Cullen, P., Soffker, J., Hopfl, M., Bremer, C., Schlaghecken, R., Mehrens, T., et al. (1999). Hypochromic red cells and reticulocyte haemglobin content as markers of iron-deficient erythropoiesis in patients undergoing chronic haemodialysis. *Nephrology, Dialysis, Transplantation, 14*, 659–665.

Dale, J. C., Burritt, M. F., & Zinsmeister, A. R. (2002). Diurnal variation of serum iron, iron-binding capacity, transferrin saturation, and ferritin levels. *American Journal of Clinical Pathology, 117*, 802–808.

Dallalio, G., Fleury, T., & Means, R. T. (2003). Serum hepcidin in clinical specimens. *British Journal of Haematology, 122*, 996–1000.

Dallman, P. R., Beutler, E., & Finch, C. A. (1978). Effects of iron deficiency exclusive of anaemia. *British Journal of Haematology, 40*, 179–184.

Dallman, P. R., & Schwartz, H. C. (1965). Myoglobin and cytochrome response during repair of iron deficiency in the rat. *The Journal of Clinical Investigation, 44*, 1631–1638.

Dantas, R. O. (1999). Iron deficiency and dysphagia. *American Journal of Gastroenterology, 94*, 3072–3073.

Davidson, W. M., & Markson, J. L. (1955). The gastric mucosa in iron-deficiency anaemia. *Lancet, 269*, 639–643.

de Lima, G. A., & Grotto, H. Z. (2003). Soluble transferrin receptor and immature reticulocytes are not useful for distinguishing iron-deficiency anemia from heterozygous beta-thalassemia. *Sao Paulo Medical Journal, 121*, 90–91.

Dennison, H. A. (1999). Limitations of ferritin as a marker of anemia in end stage renal disease. *ANNA Journal, 26*, 409–414.

Dillman, E., Gale, C., Green, W., Johnson, D. G., Mackler, B., & Finch, C. (1980). Hypothermia in iron deficiency due to altered triiodothyronine metabolism. *The American Journal of Physiology, 239*, R377–R381.

Dincol, K., & Aksoy, M. (1969). On the platelet levels in chronic iron deficiency anemia. *Acta Haematologica, 41*, 135–143.

Dreyer, M. J., Chaushev, P. G., & Gledhill, R. F. (2004). Biochemical investigations in geophagia. *Journal of the Royal Society of Medicine, 97*, 48.

Ellis, L. D., Jensen, W. N., & Westerman, M. P. (1964). Marrow iron. An evaluation of depleted stores in a series of 1,332 needle biopsies. *Annals of Internal Medicine, 61*, 44–49.

Entwistle, C. C., & Jacobs, A. (1965). Histological findings in the Paterson-Kelly syndrome. *Journal of Clinical Pathology, 18*, 408–413.

Fairbanks, V. F. (1971). Is the peripheral blood film reliable for the diagnosis of iron deficiency anemia? *American Journal of Clinical Pathology, 55*, 447–451.

Fawcett, R. S., Linford, S., & Stulberg, D. L. (2004). Nail abnormalities: Clues to systemic disease. *American Family Physician, 69*, 1417–1424.

Finch, C. A., Deubelbeiss, K., Cook, J. D., Eschbach, J. W., Harker, L. A., Funk, D. D., et al. (1970). Ferrokinetics in man. *Medicine (Baltimore), 49*, 17–53.

Finch, C. A., Gollnick, P. D., Hlastala, M. P., Miller, L. R., Dillmann, E., & Mackler, B. (1979). Lactic acidosis as a result of iron deficiency. *The Journal of Clinical Investigation, 64*, 129–137.

Follezou, J. Y., & Bizon, M. (1986). Cancer chemotherapy induces a transient increase of serum-iron level. *Neoplasma, 33*, 225–231.

Fowler, W. M. (1936). Chlorosis – An obituary. *Annals of Medical History, 8*, 168.

Friedmann, B., Weller, E., Mairbaurl, H., & Bartsch, P. (2001). Effects of iron repletion on blood volume and performance capacity in young athletes. *Medicine and Science in Sports and Exercise, 33*, 741–746.

Ganz, T. (2006). Hepcidin and its role in regulating systemic iron metabolism. *Hematology/The Education Program of the American Society of Hematology, 507*, 29–35.

Gao, X. H., Li, X., Zhao, Y., Wang, Y., & Chen, H. D. (2001). Familial koilonychia. *International Journal of Dermatology, 40*, 290–291.

Garrison, F. H. (1921). *An introduction to the history of medicine*. New York: W.B. Saunders.

Gross, S., Keefer, V., & Newman, A. J. (1964). The platelets in iron-deficiency in iron-deficiency anemia. I. The response to oral and parenteral iron. *Pediatrics, 34*, 315–323.

Haas, J. D., & Brownlie, T. (2001). Iron deficiency and reduced work capacity: A critical review of the research to determine a causal relationship. *Journal of Nutrition, 131*, 676S–688S.

Haden, R. L. (1938). Historical aspects of iron therapy in anemia. *Journal of the American Medical Association, 111*, 1059.

Hagler, L., Askew, E. W., Neville, J. R., Mellick, P. W., Coppes, R. I., Jr., & Lowder, J. F., Jr. (1981). Influence of dietary iron deficiency on hemoglobin, myoglobin, their respective reductases, and skeletal muscle mitochondrial respiration. *American Journal of Clinical Nutrition, 34*, 2169–2177.

Hamilton, L. D., Gubler, C. J., Caertwright, G. E., & Wintrobe, M. M. (1950). Diurnal variation in the plasma iron level of man. *Proceedings of the Society for Experimental Biology and Medicine, 75*, 65–68.

Hansen, T. M., & Hansen, N. E. (1986). Serum ferritin as indicator of iron responsive anaemia in patients with rheumatoid arthritis. *Annals of Rheumatic Diseases, 45*, 596–602.

Heath, C. W., Strauss, M. B., & Castle, W. B. (1932). Quantitative aspects of iron deficiency in hypochromic anemia: (The parenteral administration of iron). *The Journal of Clinical Investigation, 11*, 1293–1312.

Hershko, C., Hoffbrand, A. V., Keret, D., Souroujon, M., Maschler, I., Monselise, Y., et al. (2005). Role of autoimmune gastritis, Helicobacter pylori and celiac disease in refractory or unexplained iron deficiency anemia. *Haematologica, 90*, 585–595.

Hershko, C., Patz, J., & Ronson, A. (2007). The anemia of achylia gastrica revisited. *Blood Cells, Molecules & Diseases, 39*, 178–183.

Hinton, P. S., Giordano, C., Brownlie, T., & Haas, J. D. (2000). Iron supplementation improves endurance after training in iron-depleted, nonanemic women. *Journal of Applied Physiology, 88*, 1103–1111.

Hoffman, R. M., & Jaffe, P. E. (1995). Plummer-Vinson syndrome. A case report and literature review. *Archives of Internal Medicine, 155*, 2008–2011.

Hudson, R. P. (1977). The biography of disease: Lessons from chlorosis. *Bulletin of the History of Medicine, 51*, 448–463.

Hyslop, N. S. (1977). Pica in man and animals. *British Journal of Haematology, 37*, 154–155.

Ingram, C. F., & Lewis, S. M. (2000). Clinical use of WHO haemoglobin colour scale: Validation and critique. *Journal of Clinical Pathology, 53*, 933–937.

Ioannou, G. N., Tung, B. Y., & Kowdley, K. V. (2002). Iron in hepatitis C: Villain or innocent bystander? *Seminars in Gastrointestinal Disease, 13*, 95–108.

Jacobs, A. (1960). The buccal mucosa in anaemia. *Journal of Clinical Pathology, 13*, 463–468.

Jacobs, A., & Cavill, I. (1968). The oral lesions of iron deficiency anaemia: Pyridoxine and riboflavin status. *British Journal of Haematology, 14*, 291–295.

Jacobs, A., & Kilpatrick, G. S. (1964). The Paterson-Kelly syndrome. *British Medical Journal, 2*, 79–82.

Jessner, W., Vogelsang, H., Puspok, A., Ferenci, P., Gangl, A., Novacek, G., et al. (2003). Plummer-Vinson syndrome associated with celiac disease and complicated by postcricoid carcinoma and carcinoma of the tongue. *American Journal of Gastroenterology, 98*, 1208–1209.

Junca, J., Fernandez-Aviles, F., Oriol, A., Navarro, J. T., Milla, F., Sancho, J. M., et al. (1998). The usefulness of the serum transferrin receptor in detecting iron deficiency in the anemia of chronic disorders. *Haematologica, 83*, 676–680.

Kantor, J., Kessler, L. J., Brooks, D. G., & Cotsarelis, G. (2003). Decreased serum ferritin is associated with alopecia in women. *The Journal of Investigative Dermatology, 121*, 985–988.

Kasper, C. K., Whissell, D. Y., & Wallerstein, R. O. (1965). Clinical aspects of iron deficiency. *Journal of the American Medical Association, 191*, 359–363.

Kelly, A. B. (1919). Spasm at the entrance to the oesophagus. *The Journal of Laryngology and Otology, 34*, 285–288.

Kemna, E. H., Tjalsma, H., Podust, V. N., & Swinkels, D. W. (2007). Mass spectrometry-based hepcidin measurements in serum and urine: Analytical aspects and clinical implications. *Clinical Chemistry, 53*, 620–628.

Kettaneh, A., Eclache, V., Fain, O., Sontag, C., Uzan, M., Carbillon, L., et al. (2005). Pica and food craving in patients with iron-deficiency anemia: A case-control study in France. *The American Journal of Medicine, 118*, 185–188.

Khosla, S. N. (1984). Cricoid webs – Incidence and follow-up study in Indian patients. *Postgraduate Medical Journal, 60*, 346–348.

Kumar, G., Vaidyanathan, L., & Stead, L. G. (2007). Images in emergency medicine. Koilonychia, or spoon-shaped nails, is generally associated with iron-deficiency anemia. *Annals of Emergency Medicine, 49*, 243, 250.

Larrain, C. (2005). Pica, a strange symptom unveiled even in "Don Quixote". *Revista Medica de Chile, 133*, 609–611.

Larsson, L. G., Sandstrom, A., & Westling, P. (1975). Relationship of Plummer-Vinson disease to cancer of the upper alimentary tract in Sweden. *Cancer Research, 35*, 3308–3316.

Lee, G. R. (1998). Iron deficiency and iron-deficiency anemia. In G. R. Lee, J. Foerster, J. Lukens, F. Paraskevas, J. P. Greer, & G. M. Rodgers (Eds.), *Wintrobe's clinical hematology* (10th ed., pp. 979–1010). Baltimore, Maryland: Williams & Wilkins.

Lipschitz, D. A., Cook, J. D., & Finch, C. A. (1974). A clinical evaluation of serum ferritin as an index of iron stores. *New England Journal of Medicine, 290*, 1213–1216.

London, I. M. (1980). Iron and heme: Crucial carriers and catalysts. In M. M. Wintrobe (Ed.), *Blood, pure and eloquent* (1st ed., pp. 171–208). New York: McGraw-Hill Education.

Looker, A. C., Cogswell, M. E., & Gunter, E. W. (2002). Iron deficiency – United States, 1999–2000. *MMWR Morbidity and Mortality Weekly Report, 51*, 897–899.

Loria, A., Sanchez-Medal, L., Lisker, R., De Rodriguez, E., & Labardini, J. (1967). Red cell life span in iron deficiency anaemia. *British Journal of Haematology, 13*, 294–302.

Lu, S. Y., & Wu, H. C. (2004). Initial diagnosis of anemia from sore mouth and improved classification of anemias by MCV and RDW in 30 patients. *Oral Surgery, Oral Medicine, Oral Pathology, Oral Radiology, and Endodontics, 98*, 679–685.

Macdougall, L. G., Judisch, J. M., & Mistry, S. B. (1970). Red cell metabolism in iron deficiency anemia. II. The relationship between red cell survival and alterations in red cell metabolism. *Journal of Pediatrics, 76*, 660–675.

Mackler, B., Person, R., & Grace, R. (1985). Iron deficiency in the rat: Effects on energy metabolism in brown adipose tissue. *Pediatric Research, 19*, 989–991.

Macleod, R. I., Hamilton, P. J., & Soames, J. V. (1988). Quantitative exfoliative oral cytology in iron-deficiency and megaloblastic anemia. *Analytical and Quantitative Cytology and Histology, 10*, 176–180.

Marks, J., & Shuster, S. (1970). Anaemia and skin disease. *Postgraduate Medical Journal, 46*, 659–663.

Mast, A. E., Blinder, M. A., & Dietzen, D. J. (2007, November 20). Reticulocyte hemoglobin content. *American Journal of Hematology* (epub ahead of print).

Mast, A. E., Blinder, M. A., Lu, Q., Flax, S., & Dietzen, D. J. (2002). Clinical utility of the reticulocyte hemoglobin content in the diagnosis of iron deficiency. *Blood, 99*, 1489–1491.

Matzner, Y., Konijn, A. M., & Hershko, C. (1980). Serum ferritin in hematologic malignancies. *American Journal of Hematology, 9*, 13–22.

Medrano, M. (2002). Dysphagia in a patient with rheumatoid arthritis and iron deficiency anemia. *MedGenMed: Medscape General Medicine, 4*, 10.

Mercer, C. G., & Wangensteen, S. D. (1985). "Consumption, heart-disease, or whatever": Chlorosis, a heroine's illness in the wings of the dove. *Journal of the History of Medicine and Allied Sciences, 40*, 259–285.

Messmann, H. (2001). Squamous cell cancer of the oesophagus. *Best Practice & Research. Clinical Gastroenterology, 15*, 249–265.

Miranda, A. L., & Dantas, R. O. (2003). Esophageal contractions and oropharyngeal and esophageal transits in patients with iron deficiency anemia. *American Journal of Gastroenterology, 98*, 1000–1004.

Morgan, M. A., Hoffbrand, A. V., Laulicht, M., Luck, W., & Knowles, S. (1983). Serum ferritin concentration in Gaucher's disease. *British Medical Journal (Clinical Research Ed.)*, *286*, 1864.

Munoz, J. A., Marcos, J., Risueno, C. E., de Cos, C., Lopez, R., Capote, F. J., et al. (1998). Iron deficiency and pica. *Sangre (Barcelona)*, *43*, 31–34.

Naiman, J. L., Oski, F. A., Diamond, L. K., Vawter, G. F., & Shwachman, H. (1964). The gastrointestinal effects of iron-deficiency anemia. *Pediatrics*, *33*, 83–99.

Nordlander, N. B. (1953). Therapy in restless legs. *Acta Medica Scandinavica*, *145*, 453–457.

Nordlander, N. B. (1954). Restless legs. *The British Journal of Physical Medicine, Including its Application to Industry*, *17*, 160–162.

North, M., Dallalio, G., Donath, A. S., Melink, R., & Means, R. T., Jr. (1997). Serum transferrin receptor levels in patients undergoing evaluation of iron stores: Correlation with other parameters and observed versus predicted results. *Clinical and Laboratory Haematology*, *19*, 93–97.

Novacek, G. (2006). Plummer-Vinson syndrome. *Orphanet Journal of Rare Diseases*, *1*, 36.

Olsen, E. A., Messenger, A. G., Shapiro, J., Bergfeld, W. F., Hordinsky, M. K., Roberts, J. L., et al. (2005). Evaluation and treatment of male and female pattern hair loss. *Journal of the American Academy of Dermatology*, *52*, 301–311.

Osaki, T., Ueta, E., Arisawa, K., Kitamura, Y., & Matsugi, N. (1999). The pathophysiology of glossal pain in patients with iron deficiency and anemia. *The American Journal of Medical Sciences*, *318*, 324–329.

Osman, Y. M., Wali, Y. A., & Osman, O. M. (2005). Craving for ice and iron-deficiency anemia: A case series from Oman. *Pediatric Hematology and Oncology*, *22*, 127–131.

Paterson, D. R. (1919). A clinical type of dysphagia. *The Journal of Laryngology and Otology*, *34*, 289–291.

Patial, R. K. (1999). High altitude koilonychia. *The Journal of the Association of Physicians of India*, *47*, 406–408.

Pettersson, T., Kivivuori, S. M., & Siimes, M. A. (1994). Is serum transferrin receptor useful for detecting iron-deficiency in anaemic patients with chronic inflammatory diseases? *British Journal of Rheumatology*, *33*, 740–744.

Plummer, S. (1912). Diffuse dilatation of the esophagus without anatomic stenosis (cardiospasm). A report of ninety-one cases. *Journal of the American Medical Association*, *58*, 2013–2015.

Pollycove, M. (1966). Iron metabolism and kinetics. *Seminars in Hematology*, *3*, 235–298.

Poskitt, E. M. (2003). Early history of iron deficiency. *British Journal of Haematology*, *122*, 554–562.

Prchal, J. T. (2006). Clinical manifestations and classification of erythrocyte disorders. In M. A. Lichtman (Ed.), *Williams hematology*. In M. A. Lichtman, T. J. Kipps, K. Kaushansky, E. Beutler, U. Seligsohn, & J. T. Prchal, (Eds.), *Williams hematology* (Vo. 7[1], pp. 411–418). New York: McGraw-Hill.

Rad, R., Schmid, R. M., & Prinz, C. (2006). Helicobacter pylori, iron deficiency, and gastric autoimmunity. *Blood*, *107*, 4969–4970.

Rao, G. S. (2004). Cutaneous changes in chronic alcoholics. *Indian Journal of Dermatology, Venereology and Leprology*, *70*, 79–81.

Rasch, C. A., Cotton, E. K., Griggs, R. C., & Harris, J. W. (1976). Shortened survival of autotransfused 51Cr-labeled erythrocytes in infants with severe iron-deficiency anemia. *Seminars in Hematology*, *13*, 181–186.

Rashid, Z., Kumar, A., & Komar, M. (1999). Plummer-Vinson syndrome and postcricoid carcinoma: Late complications of unrecognized celiac disease. *American Journal of Gastroenterology*, *94*, 1991.

Reynolds, R. D., Binder, H. J., Miller, M. B., Chang, W. W., & Horan, S. (1968). Pagophagia and iron deficiency anemia. *Annals of Internal Medicine*, *69*, 435–440.

Rich, I. N., Sawatzki, G., & Kubanek, B. (1981). Specific enhancement of mouse CFU-E by mouse transferrin. *British Journal of Haematology*, *49*, 567–573.

Rodvien, R., Gillum, A., & Weintraub, L. R. (1974). Decreased glutathione peroxidase activity secondary to severe iron deficiency: A possible mechanism responsible for the shortened life span of the iron-deficient red cell. *Blood*, *43*, 281–289.

Rushton, D. H., Ramsay, I. D., James, K. C., Norris, M. J., & Gilkes, J. J. (1990). Biochemical and trichological characterization of diffuse alopecia in women. *British Journal of Dermatology*, *123*, 187–197.

Samman, P. D. (1978). *The nails in disease*. (3rd ed.). London: Heinemann Medical Books.

Sawhney, M. P. (2003). Ladakhi koilonychia. *Indian Journal of Dermatology, Venereology and Leprology*, *69*, 79–80.

Scott, J., Valentine, J. A., St. Hill, C. A., & West, C. R. (1985). Morphometric analysis of atrophic changes in human lingual epithelium in iron deficiency anaemia. *Journal of Clinical Pathology*, *38*, 1025–1029.

Seligman, P. A., & Schleicher, R. B. (1999). Comparison of methods used to measure serum iron in the presence of iron gluconate or iron dextran. *Clinical Chemistry*, *45*, 898–901.

Semenza, G. L. (2004). O2–regulated gene expression: Transcriptional control of cardiorespiratory physiology by HIF-1. *Journal of Applied Physiology, 96*, 1173–1177.

Shahidi, N. T., & Diamond, L. K. (1960). Skull changes in infants with chronic iron-deficiency anemia. *New England Journal of Medicine, 262*, 137–139.

Shapiro, J. (2007). Clinical practice. Hair loss in women. *New England Journal of Medicine, 357*, 1620–1630.

Siimes, M. A., Refino, C., & Dallman, P. R. (1980). Manifestation of iron deficiency at various levels of dietary iron intake. *American Journal of Clinical Nutrition, 33*, 570–574.

Simpson, E., Mull, J. D., Longley, E., & East, J. (2000). Pica during pregnancy in low-income women born in Mexico. *The Western Journal of Medicine, 173*, 20–24.

Sinclair, R. (2002). There is no clear association between low serum ferritin and chronic diffuse telogen hair loss. *British Journal of Dermatology, 147*, 982–984.

Soff, G. A., & Levin, J. (1988). Thrombocytopenia associated with repletion of iron in iron-deficiency anemia. *The American Journal of Medical Sciences, 295*, 35–39.

Speck, B. (1968). Diurnal variation of serum iron and the latent iron-binding in normal adults. *Helvetica Medica Acta, 34*, 231–238.

Stefansson, H., Rye, D. B., Hicks, A., Petursson, H., Ingason, A., Thorgeirsson, T. E., et al. (2007). A genetic risk factor for periodic limb movements in sleep. *New England Journal of Medicine, 357*, 639–647.

Stevens, A. R., Jr. (1956). The mechanism and treatment of iron-deficiency anemia. *AMA Archives of Internal Medicine, 98*, 550–554.

Stojceski, T. K., Malpas, J. S., & Witts, L. J. (1965). Studies on the serum iron-binding capacity. *Journal of Clinical Pathology, 18*, 446–452.

Stolz, E., Valdueza, J. M., Grebe, M., Schlachetzki, F., Schmitt, E., Madlener, K., et al. (2007). Anemia as a risk factor for cerebral venous thrombosis? An old hypothesis revisited. Results of a prospective study. *Journal of Neurology, 254*, 729–734.

Sun, E. R., Chen, C. A., Ho, G., Earley, C. J., & Allen, R. P. (1998). Iron and the restless legs syndrome. *Sleep, 21*, 371–377.

Syrkis, I., & Machtey, I. (1973). Hypoferremia in acute myocardial infarction. *Journal of the American Geriatric Society, 21*, 28–30.

Thomas, H. M., III, Lefrak, S. S., Irwin, R. S., Fritts, H. W., Jr., & Caldwell, P. R. (1974). The oxyhemoglobin dissociation curve in health and disease. Role of 2,3–diphosphoglycerate. *The American Journal of Medicine, 57*, 331–348.

Trenkwalder, C., Paulus, W., & Walters, A. S. (2005). The restless legs syndrome. *Lancet Neurology, 4*, 465–475.

Trost, L. B., Bergfeld, W. F., & Calogeras, E. (2006). The diagnosis and treatment of iron deficiency and its potential relationship to hair loss. *Journal of the American Academy of Dermatology, 54*, 824–844.

Uchida, T., Matsuno, M., Ide, M., & Kawachi, Y. (1998). The frequency and development of tissue iron deficiency in 6 iron deficiency anemia patients with plummer-vinson syndrome. *Rinsho Ketsueki, 39*, 1099–1102.

Udayakumar, P., Balasubramanian, S., Ramalingam, K. S., Lakshmi, C., Srinivas, C. R., & Mathew, A. C. (2006). Cutaneous manifestations in patients with chronic renal failure on hemodialysis. *Indian Journal of Dermatology, Venereology, Leprology, 72*, 119–125.

Vinson, P. P. (1922). Hysterical dysphagia. *Minnesota Medicine, 5*, 107.

Voigt, D., Dieterich, W. R., Brushke, G., & Herrmann, H. (1967). On blood concentrations of leukocytes and thrombocytes in iron deficiency. *Blut, 14*, 267–272.

Wagner, A., Fortier, N., Giroux, A., Lukes, J., & Snyder, L. M. (1979). Catecholamines in adult iron deficiency patients. *Experientia, 35*, 681–682.

Wheby, M. S. (1980). Effect of iron therapy on serum ferritin levels in iron-deficiency anemia. *Blood, 56*, 138–140.

Wintrobe, M. M. (1933). Idiopathic hypochromic anemia. *Medicine, 12*, 187.

Wish, J. B. (2006). Assessing iron status: Beyond serum ferritin and transferrin saturation. *Clinical Journal of the American Society of Nephrology, 1*(Suppl. 1), S4–S8.

Witts, L. J. (1931). Simple achlorhydric anemiae. *Guy's Hospital Reports, 81*, 205.

Woywodt, A., & Kiss, A. (2002). Geophagia: The history of earth-eating. *Journal of the Royal Society of Medicine, 95*, 143–146.

Wray, D., Ferguson, M. M., Hutcheon, W. A., & Dagg, J. H. (1978). Nutritional deficiencies in recurrent aphthae. *Journal of Oral Pathology, 7*, 418–423.

Yip, R., Mohandas, N., Clark, M. R., Jain, S., Shohet, S. B., & Dallman, P. R. (1983). Red cell membrane stiffness in iron deficiency. *Blood, 62*, 99–106.

Youdim, M. B., Woods, H. F., Mitchell, B., Grahame-Smith, D. G., & Callender, S. (1975). Human platelet monoamine oxidase activity in iron-deficiency anaemia. *Clinical Science and Molecular Medicine, 48*, 289–295.

Zhu, Y. I., & Haas, J. D. (1998). Altered metabolic response of iron-depleted nonanemic women during a 15-km time trial. *Journal of Applied Physiology, 84*, 1768–1775.

Zilva, J. F., & Patston, V. J. (1966). Variations in serum-iron in healthy women. *Lancet, 1*, 459–462.

# 10 Iron-Metabolism in Neurons of the Motor System of the Central Nervous System: Lessons from Iron Deficiency and Overloading Pathologies

*Torben Moos*

**Summary**

- A massive expression of the transferrin receptor ensures uptake of iron by neurons in the brain.
- Oligodendrocytes do not contain transferrin receptors, which brings into question whether they are less capable of extracting iron under conditions where there is a shortage of iron as compared to that of neurons.
- The impaired synthesis of myelin by oligodendrocytes is the key responsible factor for impaired motor function in iron deficiency.
- In conditions with iron overload in the brain, ferritin expressed by microglia, and possibly also neurons, is responsible for scavenging excess iron which causes oxidative stress and damage to brain cells.
- New objectives for understanding iron homeostasis in the brain should be directed toward iron uptake and intracellular transport in oligodendrocytes to learn more about why these cells are so affected by iron deficiency. In conditions with iron overload, relevant studies should include looking at possible scavenging processes that prevent iron toxicity, e.g., do neurons raise their levels of ferritin and ferroportin to increase storage and export of iron, respectively?

**Key Words:** Divalent metal transporter I; ferritin; ferroportin; iron; motor neuron; myelin; oligodendrocyte; Schwann cell; transferrin; transferrin receptor

## 1. INTRODUCTION

The central nervous system (CNS) attempts to maintain its concentrations of transition metals and their ions within a certain range as both low and elevated levels can be harmful; iron is a perfect example. When the CNS is deprived of iron, neurons are affected in terms of an impaired ability to synthesize important neurotransmitters like dopamine and serotonin (Ashkenazi, Ben-Shachar, & Youdim, 1982; Beard, Wiesinger, & Jones, 2006; Burhans et al., 2005; Yehuda, Youdim, & Mostofsky, 1986). Likewise, myelin-formation by oligodendrocytes, and probably also by Schwann cells, which are responsible for myelin formation in the peripheral nervous

From: *Nutrition and Health: Iron Deficiency and Overload*
Edited by: S. Yehuda and D.I. Mostofsky, DOI 10.1007/978-1-59745-462-9_10

system (PNS), is affected by iron deficiency leading to improper fatty acid synthesis detrimental to myelination of axons (Beard, Wiesinger, & Connor, 2003; Ortiz et al., 2004; Yehuda, Rabinovitz, & Mostofsky, 2006).

When biological systems are overloaded with iron, the post-transcriptional regulation of ferritin mRNA leads to an elevated concentration of the ferritin protein that serves as a significant scavenger of non-protein-bound iron (Focht et al., 1997; Rouault & Cooperman, 2006; MacKenzie, Iwasaki, & Tsuji, 2008). The body may nonetheless be forced into a state where the availability of iron becomes so high that it gradually induces severe damage, e.g., cases of hemochromatosis where iron absorption in the gut is out of control lead to a universal iron accumulation in non-neuronal tissue (MacKenzie et al., 2008). The resulting damage is attributed to an increased risk of hydroxyl radical formation as ferrous iron participates in the Fenton reaction (Crichton, Wilmet, Legssyer, & Ward, 2002). As hemochromatosis is not likely to cause significant iron accumulation in the CNS, any evidence that an anticipated iron accumulation causes damage to cells in the brain, however, still remains somewhat hypothetical (Russo, Edwards, Andrews, O'Brien, & Bhatia, 2004; Moos, Rosengren Nielsen, Skjørringe, & Morgan, 2007).

This chapter reviews the current knowledge on iron and its related expressed proteins and genes in regions involved in principal motor pathways of the CNS, such as the components of the pyramidal tract (i.e., cerebral motor cortex, motor neurons of the cranial nerve nuclei, and the motor neurons of the spinal cord) and some of the components of the pre-motor loops responsible for proper activation of the pyramidal tract (i.e., the basal ganglia, the substantia nigra, the cerebellum, and a few other relevant nuclei of the brain stem (the red nucleus and pontine nucleus)) (Fig. 1). These regions will be addressed with regard to their neuronal iron metabolism under normal conditions, and how they may be affected by iron deficiency and iron loading.

## 2. NEURONAL IRON METABOLISM IN THE NORMAL BRAIN

*Cerebral cortex*: The abundant expression of the transferrin receptor combined with the ready demonstration of its ligand, transferrin, in neurons of the cerebral cortex of the adult brain (Fig. 2) clearly indicate that neurons internalize iron throughout life (Moos, 1996; Moos & Høyer, 1996). This is confirmed by the fact that injection of $^{59}$Fe into the peripheral circulation leads to its conjugation with transferrin in the liver revealing itself as [$^{59}$Fe]transferrin in the circulation. Neurons of the cerebral cortex subsequently exhibit a substantial $^{59}$Fe uptake (Gocht, Keith, Candy, & Morris, 1993; Dwork et al., 1990). The expression of divalent metal transporter I (DMT1) involved in pumping iron from the endosome into the cytosol also confirms the role of the transferrin receptor-internalization system for iron uptake in these neurons (Fig. 3).

Neurons of the cerebral cortex also contain ferroportin (Burdo et al., 2001) that putatively plays a role in exporting iron across the cell membrane into the brain interstitial fluid (Abboud & Haile, 2000). Combined with the low content of the iron-storage protein, ferritin, there is reason to believe that the cellular concentration of iron is tightly regulated in order to maintain a certain iron level in neurons of the cerebral cortex (Benkovic & Connor, 1993; Hansen, Nielsen, Bernth, & Moos, 1999).

*Basal ganglia*: With few exceptions, iron and many of its related proteins are distributed inside neurons of the brain regions mentioned below similar to those of the cerebral cortex.

In the basal ganglia, $^{59}$Fe is probably taken up by striatal neurons via receptor-mediated internalization of iron–transferrin (Moos, 1996; Moos & Morgan, 2004a), which then leads to its redistribution with a marked appearance in the pallidum, suggesting that iron undergoes anterograde axonal transport in the striato-pallidal pathway (Dwork et al., 1990). Indicative of

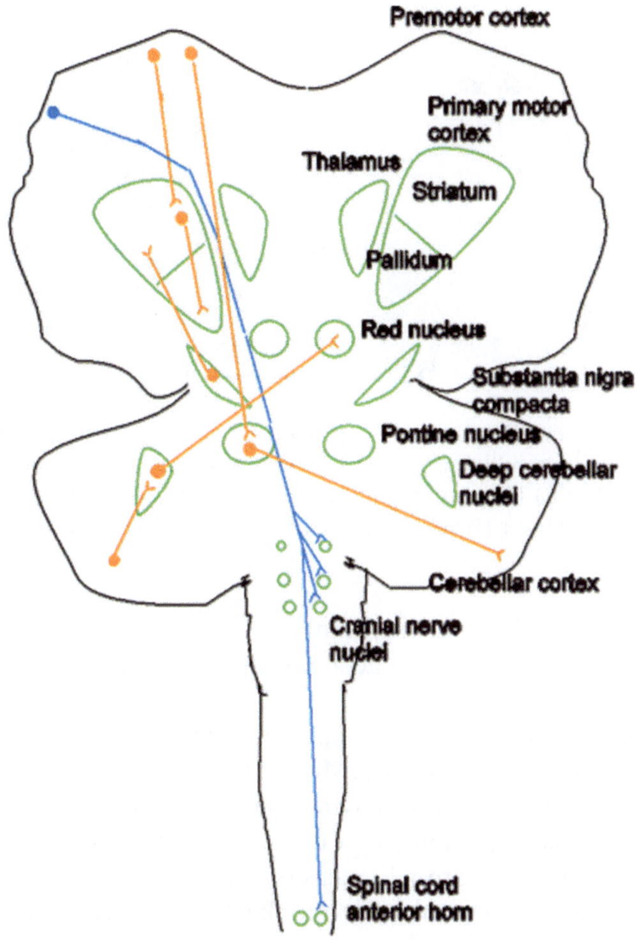


**Fig. 1.** Schematic showing brain regions involved in motor system processing. The pyramidal tract and neurons of the cerebral motor cortex, cranial motor neurons, spinal cord motor neurons are shown in blue, accessory motor regions in orange.

this hypothesis, [$^{59}$Fe]transferrin was shown to undergo axonal transport in neurons of the habenulo-interpeduncular tract (Moos & Morgan, 1998a). The content of ferritin is very high inside neurons of the pallidum, which indicates that iron is stored as ferritin–iron in these neurons. Interestingly, the level of ferroportin is not very high in neurons of the pallidum (Moos & Rosengren Nielsen, 2006), which clearly points toward the idea that the turnover of iron is much lower in these neurons as compared to those of the cerebral cortex.

*Substantia nigra*: In the substantia nigra, the neurons of the pars compacta are closely associated with a high susceptibility for oxidative stress that eventually may cause the neurons to lose their function and lead to Parkinson's disease (Russo et al., 2004; Moos et al., 2007). The fact that the concentration of iron in the substantia nigra pars compacta is significantly higher in Parkinson's disease cases as compared to that of age-matched controls may be a clue to whether iron accumulation plays a role in the pathogenesis of affected nigral neurons (Dexter et al., 1987; Sofic et al., 1988; Bartzokis et al., 1999). Exactly why iron accumulates in the Parkinsonian brain remains unexplained. Apparently, iron accumulation is not adjoined to an adequate induction of

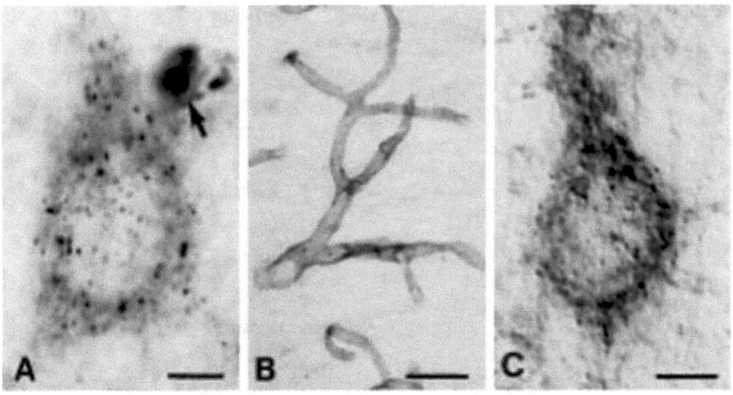


**Fig. 2.** Photomicrographs depicting Tf (**A**) and TR (**B, C**) immunoreactivity in the adult rat brain. (**A**) High-power magnification of Tf in a pyramidal neuron of the neocortex and an oligodendrocyte (*arrow*). (**B**) TR in brain capillary endothelial cells. (**C**) TR in a pyramidal neuron of the neocortex shown at high-power magnification. **A** is taken from Moos and Høyer (1996). *Scale bars*: 8 μm (**A, C**); 20 μm (**B**).

the ferritin gene (Loeffler et al., 1995; Mirza, Hadberg, Thomsen, & Moos, 2000). The expression of ferroportin by neurons of the pars compacta indicates that a delicate iron homeostasis inside these neurons is compulsory (Fig. 4).

*Cerebellum*: In cerebellum, neurons containing transferrin receptors are widespread both in the cortex and in the nuclei of its deep substance (Moos, 1996). Neurons of the cerebellar cortex are thought to take up iron-containing transferrin from both the interstitium and the cerebral ventricles, which in the latter is attributed to retrograde dendritic transport (Borges, Elliott, Gill, Iversen, & Iversen, 1985). Neuronal extensions in the molecular layer of the cerebellar cortex, probably parallel fibers of granule cells and the dendritic arbor of Purkinje cells, contain substantial amounts of ferroportin (Burdo et al., 2001).

*Cranial nerve nuclei*: In cranial nerve nuclei of the brain stem, neurons contain both transferrin receptors and their ligand transferrin. As these neurons also gain access to the periphery through their axons that project outside the CNS (Broadwell & Brightman, 1976), transferrin can also be taken up by the cells in the axonal terminal probably in a non-specific manner, and brought to the soma by retrograde axonal transport (Moos, 1995).

*Red nucleus*: The neurons of the red nucleus, particularly those in its magnocellular part, contain large amounts of iron, which is reflected by a strong expression of transferrin receptors and DMT1, suggesting continuous uptake of iron throughout life (Moos, 1996; Moos & Morgan, 2004a). By contrast, the same neurons do not contain noteworthy amounts of either ferritin or ferroportin (Hansen et al., 1999; Moos & Rosengren Nielsen, 2006).

*Pontine nucleus*: The pontine nucleus receives projections ipsilaterally from the cerebral premotor cortex. The neurons express transferrin receptors in abundance together with a coherent expression of DMT1, suggesting that they take up iron continuously (Moos, 1996; Moos & Morgan, 2004a).

*Spinal cord motor neurons*: The somata of motor neurons of the spinal cord express transferrin receptors as seen in cranial nerve nuclei (Moos, 1996). A prominent retrograde axonal transport activity of the material taken up from the extracellular phase of the synaptic cleft, however, also contributes to iron-containing transport to the motor neuron soma (Moos, 1995). This chronic

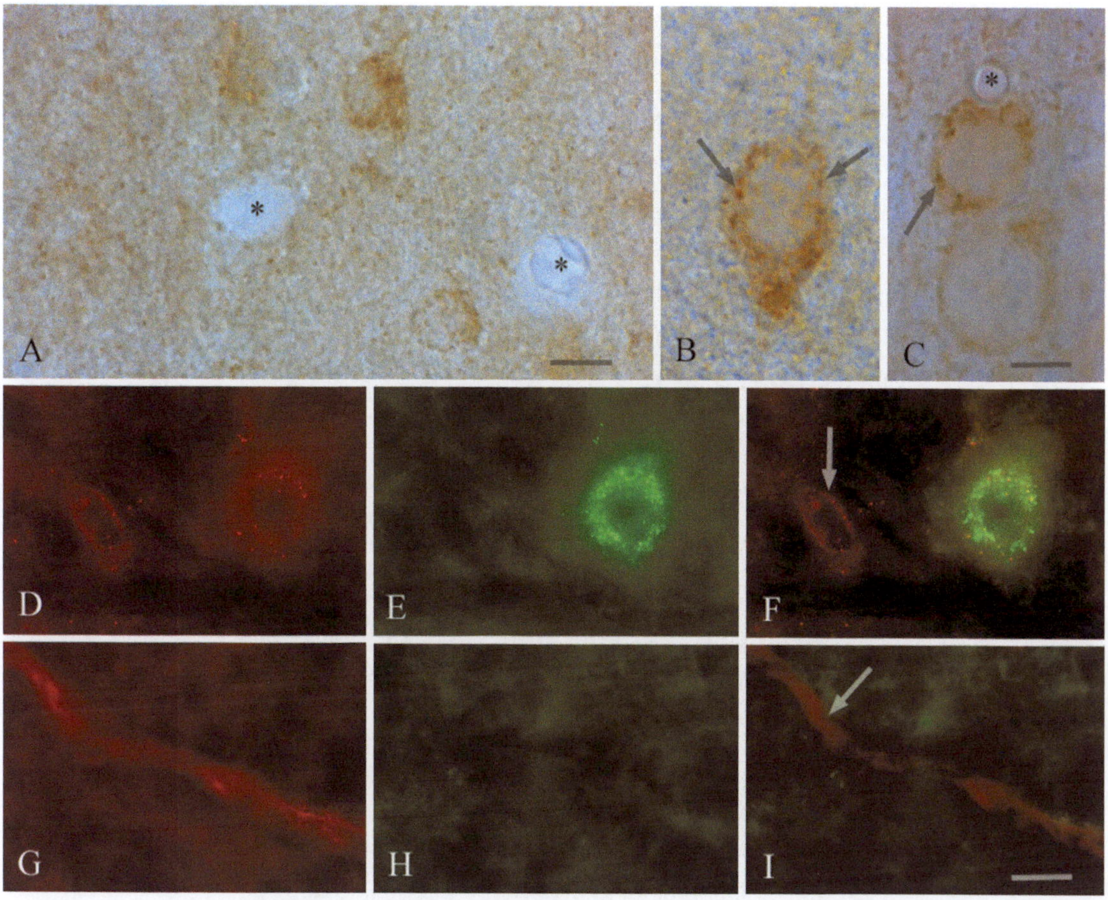


**Fig. 3.** **A–C**. DMT1 in neurons of the adult rat cerebral motor cortex. Sections from adult (**A–F**) and P0 (**G–I**) rat brain. (**A, B**) Neocortex stained for DMT1 using an antibody against exon 1A-containing sequence. (**A**) Labeling was seen in neurons, whereas brain capillary endothelial cells (*asterisks*) did not contain DMT1. (**B**) A labeled neuron shown at high-power magnification. The immunoreactivity was mainly confined to punctate, *small dots*, in the cytoplasm (*arrows*). The nucleus was unlabeled. (**C**) Neocortical neurons stained for DMT1 using an antibody that detects peptides in its fourth transmembrane loop. Labeling had a punctate appearance (*arrow*). The illustration also depicts an unlabeled brain capillary endothelial cell (*asterisk*). (**D–I**) sections of the mesencephalon of adult (**D, E, F**) and P0 (**G, H, I**) rat brain stained using antibodies raised against the transferrin receptor (**D, G**) and DMT1 (**E, H**) that were detected by fluorescent secondary antibodies and examined using epifluorescence microscopy. (**D, G**) The transferrin receptor antibody consistently labeled brain capillary endothelial cells irrespective of age, and neurons of the adult rat brain (**D**). (**E, H**) Using a DMT1 antibody detecting the sequence located near the C-terminus of the DMT1 molecule, which contains an IRE, DMT1 was not detectable in brain capillary endothelial cells but was present in neurons of the adult brain (**E**). Neuronal labeling had a punctate distribution. (**F, I**) Merged illustrations showing the absence of DMT1 from transferrin receptor–containing brain capillary endothelial cells (*arrows*), and the presence of both transferrin receptors and DMT1 in a neuron of adult rat brain. *Scale bars*: 5 μm (**B–C**); 10 μm (**A, D–I**). Permission Moos and Morgan (2004a).

and principally non-specific mechanism for deposition of material from the periphery could gradually lead to deterioration of the motor neurons. Proteins of the blood plasma, e.g., albumin and transferrin, may play an important role in this toxicity by allowing toxic metals to enter the motor neurons (Moos, 1995).

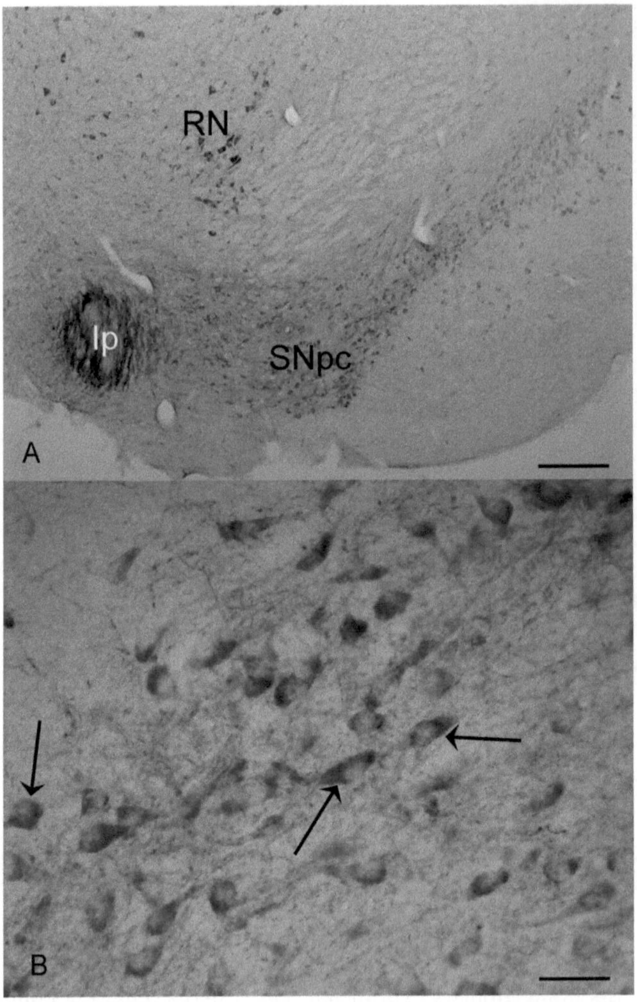


**Fig. 4.** **A**, Cross section of the mesencephalon of the adult rat brain demonstrating ferroportin immunoreactivity in substantia nigra pars compacta (SNpc). A prominent immunoreaction is also seen in the interpeduncular nucleus (Ip) and dispersely in magnocellular neurons of the red nucleus (RN). **B**, SNpc in large magnification showing ferroportin-immunoreactive dopaminergic neurons (*arrows*). *Scale bars*: 120 μm (**A**); 20 μm (**B**).

## 3. IRON HOMEOSTASIS IN MYELIN-FORMING CELLS

The expression of iron-containing proteins in oligodendrocytes of the developing brain has been thoroughly studied in the postnatal rodent brain (Connor & Fine, 1987). The uptake of iron by the developing brain is relatively high and essential for its normal growth (Taylor & Morgan, 1990). Yet, when they appear in the first postnatal week, oligodendrocytes do not express transferrin receptors or DMT1 (Moos & Morgan, 2004a). This suggests that they take up iron either from non-specific iron–transferrin that enters the developing brain, which is rich in plasma proteins derived from blood at this age (Moos & Morgan, 2002), or because they acquire iron through an uptake of non-transferrin-bound iron (Moos & Morgan, 1998b). Interestingly, oligodendrocytes initiate the expression of transferrin mRNA from the third postnatal week onward (Connor & Fine, 1987; Moos, Oates, & Morgan, 2001). The significance of the oligodendrocyte-derived transferrin is undisputed and could be related to intracellular transport of iron from the soma to the peripheral parts along the extreme extensions which envelop several axons. Oligodendrocytes increase their content of ferritin-protein with increasing age, which could reflect a deficiency in their ability to transfer iron back from the peripheral extensions to the soma (Moos et al., 2007). Oligodendrocytes also contain ferroportin (Burdo et al., 2001; Moos et al., 2007).

The iron metabolism in Schwann cells has not received much attention. Schwann cells are not protected by the blood–brain barrier and have ready access to circulating transferrin. The Schwann cells express transferrin receptors and transferrin in response to mechanical injury (Graeber, Raivich, & Kreutzberg, 1989; Salis, Setton, Soto, & Pasquini, 2007). Transferrin is particularly abundant in Schwann cells of myelinated axons, suggesting that iron and transferrin play a role in myelination of peripheral nerves (Lin, Snyder, & Connor, 1990).

## 4. CEREBRAL IRON HOMEOSTASIS IN IRON DEFICIENCY

Conditions that result in a shortage of iron in the human brain have been under scrutiny for a long time. A shortage of iron could affect the function of neurons, either directly through an impairment of neuronal dividing and differentiation during prenatal development (Yehuda et al., 1986, 2006) or indirectly through impaired myelin formation by the oligodendrocytes (Beard et al., 2003). The brain is by far most vulnerable to iron deficiency during its developmental stages, when the uptake of iron is relatively higher than later in life (Taylor & Morgan, 1990), but the impact of developmental iron deficiency on the brain can be restored by early intervention (Beard et al., 2007). Impaired myelinogenesis will affect all myelinated tracts and lead to direct detectable changes in motor behavior of experimental animals. Impaired neurotransmitter synthesis has a direct impact on neuronal functioning (Ashkenazi et al., 1982; Beard et al., 2006). Some evidence seems to indicate that neurons are impaired in both number and structure, but this statement has yet to be subjected to, e.g., an unbiased stereological counting of neurons and their processes; it would be relevant to determine whether such effects on neurons would be irreversible.

Still there is enough evidence to state that neurons respond to iron deficiency by changing their expression of transferrin receptors (Moos, Oates, & Morgan, 1998). An inadequately low availability of iron leads to higher cytosolic concentrations of iron-regulatory proteins (IRPs) (Kühn, 1998). The interaction between IRPs and the iron-responsive element (IRE) of the transferrin receptor mRNA will inhibit degradation of the transferrin receptor mRNA, thereby increasing the concentration of the mRNA and the rate of transferrin receptor protein synthesis. Variations in oxygen tension lead to an impaired interaction between IRP and IRE, which may suggest that in cases of sustained iron deficiency, where a reduced number of red cells are unable to deliver proper amounts of oxygen to the brain, the neurons' ability to extract available iron could be compromised (Meyron-Holtz, Ghosh, & Rouault, 2004).

The level of transferrin receptor protein is prominent in neurons of the developing rodent brain at approximately 3 weeks after birth, and the amount of neuronal transferrin receptor is even higher when rats have been subjected to developmental iron deficiency (Fig. 5). All neurons of the brain will be affected, but those with a high content of transferrin receptor are most easily identified, e.g., neurons of the cerebral motor cortex, red nucleus, and pontine nucleus upregulate their transferrin receptors dramatically (Moos et al., 1998). Iron deficiency, invoked by short-term changes (few weeks) in dietary iron, will induce neurons of the fully mature brain to increase their content of transferrin receptor protein. However, this change is less dramatic because the turnover of iron in the adult brain is much lower (Dallman & Spirito, 1977). The content of DMT1 in neurons does not increase with iron deficiency, which is surprising, given that DMT1

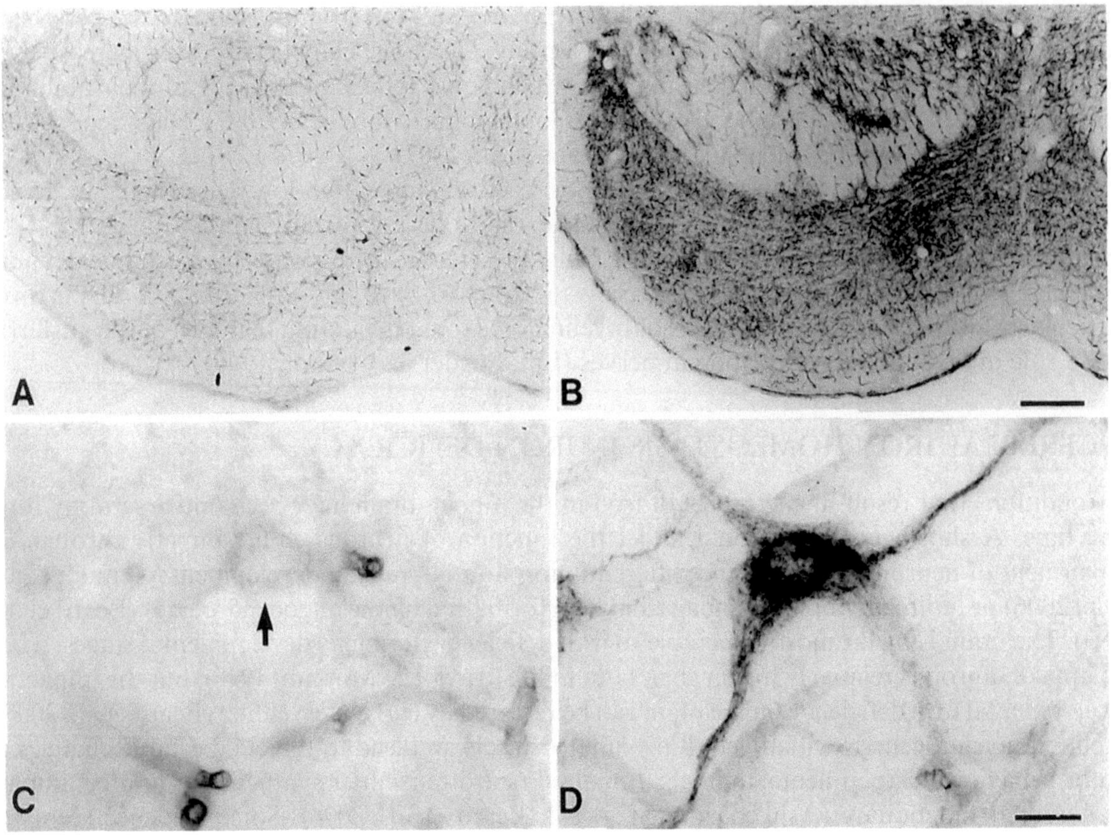


**Fig. 5.** Transferrin receptors in normal (**A, C**) and iron-deficient (**B, D**) rat brain. **A, B**, Sections taken from the brain stem. **C, D**, Neurons of the reticular formation. Neuron in **C** is marked with an *arrow*. Note the profound upregulation of the neuronal transferrin receptor in iron deficiency. *Scale bars*: 150 μm (**A, B**), 10 μm (**C, D**). Permission Moos et al. (1998).

mRNA also contains an IRE, but it is possible that the IRE only binds after a more prolonged lack of cellular iron (Burdo et al., 2001; Moos & Morgan, 2004; Ke et al., 2005). The content of ferritin is significantly lowered in neurons following iron deficiency (Hansen et al., 1999).

In contrast to the effect on neurons in iron-deficient conditions, there is solid evidence of effects on myelin formation (Beard et al., 2003; Ortiz et al., 2004; Yehuda et al., 2006). The oligodendrocytes lose their capacity to form essential fatty acids for incorporation into their membrane. Experimental studies have demonstrated that this event is irreversible which clearly underlines the significance of a proper iron supply during development. In contrast to neurons, oligodendrocytes apparently lack the ability to rescue the situation by increasing the expression of transferrin receptors (Moos et al., 1998); nor do they increase transferrin mRNA during iron deficiency (Moos et al., 2001).

## 5. MANAGEMENT OF IRON IN THE BRAIN IN CONDITIONS WITH RAISED CEREBRAL IRON

In conditions with elevated iron concentration in the bloodstream, the brain downregulates the extraction of iron by ceasing to express transferrin receptors in brain capillary endothelial cells (Taylor, Crowe, & Morgan, 1991). This mechanism begins instantly when iron availability exceeds a certain limit and explains why subjecting very large amounts of dietary iron to experimental animals does not lead to increases in cerebral iron (Lykkesfeldt, Morgan, Christen, Skovgaard, & Moos, 2007). Nonetheless, iron content clearly increases with age, which is more likely due to a reduced ability to reuse the iron, especially by the oligodendrocytes (Moos et al., 2007).

Iron is believed to play a significant role in exacerbating the degradation processes that occur in brain tissue subjected to acute damage or neurodegenerative disorders. The brain capillary endothelial cell expression of transferrin receptors upregulates in cerebral ischemia (Omori et al., 2003), which probably relies on an induction of the transferrin receptor mRNA expression by hypoxia-inducing factor (HIF) (Lok & Ponka, 2000). The damaging role of iron during ischemia probably depends on the inhibition of detoxifying enzymes responsible for catalyzing the oxidation of ferrous iron which in turn provokes formation of free radicals in the Fenton reaction (Moos & Morgan, 2004b). Provided ischemic vessels are perfused, this induction will invariably lead to increased iron transport into the brain. In brain hemorrhage, HIF is also upregulated although not to the same extent as in ischemia (Jiang et al., 2002), but it remains to be examined whether this also leads to an increased brain capillary endothelial cell transferrin receptor expression in affected regions. The main contribution of iron in hemorrhage, however, comes from lysing erythrocytes that release hemoglobin, which is taken up by microglia (cf. Wagner, Sharp, Ardizzone, Lu, & Clark, 2003). Microglia sequester heme of the hemoglobin through their expression of heme oxygenase-1 (HO-1) and ultimately store the iron in ferritin (Chi, Wang, Chen, Chau, & Lin, 2000). Ferroportin has not been studied in brains of hemorrhagic cases.

In chronic settings, there is evidence of iron accumulation in affected regions of neurodegenerative disorders like Alzheimer's disease, Parkinson's disease, and Huntington's disease (Ke & Qian, 2003; Moos & Morgan, 2004b; Dröge & Schipper, 2007), but there is no evidence that iron may directly initiate these disorders. Possibly, the deleterious effect of iron comes from the fact that the affected brain regions are chronically infested by inflammatory cells of the myelo-monocytic cell lineage, i.e., monocytes, brain macrophage, and microglia that all express ferritin probably because they carry the iron needed for free radical production as part of their oxygen burst activity. A chronic infiltration and death of these cells among affected neurons like the dopaminergic neurons in Parkinson's disease may invariably cause the level of iron to increase locally and hence increase the risks of damage to neurons. A mechanism to scavenge this resulting iron excess is to increase the number of ferritin-expressing microglia even further, but this will only increase the inflammatory process. The infiltration by microglia hence creates a vicious cycle that increases the iron deposition. For this reason, neurodegenerative disorders can be regarded as conditions with impaired iron homeostasis. Recent significant studies have identified genetic mutations associated with neurodegeneration and iron-overloading pathology (Curtis et al., 2001; Kotzbauer, Truax, Trojanowski, & Lee, 2005; Manusco et al., 2005; Morgan et al., 2006; Zhou et al., 2001). The pathogenetic potential of some of these mutations was later revealed in mutational studies in mice (Malik et al., 2008; Vidal et al., 2008), which emphasizes that single mutations may lead to phenotypes of putatively clinical relevant aspects of oxidative stress and damage due to neuronal iron excess.

The effect on oligodendrocytes has never been addressed in conditions with iron toxicity in the brain. They are known to increase their expression of transferrin mRNA after a trauma (Cook, Marcheselli, Alam, Deininger, & Bazan, 1998).

## 6. CONCLUSIONS AND OUTLOOK

Normal brain function is undisputedly dependent on an adequate uptake and transport of iron into the brain. This is especially important during the development of the brain. A lack of iron can be detrimental to the brain as it will affect myelin formation by the oligodendrocytes. This is easily recorded in iron-deficient rodents whose myelinated tracts of the motor pathways are promptly affected. It is of great importance to expand the knowledge on how oligodendrocytes metabolize iron, bearing in mind that fail to express detectable amounts of transferrin receptors during iron deficiency. Conversely, oligodendrocytes are the only cells in the CNS that contain transferrin which could serve as an intracellular supplier of iron to the extreme extensions that envelop several axons. Neurons respond to iron deficiency by increasing their expression of transferrin receptors. They reduce their production of neurotransmitters, e.g., dopamine of the nigro-striatal system, but there is no clear evidence of morphological defects in neurons of iron-deficient experimental animals.

In conditions with elevated concentrations of iron in CNS as it occurs in hemorrhages, microglia are important scavengers of excess iron that protect neurons from over-exposure. The expression of transferrin receptors in acute iron overloading has never been studied, but very likely it ceases. Conversely, neuronal ferritin levels are likely to rise. In conditions with chronic iron overload, the contribution of iron could rely on a vicious cycle that increases the iron deposition from iron-containing inflammatory cells that enter the brain to phagocytose debris of dying cells, but in turn die out and deposit their own iron. The mechanisms by which iron can cause harm in the chronic neurodegenerative brain still needs much attention.

**Acknowledgments** S Peters is thanked for revising the manuscript. Data obtained by the authors were mainly sponsored by grants from the The Lundbeck Foundation, The Danish Parkinson's Disease Organisation, and The Danish Medical Research Council.

## ABBREVIATIONS

| | |
|---|---|
| CNS | Central nervous system |
| DMT1 | Divalent metal transporter I |
| PNS | Peripheral nervous system (PNS) |

## REFERENCES

Abboud, S., & Haile, D. J. (2000). A novel mammalian iron-regulated protein involved in intracellular iron metabolism. *Journal of Biological Chemistry, 275*, 19906–19912.

Ashkenazi, R., Ben-Shachar, D., & Youdim, M. B. (1982) Nutritional iron and dopamine binding sites in the rat brain. *Pharmacology, Biochemistry, and Behavior, 17*(Suppl. 1), 43–47.

Bartzokis, G., Cummings, J. L., Markham, C. H., Marmarelis, P. Z., Treciokas, L. J., Tishler, T. A., et al. (1999). MRI evaluation of brain iron in earlier- and later-onset Parkinson's disease and normal subjects. *Magnetic Resonance Imaging, 17*, 213–222.

Beard, J. L., Wiesinger, J. A., & Connor, J. R. (2003). Pre- and postweaning iron deficiency alters myelination in Sprague-Dawley rats. *Developmental Neuroscience, 25*, 308–315.

Beard, J. L., Wiesinger, J. A., & Jones, B. C. (2006). Cellular iron concentrations directly affect the expression levels of norepinephrine transporter in PC12 cells and rat brain tissue. *Brain Research, 1092*, 47–58.

Beard, J. L., Unger, E. L., Bianco, L. E., Paul, T., Rundle, S. E., & Jones, B. C. (2007). Early postnatal iron repletion overcomes lasting effects of gestational iron deficiency in rats. *Journal of Nutrition, 137*, 1176–1182.

Benkovic, S. A., & Connor, J. R. (1993). Ferritin, transferrin, and iron in selected regions of the adult and aged rat brain. *Journal of Comperative Neurology, 338*, 97–113.

Borges, L. F., Elliott, P. J., Gill, R., Iversen, S. D., & Iversen, L. L.(1985). Selective extraction of small and large molecules from the cerebrospinal fluid by Purkinje neurons. *Science, 228*, 346–348.

Broadwell, R. D., & Brightman, M. W. (1976). Entry of peroxidase into neurons of the central and peripheral nervous systems from extracerebral and cerebral blood. *Journal of Comperative Neurology, 166*, 257–283.

Burdo, J. R., Menzies, S. L., Simpson, I. A., Garrick, L. M., Garrick, M. D., Dolan, K. G., et al. (2001). Distribution of divalent metal transporter 1 and metal transport protein 1 in the normal and Belgrade rat. *Journal of Neuroscience Research, 66*, 1198–1207.

Burhans, M. S., Dailey, C., Beard, Z., Wiesinger, J., Murray-Kolb, L., Jones, B. C., et al. (2005). Iron deficiency: Differential effects on monoamine transporters. *Nutritional Neuroscience, 8*, 31–38.

Chi, S. I., Wang, C. K., Chen, J. J., Chau, L. Y., & Lin, T. N. (2000). Differential regulation of H- and L-ferritin messenger RNA subunits, ferritin protein and iron following focal cerebral ischemia-reperfusion. *Neuroscience, 100*, 475–484.

Connor, J. R., & Fine, R. E. (1987). Development of transferrin-positive oligodendrocytes in the rat central nervous system. *Journal of Neuroscience Research, 17*, 51–59.

Cook, J. L., Marcheselli, V., Alam, J., Deininger, P. L., & Bazan, N. G. (1998). Temporal changes in gene expression following cryogenic rat brain injury. *Molecular Brain Research, 55*, 9–19.

Crichton, R. R., Wilmet, S., Legssyer, R., & Ward, R. J. (2002). Molecular and cellular mechanisms of iron homeostasis and toxicity in mammalian cells. *Journal of Inorganic Biochemistry, 91*, 9–18.

Curtis, A. R., Fey, C., Morris, C. M., Bindoff, L. A., Ince, P. G., Chinnery, P. F., et al. (2001). Mutation in the gene encoding ferritin light polypeptide causes dominant adult-onset basal ganglia disease. *Nature Genetics, 28*, 350–354.

Dallman, P. R., & Spirito, R. A. (1977). Brain iron in the rat: extremely slow turnover in normal rats may explain long-lasting effects of early iron deficiency. *Journal of Nutrition, 107*, 1075–1081.

Dexter, D. T., Wells, F. R., Agid, F., Agid, Y., Lees, A. J., Jenner, P., et al. (1987). Increased nigral iron content in postmortem parkinsonian brain. *Lancet, 2*, 1219–1220.

Dröge, W., & Schipper, H. M. (2007). Oxidative stress and aberrant signaling in aging and cognitive decline. *Aging Cell, 6*, 361–370.

Dwork, A. J., Lawler, G., Zybert, P. A., Durkin, M., Osman, M., Willson, N., et al. (1990). An autoradiographic study of the uptake and distribution of iron by the brain of the young rat. *Brain Research, 518*, 31–39.

Focht, S. J., Snyder, B. S., Beard, J. L., Van Gelder, W., Williams, L. R., & Connor, J. R. (1997). Regional distribution of iron, transferrin, ferritin, and oxidatively modified proteins in young and aged Fischer 344 rat brains. *Neuroscience, 79*, 255–261.

Gocht, A., Keith, A. B., Candy, J. M., & Morris, C. M. (1993). Iron uptake in the brain of myelin-deficient rat. *Neuroscience Letters, 154*, 187–190.

Graeber, M. B., Raivich, G., & Kreutzberg, G. W. (1989). Increase of transferrin receptors and iron uptake in regenerating motor neurons. *Journal of Neuroscience Research, 23*, 342–345.

Hansen, T. M., Nielsen, H., Bernth, N., & Moos, T. (1999). Expression of ferritin protein and subunit mRNAs in normal and iron deficient rat brain. *Molecular Brain Research, 65*, 186–197.

Jiang, Y., Wu, J., Keep, R. F., Hua, Y., Hoff, J. T., & Xi, G. (2002). Hypoxia-inducible factor-1alpha accumulation in the brain after experimental intracerebral hemorrhage. *Journal of cerebral blood flow and metabolism, 22*, 689–696.

Ke, Y., & Qian, Z. M. (2003). Iron misregulation in the brain: A primary cause of neurodegenerative disorders. *Lancet Neurology, 2*, 246–253.

Ke, Y., Chang, Y. Z., Duan, X. L., Du, J. R., Zhu, L., Wang, K., et al. (2005). Age-dependent and iron-independent expression of two mRNA isoforms of divalent metal transporter 1 in rat brain. *Neurobiology of Aging, 26*, 739–748.

Kotzbauer, P. T., Truax, A. C., Trojanowski, J. Q., & Lee, V. M. (2005). Altered neuronal mitochondrial coenzyme A synthesis in neurodegeneration with brain iron accumulation caused by abnormal processing, stability, and catalytic activity of mutant pantothenate kinase 2. *Journal of Neuroscience, 25*, 689–698.

Kühn, L. C. (1998). Iron and gene expression: Molecular mechanisms regulating cellular iron homeostasis. *Nutrition Review, 56*, s11–s19.

Lin, H. H., Snyder, B. S., & Connor, J. R. (1990). Transferrin expression in myelinated and non-myelinated peripheral nerves. *Brain Research, 526*, 217–220.

Loeffler, D. A., Connor, J. R., Juneau, P. L., Snyder, B. S., Kanaley, L., DeMaggio, A. J., et al. (1995). Transferrin and iron in normal, Alzheimer's disease, and Parkinson's disease brain regions. *Journal of Neurochemistry, 65*, 710–724.

Lok, C. N., & Ponka, P. (2000). Identification of a hypoxia response element in the transferrin receptor gene. *Journal of Biological Chemistry, 274*, 24147–24152.

Lykkesfeldt, J., Morgan, E., Christen, S., Skovgaard, L. T., & Moos, T. (2007). Oxidative stress and damage in liver, but not in brain, of Fischer 344 rats subjected to dietary iron supplementation with lipid-soluble [(3,5,5-trimethylhexanoyl)ferrocene]. *Journal of biochemical and molecular toxicology, 21*, 145–155.

MacKenzie, E. L., Iwasaki, K., & Tsuji, Y. (2008). Intracellular iron transport and storage: From molecular mechanisms to health implications. *Antioxidants & Redox Signaling, 10*, 997–1030.

Malik, I., Turk, J., Mancuso, D. J., Montier, L., Wohltmann, M., Wozniak, D. F., et al. (2008). Disrupted membrane homeostasis and accumulation of ubiquitinated proteins in a mouse model of infantile neuroaxonal dystrophy caused by PLA2G6 mutations. *American Journal of Pathology, 172*, 406–416.

Mancuso, M., Davidzon, G., Kurlan, R. M., Tawil, R., Bonilla, E., Di Mauro, S., & et al. (2005). Hereditary ferritinopathy: A novel mutation, its cellular pathology, and pathogenic insights. *Journal of Neuropathology and Experimental Neurology, 64*, 280–294.

Meyron-Holtz, E. G., Ghosh, M. C., & Rouault, T. A. (2004). Mammalian tissue oxygen levels modulate iron-regulatory protein activities in vivo. *Science, 306*, 2087–2090.

Mirza, B., Hadberg, H., Thomsen, P., & Moos, T. (2000). The absence of reactive astrocytosis is indicative of a unique inflammatory process in Parkinson's disease. *Neuroscience, 95*, 425–432.

Moos, T. (1995). Age-dependent uptake and retrograde axonal transport of exogenous albumin and transferrin in rat motor neurons. *Brain Research, 672*, 14–23.

Moos, T. (1996). Immunohistochemical localization of intraneuronal transferrin receptor immunoreactivity in the adult mouse central nervous system. *Journal of Comperative Neurology, 375*, 675–692.

Moos, T., & Høyer, P. E. (1996). Detection of plasma proteins in CNS neurons: Conspicuous influence of tissue-processing parameters and the utilization of serum for blocking nonspecific reactions. *Journal of Histochemistry and Cytochemistry, 44*, 591–603.

Moos, T., & Morgan, E. H. (1998a). Kinetics and distribution of [$^{59}$Fe-$^{125}$I]transferrin injected into the ventricular system of the rat. *Brain Research, 790*, 115–128.

Moos, T., & Morgan, E. H. (1998b). Evidence for low molecular weight, non-transferrin-bound iron in rat brain and cerebrospinal fluid. *Journal of Neuroscience Research, 54*, 486–494.

Moos, T., & Morgan, E. H. (2002). A morphological study of the developmentally regulated transport of iron into the brain. *Developmental Neuroscience, 24*, 99–105.

Moos, T., & Morgan, E. H. (2004a). The significance of the mutated divalent metal transporter (DMT1) on iron transport into the Belgrade rat brain. *Journal of Neurochemistry, 88*, 233–245.

Moos, T., & Morgan, E. H. (2004a). The metabolism of neuronal iron and its pathogenic role in neurological disease: Review. *Annals of the New York Academy of Sciences, 1012*, 14–26.

Moos, T., & Rosengren Nielsen, T. (2006). Ferroportin in the postnatal rat brain: Implications for axonal transport and neuronal export of iron. *Seminars in Pediatric Neurology, 13*, 49–57.

Moos, T., Oates, P. S., & Morgan, E. H. (1998). Expression of the neuronal transferrin receptor is age dependent and susceptible to iron deficiency. *Journal of Comperative Neurology, 398*, 420–430.

Moos, T., Oates, P. S., & Morgan, E. H. (2001). Expression of transferrin mRNA in rat oligodendrocytes is iron-independent and changes with increasing age. *Nutritional Neuroscience, 4*, 15–23.

Moos, T., Rosengren Nielsen, T., Skjørringe, T., & Morgan, E. H. (2007). Iron trafficking inside the brain. *Journal of Neurochemistry, 103*, 1730–1740.

Morgan, N. V., Westaway, S. K., Morton, J. E., Gregory, A., Gissen, P., Sonek, S., et al. (2006). PLA2G6, encoding a phospholipase A2, is mutated in neurodegenerative disorders with high brain iron. *Nature Genetics, 38*, 752–754.

Omori, N., Maruyama, K., Jin, G., Li, F., Wang, S. J., Hamakawa, Y., et al. (2003). Targeting of post-ischemic cerebral endothelium in rat by liposomes bearing polyethylene glycol-coupled transferrin. *Neurological Research, 25*, 275–279.

Ortiz, E., Pasquini, J. M., Thompson, K., Felt, B., Butkus, G., Beard, J., et al. (2004). Effect of manipulation of iron storage, transport, or availability on myelin composition and brain iron content in three different animal models. *Journal of Neuroscience Research, 77*, 681–689.

Russo, N., Edwards, M., Andrews, T., O'Brien, M., & Bhatia, K. P. (2004). Hereditary haemochromatosis is unlikely to cause movement disorders – A critical review. *Journal of Neurology, 251*, 849–852.

Rouault, T. A., & Cooperman, S. (2006). Brain iron metabolism. *Seminars in Pediatric Neurology, 13*, 142–148.

Salis, C., Setton, C. P., Soto, E. F., & Pasquini, J. M. (2007). The mRNA of transferrin is expressed in Schwann cells during their maturation and after nerve injury. *Experimental Neurology, 207*, 85–94.

Sofic, E., Riederer, P., Heinsen, H., Beckmann, H., Reynolds, G. P., Hebenstreit, G., et al. (1988). Increased iron (III) and total iron content in post mortem substantia nigra of parkinsonian brain. *Journal of Neural Transmission, 74*, 199–205.

Taylor, E. M., & Morgan, E. H. (1990). Developmental changes in transferrin and iron uptake by the brain in the rat. *Developmental Brain Research, 55*, 35–42.

Taylor, E. M., Crowe, A., & Morgan, E. H. (1991). Transferrin and iron uptake by the brain: effects of altered iron status. *Journal of Neurochemistry, 57*, 1584–1592.

Vidal, R., Miravalle, L., Gao, X., Barbeito, A. G., Baraibar, M. A., Hekmatyar, S. K., et al. (2008). Expression of a mutant form of the ferritin light chain gene induces neurodegeneration and iron overload in transgenic mice. *Journal of Neuroscience, 28*, 60–67.

Wagner, K. R., Sharp, F. R., Ardizzone, T. D., Lu, A., & Clark, J. F. (2003). Heme and iron metabolism: Role in cerebral hemorrhage. *Journal of Cerebral Blood Flow and Metabolism, 23*, 629–652.

Yehuda, S., Youdim, M. E., & Mostofsky, D. I. (1986). Brain iron-deficiency causes reduced learning capacity in rats. *Pharmacology, Biochemistry, and Behaviour, 25*, 141–144.

Yehuda, S., Rabinovitz, S., & Mostofsky, D. I. (2006). Nutritional deficiencies in learning and cognition. *Journal of pediatric gastroenterology and nutrition (Supplement), 43*(3), S22–S25.

Zhou, B., Westaway, S. K., Levinson, B., Johnson, M. A., Gitschier, J., & Hayflick, S. J. (2001). A novel pantothenate kinase gene (PANK2) is defective in Hallervorden-Spatz syndrome. *Nature Genetics, 28*, 345–349.

[illegible]

# 11 The Effects of Brain Iron Deficiency on Cognitive and Behavioral Aspects

*S. Yehuda, S. Rabinovitz, R.L. Carasso, and D.I. Mostofsky*

**Summary**

- Brain iron deficiency induced structural and functional changes in the brain.
- Brain iron deficiency reduced cognitive and learning capacities in animal and human.
- Iron deficiency is the most prevalent in the world.
- Early iron deficiency might induce longlasting behavioral consequences despite rehabilitation of the hematological values.

**Key Words:** Brain iron deficiency; dopamine; Shoham behavior

## 1. INTRODUCTION

Iron deficiency and anemia are the most common nutritional disorders in both Third World and industrial countries today. The numerous behavioral manifestations of iron deficiency in an adult or in a child may include lethargy, irritability, apathy, restlessness, fatigue, lack of concentration, pagophagia (pathological craving for ice), and pica (perverted craving for substance unfit for food), inattention, hypoactivity (or hyperactivity), and above all a decrease in mental performance. The syndromes that are associated with iron deficiency have been known for a very long time but were neglected. To be sure, iron was used as a "therapeutic agent" since the times of the ancient Egypt, yet only about 20 years ago has the scientific world become aware of this problem. The discovery of thousands of anemic children in the Third World inspired a large number of studies. Although the cases of iron deficiency are greater among the undernutritioned and malnutritioned children in the Third World, many cases can also be found in all ages even among people in rich countries (Scrimshaw, 1991, 1998). With a high-risk group for iron deficiency having been identified among the population of normal elderly people in old-age homes (Buzina, et al., 1998), the three high-risk groups for iron deficiency are children, pregnant women, and the elderly. The groups of the infants and the elderly are included in the high-risk groups, since in those two periods of life the brain structures and functions undergo rapid

From: *Nutrition and Health: Iron Deficiency and Overload*
Edited by: S. Yehuda and D.I. Mostofsky, DOI 10.1007/978-1-59745-462-9_11

changes. The number of scientific articles on iron deficiency is steadily growing, and there are now over 16,000 scientific papers cited in PubMed. The optimal solution to the problem still is not at hand.

The aim of this chapter is to highlight several aspects of the iron deficiency state mainly but not exclusively in the brain. Our working hypothesis is that iron mediates important functions in the brain, in addition to its role in oxygen delivery to the tissue. This chapter will also note recent advances in the field that might contribute to a better understanding of the phenomena and possible new avenues to treat iron deficiency.

## 2. IRON IN THE BRAIN

Age, gender, and specific body tissues determine the amount of iron in the body. The highest iron concentrations were found in the liver, with lesser iron concentrations in the lung and spleen. It appears that the skin has the lowest concentration of iron. There is no agreement about the concentration of iron in the cerebrospinal fluid (Beard, Connor, & Jones, 1993a, 1993b).

Brain tissue is very rich in iron, with significant differences between the levels of iron in the various brain areas. One of the richest areas in the brain is the basal ganglion. Two important questions need to be addressed: (1) why is the iron level in the whole brain so high and (2) why is the iron level in specific brain areas not the same. In an attempt to explain the first question, it has been postulated that the brain needs high iron levels for unique brain oxidative processes (Beard, Dawson, & Pnero, 1996). On the other hand, free iron is the substrate for free radicals' generation; therefore, non-heme iron in the brain tend to be bound to certain proteins, such as transferrin and ferritin (Connor & Menzies, 1996).

The uneven iron distribution in human and rat brain has been confirmed by using various research techniques, such as histochemical technique and MRL. Such studies show that the basal ganglia, substantia nigra, ventral pallidum caudate nucleus, globus pallidus, and putamen are among the "highest iron concentration" areas. Among the "moderate high" areas are the nucleus accumbens and the cortex (Hill, 1988). The iron "distribution map" is very similar and overlapping with other important "distribution maps," mainly of brain dopamine, and to a lesser extent to the distribution of GABA and neuropeptides (Yehuda & Youdim, 1988). The "co-localization" of iron, dopamine, and GABA is very important, because of mental, cognitive, emotional, and behavioral functions (Yehuda & Youdim, 1988; Youdim, Ben Shachar, & Yehuda, 1989; Beard et al., 1993a, 1993b). The above findings were obtained from the brain of adult rats. Examination of the iron level in the early developed brain showed that those areas are rich in iron even at such an early development period (Benkovic & Connor, 1993).

The "iron deficiency diet" (IDD) is a very powerful method to induce nutritional iron deficiency resulting in significant decreases of iron and hemoglobin levels in the periphery and brain iron levels. Dallman, Siimes, and Manies (1975) and Dallman and Spirito (1977) showed that IDD induced 27% decrease in non-heme brain iron. Youdim and Green (1977) confirmed these results and Ben Shachar, Ashkenazi, and Youdim (1986) reported that it depended on the age at which rats were made IDD (Youdim, 1990). They furthermore showed that the younger the animals the easier they became iron deficient, newborn versus adult rats. However, although brain iron in adult rats could be resorted within a few weeks when they were fed iron plus diet, the brain level of newborns could not be restored by iron repletion (Youdim & Green, 1977). They demonstrated an irreversible damage to brain functions.

## 3. THE ROLE OF IRON IN MYELINATION

The family of the cytochrome P-450 is the link between iron metabolism and fatty acids and lipids metabolism (mainly cholesterol). Iron deficiency induces modifications in the lipid metabolism. For example, the level of lipid peroxidation is much higher during iron deficiency state (Bartal, Mazor, Dvilansky, & Myerstein, 1993); the level of cytochrome *c* is reduced by iron deficiency (Parks & Wharton, 1989); and it can also induce a reduction of 60% in the level of phosphatidylinositol (Mohindra, Subramonian, & Seth, 1990). One aspect of this link is the myelin story.

Most axons in the central nervous system are covered with a special membrane called myelin, having the highest lipid:protein ratio (3:1) of all membranes. The myelin sheath isolates the axon and allows a minimal loss of the electrical potential to the surrounding areas. The myelin allows the axon to remain thin and to accelerate the speed of the propagation of nerve impulses. In addition, myelin serves to maintain the integrity of the axon. The chemical composition of the sheath is most complex. About 40% of the myelin is cholesterol, 40% phosphatides (containing fatty acids and lipids), and about 20% cerebroside (sugar-containing-fat like molecule) and 10% proteins.

Large amounts of polyunsaturated fatty acids are present in the myelin. The process of covering the axons with myelin sheaths (myelination) starts right after birth. The degree of myelination is an index of maturation. An adequate supply of iron and essential fatty acids in the developmental period is a requirement for a normal rate of myelination. In aging, the process is reversed and demyelination occurs. The effects of a fatty acid-deficient diet that was given to pregnant rats or to pups resulted in a very slow rate of myelination compared with the rate of myelination in the control group (Bourre et al., 1984). The low level of myelination observed in IDD- and FA-deficient rats (see below) was correlated with other behavioral deficits. Using Luxol fast blue stain, Yu, Steinkirchner, Rao, and Larkin (1986) confirmed earlier observations by Yehuda and Youdim (1988) that the degree of myelination is decreased in the pups or iron-deficient rats. She found that the degree of myelination of the spinal cord of 11-day-old pups and in the cortex of 17-day-old pups was very low and undeveloped. Recently, a preliminary study (Yehuda et al., unpublished results), using Luxol fast blue, showed that iron deficiency treatment in adult rats may cause demyelination. One study examined the iron and essential fatty acids on the brain development of young rats. Rats were maintained on different diets: either deficient in essential fatty acids, or low on iron, or deficient in both. The low-iron status aggravated sign of essential fatty acid deficiency (leading to decreases in both growth and brain weight), and suggesting that brain iron deficiency can produce the same effects as essential fatty acids deficiency (Oloyede, Folayan, & Odutuga, 1992).

## 4. BRAIN IRON AND BRAIN DOPAMINE

At least two scientific findings link brain iron to brain dopamine. The first finding is that iron per se is a co-factor in certain stages of catecholamine metabolism, and several iron dependent enzymes are involved in that pathway. Among them are the rate-limiting enzyme tyrosine hydroxylase and tryptophan hydroxylase and amine neurotransmitter catabolizing enzyme monoamine oxidase A and B. The other finding is that both iron and dopamine are not evenly distributed in the brain, and there is a tendency for "co-localization" of the two molecules in the brain.

The dopamine system in the brain is sensitive to iron deficiency. On the neurochemical level, Ashkenazi, Ben Shachar, and Youdim (1982) demonstrated that among all neurotransmitter systems only the dopamine D2 receptor and possibly GABA receptor system were significantly affected. The number of dopamine D2 receptor had been decreased by 40% and the affinity was very low.

On the behavioral level, Youdim and Green (1977) were first to conduct a series of studies to examine the effect of iron deficiency on the brain neurotransmitter metabolism and function and correlate them with behavior. They showed that the dopamine system was most sensitive to IDD and dopamine-dependent behaviors were affected. These studies have been summarized elsewhere (Weinberg, Dallman, & Levine, 1980; Youdim, Ben Shachar, Ashkenzi, & Yehuda, 1983).

Among the dopamine-mediated behaviors are

- *Thermoregulation in cold environments*: Iron-deficient rats cannot regulate body temperature at 4°C and hypothermic drugs worsen the regulation.
- *Circadian cycles*: The motor and thermal circadian cycles are completely reversed (dark-light periods) in iron-deficient rats. In iron deficient rats later treated with iron-enriched diet, the circadian cycles were restored to normal cycles. It should be noted that the cognitive deficits were not rehabilitated.
- *Pain*: The study of the circadian cycle of pain threshold in rats also indicated that this cycle is also reversed between light and dark periods. However, a small dose of b-endorphin was able to elevate the pain threshold in iron-deficient rats but not in control rats (Yehuda & Youdim, 1984). This finding led to another finding that iron deficiency induced modification of the blood–brain barrier (BBB). Those modifications allow peripheral b-endorphin to enter into the brain. In addition, a negative correlation between dopamine activity and b-endorphin activity was found.
- *Stereotyped behavior*: This behavior is clearly mediated by the activation of the brain dopamine system. Drug-induced stereotypy is also circadian cycle dependent. In iron-deficient rats the stereotypy cycle is also reversed, and iron-enriched diet can correct the reversed cycles.

## 5. IRON AND SCHIZOPHRENIA

The relationships between functional level of dopamine and iron can be demonstrated in acutely psychotic schizophrenic patients. The dopamine level in the brain of schizophrenic patients is very high. Abnormal iron deposits have been found in the brains of schizophrenics in CT and in post-mortem studies. Recently, the levels of serum iron were examined at 08:00, 17:00, and 24:00 in a large group of medication-free schizophrenic patients in acute psychotic relapse and were compared to the iron level of a normal control group. The results showed a significant decrease in the iron level at 17:00 and 24:00, and a non-significant drop at 08:00 o'clock levels (Weiser, Levkowitch, Neuman, & Yehuda, 1994).

## 6. IRON DEFICIENCY, LEARNING, AND HIPPOCAMPUS INTEGRITY

### 6.1. *Animal Studies*

One of the major symptoms of iron deficiency in human is a decline in cognitive IQ level capacity (see below). The ability of an IDD to modify cognitive functions, such as learning, permits the use of an animal IDD model of iron deficiency as human analog. The first report came from Weinberg's laboratory (Weinberg, Levine, & Dallman, 1979; Weinberg, Brett, Levine,

& Dallman, 1981). Learning (passive and active avoidance) was studied in offspring of iron-deficient pregnant rats or those rats exposed to an IDD at a very early age. All showed learning deficits in those tasks.

Yehuda and Youdim studied the following learning paradigms:

- *Water maze*: In this study, iron-deficient rats were very slow learners in this task. The degree of the deficit in learning is correlated with the hemoglobin level (Yehuda, Youdim, & Mostofsky, 1986). One of the striking findings was that the deficit in learning was evident even when the levels of hemoglobin did not reach a significant decreased level.
- *Morris water maze:* Iron-deficient rats are very slow learners of the task and barely learned to solve the problem. In this study, the motor activity of the iron-deficient rats was carefully studied. The significant decrease in learning capacity cannot be attributed to fatigue or muscle weakness (Yehuda & Carasso, 1993). At the end of both studies, the rats were fed with an iron-supplemented diet and were tested either in the same water maze or in the Morris Water maze 2, 4, 6, and 8 weeks later. No restoration of learning was found. It should be noted that other effects of iron deficiency could be reversed by such a treatment, e.g., hemoglobin level, reversal of motor activity, thermoregulation, and stereotype behavior and pain threshold. Lozoff, Wolf, and Jimenez (1996) reported similar results in children.
- *Electric shock:* Electric shock increased the level of the opiate system. The combination of electric shock IDD made Water maze learning impossible (Yehuda, Mei-Tal, & Youdim, 1991).

The mode of action of iron deficiency in inducing learning deficits is not known. There are at least three possible approaches to explain this effect. The first approach was proposed by several researchers, which suggested that the reversed circadian rhythm of activity and altered thermoregulation are changes which adaptively predispose different performances in a test of learning. The second approach is based on the findings that dopamine D2 receptors mediate several forms of learning (Gasbarri et al., 1997; Sigala, Missale, & Spano, 1997; Setlow & McGaugh, 1998; Smith, Niell, & Costall, 1999). The third approach considers the unique role of the hippocampus in various forms of learning and especially in spatial learning. The level of iron in the hippocampus depends upon age (Savory, Rao, Huang, Letada, & Herman, 1999) and strain (Ono & Cherian, 1999). Prenatal iron deficiency predisposes the neonatal hippocampus to a greater acute loss of neurons and neuronal metabolic activity after a hypoxic-ischemic or other stressful event (Rao et al., 1999). That the vulnerability of the iron-deficient hippocampus to stressful events leads to greater loss of hippocampal neuronal integrity suggests a site of action for iron deficiency and predicts poorer recoverability after injury or stress in the prenatal iron-deficient brain. The hippocampus is the focus of many studies today, since this brain structure is highly involved in many forms of cognitive deficits, including Alzheimer's disorder and other dementias. Recently, many studies indicated that a high level of cortisone and corticosterone is selectively toxic to the hippocampus (Yehuda et al., submitted to Nutritional Neuroscience).

We have examined the effects of IDD on the hippocampus iron metabolism and the response of hippocampus to excitatory amino acid (EAA), kainite (41a and b) neurotoxin because of the sensitivity of this region. In adult rats (6 months old), intense histochemical staining of iron was observed in the CA3 region. In young iron-supplemented rats (8 weeks old), this region did not stain for iron. In adult rats, ferritin-immunoreactive (Fr-ir) microglia formed a pattern overlapping the CA4 region and dentate gyrus. In young rats, Fr-ir microglia were observed in CA3, but their density was lower in CA4 compared to adult rats and there were no FR-ir microglia in their dentate gyrus. In iron-deficient rats, Fr-ir microglia appeared at CA3 but was not present at all in CA4 or dentate gyrus. To the best of our knowledge this is the first description of such an anatomical spread of ferritin expression in hippocampus microglia in early development in rats and retardation of this process in iron deficiency.

In both adult and young rats, transferrin immunoreactivity (Tf-ir) oligodendrocytes were distributed throughout the hippocampus. Their lower numbers in IDD may reflect poorer myelination. However, transferrin receptor immunoreactivity (TFR) changed from staining of both nerve cells and blood vessels in CA1-3 in early development to exclusive staining of blood vessels in adults. In IDD rat neurons were TFR-ir stained, but blood vessels were generally not stained. This distribution pattern coverage may indicate the retardation of hippocampus development in IDD and thus may be a site for possible mechanism of cognitive and learning deficits.

Since BBB is compromised in iron-deficit rats, the danger of dietary neurotoxins such as EAA in IDD was considered by exploring hippocampal neurotoxicity responses after systemic injection of the neurotoxin, kainite, an agonist of glutamate receptor. Six hours after kainic acid injection, morphological damage to nerve cells was observed in the hippocampus CA3 of iron-deficient rats. By contrast in iron-supplemented rats, this region was intact. Damage to the CA3 field after such a short time interval parallels the effect of kainate administration into the lateral cerebral ventricle.

Thus, the vulnerability of CA3 region in iron-deficient animals could very well reflect alteration or disruption of BBB to kainate. The implication of these findings and the permanent damage that can be done to the brain neuronal system are clear. This problem is presently being investigated since it may lead to a better understanding for prevention of diet-induced neurotoxicity in human iron deficiency (Shoham & Youdim, 1999).

### *6.2. Human Studies*

The literature of human studies with ID began with the paper by Oski and Honig (1978), which examined the effects of iron deficiency on cognitive performance. Administration of iron treatment vs. placebo was shown to improve the scores on the Bayley test. From the results on 24 infants they concluded that iron treatment is beneficial for iron-deficient infants. This study was the turning point, which produced hundreds of studies on children all over the world. This review is not the placc to summarize and evaluate those excellent studies. It is enough to mention that A. Heywood, Oppenheimer, P. Heywood, and Jolley (1989) and Lozoff (1989) studies children in Costa Rica and Guatamala, Walter (1989) studied children in Chile, and Pollitt (Soewondo, Husaini, & Pollitt, 1989) worked in Indonesia, Thailand, and Egypt.

Despite many variations in the methods, age of the subjects, and the evaluation tools between the various studies, two conclusions were found in almost all studies. There exist two important factors – the duration of the iron deficiency period and its magnitude. The combination of both factors will determine the degree of the cognitive deficit (Lozoff, Brittenham, Viteri, Wolf, & Urutia, 1982). These conclusions agree with results obtained in animal models. Duration and magnitude of iron deficiency are the factors which influence the degree of cognitive deficits in rat pups (Yehuda & Youdim, 1989; Sigala et al., 1997).

## 7. IRON DEFICIENCY AND PRETEMS

One of the critical periods for adequate iron supplies is the prenatal period. Recently, we examined the relation between iron status and neurobehavioral development in premature infants. Infants born before 34 weeks postmenstrual age and who were medically stable were studied. Anemia was defined as hemoglobin ≤10 g/dL and low iron stores as a serum ferritin concentration ≤75 μg/L. The infants were classified as anemic with low ferritin (Group 1; $n=18$), anemic with normal ferritin (Group 2; $n=14$), and non-anemic with normal ferritin (Group 3; $n=21$). A total of 18 reflexes were behaviourally evaluated at 37 weeks postmenstrual age and "reflex scores" were compared between the groups. Higher scores reflect a greater percentage of abnormal reflexes. RESULTS: Infants in Group 1 (anemia/low ferritin) had a significantly higher reflex score (51.45±18.32%) than infants in Group 3 (38.32±17.75%). Group 2 had an intermediate score (45.40±21.70%), but not different from the other two groups. These data indicate that low-iron status, both measured by anemia and ferritin levels, is related to poorer neurobehavioral status in premature infants (Armony-Sivan, Eidelman, Lanir, Sredni, & Yehuda, 2005).

## 8. LONG-TERM EFFECTS OF TRANSIENT IRON DEFICIENCY PERIOD

One important issue was the magnitude of the IDD effect. Early studies showed that an early IDD treatment had the strongest effect. IDD treatment to pregnant rats had more severe biochemical and behavioral effects than an IDD treatment at the age of 10 days (Weinberg et al., 1980). Similar findings were obtained in our study (Yehuda & Youdim, 1988) on early age effects of IDD. Additional information came very recently from a study that showed certain brain areas (such as pons, thalamus) are more resistant to an IDD treatment. Other brain areas (such as cortex and hippocampus) are very sensitive to the treatment and lose iron very quickly (Erikson, Pinero, Connor, & Beard, 1997). Similar results were reported in other studies (Li, 1998; Shukula, Agarwal, & Shukula, 1989). It is important to emphasize that while IDD treatment had a larger effect in the early developmental stages, an IDD treatment has a significant effect on human adults and other animals.

The long-term effects of rehabilitated infancy (1 year old) iron deficiency (ID) were examined at age 10. The children were examined for the following variables: auditory system function, the level of morning cortisol, IQ score (WISC-R), and behavioral profile. The results indicate that while the former ID children's hearing system appears to function well, there was a delay in brain stem processing of the auditory signals. In addition, the level of morning cortisol was reduced, the general IQ scores were lower than the normal group (mainly in the performed subtest), and more sleep disturbances and fatigue during day were reported. These outcomes are consistent with established reports on the effect of iron deficiency on the rate of myelination in selected brain areas during critical period of 1-year-olds. The findings of increased sleep disturbances and lower IQ tests require further study.

Total IQ level of both groups was in the normal range; however, the control group was at the upper limit and the former iron-deficient group was at the lower limit. In all subtests the former iron-deficient group was lower than the control group (Yehuda & Yehuda, 2006).

Recently, we created an animal to study the cognitive longlasting effects of rehabilitated early ID. Rats were given an IDD diet from day 21 for 4 weeks and that control diet. Also the hematological values of former ID rats were normal; their learning capacities were lower than control rat. They were hypothermic. Treatment with a mixture of essential fatty acids was able to restore the cognitive level (Table 1).

**Table 1**
**Longlasting Effects of Early IDD on Learning Capacity and Rehabilitation by Treatment of a Mixture of Essential Fatty Acids**

| | *Control + Saline* | *Control + SR-3* | *ID + Saline* | *ID + SR-3* | *Former ID + Saline* | *Former ID + SR-3* |
|---|---|---|---|---|---|---|
| No. of trials to reach criterion | 12.9 ± 2.8 | 6.0 ± 2.2 | 23.2 ± 3.1 | 6.8 ± 2.5 | 17.5 ± 3.0 | 8.5 ± 4.0 |
| Swimming span | 488 ± 22 | 365 ± 19 | 1344 ± 65 | 398 ± 45 | 600 ± 63 | 400 ± 44 |
| Passive avoidance (Max. 360 s) | 300 ± 29 | 357 ± 33 | 76 ± 16 | 330 ± 26 | 218 ± 60 | 348 ± 36 |
| Line crossing | 769 ± 35 | 749 ± 56 | 510 ± 28 | 720 ± 49 | 754 ± 51 | 770 ± 49 |
| Rearing | 66.6 ± 8 | 71 ± 8 | 49 ± 10 | 68 ± 9 | 64.5 ± 22 | 68.8 ± 24 |
| Body temperature (°C) | 37.8 ± 0.7 | 37.1 ± 0.8 | 35.3 ± 1.0 | 37.2 ± 0.6 | 36.0 ± 0.6 | 37.0 ± 0.8 |
| Hemoglobin level (g/100 mL) | 14.9 ± 1.4 | 13.5 ± 1.8 | 6.9 ± 0.3 | 12.3 ± 1.3 | 14.7 ± 1.9 | 14.0 ± 2.2 |
| Serum iron level (g/mL) | 3.9 ± 0.7 | 4.4 ± 1.0 | 1.9 ± 0.9 | 3.0 ± 0.9 | 3.8 ± 0.8 | 4.0 ± 0.9 |

## 9. THE AUDITORY SYSTEM AND IRON DEFICIENCY

Iron-deficient rats are much more sensitive to strong noise. Hearing loss is induced in lower magnitude of noise in iron-deficient rats compared to normal rats (Sun et al., 1991). The explanation to the finding was that iron deficiency induced changes in the inner ear. Recently, Walter and Lozoff's group (Roncagliolo, Garrido, Walter, Peirano, & Lozoff, 1998) used brain auditory responses of 6-month-old infants. They reported a delayed maturation of auditory brainstem responses in infants with iron deficiency anemia. They explained their results in a delayed brain and auditory system myelination. It seems that iron deficiency has a multiple site of action.

## 10. IRON DEFICIENCY AND THE ENDOCRINE SYSTEM

Among the multiple effects of iron deficiency on various tissues, the effects of iron deficiency state on the endocrine system have been studied. Beard, Green, Miller, and Finch (1984), Beard, Tobin, and Green (1989), Brigham and Beard (1996), and Beard, Borel, and Peterson (1997) demonstrated that iron deficiency anemia is associated with lower plasma thyroid hormone concentration in rodents and, in some studies, in humans. Another hormone that is affected by iron deficiency is cortisol. Early studies showed that the level of cortisol is decreased in the iron-deficient rat (Weinberg et al., 1979, 1981; P. R. Dallman, Refino, & M. F. Dallman, 1984). Confirmatory studies with humans demonstrated reduced cortisol secretion in patients with iron deficiency (M. J. Saad, Morais, & S. T. Saad, 1991).

## 11. IRON DEFICIENCY AND THE IMMUNE SYSTEM

It is not surprising that nutritionally induced iron deficiency causes changes in other body systems in addition to brain biochemistry. The clinical setting was the observation that most of the anemic children are sick much more often than normal children. It seems that the immune defense system is not working in those children as they had fever and inflammations, symptoms of infectious diseases.

A closer look reveals that there is a reciprocal relationship between the nutritional status and the immune system. On one hand, most inflammations caused anorexia. The more severe the inflammation, the more severe the anorexia. On the other hand, nutritional deficits may cause immunological deficits. Protein undernutrition induced a decrease in the immune cells, in the phagocytes functions, in immunoglobin A secretion, and in cytokines production. A deficit in even single nutrients (iron, copper, zinc, or certain vitamins) leads to immunological problems (Chandra, & Kumari, 1994, Chandra, 1997; Scrimshaw & SanGiovanni, 1997).

This chapter is not the place to review the vast literature on the relationships between the components of the immune system and iron deficiency, except to note the relationships between the iron system and the cytokines.

In a previous study, Yehuda (1990) showed that IDD treatment is rats induced a significant increase in IL-1 level and a significant decrease in IL-2. The levels of both cytokines were circadian cycle dependent, and IL-1 causes a decrease in serum iron (Gordeuk, Prithviraj, Dolinar, & Brittenham, 1988). Kuvibidila, Murthy, and Suskind (1992) also reported an IL-2 level decrease in iron-deficient mice. Since IL-1 is a pro-inflammatory cytokine and IL-2 is an anti-inflammatory cytokine, our finding may explain the "chronic" inflammation of iron-deficient children.

Recently, we examined the cytokines profile in iron-deficient rats (Yehuda, unpublished report). The study was instructive in that it illustrated how difficult it is to interpret results in this field. First, the body weight of the ID rats was decreased by about 30%. The spleen of the ID rats was enlarged, and the number of cells was much greater than in normal rats. Immunological comparison showed that IDD spleen cells produced per cell the same amount of IL-1 as in normal rats; however, since there are more cells, the total production is greater on the basis of lighter weight. The IDD spleen cells produced more IL-6 per cell, and there was a decrease in the secretion of IL-2 and IL-10 per cell from IDD spleen. Some of the discrepancies in this field can be attributed to the failure to take into account the factors of body weight and the number of spleen cells.

Another new issue in human studies is the immunological profile of premature babies born at week 27–34 of the pregnancy. A high percentage of them suffered from iron deficiency. The results showed that the immunological profile of the premature babies is different from the immunological profile of full-term babies and that iron-deficient premature babies have malfunctioned immune system (Yehuda et al., unpublished results).

## 12. CONCLUSION

Animal studies so far have demonstrated that the brain is sensitive to alterations (diminution or elevation) in its iron content. Increased brain is now thought to be closely linked to a number of neurodegenerative diseases, among them Parkinson's disease, Alzheimer's disease, and Hallervorden-Spatz disease to mention a few. This has been linked to the role iron plays in promoting the generation of radical oxygen species, which can result in oxidative stress and neurodegeneration (Riederer, Sofic, Rausch, Jellinger, & Youdim, 1989). On the other hand, for the present discussion the inadequate availability of brain iron is now closely associated with alterations in brain development and its neuronal system. Furthermore, deficiency of the metal can result in pathological changes where the dopamine-opiate system and hippocampus are more severely affected, with consequential cognitive impairment. These effects appear to be irreversible and more pronounced at an early age, with possible long-term consequences in adult life. The fact that BBB is also compromised has been observed in iron-deficient rats (Gerlach, Ben Shachar, Riederer, & Youdim, 1994), suggesting that the brain may also be more sensitive to dietary or environmental toxin. It may be for these reasons that the brain has such a tight regulatory mechanism for handling iron. There are a number of aspects to this. All the iron that is present in the brain is deposited before the BBB is fully developed and once formed serum iron has no access to the brain. Furthermore, the turnover of brain iron is significantly slower than other tissues, specially compared to the liver. Thus, the brain conserves its iron and in human brain iron remains constant after the age of 30.

## REFERENCES


Armony-Sivan, R., Eidelman, A. I., Lanir, A., Sredni, D., & Yehuda, S. (2004). Iron status and neurobehavioral development of premature infants. *Journal of perinatology, 24*(12), 757–762.

Ashkenazi, R., Ben Shachar, D., & Youdim, M. B.H. (1982). Nutritional iron and dopamine binding sites in the rat brain. *Pharmacology Biochemistry and Behavior, 17*(Suppl. 1), 43–47.

Bartal, M., Mazor, D., Dvilansky, A., & Myerstein, N. (1993). Iron deficiency anemia: Recovery in vitro oxidative stress. *Acta Haematologica, 90*, 94–98.

Beard, J., Borel, M., & Peterson, F. J. (1997). Changes in iron status during weight loss with very-low-energy diets. *American Journal of Clinical Nutrition, 66*(1), 104–110.

Beard, J., Green, W., Miller, L., & Finch, C. (1984). Effect of iron deficiency anemia on hormone levels and thermoregulation during cold exposure. *American Journal of Physiology, 247*(1), 114–119.

Beard, J., Tobin, G., & Green, W. (1989). Evidence for thyroid hormone deficiency in iron deficient anemic rats. *Journal of Nutrition, 119*(5), 772–778.

Beard, J. L., Connor, J. D., & Jones, B. C. (1993a). Brain iron: Location and function. *Progress in Food & Nutrition Science, 17*, 183–221.

Beard, J. L., Connor, J. R., & Jones, B. C. (1993b). Iron in the brain. *Progress in Food & Nutrition Science, 51*(6), 157–170.

Beard, J. L., Dawson, H., & Pnero, D. J. (1996). Iron metabolism: A comprehensive review. *Nutrition Reviews, 54*(10), 295–317.

Ben Shachar, D., Ashkenazi, R., & Youdim, M. B. H. (1986). Long term consequence of early iron deficiency on dopamine neurotransmitters in rats. *International Journal of Developmental Neuroscience, 4*, 81–88.

Benkovic, S., & Connor, J. R. (1993). Ferritin, transferrin and iron in normal and aged rat brains. *The Journal of Comparative Neurology, 337*, 97–113.

Bourre, J. M., Pascal, G., Durand, G., Masson, M., Dumont, O., & Piciotti, I. (1984). Alterations in the fatty acid composition of the rat brain cells (neurons, astrocytes and oligodendrocytes) and the cellular fractions (myelin and synaptosomes) induced by devoid of n-3 fatty acids. *Journal of Neurochemistry, 43*(2), 342–348.

Brigham, D., & Beard, J. (1996). Iron and thermoregulation: A review. *Critical Reviews in Food Science and Nutrition, 36*(8), 747–763.

Buzina,S. K., Buzina. R., Stavijenic, A., Farley, T. M, Haller, J., & Bergman, M., et al. (1998). Aging, multinational status and immune response. *Journal of Vitamin and Nutrition Research, 68*(2), 133–141.

Chandra, R. K. (1997). Nutrition and the immune system: An introduction. *American Journal of Clinical Nutrition, 66*(2), S460–S463.

Chandra, R. K., Kumari, S. (1994). Nutrition and immunity: an overview. *Journal of nutrition*. 124(Suppl. 8), 1433S–1435S.

Connor, J. R., & Menzies, S. L. (1996). Relationship of iron to oligodendrocytes and myelination. *Glia,17*, 83–93.

Dallman, P. R., & Spirito, R. A. (1977). Brain iron in the rat: Extremely slow turnover in normal rats may explain long lasting effects of early iron deficiency. *The Journal of Nutrition, 107*, 1075–1081

Dallman, P. R., Refino, C. A., & Dallman, M. F. (1984). The pituitary-adrenal response to stress in the iron-deficient rat. *The Journal of Nutrition, 114*(10), 1747–1753.

Dallman, P. R., Siimes, M. A., & Manies, E. C. (1975). Brain iron: Persistent deficiency following short term iron deprivation in the young rat. *British Journal of Haematology, 31*, 209–215.

Erikson, K. M., Pinero, D. J., Connor, J. R., & Beard, J. L. (1997). Regional brain iron, ferritin and transferrin concentrations during iron deficiency in developing rats. *The Journal of Nutrition, 127*(10), 2030–2038.

Gasbarri, A., Sulli, A., Pacitti, C., Puglisi Allegra, S., Cabib, S., Castellano, C., et al. (1997). Strain-dependent effects of D2 dopaminergic and muscarinic-cholinergic agonist antagonist on memory consolidation process in mice. *Behavioural Brain Research, 86*(1), 97–104.

Gerlach, M., Ben Shachar, D., Riederer, P., & Youdim, M. B. H. (1994). Altered brain metabolism of iron as a cause of neurodegenerative diseases. *Behavioural Brain Research, 63*, 793–804.

Gordeuk, V. R., Prithviraj, P., Dolinar, T., & Brittenham, G. M. (1988). Interleukin-1 administration in mice produces hypoferremia despite neutroenia. *Journal of Clinical Investigation, 82*, 1934–1938.

Heywood, A., Oppenheimer, S., Heywood, P., & Jolley, D. (1989). Behavioral effects of iron supplementation in infants in Madang, Paua New Guinea. *American Journal of Clinical Nutrition, 50*, 630–640.

Hill, J. M. (1988). The distribution of iron in the brain. In M. B. H. Youdim (Ed.), *Brain iron: Neurochemical and behavioral aspects* (pp. 1–24). London: Taylor and Francis.

Kuvibidila, S., Murthy, K. K., & Suskind, R. M. (1992). Alternation of interleukin-2 production in iron deficiency anemia. *Journal of Nutritional Immunology, 1*(1), 81–89.

Larkin, E. C., & Rao, G. A. (1990). Importance of fetal and neonatal iron: Adequacy for normal development of central nervous system. In J. Dobbing (Ed.), *Brain, behavior and iron in the infant diet* (pp. 43–62). London: Springer-Verlag.

Li, D. (1998). Effects of iron deficiency on iron distribution and gamma-aminobutyric acid (GA) in young rat brain tissue. *Hokkaido Igaku Zasshi, 73*(3), 215–225.

Lozoff, B. (1989). Methodological issues in studying behavioral effects of infant iron deficiency anemia. *American Journal of Clinical Nutrition, 50*, 641–654.

Lozoff, B., Brittenham, G. M., Viteri, F. E., Wolf, A. W., & Urutia, J. J. (1982). Developmental deficits in iron deficiency infants: Effects of age and severity of iron lack. *The Journal of Pediatrics, 101*(6), 948–952.

Lozoff, B., Wolf, A. W., & Jimenez, E. (1996). Iron deficiency anemia and infant development: Effects of extended oral iron therapy. *The Journal of Pediatrics, 129*(3), 382–389.

Mohindra, J., Subramonian, A., & Seth, P. K. (1990). Effect of iron deficiency on phosphoinositide levels in rat brain. *Indian Journal of Experimental Biology, 28*(7), 688–690.

Oloyede, O. B., Folayan, A. T., & Odutuga, A. A. (1992). Effects of low-iron status and deficiency of essential fatty acids on some biochemistry of rat brain. *Biochemistry International, 27*(5), 913–922.

Ono, S. L., & Cherian, M. G. (1999). Regional distribution of metallothionein, zinc and copper in the brain of different strains of rats. *Biological Trace Element Research, 69*(2), 151–159.

Oski, F. A., & Honig, A. S. (1978). The effects therapy on the development scores of iron deficient infants. *The Journal of Pediatrics, 92*(1), 21–25.

Parks, Y. A., & Wharton, B. A. (1989). Iron deficiency and the brain. *Acta Paediatrica Scandinavica, Supplement, 361*, 71–77.

Rao, R., de Ungria, M., Sullivan, D., Wu, P., Wobken, J. D., Nelson, C. A., et al. (1999). Perinatal brain iron increases the vulnerability of rat hippocampus to insult. *The Journal of Nutrition, 129*(1), 199–206.

Riederer, P., Sofic, E., Rausch, W. D., Jellinger, K., & Youdim, M. B. R. (1989). Transition metals, ferritin, glutathione and ascorbic acid in Parkinson brains. *Journal of Neurochemistry, 52*, 515–521.

Roncagliolo, M., Garrido, M., Walter, T., Peirano, P., & Lozoff, B. (1998). Evidence of altered central nervous system development in infants with iron deficiency anemia at 6 months. Delayed maturation of auditory brainstem responses. *The American Journal of Clinical Nutrition,, 68*, 683–690.

Saad, M. J., Morais, S. L., & Saad, S. T. (1991). Reduced cortisol secretion in patients with iron deficiency. *Annals of Nutrition and Metabolism, 35*(2), 111–115.

Savory, J., Rao, J. K. S., Huang, Y., Letada, P. R., & Herman, M. M. (1999). Age-related hippocampal associated with aluminium-induced neurodegeneration: Increased susceptibility with aging. *Neurotoxicology, 20*(5), 805–817.

Scrimshaw, N. S. (1998). Malnutrition, brain development learning and behavior. *Nutrition Research, 18*(2), 351–379.

Scrimshaw, N. S., & Giovanni, J. P. (1997). Synergism of nutrition, infection and immunity. *The American Journal of Clinical Nutrition, 66*, 464S–477S.

Scrimshaw, N. S. (1991). Iron deficiency. *Scientific American, 265*(4), 24–30.

Setlow, B., & McGaugh, J. L. (1998). Sulpride infused into the nucleus accumbens posttraining impairs memory of sp. training. *Behavioral Neuroscience, 112*(3), 603–610.

Shoham, S., & Youdim, M. B. H. (1999). Differential sensitivity of hippocampal subregions to iron deficiency and to iron and zinc nutritional therapy. *Neuroscience Letters, 54*(suppl.), S37 [abstract].

Shoham, S., & Youdim, M. B. H. (1999). Protective effects of iron deficiency and interaction with zinc in kainite model of temporal lobe epilepsy. *Neuroscience Letters, 54*(suppl.), S37–38 [abstract].

Shukula, A., Agarwal, K. N., & Shukula, G. S. (1989). Effect of latent iron deficiency on metal levels of rat brain regions. *Biological Trace Element Research, 22*(2), 141–152.

Sigala, S., Missale, C., & Spano, P. (1997). Opposite effects of dopamine D2 and D3 receptors on learning and memory in the rat. *European Journal of Pharmacology, 336*(2–3), 107–112.

Smith, A. G., Niell, J. C., & Costall, B. (1999). The dopamine D3/D2 receptor agonist 7-OH-DPAT induces cognitive impaired marmoset. *Pharmacology, Biochemistry and Behavior, 63*(2), 201–211.

Soewondo, S., Husaini, M., & Pollitt, E. (1989). Effects of iron deficiency on attention and learning process in preschool children. Bandung, Indonesia. *The American Journal of Clinical Nutrition, 50*, 667–675.

Sun, A. H., Wang, Z. M., Xiao, S. Z., Li, Z. J., Liang, Z. F., Hu, G. Y.,et al. (1991). Noise-induced hearing loss in iron deficient rats. *Acta Oto-laryngologica, 111*, 684–690.

Walter, T. (1989). Infancy: Mental and motor development. *The American Journal of Clinical Nutrition, 50*, 655–666.

Weinberg, J., Brett, L. P., Levine, S., & Dallman, P. R.(1981). Long-term effects of early iron deficiency on consummately behavior in the rat. *Pharmacology, Biochemistry and Behavior, 14*(4), 447–453.

Weinberg, J., Dallman, P. R., & Levine, S. (1980). Iron deficiency during early development in the rat: Behavioral and psychological consequences. *Pharmacology, Biochemistry and Behavior, 12*, 493–502.

Weinberg, J., Levine, S., & Dallman, P. R. (1979). Long-term consequences of early iron deficiency in the rat. *Pharmacology, Biochemistry and Behavior, 11*(6), 631–638.

Weiser, M., Levkowitch, Y., Neuman, M., & Yehuda, S. (1994). Decrease of serum iron in acutely psychotic schizophrenic patients. *The International Journal of Neuroscience, 78*(1–2), 49–52.

Yehuda, S. (1990). Neurochemical basis of behavioral effects of brain iron deficiency in anemia. In J. Dobbing, (Ed.), *Brain, behavior and iron in the infant diet* (pp. 63–81). London: Springer Verlag.

Yehuda, S., & Carasso, R. L. (1993). Modulation of learning, pain threshold and thermoregulation in the rat by preparations of free purified a-linolenic and linoleic acids: Determination of the optimal n-3 to n-6 ratio. *Proceedings National Academy of Science, USA90*, 10345–10349.

Yehuda, S., Mei-Tal, R., & Youdim, M. B. H. (1991). The effects of iron deficiency and electric shock on learning in rats. *International Journal of Neuroscience, 57*, 81–94.

Yehuda, S., & Yehuda, M. (2006). Long lasting effects of infancy iron deficiency-preliminary results. *Journal of Neural Transmission*, Suppl. 71, 197–200.

Yehuda, S., & Youdim, M. B. H. (1984). The increase opiate action of beta-endorphin in iron deficient rats: The possible involvement of dopamine. *European Journal of Pharmacology, 104*, 254–251.

Yehuda, S., & Youdim, M. B. H. (1988). Brain iron deficiency: Biochemistry and behavior. In M. B. H. Youdim (Ed.), *Brain iron: Neurochemical and behavioral aspects* (pp. 89–114). London: Taylor and Francis.

Yehuda, S., & Youdim, M. B. H. (1989). Brain iron: A lesson from animal models. *The American Journal of Clinical Nutrition, 50*, 618–629.

Yehuda, S., Youdim, M. B. H., & Mostofsky, D. I. (1986). Brain iron deficiency causes reduced learning capacity in rats. *Pharmacology, Biochemistry and Behavior, 25*, 141–144.

Youdim, M. B. H. (1990). Neuropharmacological and neurobiochemical aspects of iron deficiency. In J. Bobbing (Ed. ), *Brain, behavior, and iron in the infant diet*. London: Springer-Verlag.

Youdim, M. B. H., Ben Shachar, D., Ashkenzi, R., & Yehuda, S. (1983). Iron and dopamine receptor function. In P. Mandel & P. V. de Freudis (Eds.), *CNS receptors from molecular pharmacology to behavior* (pp. 309–322). New York: Plenum Press.

Youdim, M. B. H., Ben Shachar, D., & Yehuda, S. (1989). Putative biological mechanisms of the effect of iron deficiency on brain biochemistry and behavior. *The American Journal of Clinical Nutrition, 50*, 607–617.

Youdim, M. B. H., & Green, A. R. (1977). *Biogenic monoamine metabolism and functional activity in iron deficient rats; functional correlates.* Ciba Foundation Symposium No. 51, Elsevier, Amsterdam, pp. 201–223.

Yu, G. S. M., Steinkirchner, T. M., Rao, G. A., & Larkin, E. C. (1986). Effect of prenatal iron deficiency on myelination in rat pups. *The American Journal of Pathology, 125*(3), 620–624.

# 12 Stress, Immunology, and Cytokines

*Dvora Sredni-Kenigsbuch*

**Summary**

- Stress was considered, in general, to be immunosuppressive.
- This chapter indicates that stress hormones may influence the immune response in a different way.
- There is a close connection between stress, cytokines, and the function of T helper.
- Glucocortecoids and catecholamines, the major stress hormones, inhibit IL-12 and increase IL-10, thus causing a switch from Th1 to Th2.
- Glucocortecoids and catecholamines induced by stress inhibit IL-6 and IL-1, thus inhibiting Th17 and causing an upregulation of $T_{reg}$ cells.
- In conclusion, we suggest that stress may in fact be anti-inflammatory and may prevent manifestation of autoimmune diseases.

**Key Words:** Stress; T helpers; cytokines; inflammation; autoimmunity

## 1. CHARACTERISTICS OF STRESS

An organism is said to be in a state of *stress* when its dynamic equilibrium (homeostasis) is threatened or disrupted by external or internal forces (stressors). Stressors include changes in the environment, such as temperature extremes; physiologic difficulties, such as food or water shortage; and psychosocial burdens, such as social subordination or loneliness. Some of these stressors may be acute, imposing short-term demands on individuals; others may recur or be longlasting, creating a chronic burden on the organism.

When the stress threshold is crossed, the stress system in the brain is activated, along with its peripheral components, the hypothalamic pituitary–adrenal (HPA) axis, and the autonomic sympathetic system (ASS). A living organism responds to stress through various behavioral and physical reactions, including higher pulse and respiratory rates, and increased muscle tone (Mastorakos, Pavlatou, Diamanti-Kandarakis, & Chrousos, 2005). Both the immune and the nervous systems are designed to interact with the organism's environment by perceiving and responding to physical or chemical stimuli generated within or outside it. In animals, the central nervous system (CNS) has usually been regarded as an immunologically privileged site because it is devoid of a lymphatic system that captures potential antigens, and it is protected from circulating blood by the blood–brain barrier (BBB), a specialized vasculature consisting of endothelial cells with tight junctions. This barrier is impermeable to many soluble substances,

From: *Nutrition and Health: Iron Deficiency and Overload*
Edited by: S. Yehuda and D.I. Mostofsky, DOI 10.1007/978-1-59745-462-9_12

including immunoglobulins and growth factors, and restricts the migration of lymphoid cells. Cells of the CNS (neurons, astrocytes, oligodendrocytes, microglia) constitutionally express low levels of class I and II major histocompatibility complex (MHC) antigens, which have a fundamental role in the induction and regulation of the immune response (Benacerraf, 1981; Wong, Barteltt, Clark-Lewis, Battye, & Schrader, 1984). In addition, the CNS does manifest an innate immune reaction to systemic bacterial infection and cerebral injury (Rivest, 2003).

## 2. STRESS, THE CNS, AND THE IMMUNE SYSTEM

The nervous and immune systems form an interdependent neuroimmune network. This cross-talk mostly depends on soluble mediators released by the immune system – the cytokines – which modulate normal and pathological neurophysiological and behavioral responses. These bidirectional interactions between the CNS and the immune system become even more pronounced under pathological conditions. Striking examples include disorders such as CNS infections, autoimmune disease, traumatic CNS injury, and, especially, neurodegenerative diseases such as Alzheimer's or Parkinson's diseases.

Stress has traditionally been associated with impaired immune function and increased susceptibility to infectious and neoplastic diseases (Leonard, 1995). Studies have reported a reduction in NK cell activity and neutrophil-mediated phagocytosis- and mitogen-stimulated lymphocyte proliferation in response to stress (Connor, Kelly, & Leonard, 1997; Shavit, Lewis, Terman, Gale, & Liebeskind, 1984). In addition, stressor-induced changes in leukocyte subsets, including increased neutrophils and reduced lymphocytes in the peripheral blood, have been reported in rats (Dhabhar, Millar, Mcewen, & Spencer, 1995; Shu, Stevenson, & Zhou, 1993). This chapter discusses the evidence that stress modulates the immune system via changes in cytokines, and has an impact on human health.

## 3. CYTOKINES AS MEDIATORS OF NEUROIMMUNE COMMUNICATION

This chapter will describe what is known about the interplay and communication between the immune system and the CNS; we will concentrate mainly on cytokines that play a key role in inflammation. Both immune and inflammatory responses are regulated by cytokines, small polypeptide cell regulators that are produced by a wide range of cells during the effector phase of immunity. Most cells do not constitutionally produce cytokines; rather transcription of cytokine genes occurs in response to an activating event. In general, cytokines are secreted, but they can also be expressed on the cell surface. An individual cytokine can be produced by various cell lineages and may have multiple effects on different types of cells. Cytokines also have redundant functions; that is, several cytokines can mediate a common event. Apart from displaying pleiotropism and redundancy, cytokines also have synergistic or antagonistic effects, and can induce or inhibit the synthesis of other cytokines, resulting in complex "cytokine cascades" in immune and inflammatory responses. Although cytokines usually act locally and initiate their action by binding to specific cell-surface receptors on target cells, these receptors generally show high affinities to their ligands, and only small amounts of a cytokine are required to elicit a biological response. The ultimate response of a particular cell to a given cytokine is determined by the level of expression of the cytokine receptor, the signal transduction pathways of the target cell that are activated by that cytokine, and the target cell microenvironment (Romagnani, 1994).

Cytokines and their receptors have recently been detected in other tissues, including those of the peripheral and central nervous systems (Schobitz, De Kloet, & Holsboer, 1994). Receptors for

IL-1, IL-2, IL-6, and TNF-α and some other growth factors have been identified in rodent brains, with highest densities in the hippocampus and hypothalamus (Hopkins & Rothwell, 1995). Histochemical studies using rodent and human tissues have shown that IL-1, IL-6, and TNF-α are expressed in neurons and glial cells within the CNS under non-inflammatory conditions, albeit in small quantities. After infection or trauma, cytokines are expressed in much larger quantities, and excessive secretion of cytokines is thought to be involved in many pathological processes within the CNS (Schobitz et al., 1994). Despite a great deal of research on cytokines, the physiological roles of specific cytokines within the brain are not fully understood.

It has, however, been shown that peripheral cytokines act indirectly on the brain; they trigger the production of cytokines in the brain parenchyma itself (Laye, Parnet, Goujon, & Dantzer, 1994), and provide a possible mechanism to relay information at the interface between the internal milieu and the brain, represented by endothelial cells and circumventricular organs (Konsman, Parnet, & Dantzer, 2002). Cytokines released from activated immune cells can induce effects in the CNS by several possible mechanisms. They may, for example, enter the CNS at sites where the BBB is absent, particularly via the *organum vasculosum of the laminae terminalis* (OVLT). The circumventricular organs are areas of the brain where there is no functional BBB (Hopkins & Rothwell, 1995). In the OVLT, cytokines are thought to bind to glial cells, which in turn produce additional cytokines and other mediators such as prostaglandins, particularly prostaglandin E (PGE) (Banks & Kastin, 1985; Gutierrez, Banks, & Kastin, 1994).

It has also been shown that the peripheral administration of bacterial lipopolysaccharide (LPS) induces the expression of mRNA encoding IL-l, IL-6, and TNF-α within the CNS (Dantzer, 1994), suggesting that not only can peripherally produced cytokines act on the CNS but alsothese cytokines induce the production of other cytokines within the brain, which can directly modulate CNS function. In fact, it has been proposed that circulating IL-1 acts on cyclooxygenase-containing neurons within the OVLT to induce local prostaglandin secretion; the local diffusion of prostaglandins into the hypothalamic area, in turn, acts on IL-l secreting/producing neurons in this region, causing IL-l to be released from neuronal terminals. Thus, it has been suggested that peripheral IL-1 induces the synthesis and release of IL-1 within the brain (Saper & Breder, 1992).

Other studies have reported that IL-1 not only acts at the OVLT but also can cross the BBB via an active transport mechanism. An active transport mechanism for TNF-α has also been described (Gutierrez, Banks, & Kastin, 1993). However, the concentrations of these cytokines that cross the BBB may be so low as to be physiologically insignificant, although it has been suggested that active transport mechanisms may become an important entry route when plasma concentrations of cytokines are very high (Banks, Ortiz, Plotkin, & Kastin, 1991).

The inflammatory cytokines, IL-1β and IL-6, as well as their receptors, are expressed in the brain and by cells of the endocrine and immune systems. These shared ligands and receptors are used as a common chemical language of communication within and between the immune and the neuroendocrine systems. Such communication suggests that the CNS can influence immune function, and the immune system can regulate the state of the CNS. Interplay between the immune, nervous, and endocrine systems is commonly associated with the marked effects of stress on immunity. The hypothalamic–pituitary–adrenal (HPA) axis, the key player in stress response, is stimulated by the cytokines when the body is under stress or experiences an infection.

In summary, communication between the periphery and the brain occurs via neural and humoral pathways. Cytokines released by monocytes and lymphocytes are one means by which the immune system communicates with the CNS, and thereby influences behavior. IL-1, IL-2, IL-6, IFN-γ, and TNF-α influence activation of the HPA axis and are, in turn, influenced by glucocorticoid hormone secretion (Munck & Guyre, 1991; Sternberg, 2001). Recognition of the role played by the local production of cytokines and their downstream messengers in the CNS opens up new research possibilities for understanding and treating non-specific neurological and psychiatric symptoms of diseases.

## 4. THE INTERACTION BETWEEN CYTOKINES AND THE HPA AXIS

Many in vitro studies have shown that IL-1 and IL-6 stimulate the HPA axis (Basedovsky & del Rey, 2000). Furthermore, both IL-6 and its receptor are expressed in the adrenal glands; in vitro adrenal culture studies have shown that IL-6 may regulate steroidogenesis locally in the adrenal glands, possibly acting as a chronic regulator of the stress response (Path, Bornstein, Ehrhart-Bornstein, & Scherbaum, 1997). Systemic IL-1 or IL-6 administration synergistically increases circulating concentrations of both adrenocorticotropin (ACTH) and corticosterone in response to mild stressors in rats (Zhou, Kusnecov, Shurin, DePaoli, & Rabin, 1996), suggesting that elevated circulating levels of these proinflammatory cytokines can increase HPA-axis reactivity to mild emotional stress. Thus, the HPA-axis and the proinflammatory cytokines, IL-1 and IL-6, are involved in the response to somatic stress in health and in acute or chronic disease. It is also of interest that the acute systemic injection of either IL-l or IL-6 produces an enhancement of stressor-induced monoamine alterations (Merali, Lacosta, & Anisman, 1997), suggesting that cytokines may increase susceptibility to stressor-induced monoamine changes.

Studies have concentrated on the effects of IL-1 on the interstitial levels of various monoamines in order to assess whether IL-1 might potentiate the neurochemical response(s) to environmental stimuli (neurogenic stressors). In fact, it appeared that IL-1 elicits region-specific changes in the interstitial levels of neurotransmitters and/or their metabolites; the response to air puff stimulation is also enhanced in rats that were treated with the cytokine. It seems that although IL-1 may have only modest effects on central monoamines, this cytokine may influence neuronal reactivity, thereby leading to augmented monoamine changes upon presentation of a stressor.

More importantly, several studies have shown that IL-1 and IL-6 are secreted in response to stress in rodents. Both physical and psychological stress have been reported to increase plasma IL-6 concentrations (Takaki, Huang, Somogyvári-Vigh, & Arimura, 1994; Zhou et al., 1993). With regard to the mechanism of stressor-induced IL-6 secretion, it is of interest that adrenaline administration to rats induces a rapid increase in plasma IL-6 concentrations, an effect that is blocked by pretreatment with the *p*-adrenoceptor antagonist, I-propranolol (De Rijk, Boelen, Tilders, & Berkenbusch, 1994). This suggests that stressor-induced increases in plasma IL-6 concentrations may be mediated by increased sympathetic activity and concomitant release of adrenaline from the adrenal medulla.

To date, most experimental studies on the stress-like effects of inflammatory cytokines such as IL-1 or IL-6 on neurotransmitters, behavior, and the HPA axis were limited to the acute administration of these immunological mediators. It was demonstrated that acute pretreatment with cytokines (IL-l and IL-6) produces an enhancement of stressor-induced monoamine changes in rats (Merali et al., 1997). Future research should, therefore, focus on examining the effects of repeated cytokine administration in chronic immunological activation, on behavior, neurochemistry, and HPA-axis activity in rodents.

In humans, excessive stress may lead to depression. Depression has been associated with increases in circulating levels of the proinflammatory cytokine, IL-6, in adults with major depression (Zorrilla et al., 2001), in depressed elderly populations, and in those depressed persons with chronic medical disorders such as rheumatoid arthritis (Zautra et al., 2004), cancer (Musselman et al., 2003) and cardiovascular disease (Lesperance, Frasure-Smith, Theroux, & Irwin, 2004).

Recent data further show that depressed patients exhibit exaggerated activation of the inflammatory response following acute psychological stress, with greater increases of IL-6 as well as activation of the nuclear factor (NF)-κB, a transcription factor that signals the inflammatory cascade (Pace et al., 2006). Moreover, depressed patients with severe sleep disturbances may be at greater risk of elevated IL-6 levels and other proinflammatory markers, because sleep loss has been shown to induce acute increases in cellular and genomic markers of inflammation (Irwin, Wang, Campomayor, Collado-Hidalgo, & Cole, 2006). Collectively, these findings suggest that elevated IL-6 is associated with several conditions reflecting mental health, in general, and stress and depression, in particular.

## 5. CYTOKINES IN THE CNS

The CNS and immune system communicate bidirectionally. The neuroimmune–endocrine interface is also mediated by inflammatory cytokines, acting as auto/paracrine or endocrine factors regulating pituitary development, cell proliferation, hormone secretion, and feedback control of the HPA axis (Woiciechowsky et al., 1999; Safieh-Garabedian et al., 2002). There is growing evidence of bidirectional circuits between the CNS and the immune system.

In support of such circuits between the CNS and the immune system, Betancur, Lledo, and Guaza (1994) reported that IL-1 and glucocorticoid hormones represent two key mediators involved in the modulation of the neuroimmuno-endocrine response to stress. In the immune system, glucocorticoids modulate IL-1 production and a number of IL-1 receptors. Moreover, glucocorticoids inhibit the autoregulatory loop of IL-1 in LPS-stimulated monocytes and constitute a mechanism for controlling IL-1 feedback stimulation (Paez et al., 1996; Groujon, Layé, Parnet, & Dantzer, 1997; Plagemann et al., 1998). Stress acts to provoke the inflammatory process. Inflammatory cells respond by secreting the inflammatory cytokines, IL-1 and IL-6, that act either directly or indirectly to increase the production or release of hormones by the HPA axis, and of pituitary hormones, cortisol, and catecholamines.

The stimulation of the HPA axis by IL-1 and IL-6 is recognized as a critical component of the inflammatory response. In this respect, it was demonstrated that the administration of IL-6 alone could not duplicate the stimulatory effect of IL-1 on ACTH release (Perlstein, Mougey, Jackson, & Neta, 1991; Connor, Song, Leonard, Merali, & Anisman, 1998). On the other hand, suboptimal amounts of IL-1 and IL-6 synergize to induce the early ACTH response and produce a subsequent response that is similar to the one observed after IL-1 was administered alone, suggesting that the latter response to IL-1 may be dependent on synergy, with endogenous IL-6 induced in the CNS.

Glucocorticoids (GCs) and catecholamines (CAs), the main stress hormones, mediate an anti-inflammatory response by downregulating the expression of proinflammatory cytokines such as IL-1 and IL-6 (Fig. 1). GCs have been shown to downregulate the transcription of IL-1, to destabilize IL-1 mRNA (Groujon et al., 1997; Schmidt et al., 1999), and to downregulate IL-1 protein levels (Kunicka et al., 1993). They also upregulate the expression of the decoy IL-1 receptor, IL-1R II (Colotta et al., 1993).

GCs are crucial for balancing somatic responses to challenge, serving to both restore and maintain homeostasis. They are involved in restraining inflammatory and neuroendocrine responses, including those induced by pathogen exposure and stress (Raison & Miller, 2003). They suppress critical inflammatory signaling pathways, including that of nuclear factor-κB (NF-κB), and inhibit stress-related outflow pathways, including those related to corticotrophin-releasing hormone (CRH), the HPA axis, and the sympathetic nervous system (SNS). GCs directly and indirectly regulate IL-6 production through their effects on transcription factors

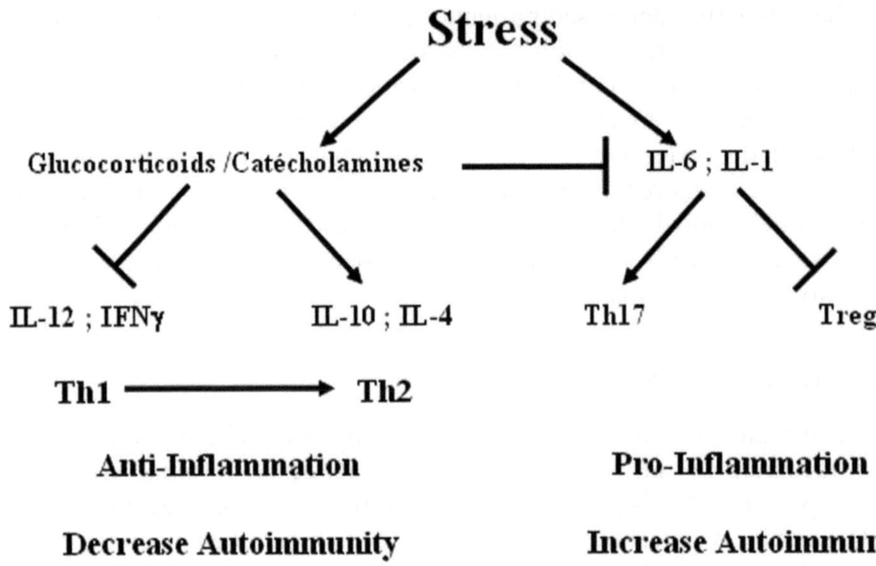


**Fig. 1.** Systemic effects of stress hormones on proinflammatory and anti-inflammatory cytokine production.

that regulate IL-6 or IL-1. Induction of IL-6 is mediated via NF-κB and by another nuclear factor, NF-IL6. The IL-1-induced induction of IL-6 can be inhibited by glucocorticoid-activated GR via protein–protein interactions at the C-terminal transactivation domain of NF-κB (De Bosscher et al., 1997; Vanden Berghe et al., 2000), whose effect does not require protein synthesis and does not affect the DNA-binding capacity of NF-κB.

## 6. INFLAMMATORY CYTOKINES, GLUCOCORTICOIDS, AND HUMAN DISEASE

The failure of GCs to inhibit IL-1 and IL-6 production has been found to contribute to disease development (Fig. 1), (Raison & Miller, 2003). Recent data indicate that excessive inflammation may play a significant role in a number of diseases, including cardiovascular disease, diabetes, and cancer (Raison, Capuron, & Miller, 2006). Moreover, excessive responses of the HPA axis, including increased production and release of CRH, and SNS hyperactivity, are hallmarks of depression. Given the central role of GCs and their signaling pathways, it is not surprising that a number of disorders characterized by excessive inflammatory responses, including rheumatoid arthritis, asthma, and inflammatory bowel disease, as well as depression, have been associated with resistance to GC (Pariante & Miller, 2001; Raison & Miller, 2003). In major depression, characterized by significant alterations in mood, neurological function, and cognition, GC resistance has been one of the most reproducible biological findings, occurring in up to 80% of patients (Holsboer, 2000; Pariante & Miller, 2001).

## 7. STRESS AND TH1/TH2 SUBSETS

Stress hormones affect major immune functions, including antigen presentation, lymphocyte proliferation and traffic, secretion of cytokines and antibodies, and selection of T helper (Th) 1 versus Th2 responses.

$CD4^+$ Th cells can be segregated into Th1 and Th2 subsets on the basis of cytokine expression, bioactivities, and helper function. Th1 cells mainly secrete IL-2, IL-3, TNF-α, and, most notably,

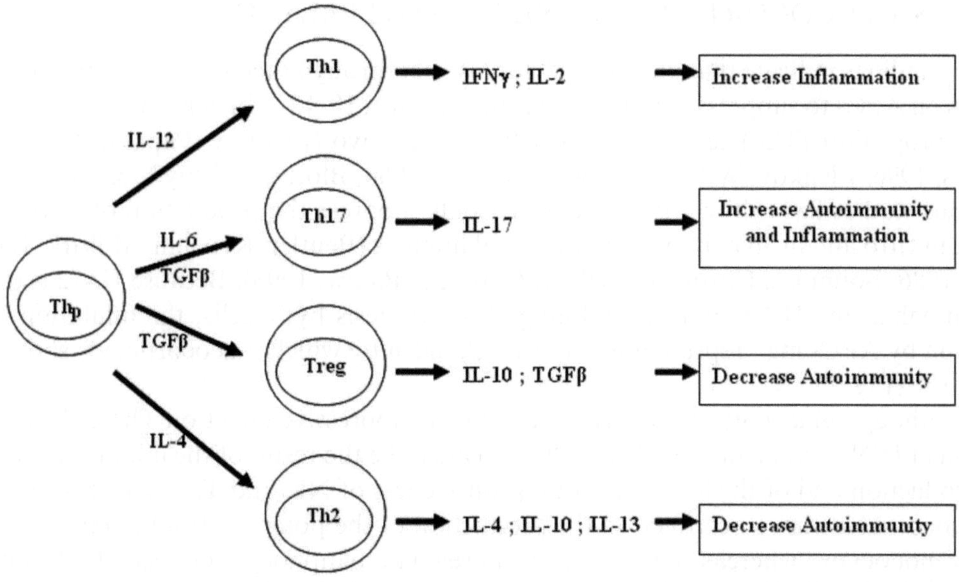


**Fig. 2.** Differentiation of naïve T cells into an effector T-cell subtype induced by cytokines.

IFN-γ (Fig. 2), and they control cell-mediated functions such as the activation of macrophages, the secretion of IL-4, IL-5, and IL-13 by Th2 cells, leading to the stimulation of humoral immunity by aiding B cell activation and class switching (Coffman, 2006). In addition, the cytokines of each Th subtype further promote the expansion of that population, while simultaneously inhibiting the development of the other subset. This allows each Th subset to produce characteristic cytokines that, in turn, provoke the development of a distinctive effector function specific to that T-cell subset. Thus, while Th1 cells induce proinflammatory responses, such as delayed-type hypersensitivity, and eliminate intracellular infections, Th2 cells mediate allergic reactions and anti-helminth responses (Moss et al., 2004).

The differentiation of lymphocytes into Th1 or Th2 cells is dependent on the production of cytokines by antigen-presenting cells (APCs) and T cells. APCs (macrophages and dendritic cells) are innate immune cells activated by microbial components via pattern-recognition receptors such as Toll-Like Receptors (TLRs). Such triggering stimulates the secretion of a precise set of cytokines that ultimately results in a T-cell-mediated antigen-specific response. It has been shown that the APC-derived cytokines, IL-12 and IL-18, are key players in the development of a Th1 cell response, and they synergize with one another by upregulating their reciprocal receptors on the surface of Th1 cells (Yoshimoto et al., 1998; Chang, Segal, Nakanishi, Okamura, & Shevach, 2000). In contrast, Th2 cell differentiation seems to be promoted mostly by T-cell-derived cytokines, in particular IL-4, subsequent to T-cell interaction with APCs (Fig. 2).

A novel concept that has emerged in the past decade indicates that stress hormones have pleiotropic effects on the immune response; systemically, they exert mostly anti-inflammatory effects and induce a Th2 shift, while in certain local responses they may induce proinflammatory activities. Thus, it is becoming increasingly clear that stress hormone-induced inhibition or upregulation of the systemic or local pro- and anti-inflammatory cytokine production and the Th1/Th2 balance may represent a major mechanism by which stress affects disease susceptibility and outcome (Fig. 1).

## 8. STRESS, GLUCOCORTICOIDS, AND TH1/TH2 BALANCE

Recent findings indicate that glucocorticoids also act through their classic cytoplasmic/nuclear receptors on APCs to suppress production of the cytokine, IL-12, which is known to differentiate T-helper progenitor (Thp) cells to Th1 in vitro and ex vivo (Elenkov, Papanicolau, Wilder, & Chrousos, 1996; Elenkov, Wilder, Chrousos, & Vizi, 2000; Blotta, Dekruyff, & Umetsu, 1997).

Previous studies have shown that glucocorticoids suppress the production of TNF-α, IFNγ, and IL-2 in vitro and in vivo, in both animals and humans (Beutler, Krochin, Milsark, Luedke, & Cerami, 1986; Boumpas, Chrousos, Wilder, Cupps, & Balow, 1993). Because IL-12 is extremely potent in enhancing IFNγ and in inhibiting IL-4 synthesis by T cells, the inhibition of IL-12 production by APCs may represent a major mechanism by which glucocorticoids shift the Th1/Th2 balance (Fig. 1).

Thus, although glucocorticoids may have a direct suppressive effect on Th1 cells, the overall inhibition of IFNγ production by these cells appears to be the result of the inhibition by APCs of IL-12 production and of the loss of IL-12 responsiveness of NK and Th1 cells. It is noteworthy that glucocorticoids have no effect on the production of the potent anti-inflammatory cytokine IL-10 by monocytes, whereas they appear to upregulate lymphocyte-derived IL-10 production (Van Der Poll, Barber, Coyle, & Lowry, 1996; Elenkov et al., 1996). The effect of dexamethasone on IL-4 production in T cells has been studied; since IL-4 is a Th2-associated cytokine, and glucocorticoids induce a shift from Th1 to Th2 immunity, one might expect dexamethasone to induce IL-4 expression. Indeed, in the mouse lymph node and spleen, IL-4 is induced in response to physiological concentrations of glucocorticoids both in vivo and in vitro (Daynes, Araneo, Dowell, Huang, & Dudley, 1990).

Thus, during immune and inflammatory responses, the activation of the stress system, through induction of a Th2 shift, in conjunction with the increase in the anti-inflammatory efferent vagus activity in visceral organs, may actually protect the organism from systemic overshooting with Th1/proinflammatory cytokines (Elenkov & Chrousos, 2002).

In conclusion, glucocorticoids and catecholamines directly inhibit the production of type-1 cytokines such as IL-12, INF-γ, which enhances cellular immunity and Th1 formation and, conversely, favors the production of type-2 cytokines such as IL-10 and IL-4, which induce humoral immunity and Th2 formation. Thus, during an immune challenge, stress causes an adaptive Th1-to-Th2 shift in order to protect the tissues from the potentially destructive actions of the proinflammatory type 1 cytokines and other products of activated macrophages. The homeostatic role of stress-induced Th2 shift against overshooting of cellular immunity often complicates pathologic conditions under which either cellular immunity is beneficial.

## 9. STRESS, INFLAMMATION, AND AUTOIMMUNE DISEASES

The effect of stress on autoimmunity is extremely complex; often stress is related to both induction/exacerbation and amelioration of disease activity (Elenkov & Chrousos, 1999; Rogers & Fozdar, 1996; Elenkov & Chrousos, 2002). The relationship between stressful life events and the onset of an autoimmune disease is probably best characterized in Graves' disease, an autoimmune inflammatory disease of the thyroid gland. Several epidemiologic studies demonstrated that patients with Graves' disease were more likely to have encountered stressful life events than control subjects immediately prior to the onset or diagnosis of disease; in addition, stress had an unfavorable effect on disease prognosis. Graves' disease is generally considered to be a Th2-mediated syndrome. Since stress hormones induce a systemic Th2 shift, as discussed above, the activation of the stress system may affect the onset or course of Graves' disease. In fact, patients with Graves' disease have significantly higher serum levels of Th2 cytokines, and the disease is frequently associated with allergic rhinitis and other Th2-predominant conditions (Mizokami, Wu, El-Kaissi, & Wall, 2004).

In multiple sclerosis (MS), there is fairly consistent support for an association between stressful life events and disease exacerbation (Gold & Irwin, 2006; Mohr & Pelletier, 2006). However, the mechanism by which the stress response may affect susceptibility to or onset of MS remains poorly understood. In MS patients, $CD8^+$ T cells are increased between two- to threefold, compared with age-matched controls. Furthermore, immune cells from MS patients are less sensitive to GC-induced suppression of IL-6 and TNF (Arnason, Brown, Maselli, Karaszewski, & Reder, 1988). Thus, a hypoactive SNS, resulting in reduced tonic inhibition of Th1/proinflammatory responses, in combination with GC resistance, may facilitate or sustain the Th1 shift in MS and contribute to overshooting inflammation during relapses. The impact of stress on MS exacerbation likely depends on the co-occurrence of stressful life events and other factors that provoke MS exacerbation.

## 10. T-HELPER CELL COMMITMENT TOWARD SPECIFIC LINEAGES: THE ROLE OF THE TH17 SUBSET IN INFLAMMATION

T-helper cell precursors (Thp) can be skewed toward mutually exclusive Th1, Th2, Th17, and T regulatory cell ($T_{reg}$) phenotypes on the basis of the cytokine environment. Presence of IL-12 promotes skewing toward Th1. Th1 cells are characterized by producing IFNγ and IL-2. Th2 cell commitment is promoted by IL-4. Th2 committed cells are characterized by producing IL-4, IL-10, and IL-13. Development of both $T_{reg}$ and Th17 phenotypes requires the presence of TGF-β, but the presence of IL-6 preferentially tends the response toward a Th17 phenotype. $T_{regs}$ are characterized in mice by producing IL-10 and TGF-β, and Th17 is characterized by producing IL-17. Th1 and Th17 are proinflammatory and increase autoimmunity, while Th2 and $T_{reg}$ decrease autoimmunity.

On the other hand, in certain local responses and under particular conditions, stress hormones may actually facilitate inflammation through redeployment of immune cells and through induction of IL-1, IL-6, IL-8, TNFα, and the recently discovered IL-17. IL-17 (also known as IL-17A) is a proinflammatory cytokine that induces the expression of IL-1, IL-6, and G-CSF by fibroblasts, stromal cells, and endothelial cells, among others (Aggarwal & Gurney, 2002; Kolls & Linden, 2004; Gaffen, Kramer, Yu, & Shen, 2006). IL-17 is secreted by $CD4^+$ Th17 cells, which characteristically also produce IL-17F, IL-6, TNF-α (Langrish et al., 2005; Infante-Duarte, Horton, Byrne, & Kamradt, 2000), and IL-22 (Liang et al., 2006; Chung et al., 2006; Zheng et al., 2006). Indeed, this Th17 subset is now considered to be the critical pathogenic population during inflammation and autoimmunity. IL-17 expression has been associated with several human autoimmune diseases, including rheumatoid arthritis (RA) (Chabaud, Kallberg, Miossec, & Natvig, 1999; Kotake et al., 1999) and multiple sclerosis (MS) (Matusevicius et al., 1999; Lock et al., 2002), and its inhibition or depletion in the corresponding animal models has been shown to provide varying degrees of protection (Langrish et al., 2005; Komiyama et al., 2006; Park et al., 2005).

As an emerging T-cell subset, Th17 can help explain some of the known discrepancies in the Th1/Th2 paradigm of autoimmunity. Uncommitted (naive) murine $CD4^+$ T-helper precursors cells (Thp) can be induced to differentiate toward Th1, Th2, Th17, and regulatory ($T_{reg}$) phenotypes depending on the local cytokine milieu (Fig. 2). The presence of interleukin (IL)-12 [which signals through signal transduction and activator of transcription (STAT)-4] tends toward Th1; IL-4 (signaling through STAT-6) induces Th2 differentiation, transforming growth factor (TGF)-β tends toward $T_{reg}$, and IL-6 and TGF-β tend toward Th17. The committed cells are characterized by the expression of specific transcription factors, *T-bet* for Th1, *GATA-3* for Th2, forkhead box P3 (FoxP3) for $T_{regs}$, and *RORγt* for Th17 cells. It was recently shown that IL-6, and not IL-23 (Bettelli et al., 2006; Veldhoen, Hocking, Atkins, Locksley, & Stockinger, 2006; Mangan et al., 2006), is critical for the induction of Th17 lineage commitment. During inflammation, Th-cell phenotypes appear to be skewed toward proinflammatory lineages (Th17 and Th1) and away from anti-inflammatory phenotypes (Fig. 2).

If stress increases IL-6 and IL-1 secretion, it is possible that this increase regulates the adaptive immune system toward IL-17 production, along with a decrease in T regulatory cells, and may thus aggravate inflammatory diseases such as RA and psoriasis. This hypothesis is supported by the evidence that stress increases inflammation, which, in turn, leads to the outbreak of these diseases. The relation of stress, the Th17 population, and IL-17 will be an important issue for future study.

In conclusion, stress upregulates the production of IL-1 and IL-6 proinflammatory cytokines by monocytes/macrophages. These cytokines skew the response toward a Th17 phenotype and inhibit $T_{reg}$ and increased autoimmunity. However, glucocorticoids and catecholamines directly inhibit the production of IL-1 and IL-6, thus preventing inflammation and decreased autoimmunity.

## 11. SUMMARY

Communication between the central nervous system and the immune system occurs via a complex network of bidirectional signals linking the nervous, endocrine, and immune systems. The field of psychoneuroimmunology (PNI) has provided new insights to help understand the pathophysiological processes that are linked to the immune system. Work in this field has established that psychological stress affects the functional interaction between the nervous and the immune systems and regulates major immune functions such as antigen presentation, antibody production, lymphocyte activity, proliferation and traffic, and the secretion of cytokines including the selection of T helper (Th)1 versus Th2 cytokine responses. During inflammation, the activation of the stress system, through induction of a Th2 shift, protects the organism from systemic "overshooting" with excessive production of Th1/proinflammatory cytokines. Under certain conditions, however, stress hormones may actually facilitate inflammation through induction of interleukin (IL)-1, IL-6, IL-8, IL-18, tumor necrosis factor (TNF)-α, and, possibly, IL-17. Better understanding of the relationship between stress and immune system may provide critical insights into a variety of human immune-related diseases.

## REFERENCES

Aggarwal, S., & Gurney, A. L. (2002). IL-17: Prototype member of an emerging cytokine family. *Journal of Leukocyte Biology, 71*, 1–8.

Arnason, B. G., Brown, M., Maselli, R., Karaszewski, J., & Reder, A. (1988). Blood lymphocyte β-adrenergic receptors in multiple sclerosis. *Annals of the New York Academy of Sciences, 540*, 585–588.

Banks, W. A., & Kastin, A. J. (1985). Permeability of the blood–brain barrier to neuropeptides: The case for penetration. *Psychoneuroendocrinology, 10*, 385–399.

Banks, W. A., Ortiz, L., Plotkin, S. R., & Kastin, A. J. (1991). Human interleukin (IL) 1 alpha, murine IL-1 alpha and murine IL-1 beta are transported from blood to brain in the mouse by a shared saturable mechanism. *The Journal of Pharmacology and Experimental Therapeutics, 259*, 988–996.

Basedovsky, H. O., & del Rey, A. (2000). The cytokine-HPA axis feedback circuit. *Zeitschrift für Rheumatologie, 59*(Suppl. 2), 26–30.

Benacerraf, B. (1981). Role of MHC gene products in immune regulation. *Science, 212*, 1229–1238.

Betancur, C., Lledo, A., Borrell, J., & Guaza, C. (1994) Corticosteroid regulation of IL-1 receptors in the mouse hippocampus: Effects of glucocorticoid treatment, stress and adrenalectomy. *Neuroendocrinology, 59*, 120–128.

Bettelli, E., Carrier, Y., Gao, W., Korn, T., Strom, T. B., Oukka, M., et al. (2006). Reciprocal developmental pathways for the generation of pathogenic effector TH17 and regulatory T cells. *Nature, 441*, 235–238.

Beutler, B., Krochin, N., Milsark, I. W., Luedke, C., & Cerami, A. (1986). Control of cachectin (tumor necrosis factor) synthesis: Mechanisms of endotoxin resistance. *Science, 232*, 977–980.

Blotta, M. H., Dekruyff, R. H., & Umetsu, D. T. (1997). Corticosteroids inhibit IL-12 production in human monocytes and enhance their capacity to induce IL-4 synthesis in CD4lymphocytes????. *The Journal of Immunology, 158*, 5589–5595.

Boumpas, D. T., Chrousos, G. P., Wilder, R. L., Cupps, T. R., & Balow, J. E. (1993). Glucocorticoid therapy for immune-mediated diseases: Basic and clinical correlates. *Annals of Internal Medicine, 119*, 1198–1208.

Chabaud, A. T., Kallberg, M., Miossec, E., & Natvig, J. B. (1999). Human interleukin-17: A T cell-derived proinflammatory cytokine produced by the rheumatoid synovium. *Arthritis & Rheumatism, 42*, 963–970.

Chang, J. T., Segal, B. M., Nakanishi, K., Okamura, H., & Shevach, E. M. (2000). The costimulatory effect of IL-18 on the induction of antigen-specific IFN-gamma production by resting T cells is IL-12 dependent and is mediated by up-regulation of the IL-12 receptor beta2 subunit. *European Journal of Immunology, 30*, 1113–1119.

Chung, Y., Yang, X., Chang, S. H., Ma, L., Tian, Q., & Dong, C. (2006). Expression and regulation of IL-22 in the IL-17-producing CD4+ T lymphocytes. *Cell Research, 16*, 902–907.

Coffman, R. L. (2006). Origins of the T(H)1-T(H)2 model: A personal perspective. *Nature Immunology, 7*, 539–541.

Colotta, F., Re, F., Muzio, M., Bertini, R., Polentarutti, N., Sironi, M., et al. (1993). Interleukin-1 type II receptor: A decoy target for IL-1 that is regulated by IL-4. *Science, 261*, 472–475.

Connor, T. J., Song, C., Leonard, B. E., Merali, Z., & Anisman, H. (1998). An assessment of the effects of central interleukin-1β, -2, -6, and tumor necrosis factor-α administration on some behavioral, neuro-chemical, endocrine and immune parameters in the rat. *Neuroscience, 84*, 923–933.

Connor, T. J., Kelly, J. P., & Leonard, B. E. (1997). Forced swim test-induced neurochemical endocrine, and immune changes in the rat. *Pharmacology Biochemistry and Behavior, 58*, 961–967.

Dantzer, R. (1994). How do cytokines say hello to the brain? Neural versus humoral mediation. *European Cytokine Network, 5*, 271–273.

Daynes, R. A., Araneo, B. A., Dowell, T. A., Huang, K., & Dudley, D. (1990). Regulation of murine lymphokine production in vivo. III. The lymphoid tissue microenvironment exerts regulatory influences over T helper cell function. *The Journal of Experimental Medicine, 171*, 979–996.

De Bosscher, K., Schmitz, M. L., Vanden Berghe, W., Plaisance, S., Fiers, W., et al. (1997). Glucocorticoid-mediated repression of nuclear factor-κB-dependent transcription involved direct interference with transactivation. *Proceedings of the National Academy of Sciences, USA, 94*, 13504–13509.

De Rijk, R., Boelen, F. J. H., Tilders, S., & Berkenbusch, F. (1994). Induction of plasma interleukin-6 by circulating adrenaline in the rat. *Psychoneuroendocrinology, 19*, 155–163.

Dhabhar, F. S., Millar, A. H., Mcewen, B. S., & Spencer, R. L. (1995). Effects of stress on immune cell distribution. Dynamics and hormonal mechanisms. *Journal of Immunology, 154*, 5511–5527.

Elenkov, I. J., & Chrousos, G. P. (2002). Stress hormones, proinflammatory and antiinflammatory cytokines, and autoimmunity. *Annals of the New York Academy of Sciences, 966*, 290–303.

Elenkov, I. J., & Chrousos, G. P. (1999). Stress hormones, Th1/Th2 patterns, pro/anti-inflammatory cytokines and susceptibility to disease. *Trends in Endocrinology and Metabolism, 10*, 359–368.

Elenkov, I. J., Wilder, R. L., Chrousos, G. P., & Vizi, E. S. (2000). The sympathetic nerve – an integrative interface between two supersystems: The brain and the immune system. *Pharmacological Reviews, 52*, 595–638.

Elenkov, I. J., Papanicolau, D. A., Wilder, R. L., & Chrousos, G. P. (1996). Modulatory effects of glucocorticoids and catecholamines on human interleukin-12 and interleukin-10 production: Clinical implications. *Proceedings of the Association of American Physicians, 108*, 374–381.

Gaffen, S. L., Kramer, J. M., Yu, J. J., & Shen, F. (2006).The IL-17 cytokine family. *Vitamins and Hormones, 74*, 255–282.

Gold, S. M., & Irwin, M. R. (2006). Depression and immunity: Inflammation and depressive symptoms in multiple sclerosis. *Neurologic clinics, 24*, 507–519.

Gold, S. M., Mohr, D. C., Huitinga, I., Flachenecker, P., Sternberg, E. M., & Heesen, C. (2005). The role of stress-response systems for the pathogenesis and progression of MS. *Trends in Immunology, 26*, 644–652.

Groujon, E., Layé, S., Parnet, P., & Dantzer, R. (1997). Regulation of cytokine gene expression in the central nervous system by glucocorticoids: Mechanisms and functional consequences. *Psychoneuroendocrinology, 22*, S75–S80.

Gutierrez, E. G., Banks, W. A., & Kastin, A. J. (1994). Blood-borne interleukin-1 receptor antagonist crosses the blood–brain barrier. *Journal of Neuroimmunology, 55*, 153–160.

Gutierrez, E. G., Banks, W. A., & Kastin, A. J. (1993). Murine tumor necrosis factor alpha is transported from blood to brain in the mouse. *Journal of Neuroimmunology, 47*, 169–176.

Holsboer, F. (2000). The corticosteroid receptor hypothesis of depression. *Neuropsychopharmacology, 23*, 477–501.

Hopkins, S. J., & Rothwell, N. J. (1995). Cytokines and the nervous system. I: Expression and recognition. *Trends in Neurosciences, 18*, 83–88.

Infante-Duarte, C., Horton, H. F., Byrne, M. C., & Kamradt, T. (2000). Microbial lipopeptides induce the production of IL-17 in Th cells. *Journal of Immunology, 165*, 6107–6115.

Irwin, M. R., Wang, M., Campomayor, C. O., Collado-Hidalgo, A., & Cole, S. (2006). Sleep deprivation and activation of morning levels of cellular and genomic markers of inflammation. *Archives of Internal Medicine, 166*, 1756–1762.

Kolls, J. K., & Lindén, A. (2004). Interleukin-17 family members and inflammation. *Immunity, 21*, 467–476.

Komiyama, Y., Nakae, S., Matsuki, T., Nambu, A., Ishigame, H., Kakuta, S., et al. (2006). IL-17 plays an important role in the development of experimental autoimmune encephalomyelitis. *Journal of Immunology, 177*, 566–573.

Konsman, J. P., Parnet, P., & Dantzer, R. (2002). Cytokine-induced sickness behaviour: mechanisms and implications. *Trends in Neurosciences, 25*, 154–159.

Kotake, S., Udagawa, N., Takahashi, N., Matsuzaki, K., Itoh, K., Ishiyama, S., et al. (1999). IL-17 in synovial fluids from patients with rheumatoid arthritis is a potent stimulator of osteoclastogenesis. *The Journal of Clinical Investigation, 103*, 1345–1352.

Kunicka, J. E., Talle, M. A., Denhardt, G. H., Brown, M., Prince, L. A., & Goldstein, G. (1993). Immunosuppression by glucocorticoids: Inhibition of production of multiple lymphokines by in vivo administration of dexamethasone. *Cellular Immunology, 149*, 39–49.

Langrish, C. L., Chen, Y., Blumenschein, W. M., Mattson, J., Basham, B., Sedgwick, J. D., et al. (2005). IL-23 drives a pathogenic T cell population that induces autoimmune inflammation. *The Journal of Experimental Medicine, 201*, 233–240.

Laye, S., Parnet, P., Goujon, E., & Dantzer, R. (1994). Peripheral administration of lipopolysaccharide induces the expression of cytokine transcripts in the brain and pituitary of mice. *Molecular Brain Research, 27*, 157–162.

Leonard B. E. (1995). Stress and the immune system: Immunological aspects of depressive illness. In B. E. Leonard & K. Miller (Eds), *Stress, the immune system and psychiatry* (pp. 114–136). Oxford: John Wiley and Sons Ltd.

Lesperance, F., Frasure-Smith, N., Theroux, P., & Irwin, M. (2004). The association between major depression and levels of soluble intercellular adhesion molecule 1, interleukin-6, and C-reactive protein in patients with recent acute coronary syndromes. *Journal of the American Psychiatric, 161*, 271–277.

Liang, S. C., Tan, X. Y., Luxenberg, D. P., Karim, R., Dunussi-Joannopoulos, K., Collins, M., et al. (2006). Interleukin (IL)-22 and IL-17 are coexpressed by Th17 cells and cooperatively enhance expression of antimicrobial peptides. *The Journal of Experimental Medicine, 203*, 2271–2279.

Lock, C., Hermans, G., Pedotti, R., Brendolan, A., Schadt, E., Garren, H., et al. (2002). Gene-microarray analysis of multiple sclerosis lesions yields new targets validated in autoimmune encephalomyelitis. *Nature Medicine, 8*, 500–508.

Mangan, P. R., Harrington, L. E., O'Quinn, D. B., Helms, W. S., Bullard, D. C., Elson, C. O., et al. (2006). Transforming growth factor-beta induces development of the T (H) 17 lineage. *Nature, 441*, 231–234.

Mastorakos, G., Pavlatou, M., Diamanti-Kandarakis, E., & Chrousos, G. P. (2005). Exercise and the stress system. *Hormones, 4*, 73–89.

Matusevicius, D., Kivisakk, P., He, B., Kostulas, N., Ozenci, V., Fredrikson, S., et al. (1999). Interleukin-17 mRNA expression in blood and CSF mononuclear cells is augmented in multiple sclerosis. *Multiple Sclerosis, 5*, 101–104.

Merali, Z., Lacosta, S., & Anisman, H. (1997). Effects of interleukin-1beta and mild stress on alterations of norepinephrine, dopamine and serotonin neurotransmission: A regional microdialysis study. *Brain Research, 761*, 225–235.

Mizokami, T., Wu Li, A, El-Kaissi, S., & Wall, J. R. (2004). Stress and thyroid autoimmunity. *Thyroid, 14*, 1047–1055.

Mohr, D. C., & Pelletier, D. (2006). A temporal framework for understanding the effects of stressful life events on inflammation in patients with multiple sclerosis. *Brain, Behavior, and Immunity, 20*, 27–36.

Mosmann, T. R., Cherwinski, H., Bond, M. W., Giedlin, M. A., & Coffman, R. L. (1986). Two types of murine helper T cell clone. I. Definition according to profiles of lymphokine activities and secreted proteins. *Journal of Immunology, 136*, 2348–2357.

Moss, R. B., Moll, T., El-Kalay, M., Kohne, C., Soo Hoo, W., Encinas, J., & et al. (2004). Thl/Th2 cells in inflammatory disease states: therapeutic implications. *Expert Opinion on Biological Therapy, 4*, 1887–1896.

Munck, A., & Guyre, P. M. (1991). Glucocorticoids and immune function. In R. Ader, D. L. Felten, & N. Cohen (Eds.), *Psychoneuroimmunology* (2nd ed., pp. 447–474). San Diego: Academic Press.

Musselman, D. L., Miller, A. H., Porter, M. R., Manatunga, A. K., Gao, F., Penna, S., et al. (2003). Suppression of immune induction of collagen-induced arthritis in IL-17-deficient mice. *Journal of Immunology, 171*, 6173–6177.

Pace, T. W., Mletzko, T. C., Alagbe, O., Musselman, D. L. Nemeroff, C. B. Miller, A. H., et al. (2006). Increased stress-induced inflammatory responses in male patients with major depression and increased early life stress. *The American Journal of Psychiatry, 163*, 1630–1633.

Paez Pereda, M., Perez Castro, C., Costas, M., Nahmod, V. E., Stalla G. K., Holsboer, F., et al. (1996). Glucocorticoids inhibit the auto-regulatory induction of interleukin-1 in monocytes after endotoxin stimulation. *Neuroimmunomodulation, 3*, 227–232.

Pariante, C. M., & Miller, A. H. (2001). Glucocorticoid receptors in major depression: Relevance to pathophysiology and treatment. *Biological Psychiatry, 49*, 391–404.

Park, H., Li, Z., Yang, X. O., Chang, S. H., Nurieva, R., Wang, Y. H., et al. (2005). A distinct lineage of CD4 T cells regulates tissue inflammation by producing interleukin 17. *Nature Immunology, 6*, 1133–1141.

Path, G., Bornstein, S. R., Ehrhart-Bornstein, M., & Scherbaum, W. A. (1997). Interleukin-6 and the interleukin-6 receptor in the human adrenal gland: Expression and effects on steroidogenesis. *Journal of Clinical Endocrinology & Metabolism, 82*, 2343–2349.

Perlstein, R. S., Mougey, E. H., Jackson, W. E., & Neta, R. (1991). Interleukin-1 and interleukin-6 act synergistically to stimulate the release of adrenocorticotropic hormone in vivo. *Lymphokine Cytokine Research, 10*, 141–146.

Plagemann, A., Staudt, A., Gotz, F., Malz, U., Rohde, W., Rake, A., et al. (1998). Long-term effects of early postnatally administered interleukin-1β on the hypothalamic–pituitary–adrenal (HPA) axis in rats. *Endocrine Regulation, 32*, 77–85.

Raison, C. L., & Miller, A. H. (2003). When not enough is too much: The role of insufficient glucocorticoid signaling in the pathophysiology of stress-related disorders. *American Journal of Psychiatry, 160*, 1554–1565.

Raison, C. L., Capuron, L., & Miller, A. H. (2006). Cytokines sing the blues: Inflammation and the pathogenesis of depression. *Trends in Immunology, 27*, 24–31.

Rivest, S. (2003). Molecular insights on the cerebral innate immune system. *Brain, Behavior, and Immunity, 17*, 13–19.

Rogers, M. P., & Fozdar, M. (1996). Psychoneuroimmunology of autoimmune disorders. *Advances in Neuroimmunology, 6*, 169–177.

Romagnani, S. (1994). Human Thl and Th2 subsets: "eppur si muove" [review]. *European Cytokine Network, 5*, 7–12.

Safieh-Garabedian, B., Poole, S., Haddad, J. J., Massaad, C. A., Jabbur, S. J., & Saadé, N. E. (2002). The role of the sympathetic efferents in endotoxin-induced localized inflammatory hyperalgesia and cytokine upregulation. *Neuropharmacology, 42*, 864–872.

Saper, C. B., & Breder, C. D. (1992). Endogenous pyrogens in the CNS: Role in the febrile response. *Progress in Brain Research, 93*, 419–428.

Schmidt, M., Pauels, H.-G., Lügering, N., Lügering, A., Domschke, W., & Kucharzik, T. (1999). Glucocorticoids induce apoptosis in human monocytes: Potential role of IL-1β. *Journal of Immunology, 163*, 3484–3490.

Schöbitz, B., De Kloet, E. R., & Holsboer, F. (1994). Gene expression and function of interleukin 1, interleukin 6 and tumor necrosis factor in the brain. *Progress in Neurobiology, 44*, 397–432.

Schöbitz, B., de Kloet, E. R., Sutanto, W., & Holsboer, F. (1993). Cellular localization of interleukin 6 mRNA and interleukin 6 receptor mRNA in rat brain. *European Journal of Neuroscience, 5*, 1426–1435.

Shavit, Y., Lewis, J. W., Terman, G. W., Gale, R. P., & Liebeskind, J. C. (1984). Opioid peptides mediate the suppressive effect of stress on natural killer cell cytotoxicity. *Science, 223*, 188–190.

Shintani, F., Nakaki, T., Kanba, S., Sato, K., Yagi, G., & Shiozawa, M., et al. (1995). Involvement of interleukin-1 in immobilization stress-induced increase in plasma adrenocorticotropic hormone and in release of hypothalamic monoamines in the rat. *The Journal of Neuroscience, 15*, 1961–1970.

Shu, J., Stevenson, J. R., & Zhou, X. (1993). Modulation of cellular immune responses by cold water swim stress in the rat. *Developmental and Comparative Immunology, 17*, 357–371.

Sternberg, E. M. (2001). Neuroendocrine regulation of autoimmune/inflammatory disease. *Journal of Endocrinology, 169*, 429–435.

Takaki, A., Huang, Q. H., Somogyvári-Vigh, A., & Arimura, A. (1994). Immobilization stress may increase plasma interleukin-6 via central and peripheral catecholamines. *Neuroimmunomodulation, 1*, 335–342.

Van Der Poll, T., Barber, A. E., Coyle, S. M., & Lowry, S. F. (1996). Hypercortisolemia increases plasma interleukin-10 concentrations during human endotoxemia – A clinical research center study. *Journal of Clinical Endocrinology & Metabolism, 81*, 3604–3606.

Vanden Berghe, W., Vermeulen, L., De Wilde, G., De Bosscher, K., Boone, E., & Haegeman, G. (2000). Signal transduction by tumor necrosis factor and gene regulation of the inflammatory cytokine interleukin-6. *Biochemical Pharmacology, 60*, 1185–1195.

Veldhoen, M., Hocking, R. J., Atkins, C. J., Locksley, R. M., & Stockinger, B. (2006). TGFbeta in the context of an inflammatory cytokine milieu supports de novo differentiation of IL-17-producing T cells. *Immunity, 24*, 179–189.

Woiciechowsky, C., Schoning, B., Daberkow, N., Asche, K., Stoltenburg, G., Lanksch, W. R., et al. (1999). Brain-IL-1β induces local inflammation but systemic anti-inflammatory response through stimulation of both hypothalamic–pituitary–adrenal axis and sympathetic nervous system. *Brain Research, 816*, 563–571.

Wong, G. H. W., Barteltt, P. F., Clark-Lewis, I., Battye, F., & Schrader, J. W. (1984). Inducible expression of H-2 and Ia antigens on brain cells. *Nature, 310*, 688–691.

Yoshimoto, T., Takeda, K., Tanaka, T., Ohkusu, K., Kashiwamura, S., Okamura, H., et al. (1998). IL-12 up-regulates IL-18 receptor expression on T cells, Th1 cells, and B cells: synergism with IL-18 for IFN-gamma production. *The Journal of Immunology, 161*, 3400–3407.

Zautra, A. J., Yocum, D. C., Villanueva, I., Smith, B., Davis, M. C., Attrep, J., et al. (2004). Immune activation and depression in women with rheumatoid arthritis. *The Journal of Rheumatology, 31*, 457–463.

Zheng, Y., Danilenko, D. M., Valdez, P., Kasman, I., Eastham-Anderson, J., Wu, J., et al. (2006). Interleukin-22, a T(H)17 cytokine, mediates IL-23-induced dermal inflammation and acanthosis. *Nature, 445*, 648–651.

Zhou, D., Kusnecov, A. W., Shurin, M. R., DePaoli, M., & Rabin, B. S. (1993). Exposure to physical and psychological stressors elevates plasma interleukin 6: Relationship to the activation of hypothalamic-pituitary-adrenal axis. *Endocrinology, 133*, 2523–2530.

Zhou, D., Shanks, N., Riechman, S. E., Liang, R., Kusnecov, A. W., & Rabin, B. S. (1996). Interleukin 6 modulates interleukin-1-and stress-induced activation of the hypothalamic-pituitary-adrenal axis in male rats. *Neuroendocrinology, 63*, 227–236.

Zlotnik, A. (1996). Mouse IL-17: A cytokine preferentially expressed by alpha beta TCR + CD4-CD8-T cells. *Journal of Interferon and Cytokine Research, 16*, 611–617.

Zorrilla, E. P., Luborsky, L., McKay, J. R., Rosenthal, R., Houldin, A., Tax, A., et al. (2001). The relationship of depression and stressors to immunological assays: A meta-analytic review. *Brain, Behavior, and Immunity, 15*, 199–226.

# III

# Diagnostic and Clinical Aspects in CNS Disorders

# 13 MRI of Brain Iron and Neurodegenerative Diseases: A Potential Biomarker

*John F. Schenck*

**Summary**

- Magnetic resonance imaging (MRI) brain imaging at high field strengths can demonstrate regions of high iron deposition in the brain.
- Iron deposits are present in all normal adult brains, but increased or decreased iron deposition may serve as a biomarker of brain diseases.
- Several rare genetic disorders are now known which have marked increases in brain iron. The specific mutations associated with these are known, and MRI can demonstrate the abnormal iron deposition with remarkable clarity.
- Brain iron may play a role in many common neurodegenerative diseases, including Alzheimer's and Parkinson's diseases. This may permit the use of MRI of brain iron as a biomarker for the presence and progression of these diseases.
- New MRI scanners operating at very high magnetic field strengths are becoming available and permit greatly improved clarity in brain iron images.

**Key Words::** Brain iron; magnetic resonance imaging; neurodegenerative diseases; aceruloplasminemia

## 1. INTRODUCTION

The purpose of this chapter is to describe recent developments in the field of brain iron and to describe the capabilities and limitations of magnetic resonance imaging (MRI) in the study of the relation between brain iron and disease. We will begin with a brief sketch of the history of brain iron research and its relation to neurological disorders. This sketch cannot come close to providing complete recognition of the many workers who have contributed to this field, but recent detailed historical reviews are available (Hill, 1988; Koeppen, 1995, 2003). More than 120 years ago, in 1886, a German researcher, S. S. Zaleski, reported on the presence of a remarkable level of iron present in the human brain. Working with a single autopsied brain, he made several observations that have stood the test of time.

- This iron is not in the form of iron salts; instead, it is bound to organic molecules. However, it is completely independent of hemoglobin.

From: *Nutrition and Health: Iron Deficiency and Overload*
Edited by: S. Yehuda and D.I. Mostofsky, DOI 10.1007/978-1-59745-462-9_13

- The iron is in the ferric not the ferrous oxidation state.
- This iron is more prevalent in gray matter than in white matter.

Decades were required for this work to be confirmed and extended. As described by Koeppen (1995, 2003), a German pathologist, Hugo Spatz, in 1922 published a detailed study of the regional distribution of brain iron. Spatz and others demonstrated the presence of ferric iron in brain sections by use of hydrochloric acid followed by potassium ferrocyanide (Perls' stain) to produce the bright blue precipitate known as Prussian blue or Berlin blue. Spatz demonstrated a strong concentration of ferric iron in the deep brain nuclei of the extrapyramidal motor system. These nuclei include the globus pallidus, the caudate nucleus, the red nucleus, the dentate nucleus, and the substantia nigra (Figs. 1 and 2A).

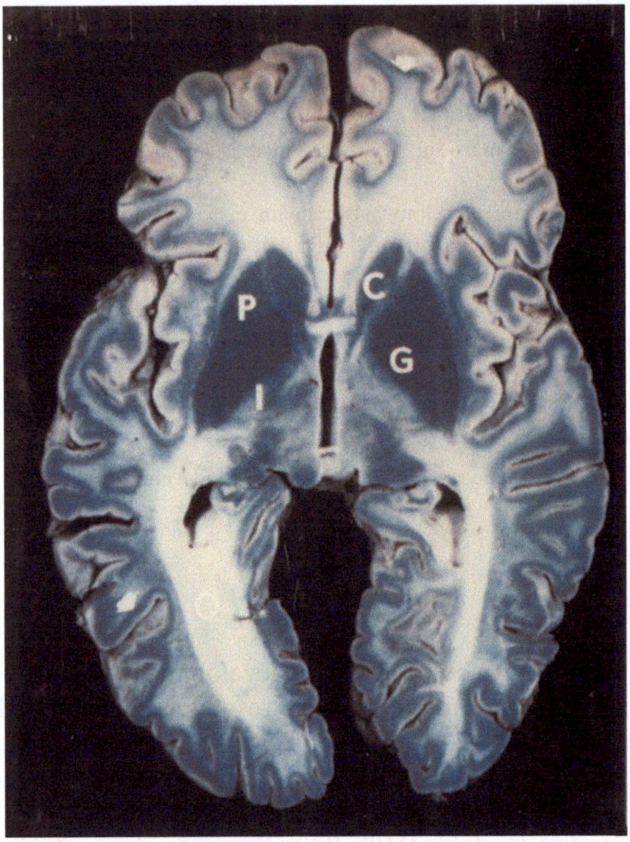


**Fig. 1.** Perls' stained brain section. The regions of highest iron concentration stain a *bright blue* and appear dark in this image. These iron-rich regions include the globus pallidus (G), the putamen (P) and the caudate nucleus (C), Additional evidence of iron staining is present in the frontal white matter (F), the optic radiation (O), the internal capsule (I), and in the subcortical U-fibers. (Reprinted from Drayer et al., 1986, with permission from the American Society of Neuroradiology.)

Also in 1922, Spatz and his student, Julius Hallervordern, described a family with several children suffering from a severe developmental disorder characterized by heavy brain iron accumulation. This disorder, known as Hallervorden-Spatz disease or syndrome, became the prototypical example of a brain disease characterized by excessive iron storage. Because of concerns regarding unethical behavior in the 1930s and 1940s, there has been a recent effort to

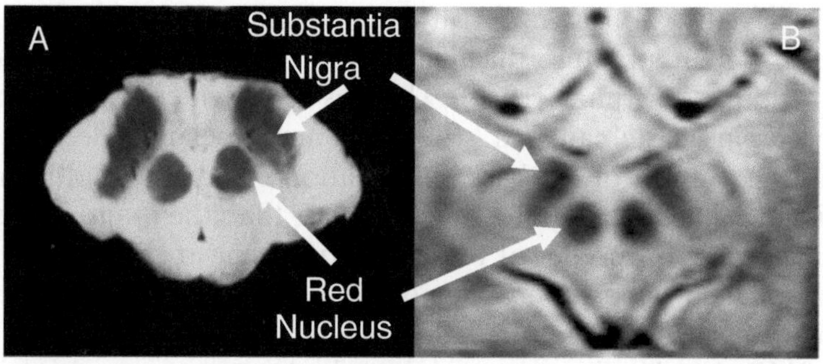


**Fig. 2.** Perls' stain and MRI of brain stem. (A) Perls' stain of brain stem showing the red nucleus (RN) and the substantia nigra (pars reticulata) of the same subject as in Fig. 1. (B) T2-weighted spin echo MR image at 4 T of the corresponding region of a healthy volunteer. Note the close correspondence between the hypointense regions of the MR image and of the regions of heavy Perls' staining. (Panel A reprinted from Drayer et al., 1986, with permission from the American Society of Neuroradiology.)

change the name of the disorder away from the Hallervorden-Spatz eponym to neurodegeneration with brain iron accumulation, Type I (NBIA1) (Geiderman, 2003; Hayflick et al., 2003). As discussed below, disorders of iron metabolism have more recently been established as a feature of a number of other rare genetic diseases.

It is important to note that, in addition to rare genetic disorders, various investigators have found a relationship between brain iron and much more common brain diseases. There were early reports of iron involvement in Alzheimer's disease (Goodman, 1953), multiple sclerosis (Craelius, Migdal, Luessenhop, Sugar, & Mihalakis, 1982), and Parkinson's disease (Dexter et al., 1987). Various technical and research advances have led to a large number of subsequent studies of iron and other metals in neurodegenerative diseases. and it is possible to list only a sample (Ye, Allen, & Martin, 1996; Bartzokis, Cummings, Markham, et al., 1999; Bartzokis, Cummings, Perlman, Hance, & Mintz, 1999; Vymazal, Urgosik, & Bulte, 2000; Rouault, 2001; Grabill, Silva, Smith, Koretsky, & Rouault, 2003; Connor et al., 2003; Perry et al., 2003; Zecca, Zucca, Wilms, & Sulzer, 2003; Schenck et al., 2006; House, St Pierre, & McLean, 2008; Adlard et al., 2008; Barnham & Bush, 2008; Shibata et al., 2008; McNeill et al., 2008) and several book-length treatments are available (Youdim, 1988; Connor, 1997; Testa, 2002; Zata, 2003; Levine, Connor, & Schipper, 2004; Crichton & Ward, 2006). High-resolution MRI of transgenic mice has recently provided evidence for the association of iron with amyloid plaques (Jack et al., 2005).

MRI entered clinical medicine in the early 1980 s and high-resolution brain images became possible at a field strength of 1.5 tesla shortly after that. In this technique image contrast depends largely on differences from one brain region to another in the relaxation times, T1 and T2, of the magnetic spins associated with the protons in the tissue water molecules (Bernstein, King, & Zhou, 2004). With the advent of high-field (1.5 tesla), whole-body superconducting magnets, it was noticed (Drayer et al., 1986) that MR images designed to emphasize contrast based on regional T2 variations (T2-weighted imaging) showed markedly decreased signal intensities (hypointensities) in the same brain regions that had previously been identified in autopsy studies as having high iron concentrations (Fig. 2).

Much of the non-heme iron in the brain is believed to be present as a mineralized iron oxide linked to protein either as ferritin or hemosiderin. The ferritin molecule is a soluble spherical protein shell surrounding a core, which can contain up to 4,500 iron atoms as the iron oxide ferrihydrite (Crichton, 2001). Hemosiderin is insoluble and is much less well characterized than ferritin. It is also believed to consist of ferrihydrite or similar iron oxide granules linked to a relatively disordered protein structure that may result from lysosomal degradation of ferritin protein (Wixom, Prutkin, & Munro, 1980). There is also evidence for additional brain iron associated with lipofuscin (Castelnau et al., 1998) and neuromelanin (Zecca et al., 2003).

It is worth noting that much of the basic information on ferritin and hemosiderin has been derived from studies in other species and on organs other than the brain. Therefore, it is possible that there are brain-specific properties of these materials that are yet to be discovered, and, at present, the details of iron deposition and mobilization and the magnetic properties of the mineralized iron oxide particles in brain remain somewhat uncertain.

The rapid loss of MR signal in tissues containing a high iron concentration is attributed to the field-induced magnetization of microscopic iron oxide particles. This produces a magnetic field of microscopic dimensions that is superimposed on the uniform magnetic field produced by the MR scanner. Water molecules diffuse through this microscopic field inhomogeneity, and the phase coherence of their spins is disrupted and this leads to the loss of MRI signal intensity from the region. Because this magnetization and the resulting field inhomogeneities increase linearly with applied field strength, iron-dependent contrast becomes much more prominent as the field strength is increased (Schenck, 1995). As mentioned above, this contrast mechanism was first observed in scanners operating at 1.5 tesla. Scanners operating at 3 tesla are becoming more common in clinical practice, and in 2008 they represent about 4% of the scanners in service. With these high-field scanners it is possible to resolve finer details of the distribution of brain iron. Theoretical analyses indicate that the effectiveness of iron deposits in reducing the T2 of the tissue is increased by the fact that these deposits form granular clusters rather than being uniformly distributed across the cells and tissues (Jensen & Chandra, 2000a, 2000b).

In addition to the use of MRI in brain iron studies, the past two decades have seen dramatic advances in the genetics, bioinorganic chemistry, and cell biology of brain iron. Also, a number of advanced x-ray and other imaging techniques have been applied to the study of brain iron in postmortem tissue (Collingwood et al., 2005; Pankhurst, Hautot, Khan, & Dobson, 2008). The result of this has been a rapid increase in the depth of knowledge and in the number of papers being published in this area (Fig. 3). In 2007, approximately one new paper on brain iron paper was published every day.

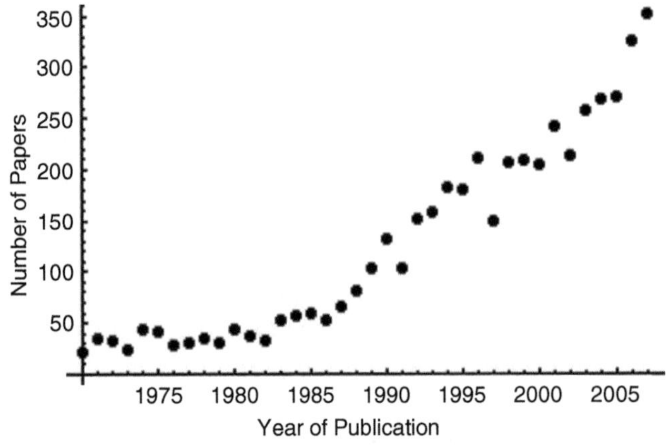


**Fig. 3.** Number of research papers published per year containing the phrase "brain iron" from 1970–2007. The data are from the PubMed database. Of the approximately 4,700 papers on this topic published during this period, more than 1,200 (26%) were published from 2004 through 2007.

## 2. OTHER FORMS OF IRON IN THE BRAIN

To avoid confusion it is important to separate clearly the phenomenon of endogenous brain iron located in the brain parenchyma, which is the subject of this chapter, from various other forms of iron found in the brain. Each of these forms of brain iron has characteristic MRI findings as well as an extensive literature. These other iron-dependent phenomena include the following:

- Iron in the blood. Each hemoglobin molecule contains four iron atoms. In the blood-oxygen-level-dependent (BOLD) contrast mechanism, deoxygenated hemoglobin produces a reduction in the MRI signal from the vicinity of the various blood vessels in the brain. This is the basis of functional magnetic resonance imaging (fMRI) (Small et al., 2000; Logothetis, 2008).
- Intracerebral hemorrhage. Also known as hemorrhagic stroke or subarachnoid hemorrhage, this condition leads to large-scale extravasation of blood into the brain tissue. As the hemorrhage is gradually resolved, the hemoglobin iron is processed into ferritin or hemosiderin forms of iron storage that produce a characteristic time sequence of MRI findings (Bradley, 1993).
- Microhemorrhage. This represents small, localized hemorrhages into brain tissue. These are associated with smoking, hypertension, aging, and other neurological conditions. They are seen as small regions of MRI signal loss on T2-weighted images that are usually less than 5 mm in diameter. (Viswanathan & Chabriat, 2006).
- Superficial siderosis. In this disorder a slow leakage of blood into the subarachnoid space is believed to lead an encrustation of hemosiderin deposits on CNS surfaces, particularly those of the brainstem, cerebellum, and spinal cord (Koeppen, Dickson, Chu, & Thach, 1993).
- Exogenous iron agents. Small iron oxide particles can be injected into the blood and targeted to specific regions of the body to provide an exogenous form of MR contrast agent (Bulte& Modo, 2008). For example, such particles, when taken up by brain macrophages, can be used to demonstrate inflammation in experimental stroke models (Tang et al., 2006).

Biological processes involving these other forms of iron need have no direct relation to the biology of endogenous brain iron, and the MRI findings in these various situations should not be confused with one another. For example, the deposition of ferritin and hemosiderin is invoked to describe both the deposition of parenchymal brain iron in the normally developing brain and the storage and detoxification of heme iron following brain hemorrhage. At a microscopic level, however, it is likely that the molecular details of the iron chemistry in these distinct processes are not closely related.

## 3. BIOLOGY OF BRAIN IRON AND COPPER

Metals are increasingly recognized to play a highly significant role in tissue and cell biology (Lippard & Berg, 1994; Williams & Silva 1996; Silva & Williams, 2001; Bertini, Gray, Stiefel, & Valentine, 2007). Consideration of the various metals and their interactions within tissues has led to the concept of a metallome within cells, analogous to the genome and the proteome (Williams, 2001), and the study of metals in brain function and disease can be considered as an emerging discipline in transitional medicine (Williams, 2003; Burdette & Lippard, 2003; Schipper, 2004; Schenck, 2005; Zecca, Youdim, Riederer, Connor, & Crichton, 2004; Bush & Curtain, 2008). In brain research, much of the recent attention has focused on the metals iron, zinc, and copper. Iron and copper each can exist in more than one charge state and readily participate in redox reactions, which lead to tissue damage through the generation of toxic free radicals (Halliwell & Gutteridge,

1999; Perry et al., 2002, 2003). They can each carry magnetic moments and, unlike zinc, they can potentially affect the nuclear magnetic signal produced by the water protons within tissues. Metal chelation is a potential mode of treatment for these brain disorders (Richardson, 2004; Zecca et al., 2004).

A uniformly distributed background iron concentration, identical in all regions of the brain, would give only a uniform contribution to the T2 relaxation and would be superimposed on the relaxation produced by many other water interactions within the tissues. As a result, such a uniform concentration would be of little interest in MRI other than to comprise one of many contributions to the T2 values of the cells and tissues of interest. However, when there is a significant variation in iron concentration from cell to cell and region to region, the iron contribution to T2 relaxation will also vary and will produce an endogenous contrast mechanism that can function as a biomarker of brain diseases (Schenck & Zimmerman, 2004; Haacke et al., 2005).

Iron and copper are essential for basic cell functions such as electron transport in mitochondria and as active elements in a very large number of metalloproteins such as ribonucleotide reductase. Therefore, it is expected that there will be a baseline cellular concentration of the essential metals required to meet housekeeping functions required of all cells. Studies on yeast and bacteria indicate that the baseline concentration for iron is approximately 0.1 mM and for copper it is approximately 0.01 mM (Outten & O'Halloran, 2001; Finney & O'Halloran, 2003).

Quantitative measurements of parenchymal brain copper and iron content have been reported by a few investigators. Cumings (1948) reviewed earlier studies and also reported iron and copper content in six normal brains. Hallgren and Sourander (1958) reported the non-heme iron concentrations in various brain regions from a series of 98 autopsies of people who died without evidence of neuropsychiatric or cerebrovascular disease and whose ages ranged up to 100 years. They did not report on copper concentration. Some results of these studies are given in Table 1. For reference convenience, these concentration values are given in various units: mg/cc, mM, and iron or copper atoms/cc.

Table 1 suggests that, averaged over the entire brain, there are approximately 8 iron atoms for every copper atom and there is a significant variation in the concentration of both elements from one brain region to another. The concentrations in Table 1 should be viewed as approximate for several reasons; (i) the conversion factor between dry and wet tissue concentrations is only an estimate and would be expected to vary from one laboratory's protocol to another, (ii) age and gender of the subjects are not accounted for in this table, (iii) an uncertain amount of iron and copper will inevitably be lost during sample preparation and (iv) the subjects studied were from localized populations (Sweden, Japan and the United Kingdom). Furthermore, there is good evidence that the iron concentration can vary strongly from one cell to its nearest neighbors (Morris, et al., 1992). This suggests that in a given brain region there are some cells with much higher than average iron concentration and vice versa.

Table 2 summarizes these findings to provide baseline values for iron and copper in normal adult human brains which have had all blood removed and which have not experienced pre-mortem bleeding into the brain. In using these values it should be remembered that the results were obtained from difficult measurements on a limited number of cases. The results on individual brains showed a substantial variation and the tabulated results should be viewed as approximations. It is seen that, for both iron and copper in the brain, the overall concentrations are well above the minimal housekeeping levels, indicating that the brain has a specific affinity for these elements, presumably reflecting specific metabolic requirements.

Table 1

**Tissue Iron and Copper Concentrations in Normal Adult Humans. The adult brain mass is taken as 1,470 g (Blinkov & Glezer, 1968). Values reported in terms of brain dry weight were divided by 5.65 to convert to estimated wet weight values (Koeppen, 1995). The relatively wide range of values reported by different investigators for some regions may result from differing techniques or from individual differences in the brains studied.**

| | *Iron* | | | *Copper* | | |
|---|---|---|---|---|---|---|
| *Brain Region* | *Density (mg/cc)* | *Molarity (mM)* | *Density ($10^{16}$ Fe atoms/cc)* | *Density (mg/cc)* | *Molarity (mM)* | *Density ($10^{16}$ Cu atoms/cc)* |
| Whole Brain[2] | 0.041 | 0.73 | 44 | – | – | – |
| Whole Brain[1,4] | – | – | – | 0.0057 | 0.089 | 5.4 |
| Cortex[1,4] | 0.064 | 1.1 | 69 | 0.0084 | 0.13 | 8.0 |
| Cortex[2,5] | 0.041 | 0.73 | 44 | – | – | – |
| Globus Pallidus[1] | 0.20 | 3.6 | 215 | 0.026 | 0.415 | 25.0 |
| Globus Pallidus[2] | 0.21 | 3.8 | 230 | – | – | – |
| Globus Pallidus[3] | 0.13 | 2.3 | 140 | 0.0043 | 0.067 | 4.0 |
| Putamen[1] | 0.12 | 2.2 | 130 | 0.016 | 0.26 | 16 |
| Putamen[2] | 0.13 | 2.4 | 140 | – | – | – |
| Putamen[3] | 0.115 | 2.1 | 120 | 0.0045 | 0.070 | 4.2 |
| Thalamus[1] | 0.073 | 1.3 | 79 | 0.010 | 0.16 | 9.9 |
| Thalamus[2] | 0.048 | 0.86 | 52 | – | – | – |
| Thalamus[3] | 0.070 | 1.25 | 75 | 0.0048 | 0.076 | 4.6 |
| Caudate[1] | 0.099 | 1.8 | 107 | 0.012 | 0.20 | 12 |
| Caudate[2] | 0.093 | 1.7 | 100 | – | – | – |
| Substantia Nigra[2] | 0.18 | 3.3 | 190 | – | – | – |
| Hippocampus[3] | 0.048 | 0.86 | 52 | 0.0061 | 0.096 | 5.8 |
| Frontal White Matter[2] | 0.042 | 0.75 | 45 | – | – | – |
| Liver[1] | 0.18 | 3.3 | 200 | 0.019 | 0.30 | 18.0 |
| Liver[2] | 0.13 | 2.3 | 140 | – | – | – |
| Liver[3] | 0.135 | 2.4 | 145 | 0.0054 | 0.084 | 5.1 |
| Pancreas[3] | 0.019 | 0.34 | 21 | 0.0011 | 0.018 | 1.1 |
| Heart[3] | 0.060 | 1.1 | 64.5 | 0.0030 | 0.047 | 2.9 |

[1]Calculated from Cumings (1948); [2]Calculated from Hallgren and Sourander (1958); [3]Calculated from Miyajima, Takahashi, and Kono (2003); [4]Average of two locations; [5]Average of five locations

mM = millimol/liter; 1 mg Fe/cc = 17.91 mM; 1 mg Cu/cc = 15.74 mM; 1 mM = 60.22 $10^{16}$ atoms/cc

There is an approximate average total of 60 mg of iron and 5.6 mg of copper in the normal adult human brain parenchyma. These total amounts of iron and copper are not distributed uniformly across the brain as is indicated by the large local concentrations in the globus pallidus. There is a tendency for regions with high iron concentrations to also have high copper concentrations although this has not been examined in detail throughout brain. The reason or reasons for

Table 2
**Parenchymal Iron and Copper in the Normal Adult Human Brain. These values are taken from Cumings (1948) and Hallgren and Sourander (1958) as reported in Table 1. Because of the variations reported between individual brains and differences in the experimental techniques, these results should be considered as first approximations rather than precise absolute values**

| *Metal* | *Baseline** (*mM*) | *Average* (*mM*) | *Total* (*mg*) | *Globus Pallidus* (*mM*) | *Frontal White Matter* (*mM*) |
|---|---|---|---|---|---|
| Iron | 0.1 | 0.73 | 60 | 3.7 | 0.75 |
| Copper | 0.01 | 0.06 | 5.6 | 0.41 | – |

*Finney and O'Halloran (2003)

these localized high brain concentrations are not thoroughly understood although many potential metabolic explanations have been proposed. These include a possible need for iron in the metabolism of the neurotransmitter gamma aminobutyric acid (GABA) (Hill & Switzer, 1984; Hill, 1988), a possible need for iron in myelin synthesis (Benkovic & Connor, 1993; Levine & Chakrabarty, 2004), and the production of iron at specific locations within the brain by the enzyme heme oxygenase-1 (Schipper, 2004).

Morris, Candy, Oakley, Bloxham, & Edwardson (1992) carried out the most detailed anatomical study of human brain iron. They characterized more than 65 specific brain regions with detectable iron staining ranging from moderate to intense. Some of these regions are quite small. The authors note that "microscopically the iron appears to be found predominantly in glial cells as fine granules which in heavily stained areas coalesce to fill the entire cell." They also note that neurons generally contain less iron than glial cells, but in some highly stained regions neurons are found to stain for iron as intensely as the local glial cells. Iron deposition is found in other mammals and the pattern of iron distribution is similar to that in humans. Detailed studies on rat brains identified more than 55 brain regions that exhibit moderate to very high iron staining, and these regions correspond well with the comparably staining regions in the human brain (Hill & Switzer, 1984; Hill, 1988). Hallgren and Sourander (1958) and others have demonstrated that the total brain iron concentration is very low at birth and gradually increases to a more or less stable constant level reached by age 30 in the globus pallidus and at 50–60 years in the putamen.

The iron detected by Perls' staining or by MRI is likely to be in the form of granular aggregates of iron oxide particles associated with ferritin and hemosiderin. Iron atoms in this mineralized state would require mobilization before they could participate in cellular chemical processes such as the formation of active metalloenzymes by insertion of iron into apoenzyme proteins. There are two general models of metabolically active intracellular iron and copper. In one model it is postulated that there is a labile iron pool (LIP) (Jacobs, 1977; Crichton, 2001; Cabantchik, Kakhlon, Epsztejn, Zanninelli, & Breuer, 2002; Kakhlon & Cabantchik, 2002) at a very low concentration (~0.001 mM), which is in some form of chemical exchange with the much larger storage iron pool (~0.7–3.6 mM). The LIP is envisioned to consist of a mixture of free, hydrated metal iron ions (aqua ions) as well as iron ions bound to a heterogeneous population of organic anion groups such as carboxylates and phosphates, small peptides, and membrane surface components (Cabantchik et al., 2002). In this form the iron ions are capable of participating in chelation reactions, redox reactions, and other cellular metabolic processes.

In another model the metal ions are considered as bound not to small molecular weight ligands but to specific proteins called metal chaperones (Pufahl et al., 1997; Valentine & Gralla, 1997; Finney & O'Halloran, 2003). This work has been primarily carried out for copper ions and their chaperones in yeast. These chaperones have a dual functionality: (i) they tightly bind the copper ions to prevent copper toxicity and (ii) they are capable of recognizing and docking with target proteins and then transferring the copper ions to these targets. This model suggests that in many cases on average there may be less than a single free, hydrated copper ion present in the cytoplasm of a given cell. In addition to this work on copper chaperones, an iron chaperone protein has recently been identified in yeast, with the role of delivering iron atoms to ferritin (Shi, Bencze, Stemmler, & Philpott, 2008).

Using either model we may form a picture of iron in the brain that includes a metabolically inert storage pool present in a relatively high concentration and capable of being visualized by MRI or postmortem Perls' staining. This storage pool interacts and exchanges iron, in a poorly understood manner, with a metabolically active iron pool (MAP). The MAP may exist as a pool of iron ions bound to small molecular weight ligands (LIP) or in the form of iron ions bound to chaperone proteins. Perhaps, a combination of these iron models is appropriate when considering different subcellular regions such as mitochondria and synaptic vesicle. Recently, iron accumulation has been demonstrated in dopamine-containing vesicles within neurons by x-ray techniques (Ortega, Cloetens, Deves, Carmona, & Bohic, 2007). Tomography based on optical and electron microscopy has also recently shown a role for ferritin mediation of axonal degeneration in knockout mice that lack normal levels of iron-responsive proteins (IRPs) (Zhang et al., 2005). The development of fluorescent probes capable of real-time studies of intracellular metal pools is providing new opportunities for observing these processes (Domaille et al., 2008).

It is clear that further elucidation of the interactions between the metabolically active iron and the storage iron would greatly enhance the interpretation and utility of clinical brain iron imaging. In the absence of this understanding, the utilization of brain iron MRI will have to continue being based on empirical clinical studies that attempt to relate MRI-based iron measures to the clinical status of patients with specific neurodegenerative diseases.

## 4. INBORN ERRORS OF BRAIN IRON METABOLISM

It has often been proposed, but not rigorously established, that errors in iron metabolism are involved in very common neurodegenerative diseases such as Alzheimer's and Parkinson's diseases and multiple sclerosis. However, as indicated in Table 3, several rare

**Table 3**
**Inherited Neurological Diseases with Brain Iron Accumulation. All These Diseases Except Neuroferritinopathy Are Autosomal Recessive**

| *Disease* | *Date Described* | *Gene* | *Reference* |
|---|---|---|---|
| Hallervorden-Spatz DISEASE (HSD or NBIA1) | 1922 | Pantothenate Kinase (PANK2) | Hayflick et al. (2003) |
| Aceruloplasminemia (aCp) | 1987 | Ceruloplasmin | Miyajima et al. (2003) |
| Neuroferritinopathy (autosomal dominant) | 2001 | Ferritin Light Chain, *FTL1* 460InsA | Chinnery et al. (2007) |
| Friedreich's ataxia | 1863 | Frataxin, FXN (formerly X25, FARR, FRDA) | Delatycki, Williamson, and Forrest (2000); Koeppen et al. (2007) |

inherited brain diseases, unequivocally associated with brain iron accumulation, have now been identified and the genetic defects have been established (Madsen & Gitlin, 2007). Even in these disorders, however, it is not known with certainty the extent to which the abnormal iron accumulations cause the pathological symptoms or whether they merely are a result of the underlying genetic pathology. In either instance, MRI, particularly at high field strength, provides a means of diagnosing the disorder based on the finding of iron accumulation. It is now common for T2-weighted MRI to be a crucial factor in the initial diagnoses of new cases of these disorders.

## 5. MRI TECHNIQUES FOR IMAGING BRAIN IRON

The MR signal arises from the precession of the spins present in the protons of the water molecules within the tissues. This precession is driven a rate determined by the magnetic field. The MR magnet produces a very uniform magnetic field, and when it is the only field driving this precession, the spins all remain locked in phase with one another and produce a strong total signal. The presence of iron-rich regions within the brain leads to regions of microscopic variations in the magnetic field. Therefore, different water molecules experience slightly different magnetic fields as they diffuse through the brain (Brooks, Vymazal, Goldfarb, Bulte, & Aisen, 1998). These field inhomogeneities lead to a dephasing of the spin precession and to a decrease in the overall MR signal.

In the simplest models, the MR signal is assumed to decay exponentially with a time constant, T2. In iron-rich regions this relaxation time, T2 will be shortened either if the iron concentration is increased or if the magnetic field of the scanner is increased. This is because either of these changes increases the magnitude of the field inhomogeneity and the rate of spin dephasing. In practice, many different MRI sequences may be used to produce MR images with iron-dependent contrast. Different research groups have developed several imaging pulse sequences to optimize one or another aspect of brain iron imaging (Table 4). They have also developed a variety of notations for the decay constants that characterize the loss of signal found with specific pulse sequences. These symbols are usually some variations on the standard symbol T2 that is used in straightforward spin echo imaging. This can be a significant source of confusion, especially to investigators who have only a secondary interest in the details of the MRI technology. For this reason the symbols conventionally used with various pulse sequences are also indicated Table 4. The relaxation rate R2, which is the reciprocal of the decay constant ($R2 = 1/T2$), is also often used to characterize this effect.

The simplest approach to demonstrating iron-dependent contrast is to make a single image with a relatively long duration, called the echo time or TE, between the spin excitation pulse and the acquisition of the signal. This technique is called T2-weighted imaging, and the long TE time permits regions with relatively rapid signal decay to be differentiated from neighboring tissues by appearing relatively dark (hypointense). This approach is useful for qualitative studies (Fig. 2B). However, the results are dependent on machine parameters, such as the echo time, and the technique does not lend itself to quantitative tissue characterization.

If a second set of images is taken, using a different TE value, an exponential decay formula can be used to calculate a relaxation time T2 for each voxel in the imaging volume. This T2 value is, ideally, a property of the tissue and is independent of machine parameters. However, this approach obviously doubles the time required to complete the imaging session and requires the subject to keep his or her head immobile for the full duration of the two scans. Alternatively, by using applied gradient fields and a 180° refocusing pulse, both echoes can be produced from a

Table 4

**Comparison of various pulse sequences for imaging and quantifying brain iron effects. The references indicate authors who have used or described particular sequences. They are not intended to be complete or to describe the earliest use of a technique**

| *Pulse Sequence* | *Symbol for Decay Time Constant* | *Symbol for Decay Rate* | *References* |
|---|---|---|---|
| Single T2-weighted image | – | – | Drayer et al. (1986) |
| Repeated single spin echo (SE) | T2 | R2 | Schenck (1995) |
| Dual spin echo (DSE) | T2 | R2 | Schenck et al. (2006) |
| Multiple spin echo (CPMG)[1] | T2 | R2 | Ye et al. (1996a); Jensen, Chandra, and Yu (2001) |
| Fast spin echo (FSE) | T2 | R2 | Allkemper, Schwindt, Maintz, Heindel, and Tombach (2004) |
| Gradient recalled echo (GRE) | T2* | R2* | Duewell, Wolff, Wen, Balaban, and Jezzard (1996) |
| Magnetic field correlation (MFC) | – | – | Jensen et al. (2006) |
| Variable interecho times | – | $\Delta R2_{app}$ | Ye et al. (1996a); Ye, Allen, et al. (1996) |
| Field-dependent R2 increase (FDRI) | – | – | Bartzokis (1993) |
| Susceptibility weighted imaging (SWI) | – | – | Haacke, Xu, Cheng, and Reichenbach (2004) |
| Gradient echo sampling of free induction decay and echo (GEFSIDE) | $T2' = 1/R2'$ | $R2' = R2^* - R2$ | Ordidge, Gorell, Deniau, Knight, and Helpern (1994); Ma and Wehrli (1996); Gelman et al. (1999) |
| Multiecho adiabatic spin echo (MASE) | $T2^{\dagger}$ | $1/T2^{\dagger}$ | Mitsumori, Watanabe, Takaya, and Garwood (2007) |
| Phase-sensitive imaging | – | – | Duyn et al. (2007) |

[1]CPMG – Carr, Purcell, Meiboom, Gill (Bernstein et al., 2004)

single excitation pulse. This permits the measurement of T2 value in the same time it takes to acquire a single image. This is called dual spin echo imaging (Bernstein et al., 2004). However, imperfections in the 180° pulse across the imaging field of view are inevitable, particularly at high field strengths. Therefore, although T2 values measured by the dual spin echo method are usually in reasonable agreement with results found using two successive images made with different TE values, they are not identical to them.

The use of the 180° radiofrequency pulses cancels out a portion of the spin dephasing produced by the microscopic field inhomogeneities, and thereby reduces somewhat the total rate of signal loss. As described by Bernstein et al. (2004) a gradient-induced echo, rather than a radiofrequency pulse, may be used to refocus the spins. This is called gradient-recalled echo (GRE) imaging. In this case, there is no partial refocusing and the full spin dephasing caused by the iron deposits is maintained. This results in a shortened relaxation time that is usually called T2*.

The relaxation of the spins of the water molecules diffusing within the voxels is determined both by the combined effect of the iron-related magnetic field inhomogeneities and by a host of interactions between the water molecules and the various macromolecules present in the tissue. The relaxation rate for brain tissue has been effectively modeled in terms of a constant background relaxation rate added to an iron-dependent rate that is, to a good approximation, linearly proportional to the iron concentration (Gelman et al., 1999).

A large number of additional techniques listed in Table 4 have been devised to achieve some benefit in the imaging of brain iron. The factors to be considered in choice of a technique include the time to complete the scan, which is important for both patient's comfort and economic factors. It is also important to consider the susceptibility of the technique to machine- and field-dependent factors such as the uniformity of the 180° pulse and the amount of radiofrequency energy deposited in the patient by these pulses. Some techniques, such as FSE, have advantages of very short scan time but do not produce images with the same degree of image sharpness as single echo scans. It is also important to consider whether an imaging sequence will cover the entire brain or only a restricted region of it.

If data from several echo times are available, a multi-exponential decay model may be used to fit the image intensity data (Whittall, MacKay, & Li, 1999). This technique may require long acquisition times. If the model includes a physical basis for multiple T2 times, and is not just simple curve fitting, this approach may provide additional useful information on tissue properties.

## 6. BRAIN IRON IMAGING AT SEVEN TESLA

As expected, iron-dependent contrast has been found to increase as the field strength of the imaging system is increased. Several whole-body scanners capable of brain imaging at 7 tesla have recently been introduced. In 2009 there were approximately 30 of these research scanners in operation (Fig. 4). There are also a very few scanners operating at 9.4 tesla. These very high field devices have shown, as expected, even stronger iron-dependent contrast (Fig. 5). The very high

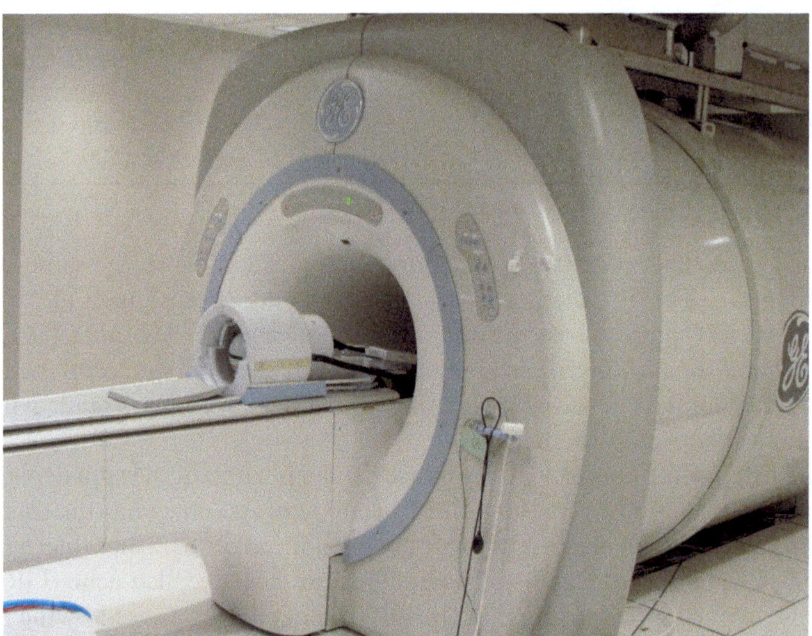

**Fig. 4.** Seven-tesla research magnet. Approximately 30 of these research systems are now available worldwide. (Courtesy of Dr. D. A. C. Kelley, General Electric Healthcare and the University of California at San Francisco.)

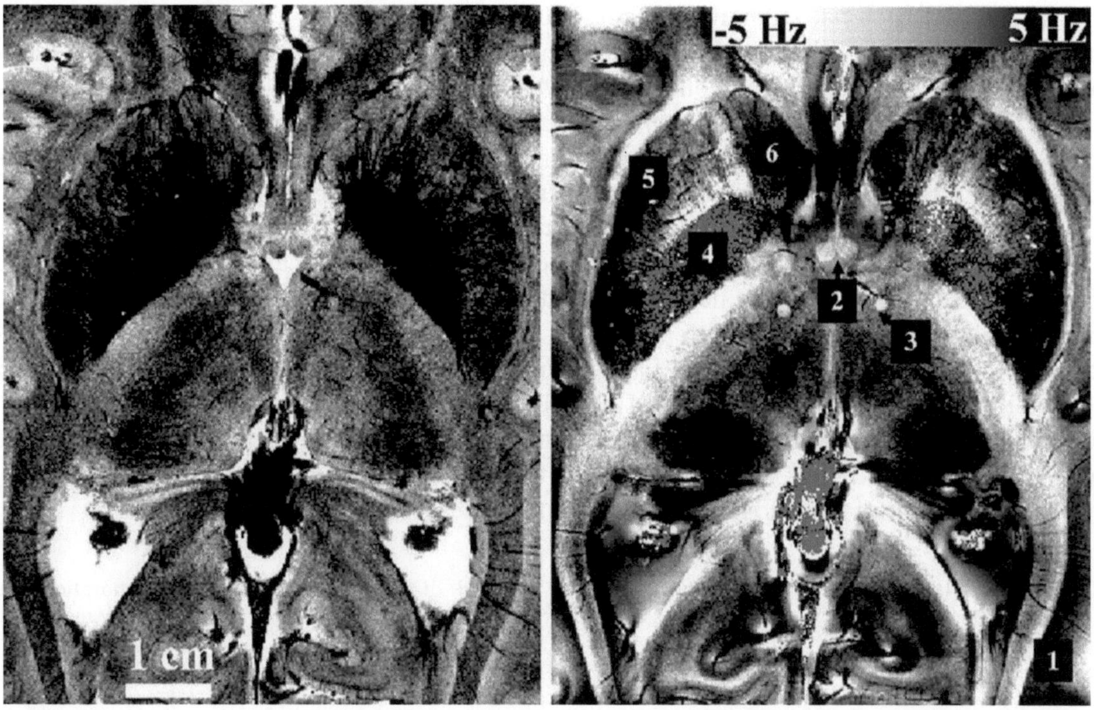


**Fig. 5.** High-resolution MR brain imaging at 7 tesla. A number of anatomical structures either not seen or seen indistinctly at lower field strengths are evident at this resolution. These include veins crossing the optic radiations (1), the columns of the fornix (2), the mamillothalamic tract (3), the globus pallidus (4), the putamen (5), putamen, and the head of the caudate nucleus (6). (Reprinted with permission from Duyn et al., 2007. Copyright 2007, National Academy of Sciences, USA.)

resolution possible at these high field strengths permits imaging of ever-finer details of brain iron distribution. A phase-dependent imaging sequence has been developed, which overcomes some limitations associated with non-uniform radiofrequency excitation fields. These images demonstrate vividly the granularity of brain iron deposition (Duyn et al., 2007). The availability of these high-performance scanners will provide additional impetus to the field of iron-dependent brain imaging. These authors are careful to acknowledge that iron deposition is not the only process that can lead shortened T2 times in brain. Other processes, such as water proton exchange with macromolecules, need to be considered to fully understand the high localized imaging of shortened T2 values that are now available (Zhong, Leupold, von Elverfeldt, & Speck, 2008).

## 7. CONCLUSION

Our current understanding of brain iron physiology and pathology is of an intermediate nature. We obviously know much more about this than our predecessors in the early 20th century; however, most details of brain iron metabolism are currently known only in an approximate way. In particular, the transport of iron between the high-density storage sites present in some brain cells and the metabolically active cellular regions has not been elucidated with precision. It is not obvious, therefore, whether increases or decreases in brain iron observed with MRI are directly responsible for the development of disease or if they are a more passive consequence of disease processes. Many of the most productive studies on iron metabolism have been done on organisms such as yeast and bacteria. Human studies have concentrated on iron absorption in the gut, iron transport (transferrin) in the blood, and the formation and resorption of hemoglobin for the red blood cells in the liver, spleen, and bone marrow. All of these processes take place outside the brain and it is likely that unique processes of iron metabolism occur in the brain. These could include axonal transport, intracellular and extracellular signaling, and vesicular storage and release. Because of this, there is a great opportunity for further brain-specific studies of iron physiology.

There is ample evidence of a profound role for iron in several rare genetic diseases and also in many highly prevalent neurodegenerative disorders (e.g., Alzheimer's and Parkinson's diseases). Because of the enormous burden neurodegenerative diseases place on society, research on brain iron metabolism deserves a very high priority as a translational research area in human biology and medicine. MRI is of limited spatial and temporal resolution and certainly cannot, by itself, resolve all these open issues. However, MRI has the great advantage of providing non-invasive information derived from the brains of living human beings. Because of this, it has an important role to play in advancing our knowledge of brain iron metabolism and in utilizing this knowledge for the management of neurological and psychiatric diseases.

**Acknowledgments** It is a pleasure to acknowledge many helpful discussions and research collaborations with Drs. E. A. Zimmerman, A. H. Koeppen, D. L. Henderson, S. J. Kalia, D. E. Farrell, and with many other colleagues.

## REFERENCES

Adlard, P. A., Cherny, R. A., Finkelstein, D. I., Gautier, E., Robb, E., Cortes, M., et al. (2008). Rapid restoration of cognition in Alzheimer's transgenic mice with 8-hydroxy quinoline analogs is associated with decreased interstitial Abeta. *Neuron, 59*(1), 43–55.

Allkemper, T., Schwindt, W., Maintz, D., Heindel, W., & Tombach, B. (2004). Sensitivity of T2-weighted FSE sequences towards physiological iron depositions in normal brains at 1.5 and 3.0 T. *European Radiology, 14*(6), 1000–1004.

Barnham, K. J., & Bush, A. I. (2008). Metals in Alzheimer's and Parkinson's diseases. *Current Opinion in Chemical Biology, 12*(2), 222–228.

Bartzokis, G., Aravagiri, M., Oldendorf, W. H., Mintz, J., & Marder, S. R. (1993). Field dependent transverse relaxation rate increase may be a specific measure of tissue iron stores. *Magnetic Resonance in Medicine, 29*(4), 459–464.

Bartzokis, G., Cummings, J. L., Markham, C. H., Marmarelis, P. Z., Treciokas, L. J., Tishler, T. A., et al. (1999). MRI evaluation of brain iron in earlier- and later-onset Parkinson's disease and normal subjects. *Magnetic Resonance Imaging, 17*(2), 213–222.

Bartzokis, G., Cummings, J., Perlman, S., Hance, D. B., & Mintz, J. (1999). Increased basal ganglia iron levels in Huntington disease. *Archives of Neurology, 56*(5), 569–574.

Benkovic, S. A., & Connor, J. R. (1993). Ferritin, transferrin, and iron in selected regions of the adult and aged rat brain. *Journal of Comparative Neurology, 338*(1), 97–113.

Bernstein, M. A., King, K. F., & Zhou, Z. J. (2004). *Handbook of MRI pulse sequences*. Amsterdam, Boston: Academic Press.

Bertini, I., Gray, H. B., Stiefel, E. I., & Valentine, J. S. (2007). *Biological inorganic chemistry: Structure and reactivity*. Sausalito, California: University Science Books.

Blinkov, S. M., & Glezer, I. I. (1968). *The human brain in figures and tables: A quantitative handbook*. New York: Basic Books.

Bradley, W. G., Jr. (1993). MR appearance of hemorrhage in the brain. *Radiology, 189*(1), 15–26.

Brooks, R. A., Vymazal, J., Goldfarb, R. B., Bulte, J. W., & Aisen, P. (1998). Relaxometry and magnetometry of ferritin. *Magnetic Resonance in Medicine, 40*(2), 227–235.

Bulte, J. W. M., & Modo, M. M. J. J. (2008). *Nanoparticles in biomedical imaging: Emerging technologies and applications*. New York: Springer.

Burdette, S. C., & Lippard, S. J. (2003). Meeting of the minds: Metalloneurochemistry. *Proceedings of the National Academy of Sciences of the United States of America, 100*(7), 3605–3610.

Bush, A. I., & Curtain, C. C. (2008). Twenty years of metallo-neurobiology: Where to now? *European Biophysics Journal, 37*(3), 241–245.

Cabantchik, Z. I., Kakhlon, O., Epsztejn, S., Zanninelli, G., & Breuer, W. (2002). Intracellular and extracellular labile iron pools. *Advances in Experimental Medicine and Biology, 509*, 55–75.

Castelnau, P. A., Garrett, R. S., Palinski, W., Witztum, J. L., Campbell, I. L., & Powell, H. C. (1998). Abnormal iron deposition associated with lipid peroxidation in transgenic mice expressing interleukin-6 in the brain. *Journal of Neuropathology and Experimental Neurology, 57*(3), 268–282.

Connor, J. R. (1997). *Metals and oxidative damage in neurological disorders.* New York: Plenum Press.

Chinnery, P. F., Crompton, D. E., Birchall, D., Jackson, M. J., Coulthard, A., Lombes, A., et al. (2007). Clinical features and natural history of neuroferritinopathy caused by the FTL1 460InsA mutation. *Brain, 130*(Pt. 1), 110–119.

Collingwood, J. F., Mikhaylova, A., Davidson, M., Batich, C., Streit, W. J., Terry, J., et al. (2005). In situ characterization and mapping of iron compounds in Alzheimer's disease tissue. *Journal of Alzheimers Disease, 7*(4), 267–272.

Connor, J. R., Boyer, P. J., Menzies, S. L., Dellinger, B., Allen, R. P., Ondo, W. G., et al. (2003). Neuropathological examination suggests impaired brain iron acquisition in restless legs syndrome. *Neurology, 61*(3), 304–309.

Craelius, W., Migdal, M. W., Luessenhop, C. P., Sugar, A., & Mihalakis, I. (1982). Iron deposits surrounding multiple sclerosis plaques. *Archives of Pathology and Laboratory Medicine, 106*(8), 397–399.

Crichton, R. R. (2001). *Inorganic biochemistry of iron metabolism: From molecular mechanisms to clinical consequences* (2nd ed.). Chichester, New York: Wiley.

Crichton, R. R., & Ward, R. J. (2006). *Metal-based neurodegeneration: From molecular mechanisms to therapeutic strategies.* Chichester, Hoboken, NJ: John Wiley & Sons.

Cumings, J. N. (1948). The copper and iron content of brain and liver in the normal and in hepato-lenticular degeneration. *Brain, 71*(Pt. 4), 410–415.

Delatycki, M. B., Williamson, R., & Forrest, S. M. (2000). Friedreich ataxia: An overview. *Journal of Medical Genetics, 37*(1), 1–8.

Dexter, D. T., Wells, F. R., Agid, F., Agid, Y., Lees, A. J., Jenner, P., et al. (1987). Increased nigral iron content in postmortem parkinsonian brain. *Lancet, 2*(8569), 1219–1220.

Domaille, D. W., Que, E. L., & Chang, C. J. (2008). Synthetic fluorescent sensors for studying the cell biology of metals. *Nature Chemical Biology, 4*(3), 168–175.

Drayer, B., Burger, P., Darwin, R., Riederer, S., Herfkens, R., & Johnson, G. A. (1986). Magnetic resonance imaging of brain iron. *American Journal of Roentgenology, 147*(1), 103–110.

Duewell, S., Wolff, S. D., Wen, H., Balaban, R. S., & Jezzard, P. (1996). MR imaging contrast in human brain tissue: Assessment and optimization at 4 T. *Radiology, 199*(3), 780–786.

Duyn, J. H., van Gelderen, P., Li, T. Q., de Zwart, J. A., Koretsky, A. P., & Fukunaga, M. (2007). High-field MRI of brain cortical substructure based on signal phase. *Proceedings of the National Academy of Sciences of the United States of America, 104*(28), 11796–11801.

Finney, L. A., & O'Halloran, T. V. (2003). Transition metal speciation in the cell: Insights from the chemistry of metal ion receptors. *Science, 300*(5621), 931–936.

Geiderman, J. M. (2003). Hallervorden and history. *New England Journal of Medicine, 348*(17), 1725–1726; author reply 1725–1726.

Gelman, N., Gorell, J. M., Barker, P. B., Savage, R. M., Spickler, E. M., Windham, J. P., et al. (1999). MR imaging of human brain at 3.0 T: preliminary report on transverse relaxation rates and relation to estimated iron content. *Radiology, 210*(3), 759–767.

Goodman, L. (1953). Alzheimer's disease: A clinico-pathologic analysis of twenty-three cases with a theory on pathogenesis. *Journal of Nervous and Mental Disorders, 118*, 97–130.

Grabill, C., Silva, A. C., Smith, S. S., Koretsky, A. P., & Rouault, T. A. (2003). MRI detection of ferritin iron overload and associated neuronal pathology in iron regulatory protein-2 knockout mice. *Brain Research, 971*(1), 95–106.

Haacke, E. M., Xu, Y., Cheng, Y. C., & Reichenbach, J. R. (2004). Susceptibility weighted imaging (SWI). *Magnetic Resonance in Medicine, 52*(3), 612–618.

Haacke, E. M., Cheng, N. Y., House, M. J., Liu, Q., Neelavalli, J., Ogg, R. J., et al. (2005). Imaging iron stores in the brain using magnetic resonance imaging. *Magnetic Resonance Imaging, 23*(1), 1–25.

Hallgren, B., & Sourander, P. (1958). The effect of age on the non-haemin iron in the human brain. *Journal of Neurochemistry, 3*(1), 41–51.

Halliwell, B., & Gutteridge, J. M. C. (1999). *Free radicals in biology and medicine* (3rd ed.). Oxford, New York: Clarendon Press; Oxford University Press.

Hayflick, S. J., Westaway, S. K., Levinson, B., Zhou, B., Johnson, M. A., Ching, K. H., et al. (2003). Genetic, clinical, and radiographic delineation of Hallervorden-Spatz syndrome. *New England Journal of Medicine, 348*(1), 33–40.

Hill, J. M., & Switzer, R. C., III. (1984). The regional distribution and cellular localization of iron in the rat brain. *Neuroscience, 11*(3), 595–603.

Hill, J. M. (1988). The distribution of iron in the brain. In M. B. H. Youdim (Ed.), *Brain iron: Neurochemical and behavioural aspects* (pp. 1–24). London: Taylor and Francis.

House, M. J., St Pierre, T. G., & McLean, C. (2008). 1.4T study of proton magnetic relaxation rates, iron concentrations, and plaque burden in Alzheimer's disease and control postmortem brain tissue. *Magnetic Resonance in Medicine, 60*(1), 41–52.

Jack, C. R., Jr., Wengenack, T. M., Reyes, D. A., Garwood, M., Curran, G. L., Borowski, B. J., et al. (2005). In vivo magnetic resonance microimaging of individual amyloid plaques in Alzheimer's transgenic mice. *Journal of Neuroscience, 25*(43), 10041–10048.

Jacobs, A. (1977). Low molecular weight intracellular iron transport compounds. *Blood, 50*(3), 433–439.

Jensen, J. H., & Chandra, R. (2000). Strong field behavior of the NMR signal from magnetically heterogeneous tissues. *Magnetic Resonance in Medicine, 43*(2), 226–236.

Jensen, J. H., & Chandra, R. (2000). NMR relaxation in tissues with weak magnetic inhomogeneities. *Magnetic Resonance in Medicine, 44*(1), 144–156.

Jensen, J. H., Chandra, R., & Yu, H. (2001). Quantitative model for the interecho time dependence of the CPMG relaxation rate in iron-rich gray matter. *Magnetic Resonance in Medicine, 46*(1), 159–165.

Jensen, J. H., Chandra, R., Ramani, A., Lu, H., Johnson, G., Lee, S. P., et al. (2006). Magnetic field correlation imaging. *Magnetic Resonance in Medicine, 55*(6), 1350–1361.

Kakhlon, O., & Cabantchik, Z. I. (2002). The labile iron pool: Characterization, measurement, and participation in cellular processes (1). *Free Radical Biology and Medicine, 33*(8), 1037–1046.

Koeppen, A. H., Dickson, A. C., Chu, R. C., & Thach, R. E. (1993). The pathogenesis of superficial siderosis of the central nervous system. *Annals of Neurology, 34*(5), 646–653.

Koeppen, A. H. (1995). The history of iron in the brain. *Journal of the Neurological Sciences, 134*(Suppl.), 1–9.

Koeppen, A. H. (2003). A brief history of brain iron research. *Journal of the Neurological Sciences, 207*(1–2), 95–97.

Koeppen, A. H., Michael, S. C., Knutson, M. D., Haile, D. J., Qian, J., Levi, S., et al. (2007). The dentate nucleus in Friedreich's ataxia: The role of iron-responsive proteins. *Acta Neuropathol, 114*(2), 163–173.

LeVine, S. M., Connor, J. R., & Schipper, H. M. (2004). *Redox-active metals in neurological disorders*. New York: New York Academy of Sciences.

Levine, S. M., & Chakrabarty, A. (2004). The role of iron in the pathogenesis of experimental allergic encephalomyelitis and multiple sclerosis. *Annals of the New York Academy of Sciences, 1012*, 252–266.

Lippard, S. J., & Berg, J. M. (1994). *Principles of bioinorganic chemistry*. Mill Valley, California: University Science Books.

Logothetis, N. K. (2008). What we can do and what we cannot do with fMRI. *Nature, 453*(7197), 869–878.

Ma, J., & Wehrli, F. W. (1996). Method for image-based measurement of the reversible and irreversible contribution to the transverse-relaxation rate. *Journal of Magnetic Resonance. Series B, 111*(1), 61–69.

Madsen, E., & Gitlin, J. D. (2007). Copper and iron disorders of the brain. *Annual Review of Neuroscience, 30*, 317–337.

McNeill, A., Birchall, D., Hayflick, S. J., Gregory, A., Schenck, J. F., Zimmerman, E. A., et al. (2008). T2* and FSE MRI distinguishes four subtypes of neurodegeneration with brain iron accumulation. *Neurology, 70*(18), 1614–1619.

Mitsumori, F., Watanabe, H., Takaya, N., & Garwood, M. (2007). Apparent transverse relaxation rate in human brain varies linearly with tissue iron concentration at 4.7 T. *Magnetic Resonance in Medicine, 58*(5), 1054–1060.

Miyajima, H., Takahashi, Y., & Kono, S. (2003). Aceruloplasminemia, an inherited disorder of iron metabolism. *Biometals, 16*(1), 205–213.

Morris, C. M., Candy, J. M., Oakley, A. E., Bloxham, C. A., & Edwardson, J. A. (1992). Histochemical distribution of non-haem iron in the human brain. *Acta Anatomica, 144*(3), 235–257.

Ordidge, R. J., Gorell, J. M., Deniau, J. C., Knight, R. A., & Helpern, J. A. (1994). Assessment of relative brain iron concentrations using T2-weighted and T2*-weighted MRI at 3 Tesla. *Magnetic Resonance in Medicine, 32*(3), 335–341.

Ortega, R., Cloetens, P., Deves, G., Carmona, A., & Bohic, S. (2007). Iron storage within dopamine neurovesicles revealed by chemical nano-imaging. *PLoS ONE, 2*(9), e925.

Outten, C. E., & O'Halloran, T. V. (2001). Femtomolar sensitivity of metalloregulatory proteins controlling zinc homeostasis. *Science, 292*(5526), 2488–2492.

Pankhurst, Q., Hautot, D., Khan, N., & Dobson, J. (2008). Increased levels of magnetic iron compounds in Alzheimer's disease. *Journal of Alzheimer's Disease, 13*(1), 49–52.

Perry, G., Nunomura, A., Hirai, K., Zhu, X., Prez, M., Avila, J., et al. (2002). Is oxidative damage the fundamental pathogenic mechanism of Alzheimer's and other neurodegenerative diseases? *Free Radical Biology and Medicine, 33*(11), 1475–1479.

Perry, G., Taddeo, M. A., Petersen, R. B., Castellani, R. J., Harris, P. L., Siedlak, S. L., et al. (2003). Adventiously-bound redox active iron and copper are at the center of oxidative damage in Alzheimer disease. *Biometals, 16*(1), 77–81.

Pufahl, R. A., Singer, C. P., Peariso, K. L., Lin, S. J., Schmidt, P. J., Fahrni, C. J., et al. (1997). Metal ion chaperone function of the soluble Cu(I) receptor Atx1. *Science, 278*(5339), 853–856.

Richardson, D. R. (2004). Novel chelators for central nervous system disorders that involve alterations in the metabolism of iron and other metal ions. *Annals of the New York Academy of Sciences, 1012*, 326–341.

Rouault, T. A. (2001). Iron on the brain. *Nature Genetics, 28*(4), 299–300.

Schenck, J. F. (1995). Imaging of brain iron by magnetic resonance: T2 relaxation at different field strengths. *Journal of the Neurological Sciences, 134*(Suppl.), 10–18.

Schenck, J. F., & Zimmerman, E. A. (2004). High-field magnetic resonance imaging of brain iron: Birth of a biomarker? *NMR in Biomedicine, 17*(7), 433–445.

Schenck, J. F. (2005). Brain iron as an endogenous contrast agent in high-field MRI. In J. L. Sessler, S. R. Doctorow, T. J. McMurray, & S. J. Lippard (Eds.), *Medicinal inorganic chemistry* (pp. 44–61). Washington, DC: American Chemical Society.

Schenck, J. F., Zimmerman, E. A., Li, Z., Adak, S., Saha, A., Tandon, R., et al. (2006). High-field magnetic resonance imaging of brain iron in Alzheimer disease. *Topics in Magnetic Resonance Imaging, 17*(1), 41–50.

Schipper, H. M. (2004). Redox neurology: Visions of an emerging subspecialty. *Annals of the New York Academy of Sciences, 1012*, 342–355.

Shi, H., Bencze, K. Z., Stemmler, T. L., & Philpott, C. C. (2008). A cytosolic iron chaperone that delivers iron to ferritin. *Science, 320*(5880), 1207–1210.

Shibata, E., Sasaki, K., Tohyama, K., Otsuka, K., Endoh, J., Terayama, Y., et al. (2008). Use of neuromelanin-sensitive MRI to distinguish schizophrenic and depressive patients and healthy individuals based on signal alterations in the substantia nigra and the locus ceruleus. *Biological Psychiatry*, *64*(5), 401–406.

Silva, J. J. R. F. d., & Williams, R. J. P. (2001). *The biological chemistry of the elements: The inorganic chemistry of life* (2nd ed.). Oxford, New York: Oxford University Press.

Small, S. A., Wu, E. X., Bartsch, D., Perera, G. M., Lacefield, C. O., DeLaPaz, R., et al. (2000). Imaging physiologic dysfunction of individual hippocampal subregions in humans and genetically modified mice. *Neuron, 28*(3), 653–664.

Tang, T., Howarth, S. P., Miller, S. R., Trivedi, R., Graves, M. J., King-Im, J. U., et al. (2006). Assessment of inflammatory burden contralateral to the symptomatic carotid stenosis using high-resolution ultrasmall, superparamagnetic iron oxide-enhanced MRI. *Stroke, 37*(9), 2266–2270.

Testa, U. (2002). *Proteins of iron metabolism.* Boca Raton, FL: CRC Press.

Valentine, J. S., & Gralla, E. B. (1997). Delivering copper inside yeast and human cells. *Science, 278*(5339), 817–818.

Viswanathan, A., & Chabriat, H. (2006). Cerebral microhemorrhage. *Stroke, 37*(2), 550–555.

Vymazal, J., Urgosik, D., & Bulte, J. W. (2000). Differentiation between hemosiderin- and ferritin-bound brain iron using nuclear magnetic resonance and magnetic resonance imaging. *Cellular and Molecular Biology (Noisy-le-grand), 46*(4), 835–842.

Whittall, K. P., MacKay, A. L., & Li, D. K. (1999). Are mono-exponential fits to a few echoes sufficient to determine T2 relaxation for in vivo human brain? *Magnetic Resonance in Medicine, 41*(6), 1255–1257.

Williams, R. J. P., & Silva, J. R. R. F. d. (1996). *The natural selection of the chemical elements: The environment and life's chemistry*. Oxford, New York: Clarendon Press; Oxford University Press.

Williams, R. J. P. (2001). Chemical selection of elements by cells. *Coordination Chemistry Reviews, 216–217*, 583–595.

Williams, R. J. P. (2003). The biological chemistry of the brain and its possible evolution. *Inorganica Chimica Acta, 356*, 27–40.

Wixom, R. L., Prutkin, L., & Munro, H. N. (1980). Hemosiderin: Nature, formation, and significance. *International Review of Experimental Pathology, 22*, 193–225.

Ye, F. Q., Martin, W. R., & Allen, P. S. (1996a). Estimation of brain iron in vivo by means of the interecho time dependence of image contrast. *Magnetic Resonance in Medicine, 36*(1), 153–158.

Ye, F. Q., Martin, W., & Allen, P. S. (1996b). Estimation of the iron concentration in excised gray matter by means of proton relaxation measurements. *Magnetic Resonance in Medicine, 35*(3), 285–289.

Ye, F. Q., Allen, P. S., & Martin, W. R. (1996). Basal ganglia iron content in Parkinson's disease measured with magnetic resonance. *Movement Disorders, 11*(3), 243–249.

Youdim, M. B. H. (1988). *Brain iron: Neurochemical and behavioural aspects.* London, New York: Taylor & Francis.

Zatta, P. (2003). *Metal ions and neurodegenerative disorders.* London: World Scientific.

Zecca, L., Zucca, F. A., Wilms, H., & Sulzer, D. (2003). Neuromelanin of the substantia nigra: A neuronal black hole with protective and toxic characteristics. *Trends in Neurosciences, 26*(11), 578–580.

Zecca, L., Youdim, M. B., Riederer, P., Connor, J. R., & Crichton, R. R. (2004). Iron, brain ageing and neurodegenerative disorders. *Nature Reviews Neurosciences, 5*(11), 863–873.

Zhang, P., Land, W., Lee, S., Juliani, J., Lefman, J., Smith, S. R., et al. (2005). Electron tomography of degenerating neurons in mice with abnormal regulation of iron metabolism. *Journal of Structural Biology, 150*(2), 144–153.

Zhong, K., Leupold, J., von Elverfeldt, D., & Speck, O. (2008). The molecular basis for gray and white matter contrast in phase imaging. *Neuroimage, 40*(4), 1561–1566.

# 14 Alzheimer's Dementia

*Seema Gulyani and Mark P. Mattson*

**Summary**

- The disability caused by Alzheimer's disease (AD) is increasing worldwide with 4.6 million newly diagnosed patients every year.
- Age-related oxidative stress appears to be an important contributor to the amyloid pathology and neuronal degeneration of AD.
- Iron homeostasis is altered in AD patients.
- Iron promotes the formation of amyloid plaques and neurofibrillary tangles, which are the hallmarks of the disease.
- Iron also causes synaptic dysfunction by altering cell membrane integrity and impairing the function of membrane-bound proteins.
- Future treatments for AD may include dietary modifications and drugs that reduce the amount of toxic free iron, or that protect cells against iron toxicity.

**Key Words:** Alzheimer's disease; amyloid; cognitive impairment; hydroxynonenal; neurofibrillary tangles; presenilin-1; synaptic dysfunction

## 1. CLINICAL AND PATHOLOGICAL FEATURES OF ALZHEIMER'S DISEASE

Alois Alzheimer in 1907 provided the first description of a case of the disease in a 51-year-old woman with 5-year history of progressive cognitive impairment, hallucinations, delusions, and memory disturbance. After her death Alzheimer identified in her brain neuropathology of plaques and dense bundles of fibrils (tangles) (Moller & Graeber, 1998). Later, these characteristics were given the name of Alzheimer's disease (AD), defined by the progressive loss of cognitive capacities, and the accumulations of amyloid plaques and neurofibrillary tangles in affected brain regions. AD accounts for more than 60% of all cases of dementia and is the major cause of disability (11.2%) in people aged 60 years and older [compared with stroke (9.5%), musculoskeletal disorders (8.9%), cardiovascular diseases (5.0%), and all forms of cancer (2.4%) (WHO, 2003)]. Recent systematic review of published studies by international experts (Ferri et al., 2005) concluded that an estimated 24.3 million people in the world have AD today, with 4.6 million new cases every year. By 2040, the number of people with AD will be 81 million. This study also reported the prevalence of dementia shows an exponential increase with age such

From: *Nutrition and Health: Iron Deficiency and Overload*
Edited by: S. Yehuda and D.I. Mostofsky, DOI 10.1007/978-1-59745-462-9_14

that in people aged 85 and older the prevalence is greater than 40% in the Western world. In addition to aging, other risk factors for AD include hypertension, coronary artery disease, smoking, obesity, and diabetes (Mayeux, 2003).

AD is a heterogeneous disorder with both familial and sporadic forms, though the prevalence of familial forms is less than 1% (Blennow, de Leon, & Zetterberg, 2006). Mutations in amyloid precursor protein (APP) gene on chromosome 21 were the first to be identified as causing an early onset autosomal dominant familial form of the disease (Fidani & Goate, 1992; Goate et al., 1991), but account for only a few familial cases. Instead, mutations in the presenilin-1 gene account for most of the cases of familial disease (Levy-Lahad & Bird, 1996). Two independent studies reported associations between the apolipoprotein E (ApoE) $\epsilon 4$ allele and the risk of late-onset sporadic AD (Corder et al., 1993; Poirier et al., 1993).

The key features of the lesions in AD are senile plaques, consisting of extracellular insoluble amyloid β-peptide (Aβ) aggregates, and neurofibrillary tangles, consisting of intracellular filamentous aggregates of the microtubule-associated protein tau; both Aβ and tau pathologies are associated with synaptic degeneration and neuronal death in medial temporal lobe structures and cortical areas of the brain (Hardy & Selkoe, 2002; Masters et al., 1985; Selkoe, 1991b). Aβ, the primary component of the plaques of AD, is a cleavage product of APP and is formed by the actions of two proteases, the β- and γ-secretases (Hardy & Allsop, 1991; Selkoe, 1991a). Mutations in APP and presenilin-1 increase the production of Aβ and, in particular, the longer Aβ42 peptide. Aβ, which is constitutively produced in the cell, is degraded under normal conditions in brain by peptidases including neprilysin and insulin-degrading enzyme (Carson & Turner, 2002) and is also cleared by efflux across blood–brain barrier by low-density lipoprotein receptor relate protein.(Tanzi, Moir, & Wagner, 2004). There is as yet no direct evidence for any impairment in these proteolytic or transport mechanisms for Aβ clearance in AD. The mechanism by which APOE, a cholesterol transport protein, increases the risk of AD is unknown, but possibilities included a direct interaction with Aβ and diminished antioxidant properties of ApoE4 compared to the protective ApoE2 and ApoE3 isoforms (Holtzman et al., 2000; Pedersen, Chan, & Mattson, 2000; Raber, Huang, & Ashford, 2004).

Hardy and Selkoe proposed the amyloid cascade hypothesis which states that an imbalance between the production and the clearance of Aβ in the brain is the initiating event ultimately leading to neuronal degeneration and dementia (Hardy & Selkoe, 2002). This hypothesis was supported by many studies reporting that APP and presenilin mutations increase Aβ production and also duplication of the APP locus in familial AD results in APP overexpression and Aβ deposition (Rovelet-Lecrux et al., 2006). Aβ may damage and kill neurons by inducing membrane-associated oxidative stress (lipid peroxidation) which impairs the function ion-motive ATPases and glutamate and glutamate transporters, thereby destabilizing cellular calcium homeostasis and promoting excitotoxicity and apoptosis (Mattson, 2004a). Neurofibrillary tangles are made of hyperphosphorylated tau protein (Iqbal & Grundke-Iqbal, 2007). Hyperphosphorylation of tau causes disassembly of microtubules and thus impaired axonal transport, resulting in neurotransmitter deficits with neuronal and synaptic dysfunction (Iqbal et al., 2005). Presenilin mutations may cause AD by altering the activity of γ-secretase (Rogaeva, 2002) and by disrupting cellular calcium homeostasis (Guo et al., 1997, 1999; Tu et al., 2006).

## 2. IRON AND THE PATHOGENESIS OF ALZHEIMER'S DISEASE

Iron is an essential transition metal in the body because there are many iron-containing proteins that serve major functions including electron transfer, DNA synthesis, and oxygen transport. In the brain it plays additional roles in neurotransmitter and myelin synthesis (Burdo & Connor,

2003). Though iron is essential for cellular functioning, its dysregulation can result in cellular toxicity. Ferrous iron ($Fe^{2+}$) interacts with hydrogen peroxide to generate hydroxyl radical, which is a highly reactive oxygen species (ROS) that attacks the double bonds of membrane lipids, resulting in the autocatalyic process called lipid peroxidation (Mattson, 2004b). The strong redox activity of free iron can also damage DNA and proteins resulting in mutations, protein dysfunction, and cell damage and death (Castellani et al., 2007; Smith, Cappai, & Barnham, 2007).

## 3. EVIDENCE FOR DYSREGULATION OF BRAIN IRON HOMEOSTASIS IN AD PATIENTS

The levels of iron in the brain are normally tightly regulated and, as in other tissues, iron is normally bound to proteins and so not available for ROS production. Several studies have suggested iron metabolism and homeostasis are altered in AD. Analysis of postmortem brain tissue samples from AD patients and control subjects has demonstrated the presence of increased amounts of iron in vulnerable brain regions such as the hippocampus in AD where the iron is associated with Aβ plaques (Jellinger, Paulus, Grundke-Iqbal, Riederer, & Youdim, 1990; Deibel, Ehmann, & Markesbery, 1996; Thompson, Markesbery, Ehmann, Mao, & Vance, 1988; Lovell, Robertson, Teesdale, Campbell, & Markesbery, 1998). Iron is associated with cells containing neurofibrillary tangles (NFT) and is also present in glial cells and neurites of senile plaques in the hippocampus in AD (Morris, Kerwin, & Edwardson, 1994). The iron associated with plaques and tangles is capable of in situ redox reaction with hydrogen peroxidation (Smith, Harris, Sayre, & Perry, 1997), demonstrating its potential cytotoxic activity. Using nano SIMS (secondary ion mass spectroscopy) the distribution of iron in AD brain was evaluated at the ultra structural level (Quintana et al., 2006). Iron was present in relatively high amounts in the periphery of plaques and in dystrophic neurites and oligodendrocytes, suggesting a role for iron in white matter damage in AD. Iron levels were not significantly altered in the cerebellum, a brain region that is minimally affected in AD.

In addition to the association of iron with degenerating neurons, alterations in the levels of several different iron-regulating proteins in AD have been reported. Elevated ferritin immunoreactivity was seen in and around senile plaques and blood vessels in the AD brain tissue (Connor, Menzies, St Martin, & Mufson, 1992). Iron and iron reaction products were observed both in proximity of the plaques and in cells associated with the plaques (Connor, Snyder, Beard, Fine, & Mufson, 1992). In AD brains, transferrin is decreased in the white matter of the various cerebral cortical regions (Grundke-Iqbal et al., 1990; Connor, Snyder et al., 1992). Iron-regulatory protein (IRP-2) was significantly different in AD brains as compared to controls, and it was found in intraneuronal lesions including neurofibrillary tangles, senile plaque neurites, and neuropil threads. Since IRP-2 colocalizes with redox-active iron, it was suggested that alterations in IRP-2 might be directly linked to impaired iron homeostasis in Alzheimer's disease.(Smith et al., 1998).

## 4. EXPERIMENTAL EVIDENCE FOR A PATHOGENIC ROLE FOR IRON IN AD

Studies of cell culture and animal models have provided evidence for mechanisms by which iron might contribute to Aβ accumulation, neurotoxicity, and neurofibrillary pathology in AD. Iron may alter APP processing so as to increase the production and accumulation of Aβ, as suggested from studies of vascular smooth muscle cells (Mazur-Kolecka, Kowal, Sukontasup, Dickson, & Frackowiak, 2004). The aggregation of Aβ is enhanced by even very low amounts of free iron (Dyrks, Dyrks, Hartmann, Masters, & Beyreuther, 1992; Mantyh et al., 1993), and iron may interact with Aβ in ways that result in the production of hydrogen peroxide, suggesting that Aβ may itself be a major source of ROS in AD (Hensley et al., 1994; Rottkamp et al., 2001). Indeed, Aβ may impair synaptic function, and damage and kills neurons, by causing membrane lipid peroxidation and production of toxic aldehydes that impair the function of membrane ion-motive ATPases and glucose and glutamate transporters (Mark, Hensley, Butterfield, & Mattson, 1995; Mark, Pang, Geddes, Uchida, & Mattson, 1997; Keller et al., 1997). Consistent with the latter pathogenic mechanism, infusion of iron or the lipid peroxidation product 4-hydroxynonenal into the basal forebrain impairs learning and memory in rats (Bruce-Keller et al., 1998). Iron potentiates the neurotoxic actions of Aβ, and the α-secretase secreted APP product (sAPPα) protects neurons against Aβ and iron toxicities (Goodman & Mattson, 1994). The role of iron as one of the factors involved in the pathogenesis of AD is further suggested from recent studies showing that APP is a metalloprotein, and that iron interacts specifically with the 5′-untranslated region (5′UTR) of the mRNA encoding APP (Rogers et al., 2002). The APP 5′ UTR fold into a stable RNA secondary structure and is an important regulator of the amount of APP translated in response to iron (Fig. 1).

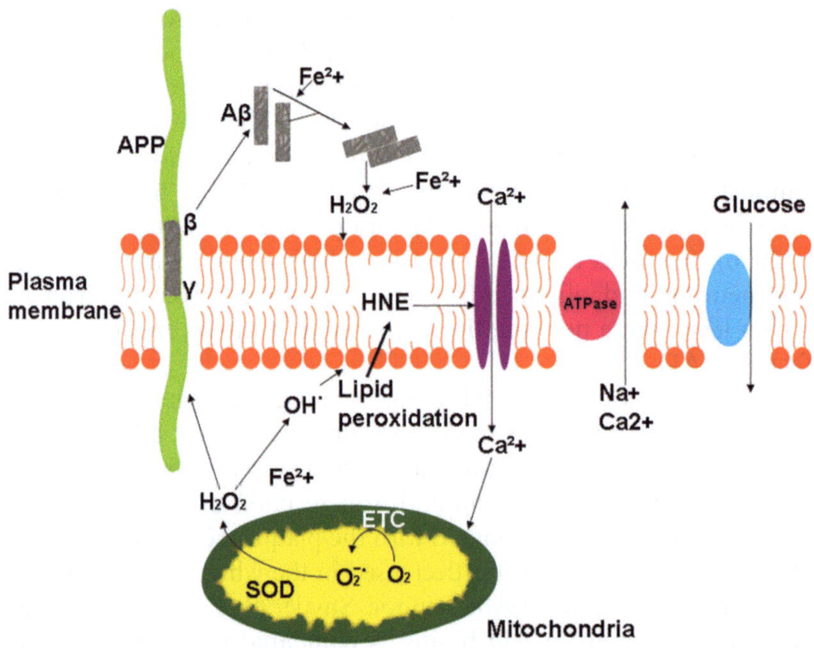


**Fig. 1.** Mechanisms by which iron may contribute to neuronal dysfunction and degeneration in Alzheimer's disease. Extracellular redox-active iron ($Fe^{2+}$) present in the vicinity of Aβ plaques may promote Aβ aggregation. $Fe^{2+}$ interacts with Aβ to promote hydrogen peroxide ($H_2O_2$) formation and also with $H_2O_2$ to generate hydroxyl radical, which in turn causes lipid peroxidation and toxic aldehyde formation. The lipid peroxidation product 4-hydroxynoneal (HNE) alters synaptic function by impairing ATP-driven ionic pumps ($Ca^{2+}$ and $Na^+/K^+$ ATPases) and glucose and glutamate transporters. As a result, a cellular energy-deficit, excessive elevation of intracellular $Ca^{2+}$ levels and excitotoxicity and apoptosis may ensue. Contributing to increased oxidative stress is mitochondrial production of superoxide anion radical ($O_2^{-}$), which is converted to $H_2O_2$ and, in the presence of $Fe^{2+}$, generates hydroxyl radical. Membrane-associated oxidative stress induced by $Fe^{2+}$ may also alter proteolytic processing of the amyloid precursor protein (APP), resulting in increased Aβ production. Thus iron plays important roles in Aβ production, aggregation, and cytotoxicity. Intracellular iron may also contribute to the formation of neurofibrillary tangles (NFT) by promoting hyperphosphorylation of the microtubule-associated protein tau.

By promoting membrane lipid peroxidation, iron may also contribute to the formation of neurofibrillary tangles. As evidence, the lipid peroxidation product 4-hydroxynonenal is increased in the brain in mild cognitive impairment and AD (Williams, Lynn, Markesbery, & Lovell, 2006), and covalently modifies tau in a manner that results in tau hyperphosphorylation (Mattson, Fu, Waeg, & Uchida, 1997). In addition, the exposure of cultured cortical neurons to iron resulted in increased activity of glycogen synthase kinase-3 and a corresponding increase in tau phosphorylation (Lovell, Xiong, Xie, Davies, & Markesbery, 2004).

The anti-diabetic hormone glucagon-like peptide 1 (GLP-1) can protect cultured neurons from being damaged and killed by iron and Aβ (Perry et al., 2003). The latter findings are of interest because increasing evidence suggests that diabetes is a risk factor for cognitive impairment in aging and AD (Pasquier, Boulogne, Leys, & Fontaine, 2006; Stranahan et al., 2008). Impaired iron regulation in diabetes could therefore conceivably play a role in promoting amyloidogenic and neurofibrillary pathologies. Transgenic mouse models of AD (mice expressing APP, presenilin-1, and/or tau mutations) are providing novel insight into the cellular and molecular alterations underlying AD pathogenesis. Falangola, Lee, Nixon, Duff, and Helpern (2005) reported that iron accumulates in Aβ plaques in the brains of APP/presenilin-1 double-mutant mice. Treatment of AD mice with antioxidant chemicals such as curcumin and DHA (Lim et al., 2001; Calon et al., 2004), or maintaining the mice on low-energy diets (Halagappa et al., 2007), can suppress Aβ and tau pathology and improve cognitive function, consistent with a role for oxidative stress and possibly iron in these models.

## 5. THERAPEUTIC IMPLICATIONS OF IRON IN AD PATHOGENESIS

The association of iron with the amyloid and neurofibrillary pathologies in the brains of AD patients and the experimental evidence that iron promotes Aβ aggregation, membrane lipid peroxidation, and neuronal death have resulted in the development of iron chelators as a new therapeutic strategy for the treatment of AD (Bandyopadhyay et al., 2006; Liu et al., 2006; Rogers et al., 2002). Treatment of cultured neuroblastoma cells with novel iron chelators and the green tea polyphenol-epigallocatechin-3-gallate resulted in a decrease in the production of Aβ (Avramovich-Tirosh et al., 2007). The rationale for the potential effectiveness of iron chelators in the treatment of AD is described above and reviewed in more detail elsewhere (Bush, 2002; Crouch, White, & Bush, 2007).

The first clinical study in which AD patients were administered an iron chelator was, in fact, intended to test the hypothesis that chelation of aluminum would be beneficial in AD (Crapper McLachlan et al., 1991). Forty eight patients with probable AD were randomly assigned to receive the iron chelator desferrioxamine (125 mg intramuscularly twice daily, 5 days per week), oral placebo (lecithin), or no treatment for 24 months. Subjects treated with desferrioxamine exhibited a rate of decline of daily living skills that was significantly less than both of the control groups. In more recent studies a metal chelator called clioquinol (iodochlorhydroxyquin), which had previously been used as an antibiotic for the treatment of traveler's diarrhea, was effective in decreasing the amyloid deposits in APP mutant transgenic mice (Cherny et al., 2001). A phase 2 clinical trial of clioquinol in 36 AD patients indicated that it was safe and possibly effective in slowing disease progression (Ritchie et al., 2003). However, there appears to be a very narrow therapeutic window for clioquinol and the potential for considerable toxicity with long-term treatments (Schäfer, Pajonk, Multhaup, & Bayer, 2007).

Finally, preventative approaches that enhance intrinsic antioxidant and anti-amyloidogenic mechanisms might be expected to protect against intrinsic iron-mediated neurotoxicity. Exercise, cognitive stimulation, and dietary energy restriction may all reduce the risk of AD, and each of these lifestyle factors has been shown to stimulate the production of neurotrophic factors and antioxidant defense systems in neurons (see Arumugam, Gleichmann, Tang, & Mattson, 2006 for review). Treatments that target Aβ production and aggregation, such as γ-secretase inhibitors (Pissarnitski, 2007) and immunotherapy (Weiner & Frenkel, 2006), would be expected to protect against iron-induced Aβ aggregation and neurotoxicity.

## REFERENCES


Arumugam, T. V., Gleichmann, M., Tang, S. C., & Mattson, M. P. (2006). Hormesis/preconditioning mechanisms, the nervous system and aging. *Ageing Research Reviews, 5*(2), 165–178.

Avramovich-Tirosh, Y., Reznichenko, L., Mit, T., Zheng, H., Fridkin, M., Weinreb, O., et al. (2007). Neurorescue activity, APP regulation and amyloid-beta peptide reduction by novel multi-functional brain permeable iron-chelating- antioxidants, M-30 and green tea polyphenol, EGCG. *Current Alzheimer Research, 4*(4), 403–411.

Bandyopadhyay, S., Huang, X., Cho, H., Greig, N. H., Youdim, M. B., & Rogers, J. T. (2006). Metal specificity of an iron-responsive element in Alzheimer's APP mRNA 5'untranslated region, tolerance of SH-SY5Y and H4 neural cells to desferrioxamine, clioquinol, VK-28, and a piperazine chelator. *Journal of Neural Transmission Supplement 71*, 237–247.

Blennow, K., de Leon, M. J., & Zetterberg, H. (2006). Alzheimer's disease. *Lancet, 368*(9533), 387–403.

Bruce-Keller, A. J., Li, Y. J., Lovell, M. A., Kraemer, P. J., Gary, D. S., Brown, R. R., et al. (1998). 4-Hydroxynonenal, a product of lipid peroxidation, damages cholinergic neurons and impairs visuospatial memory in rats. *Journal of Neuropathology and Experimental Neurology, 57*(3), 257–267.

Burdo, J. R., & Connor, J. R. (2003). Brain iron uptake and homeostatic mechanisms: An overview. *Biometals, 16*(1), 63–75.

Bush, A. I. (2002). Metal complexing agents as therapies for Alzheimer's disease. *Neurobiology of Aging, 23*(6), 1031–1038.

Calon, F., Lim, G. P., Yang, F., Morihara, T., Teter, B., Ubeda, O., et al. (2004). Docosahexaenoic acid protects from dendritic pathology in an Alzheimer's disease mouse model. *Neuron, 43*(5), 633–645.

Carson, J. A., & Turner, A. J. (2002). Beta-amyloid catabolism: Roles for neprilysin (NEP) and other metallopeptidases? *Journal of Neurochemistry, 81*(1), 1–8.

Castellani, R. J., Moreira, P. I., Liu, G., Dobson, J., Perry, G., Smith, M. A., et al. (2007). Iron: The Redox-active center of oxidative stress in Alzheimer disease. *Neurochemical Research, 32*(10), 1640–1645.

Cherny, R. A., Atwood, C. S., Xilinas, M. E., Gray, D. N., Jones, W. D., McLean, C. A, et al. (2001) Treatment with a copper-zinc chelator markedly and rapidly inhibits beta-amyloid accumulation in Alzheimer's disease transgenic mice. *Neuron, 30*(3), 665–676.

Connor, J. R., Menzies, S. L., St Martin, S. M., & Mufson, E. J. (1992). A histochemical study of iron, transferrin, and ferritin in Alzheimer's diseased brains. *Journal of Neuroscience Research, 31*(1), 75–83.

Connor, J. R., Snyder, B. S., Beard, J. L., Fine, R. E., & Mufson, E. J. (1992). Regional distribution of iron and iron-regulatory proteins in the brain in aging and Alzheimer's disease. *Journal of Neuroscience Research, 31*(2), 327–335.

Corder, E. H., Saunders, A. M., Strittmatter, W. J., Schmechel, D. E., Gaskell, P. C., Small, G. W., et al. (1993). Gene dose of apolipoprotein E type 4 allele and the risk of Alzheimer's disease in late onset families. *Science, 261*(5123), 921–923.

Crapper McLachlan, D. R., Dalton, A. J., Kruck, T. P., Bell, M. Y., Smith, W. L., Kalow, W., et al. (1991). Intramuscular desferrioxamine in patients with Alzheimer's disease. *Lancet, 337*(8753), 1304–1308.

Crouch, P. J., White, A. R., & Bush, A. I. (2007). The modulation of metal bio-availability as a therapeutic strategy for the treatment of Alzheimer's disease. *FEBS Journal, 274*(15), 3775–3783.

Deibel, M. A., Ehmann, W. D., & Markesbery, W. R. (1996). Copper, iron, and zinc imbalances in severely degenerated brain regions in Alzheimer's disease: Possible relation to oxidative stress. *Journal of Neurological Sciences, 143*(1–2), 137–142.

Dyrks, T., Dyrks, E., Hartmann, T., Masters, C., & Beyreuther, K. (1992). Amyloidogenicity of beta A4 and beta A4-bearing amyloid protein precursor fragments by metal-catalyzed oxidation. *Journal of Biological Chemistry, 267*(25), 18210–18217.

Falangola, M. F., Lee, S. P, Nixon, R. A., Duff, K., & Helpern, J. A. (2005) Histological co-localization of iron in Abeta plaques of PS/APP transgenic mice. *Neurochemical Research, 30*(2), 201–205.

Ferri, C. P., Prince, M., Brayne, C., Brodaty, H., Fratiglioni, L., Ganguli, M., et al. (2005). Global prevalence of dementia: A Delphi consensus study. *Lancet, 366*(9503), 2112–2117.

Fidani, L., & Goate, A. (1992). Mutations in APP and their role in beta-amyloid deposition. *Progress in Clinical & Biological Research, 379*, 195–214.

Goate, A., Chartier-Harlin, M. C., Mullan, M., Brown, J., Crawford, F., Fidani, L., et al. (1991). Segregation of a missense mutation in the amyloid precursor protein gene with familial Alzheimer's disease. *Nature, 349*(6311), 704–706.

Goodman, Y., & Mattson, M. P. (1994). Secreted forms of beta-amyloid precursor protein protect hippocampal neurons against amyloid beta-peptide-induced oxidative injury. *Experimental Neurology, 128*(1), 1–12.

Grundke-Iqbal, I., Fleming, J., Tung, Y. C., Lassmann, H., Iqbal, K., & Joshi, J. G. (1990). Ferritin is a component of the neuritic (senile) plaque in Alzheimer dementia. *Acta Neuropathologica, 81*(2), 105–110.

Guo, Q., Sopher, B. L., Furukawa, K., Pham, D. G., Robinson, N., Martin, G. M., et al. (1997). Alzheimer's presenilin mutation sensitizes neural cells to apoptosis induced by trophic factor withdrawal and amyloid beta-peptide: Involvement of calcium and oxyradicals. *Journal of Neuroscience, 17*(11), 4212–4222.

Guo, Q., Fu, W., Sopher, B. L., Miller, M. W., Ware, C. B., Martin, G. M., et al. (1999). Increased vulnerability of hippocampal neurons to excitotoxic necrosis in presenilin-1 mutant knock-in mice. *Nature Medicine, 5*(1), 101–106.

Halagappa, V. K., Guo, Z., Pearson, M., Matsuoka, Y., Cutler, R. G., Laferla, F. M., et al. (2007) Intermittent fasting and caloric restriction ameliorate age-related behavioral deficits in the triple-transgenic mouse model of Alzheimer's disease. *Neurobiology of Disease, 26*(1), 212–220.

Hardy, J., & Allsop, D. (1991). Amyloid deposition as the central event in the aetiology of Alzheimer's disease. *Trends in Pharmacological Sciences, 12*(10), 383–388.

Hardy, J., & Selkoe, D. J. (2002). The amyloid hypothesis of Alzheimer's disease: Progress and problems on the road to therapeutics. *Science, 297*(5580), 353–356.

Hensley, K., Carney, J. M., Mattson, M. P., Aksenova, M., Harris, M., Wu, J. F., et al. (1994) A model for beta-amyloid aggregation and neurotoxicity based on free radical generation by the peptide: Relevance to Alzheimer disease. *Proceedings of the National Academy of Sciences United States of America, 91*(8), 3270–3274.

Holtzman, D. M., Bales, K. R., Tenkova, T., Fagan, A. M., Parsadanian, M., Sartorius, L. J., et al. (2000). Apolipoprotein E isoform-dependent amyloid deposition and neuritic degeneration in a mouse model of Alzheimer's disease. *Proceedings of the National Academy of Sciences United States of America, 97*(6), 2892–2897.

Iqbal, K., Alonso Adel, C., Chen, S., Chohan, M. O., El-Akkad, E., Gong, C. X., et al. (2005). Tau pathology in Alzheimer disease and other tauopathies. *Biochimica et Biophysica Acta, 1739*(2–3), 198–210.

Iqbal, K., & Grundke-Iqbal, I. (2007, January 9). Alzheimer neurofibrillary degeneration: Significance, etiopathogenesis, therapeutics and prevention. *Journal of Cellular and Molecular Medicine Jan–Feb, 12*(1), 38–35.

Jellinger, K., Paulus, W., Grundke-Iqbal, I., Riederer, P., & Youdim, M. B. (1990) Brain iron and ferritin in Parkinson's and Alzheimer's diseases. *Journal of Neural Transmission Parkinson's Disease and Dementia Section, 2*(4), 327–340.

Keller, J. N., Mark, R. J., Bruce, A. J., Blanc, E., Rothstein, J. D., Uchida, K., et al. (1997). 4-Hydroxynonenal, an aldehydic product of membrane lipid peroxidation, impairs glutamate transport and mitochondrial function in synaptosomes. *Neuroscience, 80*(3), 685–696.

Levy-Lahad, E., & Bird, T. D. (1996). Genetic factors in Alzheimer's disease: A review of recent advances. *Annals of Neurology, 40*(6), 829–840.

Lim, G. P., Chu, T., Yang, F., Beech, W., Frautschy, S. A., & Cole, G. M. (2001). The curry spice curcumin reduces oxidative damage and amyloid pathology in an Alzheimer transgenic mouse. *Journal of Neuroscience, 21*(21), 8370–8377.

Liu, G., Huang, W., Moir, R. D., Vanderburg, C. R., Lai, B., Peng, Z., et al. (2006). Metal exposure and Alzheimer's pathogenesis. *Journal of Structural Biology, 155*(1), 45–51.

Lovell, M.A., Robertson, J.D., Teesdale, W.J., Campbell, J.L., & Markesbery, W.R. (1998). Copper, iron and zinc in Alzheimer's disease senile plaques. *Journal of the Neurological Sciences, 158*(1), 47–52.

Lovell, M. A., Xiong, S., Xie, C., Davies, P., & Markesbery, W. R. (2004). Induction of hyperphosphorylated tau in primary rat cortical neuron cultures mediated by oxidative stress and glycogen synthase kinase-3. *Journal of Alzheimer's Disease, 6*(6), 659–671.

Mantyh, P. W., Ghilardi, J. R., Rogers, S., DeMaster, E., Allen, C. J., Stimson, E. R., et al. (1993). Aluminum, iron, and zinc ions promote aggregation of physiological concentrations of beta-amyloid peptide. *Journal of Neurochemistry, 61*(3), 1171–1174.

Mark, R. J., Hensley, K., Butterfield, D. A., & Mattson, M. P. (1995). Amyloid beta-peptide impairs ion-motive ATPase activities: Evidence for a role in loss of neuronal $Ca2+$ homeostasis and cell death. *Journal of Neuroscience, 15*(9), 6239–6249.

Mark, R. J., Pang, Z., Geddes, J. W., Uchida, K., & Mattson, M. P. (1997). Amyloid beta-peptide impairs glucose transport in hippocampal and cortical neurons: Involvement of membrane lipid peroxidation. *Journal of Neuroscience, 17*(3), 1046–1054.

Masters, C. L., Multhaup, G., Simms, G., Pottgiesser, J., Martins, R. N., & Beyreuther, K. (1985). Neuronal origin of a cerebral amyloid: Neurofibrillary tangles of Alzheimer's disease contain the same protein as the amyloid of plaque cores and blood vessels. *EMBO Journal, 4*(11), 2757–2763.

Mattson, M. P., Fu, W., Waeg, G., & Uchida, K. (1997). 4-Hydroxynonenal, a product of lipid peroxidation, inhibits dephosphorylation of the microtubule-associated protein tau. *Neuroreport, 8*(9–10), 2275–22781.

Mattson, M. P. (2004a). Pathways towards and away from Alzheimer's disease. *Nature, 430*(7000), 631–639.

Mattson, M. P. (2004b) Metal-catalyzed disruption of membrane protein and lipid signaling in the pathogenesis of neurodegenerative disorders. *Annals of New York Academy of Sciences, 1012*, 37–50.

Mayeux, R. (2003). Epidemiology of neurodegeneration. *Annual Review of Neurosciences, 26*, 81–104.

Mazur-Kolecka, B., Kowal, D., Sukontasup, T., Dickson, D., & Frackowiak, J. (2004). The effect of oxidative stress on amyloid precursor protein processing in cells engaged in beta-amyloidosis is related to apolipoprotein E genotype. *Acta Neuropathologica, 108*(4), 287–294.

Moller, H. J., & Graeber, M. B. (1998). The case described by Alois Alzheimer in 1911. Historical and conceptual perspectives based on the clinical record and neurohistological sections. *European Archives of Psychiatry and Clinical Neurosciences, 248*(3), 111–122.

Morris, C. M., Kerwin, J. M., & Edwardson, J. A. (1994). Non-haem iron histochemistry of the normal and Alzheimer's disease hippocampus. *Neurodegeneration, 3*(4), 267–275.

Pasquier, F., Boulogne, A., Leys, D., & Fontaine, P. (2006). Diabetes mellitus and dementia. *Diabetes and Metabolism, 32*(5 Pt 1), 403–414.

Pedersen, W. A., Chan, S. L., & Mattson, M. P. (2000). A mechanism for the neuroprotective effect of apolipoprotein E: Isoform-specific modification by the lipid peroxidation product 4-hydroxynonenal. *Journal of Neurochemistry, 74*(4), 1426–1433.

Perry, T., Lahiri, D. K., Sambamurti, K., Chen, D., Mattson, M. P., Egan, J. M., et al. (2003). Glucagon-like peptide-1 decreases endogenous amyloid-beta peptide (Abeta) levels and protects hippocampal neurons from death induced by Abeta and iron. *Journal of Neuroscience Research, 72*(5), 603–612.

Pissarnitski, D. (2007). Advances in gamma-secretase modulation. *Current Opinions in Drug Discovery and Development, 10*, 392–402.

Poirier, J., Davignon, J., Bouthillier, D., Kogan, S., Bertrand, P., & Gauthier, S. (1993). Apolipoprotein E polymorphism and Alzheimer's disease. *Lancet, 342*(8873), 697–699.

Quintana, C., Bellefqih, S., Laval, J.Y., Guerquin-Kern, J.L., Wu, T.D., Avila, J., et al. (2006). Study of the localization of iron, ferritin, and hemosiderin in Alzheimer's disease hippocampus by analytical microscopy at the subcellular level. *Journal of Structural Biology, 153*(1), 42–54.

Raber, J., Huang, Y., & Ashford, J. W. (2004). ApoE genotype accounts for the vast majority of AD risk and AD pathology. *Neurobiology of Aging, 25*(5), 641–650.

Ritchie, C. W., Bush, A. I., Mackinnon, A., Macfarlane, S., Mastwyk, M., MacGregor, L., et al. (2003) Metal-protein attenuation with iodochlorhydroxyquin (clioquinol) targeting Abeta amyloid deposition and toxicity in Alzheimer disease: A pilot phase 2 clinical trial. *Archives of Neurology, 60*(12), 1685–1691.

Rogaeva, E. (2002) The solved and unsolved mysteries of the genetics of early-onset Alzheimer's disease. *Neuromolecular Medicine, 2*(1), 1–10.

Rogers, J. T., Randall, J. D., Cahill, C. M., Eder, P. S., Huang, X., Gunshin, H., et al. (2002). An iron-responsive element type II in the 5'-untranslated region of the Alzheimer's amyloid precursor protein transcript. *Journal of Biological Chemistry, 277*(47), 45518–45528.

Rottkamp, C. A., Raina, A. K., Zhu, X., Gaier, E., Bush, A. I., Atwood, C. S., et al. (2001). Redox-active iron mediates amyloid-beta toxicity. *Free Radical Biology and Medicine, 30*(4), 447–450.

Rovelet-Lecrux, A., Hannequin, D., Raux, G., Le Meur, N., Laquerriere, A., Vital, A., et al. (2006). APP locus duplication causes autosomal dominant early-onset Alzheimer disease with cerebral amyloid angiopathy. *Nature Genetics, 38*(1), 24–26.

Schäfer, S., Pajonk, F. G., Multhaup, G., & Bayer, T. A. (2007). Copper and clioquinol treatment in young APP transgenic and wild-type mice: Effects on life expectancy, body weight, and metal-ion levels. *Journal of Molecular Medicine, 85*, 405–413.

Selkoe, D. J. (1991a). Amyloid protein and Alzheimer's disease. *Scientific American, 265*(5), 68–71, 74–66, 78.

Selkoe, D. J. (1991b). The molecular pathology of Alzheimer's disease. *Neuron, 6*(4), 487–498.

Smith, M.A., Harris, P.L., Sayre, L.M., & Perry, G. (1997) Iron accumulation in Alzheimer disease is a source of redox-generated free radicals. *Proceedings of National Academy of Sciences United States of America, 94*(18), 9866–9868.

Smith, M. A., Wehr, K., Harris, P. L., Siedlak, S. L., Connor, J. R., & Perry, G. (1998). Abnormal localization of iron regulatory protein in Alzheimer's disease. *Brain Research, 788*(1–2), 232–236.

Smith, D. G., Cappai, R., & Barnham, K. J. (2007). The redox chemistry of the Alzheimer's disease amyloid beta peptide. *Biochimica et Biophysica Acta, 1768*(8), 1976–1990.

Stranahan, A. M., Arumugam, T. V., Cutler, R. G., Lee, K., Egan, J. & Mattson, M. P. (2008). Diabetes impairs hippocampal function via glucocorticoid–mediated effects on new and mature neurons. *Nature Neuroscience Mar, 11*(3), 309–317.

Tanzi, R. E., Moir, R. D., & Wagner, S. L. (2004). Clearance of Alzheimer's Abeta peptide: The many roads to perdition. *Neuron, 43*(5), 605–608.

Thompson, C. M., Markesbery, W. R., Ehmann, W. D., Mao, Y. X., & Vance, D. E. (1988). Regional brain trace-element studies in Alzheimer's disease. *Neurotoxicology, 9*(1), 1–7.

Tu, H., Nelson, O., Bezprozvanny, A., Wang, Z., Lee, S. F., Hao, Y. H., et al. (2006). Presenilins form ER Ca2+ leak channels, a function disrupted by familial Alzheimer's disease-linked mutations. *Cell, 126*(5), 981–993.

Weiner, H. L., & Frenkel, D. (2006) Immunology and immunotherapy of Alzheimer's disease. *Nature Reviews Immunology, 6*(5), 404–416.

World Health Organisation report-Neurological disorders: Public health Challenges. (2007). http://www.who.int/mental_health/neurology/neurodiso/en/index.html.

Williams, T. I., Lynn, B. C., Markesbery, W. R., & Lovell, M. A. (2006). Increased levels of 4-hydroxynonenal and acrolein, neurotoxic markers of lipid peroxidation, in the brain in Mild Cognitive Impairment and early Alzheimer's disease. *Neurobiology of Aging, 27*(8), 1094–1099.

# 15 Inherited Disorders of Brain Iron Homeostasis

*Hyman M. Schipper and Prem Ponka*

**Summary**

- Iron is indispensable for oxidation–reduction catalysis and bioenergetics but, unless appropriately handled, may generate highly toxic reactive oxygen species.
- Organisms are endowed with a panoply of proteins that mediate acquisition, export, transport and storage of the transition metal, and mechanisms that maintain the intracellular labile iron pool at physiological levels.
- In humans and other organisms, inherited or acquired disruption of these highly coordinated pathways may promote illness as a consequence of tissue iron deficiency or overload.
- A number of hereditary conditions perturb iron homeostasis and promote pathological deposition of the metal predominantly or exclusively within the central nervous system.
- Hereditary disorders of brain iron overload include aceruloplasminemia, neuroferritinopathy, Friedreich's ataxia, pantothenate kinase-2-associated neurodegeneration, and possibly X-linked sideroblastic anemia with ataxia in humans, and iron-regulatory protein-2 (IRP2) deficiency in mice.
- Gene mutations responsible for hemochromatosis, a genetic disorder of systemic iron homeostasis, may be risk factors or modulators of common degenerative (Alzheimer's disease, Parkinson's disease, amyotrophic lateral sclerosis) and vascular (ischemic stroke) CNS disorders.

**Key Words:** ABCB7; aceruloplasminemia; Alzheimer's disease; amyotrophic lateral sclerosis; ceruloplasmin; frataxin; ferritin; hemochromatosis; Hfe; iron; iron-regulatory protein (IRP1, IRP2); ischemic stroke; neurodegeneration with brain iron accumulation (NBIA); neuroferritinopathy; Friedreich's ataxia; pantothenate kinase-2-associated neurodegeneration; Parkinson's disease; X-linked sideroblastic anemia with ataxia

## 15.1. HUMAN IRON PHYSIOLOGY: AN OVERVIEW

Iron (Fe), the fourth most abundant element in the earth's crust, is an essential constituent of many structural proteins and enzymes and participates in a wide range of vital biological functions, including oxygen delivery (hemoglobin), electron transport (mitochondrial heme and non-heme iron proteins), and DNA synthesis (ribonucleotide reductase). In the developing and mature mammalian nervous system, iron is fundamental to oligodendroglial function and myelination, cellular proliferation, and biogenic amine metabolism. Paradoxically, the chemical properties of iron which permit this bioversatility also enable the metal to participate in Fenton and other reactions that generate reactive oxygen species inimical to proteins, lipids, nucleic acids,

From: *Nutrition and Health: Iron Deficiency and Overload*
Edited by: S. Yehuda and D.I. Mostofsky, DOI 10.1007/978-1-59745-462-9_15

and other oxidizable cellular substrates (Halliwell, 2001; McCord, 1998). Chemical pathways implicated in iron-mediated neurotoxicity are described in Chapter 7. To prevent or ameliorate such toxicity, organisms have evolved a host of specialized molecules for the safe acquisition, export, transport, and storage of tissue iron. These and other elaborate regulatory mechanisms prevent the expansion of the catalytically active intracellular labile iron pool while maintaining sufficient concentrations of the metal for metabolic use (Aisen, Enns, & Wessling-Resnick, 2001; De Domenico, McVey Ward, & Kaplan, 2008; Hentze, Muckenthaler, & Andrews, 2004; Ponka, Beaumont, & Richardson, 1998; Richardson & Ponka, 1997). Transferrin, transferrin receptor, and ferritin are "classical" proteins mediating the transport and storage of iron in humans and other mammals. More recently, a much broader array of novel genes has been implicated in tissue iron homeostasis (Table 1) and many, if not all, of the proteins coded by these genes are expressed in the brain (Burdo & Connor, 2003; Connor, 2003).

**Table 1**
**Proteins Implicated in Mammalian Iron Homeostasis**

| *Protein* | *Function* |
|---|---|
| ABC7 | Non-heme Fe export from mitochondria (?) |
| ABC-me | Mitochondrial transport related to heme synthesis |
| Ceruloplasmin (Cp) | Ferroxidase activity/cellular Fe export |
| DMT1/Nramp2 | Membrane transport for $Fe^{2+}$ |
| Duodenal cytochrome b (Dcytb) | Ferric reductase (provides $Fe^{2+}$ for DMT1 in duodenum) |
| Ferritin (H and L) | Cellular Fe storage |
| Ferrochelatase | $Fe^{2+}$ insertion into protoporphyryin IX (heme synthesis) |
| Ferroportin 1/MTP1/ Iregl | Cellular Fe export |
| Frascati | Mitochondrial Fe transport |
| Frataxin | [Fe–S] cluster synthesis |
| Heme oxygenase (1 and 2) | Recycling of heme Fe / Cell survival |
| Hemojuvelin (Repulsive Guidance Molecule C) | Unknown/cardiac and striated muscle Fe metabolism? |
| Hepcidin | Inhibitor of intestinal Fe absorption and macrophage heme Fe recycling |
| Hephaestin | Ferroxidase activity/enterocyte Fe export |
| HFE | Modulates tissue Fe uptake via interaction with TfR (?) |
| IRP (1 and 2) | Cellular Fe sensors/regulators of Fe uptake and storage proteins |
| Lactoferrin | Fe binding protein/anti-bacterial and anti-viral activities |
| Melanotransferrin | Unknown/Fe binding protein |
| Mitochondrial ferritin | Mitochondrial Fe storage (?) |
| Mitoferrin | Fe transport to mitochondria |
| Sideroflexin 1 | Mitochondrial transport related to Fe metabolism |
| Steap3 | Endosomal ferrireductase |
| Transferrin (Tf) | Plasma Fe(III)-carrier |
| Tf receptor 1 | Membrane receptor for $Fe_2$-Tf |
| Tf receptor 2 | Unknown |

Modified from Ponka (2004), with permission

Total body iron content in humans is normally maintained within narrow limits by the regulation of iron uptake in the gut (Miret, Simpson, & McKie, 2003). Both inorganic iron and heme are absorbed through the brush border of the proximal small intestine. Heme is more readily available for absorption but usually constitutes only a small fraction of dietary iron. Heme is absorbed intact, probably via specific high-affinity heme-binding sites in the mucosal brush border (Grasbeck, Majuri, Kouvonen, & Tenhunen, 1982; Worthington, Cohn, Miller, Luo, & Berg, 2001). Within the intestinal epithelium, iron is enzymatically liberated from heme by the action of heme oxygenase 1. Divalent metal transporter 1 (DMT1) (Fleming et al., 1997; Gunshin et al., 1997) is the principal transporter of inorganic iron in the intestinal mucosa. DMT1 only transports iron in the $Fe^{2+}$ state, explaining why reducing agents (e.g., ascorbate) enhance iron absorption. The duodenal brush border contains a ferric reductase (Dcytb) (McKie et al., 2001) which converts $Fe^{3+}$ to $Fe^{2+}$ prior to its transport into the enterocyte. Iron release from enterocytes and other "donor cells" (e.g., macrophages) to plasma transferrin is not fully understood, but a number of recent studies have provided new clues in this important area of iron metabolism. It is now well established that iron is exported from cells via ferroportin (Donovan et al., 2000), also known as MTP (Abboud & Haile, 2000) or Ireg (McKie et al., 2000), and the ferroxidase activity of hephaestin (Vulpe et al., 1999) and ceruloplasmin (Hellman & Gitlin, 2002; Nittis & Gitlin, 2002) facilitate the movement of iron across the membranes of enterocytes and macrophages, respectively. Ceruloplasmin and hephaestin exhibit a high degree of homology; both proteins contain several copper atoms that are necessary for their ferroxidase (i.e., oxidation of $Fe^{2+}$ to $Fe^{3+}$) activity.

In humans, the turnover of transferrin iron is ~30 mg/24 hr. Normally, ~80% of this iron is transported to the bone marrow for hemoglobin synthesis in developing red blood cells. Senescent erythrocytes are phagocytosed by macrophages of the reticuloendothelial system where the heme moiety dissociates from hemoglobin and is catabolized via heme oxygenase 1 to free iron, biliverdin, and carbon monoxide (Maines, 1997). The heme-derived iron is returned almost quantitatively to the circulation. The remaining 5 mg of the daily plasma iron turnover is exchanged with nonerythroid tissues, principally the liver. About 1 mg of dietary iron is absorbed per 24 hr, and total organismal iron balance is maintained by loss of 1 mg/day via nonspecific mechanisms (mainly cell desquamation) (Aisen et al., 2001; Ponka et al., 1998; Richardson & Ponka, 1997).

Delivery of iron to most mammalian tissues occurs following the binding of diferric transferrin to cell membrane transferrin receptors. The transferrin–transferrin receptor complexes are internalized within endosomes by endocytosis; $Fe^{3+}$ is released from transferrin by a process involving endosomal acidification (Aisen et al., 2001; Richardson & Ponka, 1997) and is then transported across the endosomal membrane by DMT1. Since the substrate for DMT1 is ferrous iron (Gunshin et al., 1997), reduction of transferrin-borne $Fe^{3+}$ must occur in endosomes. Importantly, Ohgami et al. (2005) have recently identified a gene, *Steap3* (six-transmembrane, epithelial antigen of the prostate 3), the product of which is a prime candidate for endosomal ferric reductase. The protein coded by this gene is present in endosomes and colocalizes with transferrin, transferrin receptors, and DMT1. Following its release from endosomes, iron is conveyed to various intracellular compartments for metabolic use or storage (as $Fe^{3+}$) within the high-capacity iron-sequestering protein ferritin (described in more detail below). Cells are endowed with an exquisite regulatory system that tightly controls iron levels in the "labile iron pool" (LIP), i.e., metabolically available iron in transit among various intracellular compartments. In general, expansion of the LIP stimulates ferritin synthesis and diminishes expression of transferrin receptors; the opposite occurs when this pool is depleted of the metal. Iron levels in the

LIP are "sensed" by iron-regulatory proteins, IRP1 and IRP2. IRPs control the synthesis of transferrin receptors and ferritin by binding to iron-responsive elements (IREs) located in the 3′ untranslated region (UTR) and the 5′ UTR of their respective mRNAs. When cellular iron is scarce, IRPs bind to IREs, and this association stabilizes transferrin receptor mRNA and blocks the translation of ferritin mRNA. Enlargement of the LIP inactivates IRP1 binding to the IREs and promotes proteosomal catabolism of IRP2, resulting in augmented translation of ferritin and rapid degradation of transferrin receptor mRNA (Aisen et al., 2001; Cairo & Pietrangelo, 2000; Mikulits, Schranzhofer, Beug, & Mullner, 1999; Richardson & Ponka, 1997). Nitric oxide (NO) and oxidative stress (OS) impact cellular iron metabolism, in part, by modulating the binding of IRPs to IREs (Hentze & Kuhn, 1996; Kim & Ponka, 2000; Pantopoulos, Weiss, & Hentze, 1996). Finally, mRNAs for both DMT1 and ferroportin contain IREs in their untranslated regions and are likely regulated by the IRE/IRP system.

The CNS maintains strict and fairly autonomous control of its chemical microenvironment (Zlokovic, 2008) and iron is no exception. The blood–brain barrier (BBB) precludes free passage of transferrin, ceruloplasmin, and other proteins from the systemic circulation to the CNS. Circulating diferric transferrin binds to transferrin receptors expressed by cerebrovascular endothelial cells at the BBB and the resulting complexes are internalized as described above. After dissociation of the complex within endothelial endosomes, apotransferrin is recycled to the blood and iron is exported, likely via ferroportin, across the abluminal membrane to the interstitial space. Readers are referred to a recent review by Moos, Rosengren Nielsen, Skjorringe, and Morgan (2007) for further details of iron trafficking within and among the various CNS compartments.

In humans and other mammals, brain iron uptake is maximal during periods of rapid CNS development, but neural uptake of the metal continues throughout life (Morgan & Moos, 2002). The actual daily rate of iron exchange between plasma transferrin and the CNS is uncertain, but likely does not exceed 3 mg Fe/24hr (Ponka, 2004). Far less is known regarding iron-transfer kinetics among the various CNS compartments and mechanisms governing extrusion of the metal from the brain parenchyma to the systemic circulation. As discussed in the following sections, recent years have witnessed a growing awareness of heritable disorders of iron homeostasis, characterized by pathological brain iron deposition and severe neurological morbidity. Delineation of the precise cellular and molecular pathways mediating brain iron homeostasis in health and disease should greatly inform our understanding and management of these debilitating conditions.

## 15.2. GENETIC DISORDERS OF CNS IRON HOMEOSTASIS

### *15.2.1. Friedreich's Ataxia*

Friedreich's ataxia (FA) is an autosomal recessive neurodegenerative disease and the most common of the heritable human ataxias. Disease onset is generally before age 25 and clinical manifestations include progressive limb and gait ataxia, dysarthria, areflexia, epicritic sensory loss, and cardiomyopathy (Fig. 1). The defective gene in this disease is *FRDA* (encoded by a nuclear gene) which codes for the mitochondrial protein, frataxin. About 98% of mutant alleles have an expansion of the GAA trinucleotide repeat in intron 1, resulting in a marked reduction in frataxin levels (Babady et al., 2007; Pandolfo, 1999). Frataxin is normally highly expressed in mitochondria-rich tissues such as heart, liver, and skeletal muscle, and cells from FA patients exhibit defective mitochondrial respiration (Becker & Richardson, 2001). Mitochondrial iron overload develops in the CNS and myocardium of FA patients (Babady et al., 2007; Lamarche,

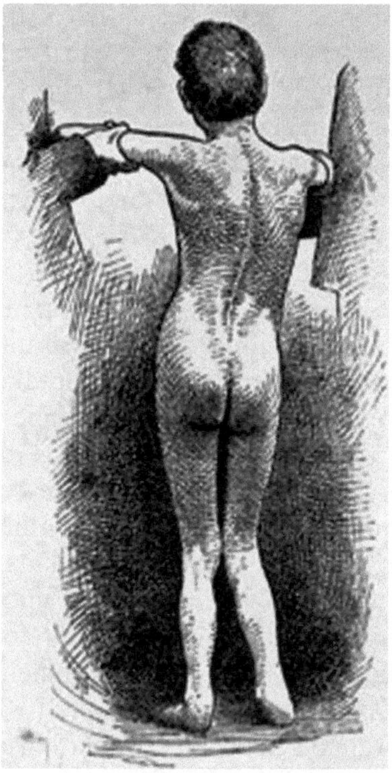

**Fig. 1.** Friedreich's ataxia. From www.neuro.wustl.edu/.../patients/fapix2sm.jpg.

Cote, & Lemieux, 1980) and mice with conditional knockout of the frataxin gene (Puccio et al., 2001). Importantly, intramitochondrial iron accumulation in frataxin-deficient mice occurs only after onset of the pathology and following inactivation of iron–sulfur (Fe–S)-dependent enzymes such as complexes I–III of the respiratory chain and the aconitases (Puccio et al., 2001). This finding suggests that iron per se may play a secondary or downstream role in the pathophysiology of FA. Unlike patients with sideroblastic anemia, another condition featuring intramitochondrial iron sequestration (Ponka, 1997), FA erythroblasts do not contain iron-overloaded mitochondria. Indeed, frataxin expression may be downregulated in differentiating erythroid cells under physiological conditions in order to allow active heme biosynthesis (Becker, Greer, Ponka, & Richardson, 2002; Welch et al., 2004). So what is the function of frataxin? Important clues to the role of frataxin in iron metabolism emerged from studies on the yeast *FRDA* ortholog, *Yfh1* (Becker & Richardson, 2001). Mitochondria in *Yfh1* mutants accumulate approximately an order of magnitude more iron than do wild-type mitochondria (Babcock et al., 1997). This process appears to be reversible as re-introduction of wild-type *Yfh1* results in the rapid export of mitochondrial non-heme iron to the cytosolic compartment (Radisky, Babcock, & Kaplan, 1999). Frataxin does not contain a trans-membrane domain, rendering it unlikely that it serves as a membrane metal transporter. It has been proposed that frataxin may assist in the assembly or export of Fe–S clusters from mitochondria or participate in mitochondrial iron storage (Becker & Richardson, 2001). Reports by Lill and co-workers (Gerber, Muhlenhoff, & Lill, 2003; Lill & Muhlenhoff, 2006; Muhlenhoff, Gerber, Richhardt, & Lill, 2003; Stehling, Elsasser, Bruckel, Muhlenhoff, & Lill, 2004) bolster the notion that frataxin is an essential component of a complex machinery responsible for the synthesis of Fe–S clusters in mitochondria. Their studies have revealed that depletion of the yeast frataxin homolog, Yfh1p, decreases Fe–S cluster biogenesis on the scaffold protein Isu1p (Muhlenhoff et al., 2003) and that Yfh1p interacts directly with Isu1p (Gerber et al., 2003). Similarly, frataxin depletion by RNAi in HeLa cells decreases the enzymatic activities of the mitochondrial Fe–S proteins, aconitase and succinate dehydrogenase, whereas the activities of non-Fe–S proteins remain constant. Furthermore, Fe–S cluster association with cytosolic IRP1 was diminished in the frataxin-deficient cells (Stehling et al., 2004). These observations indicate that frataxin is not involved in the export of Fe–S clusters from mitochondria, and raise the question as to why frataxin deficiency engenders iron trapping by this organelle. When 5-aminolevulinic acid dehydratase (second enzyme of the heme biosynthetic pathway) is inhibited in erythroblasts, iron uptake by mitochondria (where ferrochelatase inserts $Fe^{2+}$ into protoporphyrin IX to form heme) is uninterrupted and the metal accumulates in a non-heme form. When the enzyme block is relieved, mitochondrial non-heme iron is rapidly incorporated into heme, which is then released to the cytosol (Ponka, Wilczynska, & Schulman, 1982). Thus, iron might only exit mitochondria effectively bound to molecules destined for delivery to other cellular compartments. For example, the ATP-binding cassette protein B7 (ABCB7), mutant in X-linked sideroblastic anemia with ataxia (see below), is absolutely required for extramitochondrial Fe–S cluster formation (Csere, Lill, & Kispal, 1998; Kispal, Csere, Guiard, & Lill, 1997; Lill & Muhlenhoff, 2006; Napier, Ponka, & Richardson, 2005). Conceivably, in a manner analogous to blockade of heme biosynthesis, faulty Fe–S cluster assembly in frataxin-deficient mitochondria impedes an important conduit for the export of mitochondrial iron in FA cells. Of note, frataxin has recently been shown to also play a cardinal role in the assembly of extramitochondrial Fe–S clusters (Martelli et al., 2007).

A link has also been established between frataxin and mitochondrial ferritin, an iron-storage protein abundant in the testis and in sideroblasts (pathological erythroblasts with iron-laden mitochondria) of patients with sideroblastic anemia. Arosio's group silenced frataxin in HeLa cells and showed that this leads to impaired growth, inhibition of aconitase and superoxide dismutase-2 activities, and a reduction in cytosolic ferritins. Interestingly, these changes were abrogated when frataxin silencing was performed in cells expressing human mitochondrial ferritin (Zanella et al., 2008). The authors conjectured that distinct but overlapping pools of mitochondrial iron may be co-regulated by frataxin and mitochondrial ferritin, and that deficiencies in one protein (frataxin) may be offset by over-expression of the other (mitochondrial ferritin), a proposal with potentially important therapeutic implications for FA.

*Treatment of Friedreich's ataxia:* Orally administered co-enzyme Q and idebenone, respiratory chain antioxidants, have met with some minor success in improving certain cardiac parameters in FA, but have had no appreciable impact on the neurological manifestations of the disease (Hart et al., 2005). Some potentially important inroads into the management of the latter have recently been reported by Cabantchik's group (Boddaert et al., 2007) in a phase 1–2 study using the orally active, membrane-permeant iron chelator, deferiprone (3-hydroxy-1,2-dimethylpyridin-4-one). After a 6-month treatment period with 20–30 mg/kg/d, there was a significant reduction in the mean $R2^*$ signal in the cerebellar dentate nuclei on magnetic resonance imaging (MRI), an index of tissue iron stores, among nine adolescent FA patients with no overt cardiomyopathy. Moreover, there appeared to be unprecedented and clinically meaningful amelioration of ataxic gait and peripheral neuropathy in the youngest subjects, without evidence of significant adverse neurological or hematological effects.

### *15.2.2. Pantothenate Kinase-2-Associated Neurodegeneration*

Pantothenate kinase-2-associated neurodegeneration (PKAN), formerly known as the Hallervorden-Spatz syndrome and a form of neurodegeneration with brain iron accumulation (NBIA), is caused by autosomal recessive, loss-of-function mutations in the gene encoding brain-specific mitochondrial pantothenate kinase-2 (*PANK2)* at locus 20p13-p12.3 (Hayflick, 2006; Johnson et al., 2004; Zhou et al., 2001). The majority of patients present in childhood or young adulthood with combinations of dysarthria, dystonia, choreoathetosis, parkinsonism, spasticity, seizures, mental retardation, dementia, optic atrophy, and pigmentary retinopathy (Hayflick, 2003, 2006; Swaiman, 2001). On MRI, many affected and pre-symptomatic subjects exhibit the "eye-of-the-tiger sign," a hyperintense signal surrounded by a ring of hypointensity in globus pallidus attributed respectively to tissue vacuolization/gliosis and pathological iron deposits (Fig. 2) (Savoiardo et al., 1993). At autopsy, there is brownish discoloration of the basal ganglia due to the excessive iron stores. The latter can be readily visualized in sections stained for iron with Perls' method as granular deposits scattered about the neuropil and within astrocytes and microglial cells of the globus pallidus and substantia nigra pars reticulata. Similar concretions and spheroid bodies (focal axonal swellings) are encountered in cerebral white and gray matter and in the

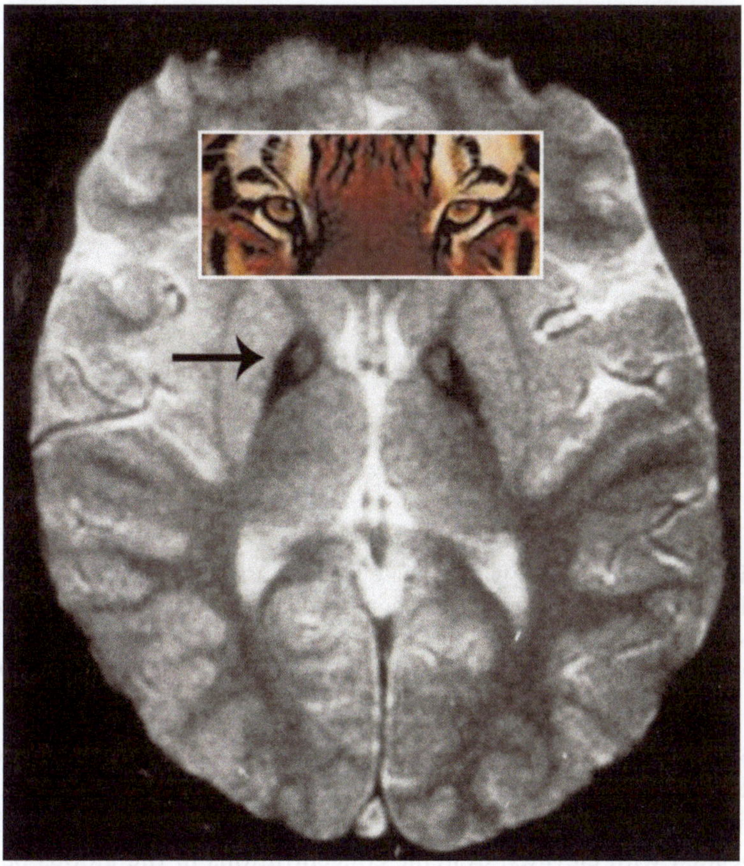

**Fig. 2.** Brain MRI of patient with pantothenate kinase-2-associated neurodegeneration (PKAN). T2*-weighted echo-planar sequences demonstrate "eye-of-the-tiger" sign in the globus pallidus (*arrow*). Inset: Tiger (*Panthera tigris*). Modified from Castelnau et al. (2001), with permission.

subthalamic nucleus of Luys (Fig. 3). Electron microscopy of vacuolated circulating lymphocytes may additionally disclose fingerprint, granular, and multilamellar bodies reminiscent of ceroid-lipofuscin (Swaiman, Smith, Trock, & Siddiqui, 1983; Zupanc, Chun, & Gilbert-Barness, 1990).

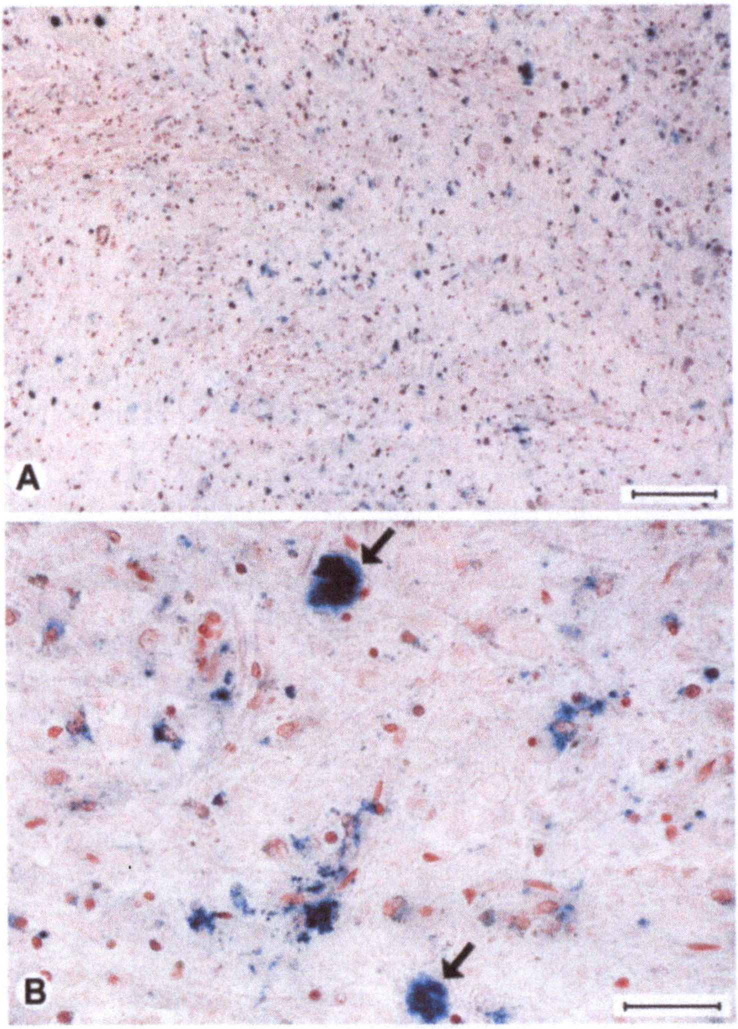


**Fig. 3.** Globus pallidus of a patient with pantothenate kinase-2-associated neurodegeneration. Perls' method reveals pathological iron deposits (*blue*) scattered about the neuropil at low (**A**) and high (**B**) magnification. Punctate staining may represent glial iron deposits, whereas globular reaction product (**B**, *arrows*) likely denotes dystrophic axons. Bars = 100 μm in **A** and 50 μm in **B**. From Koeppen and Dickson (2001), with permission.

PANK2 is essential for the synthesis of coenzyme A, catalyzing the phosphorylation of pantothenate (vitamin $B_5$). The product of the reaction, phosphopantothenate, normally condenses with cysteine in the next step of coenzyme A biosynthesis (Fig. 4). Pantothenate kinase-2 deficiency is associated with elevated cysteine concentrations in the globus pallidus of affected individuals (Perry et al., 1985). Cysteine has iron-chelating properties that might account for the regional iron accumulation observed in patients with PANK2 deficiency. Moreover, cysteine undergoes rapid autoxidation in the presence of transition metals, resulting in the generation of

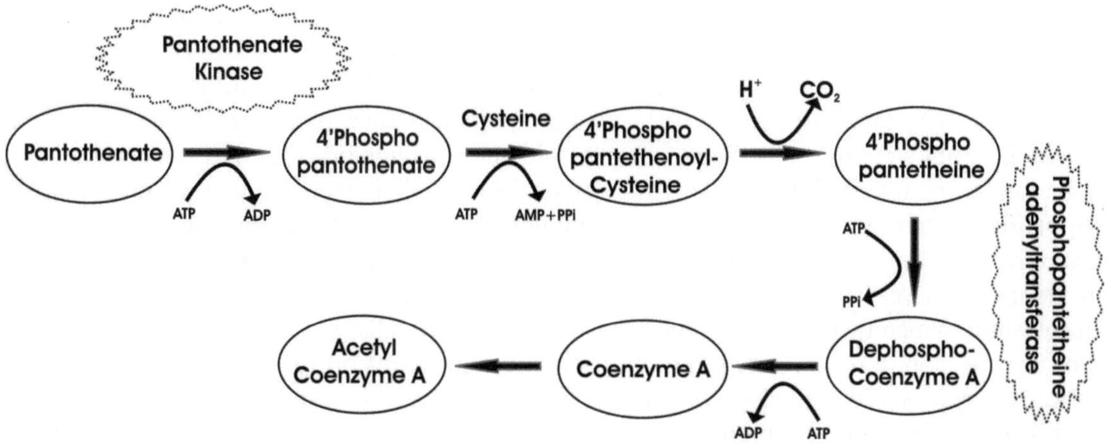


**Fig. 4.** Pantothenate kinase and the co-enzyme A biosynthetic pathway. Modified from Grimes, Lang, and Bergeron (2000), with permission.

reactive oxygen and sulfur species (Berg & Hochstrasser, 2006; Yoon, Koh, Floyd, & Park, 2000). Cysteine-bound iron may thereby promote oxidative neuronal injury in the basal ganglia of PKAN subjects with attendant clinical deterioration (Hayflick, 2003; Zhou et al., 2001).

Differential diagnosis and recommended work-up for suspected PKAN have recently been reviewed by Zimmerman & Schenck (2007). Suffice it to say that genetic lesions other than *PANK2* mutations may present a neurological picture phenotypically indistinguishable from PKAN. For example, mutations in the gene encoding a calcium-independent group VI phospholipase $A_2$ (*PLA2G6*) have been implicated in some children with NBIA (Hayflick, 2006; Morgan et al., 2006). PLA2G6 plays an important role in phospholipid remodeling, arachidonic acid release, leukotriene and prostaglandin synthesis, and apoptosis (Balsinde & Balboa, 2005). Whether pathological brain iron deposition in this condition is related to aberrant lipid neurochemistry or to some hitherto unidentified action of the mutant enzyme remains to be determined.

Unfortunately, there is no specific treatment currently available for victims of PKAN. Administration of vitamin $B_5$ and iron chelation therapy with deferoxamine have been attempted without evidence of benefit. Symptomatic relief may be obtained with dopaminergic agents, oral or intrathecal baclofen, and stereotactic pallidotomy (Justesen, Penn, Kroin, & Egel, 1999; Zimmerman & Schenck, 2007).

### *15.2.3. Aceruloplasminemia*

Ceruloplasmin is an abundant plasma $\alpha_2$-glycoprotein that has sky-blue color in its purified form and is synthesized primarily, but not exclusively, in the liver. Ceruloplasmin is composed of 1046 amino acids and contains six copper atoms. Three of these copper atoms form a trinuclear cluster that activates oxygen needed for the catalytic activity of ceruloplasmin. The substrate for ceruloplasmin is ferrous ion ($Fe^{2+}$), which becomes oxidized to $Fe^{3+}$ with concomitant complete reduction of molecular oxygen. Although ceruloplasmin can oxidize multiple substrates in vitro, the only clearly defined physiological function of ceruloplasmin is its ferroxidase activity (Hellman & Gitlin, 2002; Nittis & Gitlin, 2002).

Studies employing perfused livers (Osaki, Johnson, & Frieden, 1971) and ceruloplasmin knockout mice (Harris, Durley, Man, & Gitlin, 1999) implicated the cuproprotein in iron release from tissues. The precise mechanism by which ceruloplasmin promotes iron efflux from macrophages and other cells remains uncertain. A prevailing opinion is that the ferroxidase activity of ceruloplasmin is required for efficient insertion of iron into apotransferrin, as the transferrin binds the metal in the oxidized valence (ferric) state. However, transferrin has its own ferroxidase activity and can oxidize $Fe^{2+}$ to $Fe^{3+}$ which is then incorporated to generate the holoprotein (Ponka et al., 1998). Thus, it is possible that the ferroxidase activity of ceruloplasmin may be necessary for oxidation of ferrous ions following their transfer to the cell surface via ferroportin; the ferroxidation may foster shedding of iron from the cell membrane and "drive" the egress of ferrous ions from the intracellular milieu. Of interest, a multi-copper oxidase, Fet3, has been identified in yeast with homology to ceruloplasmin (Askwith et al., 1994). In contrast to ceruloplasmin, which facilitates iron release from vertebrate cells, Fet3 is required for the oxidation of ferrous iron in the extracellular environment in preparation for iron uptake by the yeast membrane permease Ftr1 (Stearman, Yuan, Yamaguchi-Iwai, Klausner, & Dancis, 1996).

Within the CNS, relatively high levels of ceruloplasmin expression have been documented in astrocytes, particularly those investing the microvasculature and surrounding dopaminergic neurons in the substantia nigra. Ceruloplasmin immunoreactivity is also apparent in pial epithelium, ventricular ependymocytes, and choroid plexus (Klomp, Farhangrazi, Dugan, & Gitlin, 1996). David and co-workers described a form of ceruloplasmin that is bound to astrocyte cell membranes by a glycosylphosphatidylinositol (GPI) anchor (Patel & David, 1997). This group identified a novel, alternatively spliced transcript that codes for the GPI-anchored ceruloplasmin, and demonstrated that this is the major isoform of ceruloplasmin in brain (Patel, Dunn, & David, 2000). More recently, Jeong and David (2003) provided evidence that the capacity of astrocytes isolated from ceruloplasmin-deficient mice to purge themselves of iron is compromised, tagging GPI-anchored ceruloplasmin as an important player in the maintenance of CNS iron homeostasis.

Hepatic macrophages in ceruloplasmin knockout mice develop iron overload secondary to inefficient recycling of hemoglobin iron (Harris et al., 1999). Following the administration of ceruloplasmin to these knockout mice, iron is mobilized from the liver with concomitant increases in plasma iron levels (Harris et al., 1999). Adult aceruloplasminemic mice exhibit aberrant iron deposits in cerebellum, spinal cord, and retina. Lipid peroxidation is augmented in affected brain regions indicative of free radical-mediated injury (Patel et al., 2002). Jeong and David (2006) demonstrated neuronal loss in aceruloplasminemic mice which, ironically, may have arisen from neuronal iron *deficiency* secondary to impaired iron mobilization from the astroglial compartment.

The first case of human aceruloplasminemia was reported by Miyajima et al. (1987). The patient was a 52-year-old Japanese woman who presented with diabetes mellitus, retinal degeneration, extrapyramidal symptoms, and undetectable serum ceruloplasmin. She exhibited mild anemia, low plasma iron levels, elevated plasma ferritin concentrations, severe hepatic iron overload, and signal attenuation of the basal ganglia and cerebellum on MRI compatible with excessive iron accumulation (Fig. 5). A nucleotide sequence analysis demonstrated a loss-of-function mutation in the ceruloplasmin gene (Harris et al., 1995). Additional cases have since come to light bearing distinct point mutations and splice-variants in the ceruloplasmin gene on chromosome 3q25. In most subjects evaluated to date, there is alteration in the amino acid ligands within the carboxy terminal region essential for the formation of the trinuclear copper cluster (Daimon et al., 1995; Okamoto et al., 1996; Yoshida et al., 1995). Patients homozygous for this defect manifest serious parenchymal iron overload affecting the CNS (Fig. 6), liver, and pancreas. CNS involvement is often diagnosed in middle age, is progressive, and targets the basal ganglia (dysarthria, choreathetosis, dystonia, dementia), the cerebellum (ataxia), and retina (pigmentary degeneration with visual impairment). Circulating ceruloplasmin levels and attendant ferroxidase activity in these persons are nil or negligible. Patients *heterozygous* for mutant ceruloplasmin,

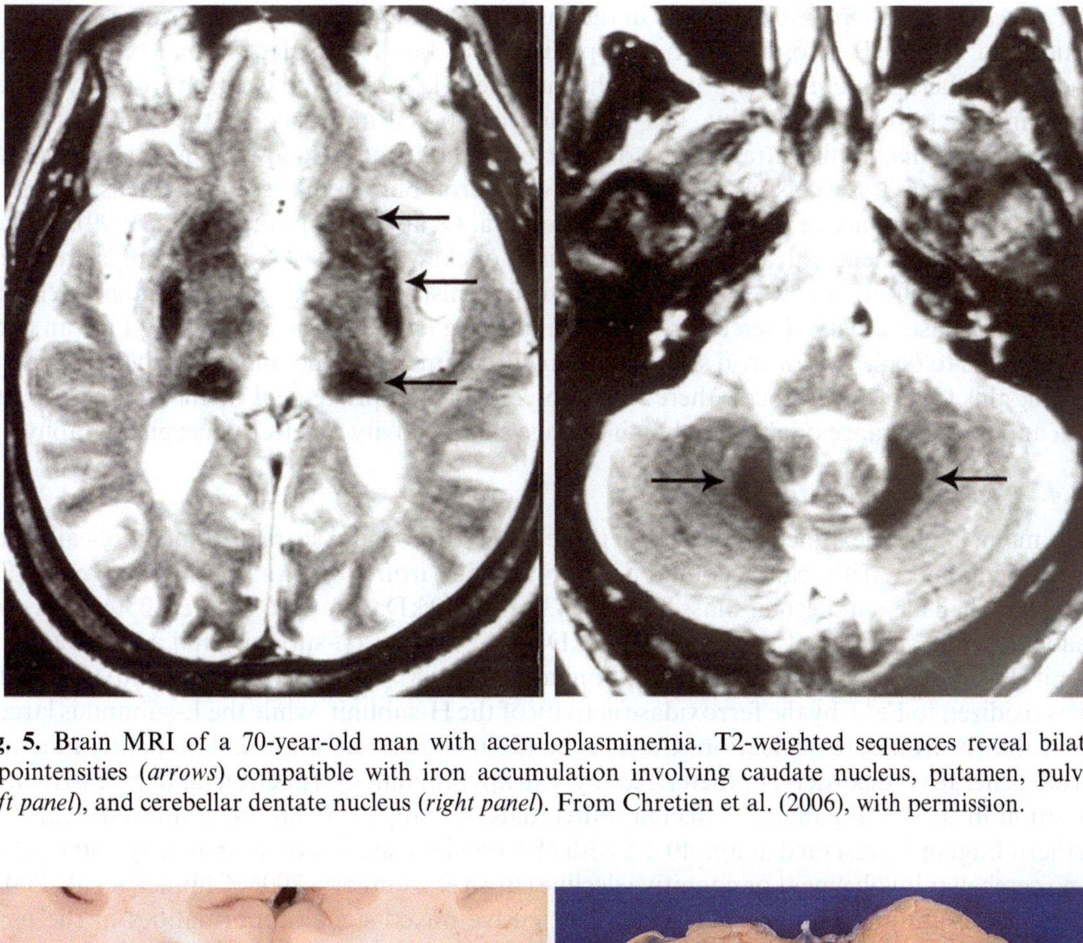

**Fig. 5.** Brain MRI of a 70-year-old man with aceruloplasminemia. T2-weighted sequences reveal bilateral hypointensities (*arrows*) compatible with iron accumulation involving caudate nucleus, putamen, pulvinar (*left panel*), and cerebellar dentate nucleus (*right panel*). From Chretien et al. (2006), with permission.

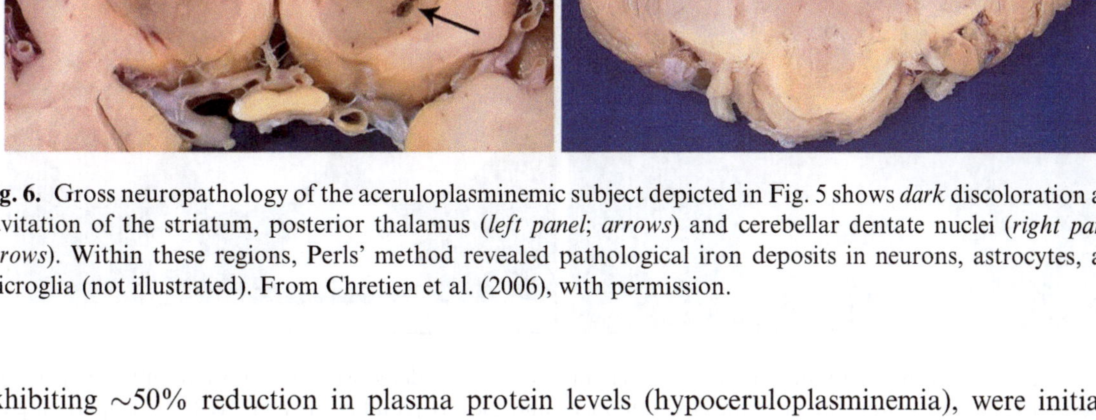

**Fig. 6.** Gross neuropathology of the aceruloplasminemic subject depicted in Fig. 5 shows *dark* discoloration and cavitation of the striatum, posterior thalamus (*left panel*; *arrows*) and cerebellar dentate nuclei (*right panel*; *arrows*). Within these regions, Perls' method revealed pathological iron deposits in neurons, astrocytes, and microglia (not illustrated). From Chretien et al. (2006), with permission.

exhibiting ~50% reduction in plasma protein levels (hypoceruloplasminemia), were initially regarded as unaffected; more careful testing revealed, however, that hypoceruloplasminemic individuals may present with subtle signs of cerebellar dysfunction (Miyajima et al., 2001).

*Treatment of aceruloplasminemia*: As in the case of most human neurodegenerative conditions, genetic (and acquired) disorders featuring pathological brain iron deposition are notoriously refractory to therapeutic intervention. Insight into the role of ceruloplasmin in iron physiology, particularly its ferroxidase activity, has suggested a rational approach to the management of aceruloplasminemia. Initial attempts to deplete brain and body iron with the $Fe^{3+}$ chelator, deferoxamine, were unsuccessful, possibly because the iron burden in these individuals favors the $Fe^{2+}$ state in the absence of ceruloplasmin (Yonekawa, Okabe, Asamoto, & Ohta, 1999). In their management of a patient with aceruloplasminemia, Yonekawa et al. (1999) first administered fresh frozen plasma (450 mL i.v./week) for 6 weeks to replenish circulating ceruloplasmin levels and restore ferroxidase activity. Thereafter, deferoxamine (1 g i.v./day) was administered for an additional 6 weeks to deplete *ferric* iron stores. Although MR images of the brain remained unchanged following this treatment protocol, there was unprecedented improvement in choreoathetosis and ataxia and disappearance of abnormal high-voltage sharp activity on electroencephalography.

### *15.2.4. Neuroferritinopathy*

The main, likely sole, function of ferritin is the sequestration and storage of metabolically inert iron. Mammalian ferritin can accommodate up to 4,500 iron atoms in its internal cavity. The apoprotein shell has a molecular mass between 430 and 460 kDa, is approximately 25 Å thick, and is made up of 24 subunits of two types, a 19 kDa light subunit (L-subunit) and a 21 kDa heavy subunit (H-subunit) (Arosio & Levi, 2002; Ponka et al., 1998). $Fe^{2+}$ incorporated into the ferritin shell is oxidized to $Fe^{3+}$ by the ferroxidase activity of the H-subunit, while the L-subunit is largely responsible for iron-core nucleation. Curtis et al. (2001) described a novel, dominantly inherited neurodegenerative disorder characterized by extrapyramidal dysfunction and excessive iron deposition in the basal ganglia. Affected individuals, initially all from the Cumbrian region of Northern England, presented at age 40–55 with choreoathetosis, dystonia, spasticity and rigidity, but no cerebellar involvement or cognitive decline (Burn & Chinnery, 2006; Chinnery et al., 2007). MRI of the brain in these patients revealed extensive mixed-signal abnormalities in the basal ganglia and red nuclei (Fig. 7A) (Curtis et al., 2001).

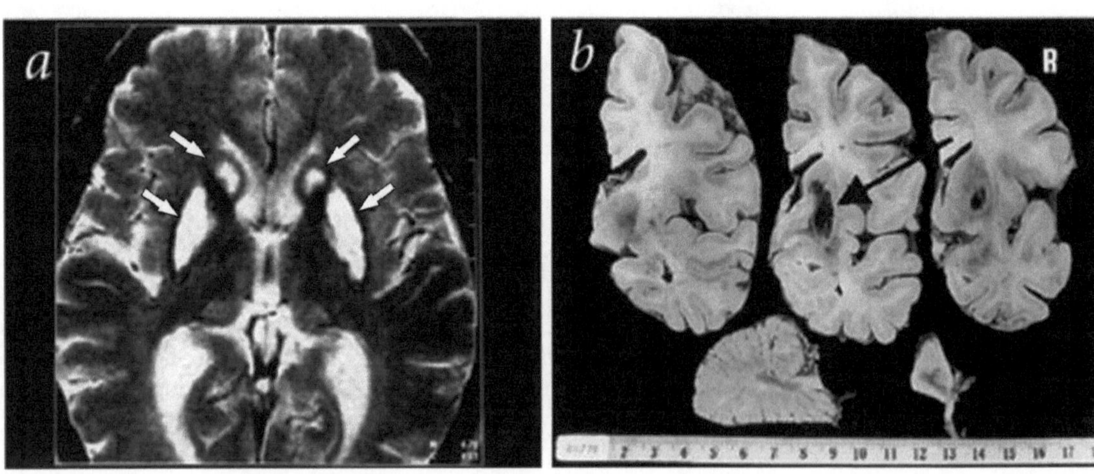


**Fig. 7.** A case of neuroferritinopathy. (**A**) T2-weighted MR image demonstrates abnormal mixed hyper- and hypointense signals in the caudate nucleus, putamen, and globus pallidus (*arrows*). (**B**). Neuropathological evaluation reveals a cystic cavity (*arrow*) in the region of the globus pallidus with extension to the putamen, internal capsule, and caudate nucleus. From Curtis et al. (2001), with permission.

In the Cumbrian cohort, the genetic defect was mapped by linkage analysis to locus 19q13.3 containing the gene for ferritin L-chain. The condition, termed "neuroferritinopathy" (Curtis et al., 2001), featured a heterozygous adenine insertion at position 460–461 in the L-ferritin gene. This insertion is predicted to alter 22 C-terminal residues of L-ferritin and extend the light chain by four amino acids (Curtis et al., 2001). Interestingly, the same mutation appears to have arisen independently in France (Chinnery et al., 2003). More recently, three additional families with neuroferritinopathy have been identified. In one kindred, insertion of two nucleotides (thymidine and cytidine) at position 498–499 in the L-ferritin gene was discovered. This mutation replaces the last nine wild-type amino acid residues with a 25 amino acid sequence, yielding a novel 191 amino acid polypeptide (Vidal et al., 2004). In the second family, a cytidine insertion was found at nucleotide 646 in exon 4 of L-ferritin mRNA. The open reading frame of this mutant L-ferritin is predicted to be translated into a 179 amino acid protein with substitutions at residues 148–175 (Mancuso et al., 2005). An A96T mutation in the L-ferritin gene was discovered in the third kindred and was associated with an earlier age of symptom onset (Maciel et al., 2005).

Gross examination of the brain in cases of neuroferritinopathy reveals cystic necrosis of the globus pallidus with variable extension into surrounding structures (Fig. 7B). A prominent histopathological feature is the marked accumulation of stainable iron and ferritin in neurons of the globus pallidus. Iron- and ferritin-positive inclusions have also been described extracellularly and within microglia and oligodendrocytes of the forebrain and cerebellum. Interestingly, the patients from Cumbria showed no evidence of systemic iron overload or diabetes, and their serum ferritin levels were surprisingly low. Hypoferritinemia was also found in an asymptomatic member of the family harboring the A96T mutation (Maciel et al., 2005). Although liver function tests in the patients from Cumbria were normal (Curtis et al., 2001), unique hepatocytic inclusions have been noted on biopsy (Professor John Burn, personal communication to PP). Patients with the TC insertion in the L-ferritin gene displayed abundant intranuclear and intracytoplasmic bodies replete with ferritin and iron in astrocytes, oligodendroglia, dermal fibroblasts, renal tubular epithelium, and muscle capillary endothelial cells (Vidal et al., 2004). These structures contained wild-type and mutant L-ferritin as well as ferritin heavy chain. One investigator has advocated muscle biopsy as a potential diagnostic test for neuroferritinopathy (Schroder, 2005).

Vidal et al. (2008) recently generated transgenic mice expressing a human cDNA carrying the thymidine and cytidine insertion at position 498–499 in the L-ferritin gene. As in human neuroferritinopathy, nuclear and cytoplasmic ferritin inclusion bodies were found in neurons and glia throughout the CNS as well as in cells of other organ systems. Expression of the transgene also promoted the sequestration of ubiquitinated proteins and proteasomal elements within the nascent inclusions, akin to the pathology of human neuroferritinopathy (Vidal et al., 2004). Importantly, mice carrying the mutant L-ferritin transgene exhibited impaired motor performance and shortened life span.

The molecular pathophysiology of neuroferritinopathy is unclear. Curtis et al. (2001) suggested that the neuroferritinopathy mutations disrupt the C-terminus of L-ferritin, thereby attenuating the protein's stability and function. It has also been proposed (Rouault, 2001) that the C-terminus of the mutated L-chain might interfere with the formation of holoferritin, causing inappropriate release of iron from iron-laden ferritin. Further studies by Levi, Cozzi, and Arosio (2005) confirmed that both the Cumbrian and the French mutations affect protein folding and stability. It was postulated that "unshielded" cytosolic iron accruing from the assembly of incompetent holoferritin might promote oxidative tissue damage in patients with neuroferritinopathy. It is also conceivable that mutant L-ferritin acquires a toxic gain-of-function unrelated to its native biology, as witnessed in other dominantly inherited neurodegenerations (Curtis et al., 2001).

### *15.2.5. X-Linked Sideroblastic Anemia with Ataxia*

The sideroblastic anemias are a heterogeneous group of disorders, which may be inherited or acquired (Fitzsimons & May, 1996). Of the relatively rare inherited forms, X-linked sideroblastic anemia, caused by mutations of erythroid-specific 5-aminolevulinate synthase (ALAS-2; the first enzyme in heme biosynthesis), is the most common (Bottomley, 2006). The hallmark of sideroblastic anemia is the ring sideroblast, a pathological erythroid precursor containing excessive deposits of non-heme iron within mitochondria encircling the nucleus. Ringed sideroblasts arise in patients with ALAS-2 gene mutations because (1) iron is specifically targeted to erythroid mitochondria; (2) mitochondrial iron cannot be adequately utilized due to lack of protoporphyrin IX; (3) heme, a negative regulator of iron uptake, is deficient; and (4) iron normally exits erythroid mitochondria after being inserted into protoporphyrin IX (Ponka, 1997). Unexpectedly, a distinct form of X-linked sideroblastic anemia with ataxia (XLSA/A) was described in several families with putative mutations mapped by linkage analysis to region Xq13 (Pagon, Bird, Detter, & Pierce, 1985). In contrast to ALAS-2-associated disease, the XLSA/A syndrome is characterized by non-progressive cerebellar ataxia and atrophy (Fig. 8) in early childhood, mild anemia with hypochromia and microcytosis, and *elevated* erythrocyte protoporphyrin levels. XLSA/A is characterized by the formation of ringed sideroblasts, but mitochondrial iron trapping in other tissues has not been documented. Allikmets et al. (1999) demonstrated that mutations in the *ABCB7* gene is responsible for XLSA/A. These authors detected a sequence variant (T1200G) in the *ABCB7* gene that substitutes methionine (ATG) for isoleucine (ATT) at position 400 (I400M). This residue is within the predicted fifth transmembrane domain of the ABCB7 protein (Allikmets et al., 1999).

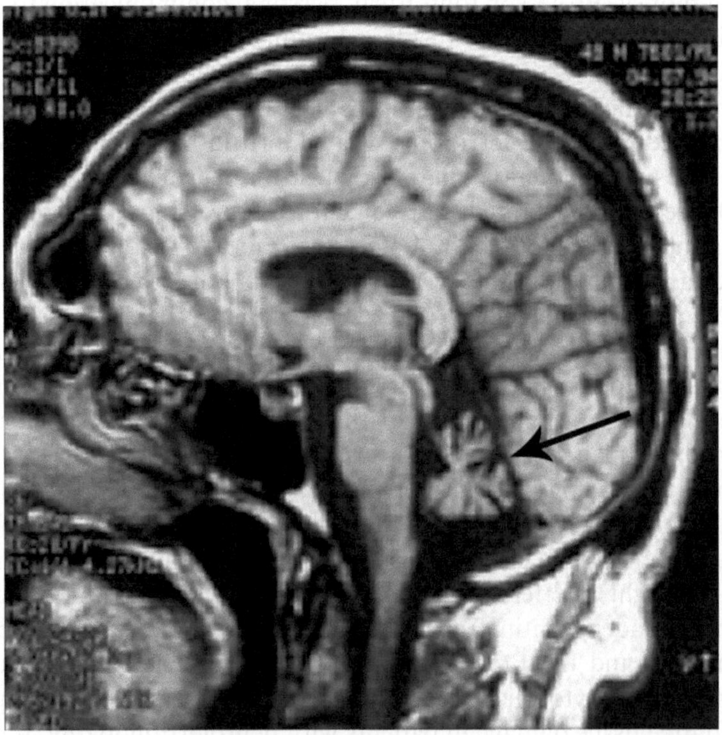

**Fig. 8.** Sagittal T1-weighted MR image of patient with X-linked sideroblastic anemia with ataxia, demonstrating prominent cerebellar atrophy (*arrow*). From Hellier et al. (2001), with permission.

Subsequently, Bekri et al. (2000) found a single missense mutation in exon 10 of the *ABCB7* gene in two brothers with XLSA/A. The mutation was a G-to-A transition at nucleotide 1305 of the full-length cDNA. The transition yields a charge inversion caused by the substitution of lysine for glutamate at residue 433, C-terminal to the putative sixth transmembrane domain of the ABCB7 protein. Maguire, Hellier, Hammans, and May (2001) reported hemizygosity in two brothers with XLSA/A, and heterozygosity in their unaffected mother, for a G→C transversion at position 1299 of the *ABCB7* cDNA. The latter predicts a V411L substitution in the proximal part of the sixth putative transmembrane region of the protein.

The ABCB7 protein is thought to transfer Fe–S clusters from mitochondria to the cytosol although formal proof of this is still required (Csere et al., 1998; Lill & Muhlenhoff, 2006; Napier et al., 2005). The presence of hypochromic microcytic erythrocytes denotes a decrease in heme synthesis in developing erythroid cells of XLSA/A patients. It is not immediately obvious, however, how the disruption of Fe–S cluster export might impede heme biosynthesis. Significantly, microcytic anemia in XLSA/A is accompanied by the accumulation of erythrocyte zinc–protoporphyrin IX (Allikmets et al., 1999; Maguire et al., 2001; Pagon et al., 1985). Additionally, mouse erythrocytes expressing mutated (E433K) ABCB7 exhibit an increase in zinc–protoporphyrin IX/heme ratios in proportion to the expression levels of $ABCB7^{E433K}$ (Pondarre et al., 2007). Since the formation of zinc–protoporphyrin IX requires ferrochelatase, the ABCB7 mutations cannot be interfering with the activity of this enzyme. Thus, the loss of function of ABCB7 might somehow diminish the availability of reduced iron (the physiological substrate for ferrochelatase) required for the assembly of heme from protoporphyrin IX. Little is known concerning the status of brain iron in XLSA/A, or the mechanism by which mutant ABCB7 predisposes to cerebellar hypoplasia or atrophy in this condition.

### *15.2.6. IRP2 Deficiency*

LaVaute et al. (2001) have generated mice with a targeted disruption of the gene encoding IRP2 (*ireb2*). These animals exhibit profound dysregulation of iron metabolism in the CNS and intestinal mucosa. It has been suggested that the over-expression of both ferritin subunits, accruing from lack of the translational repressor IRP2, plays a major role in the pathogenesis of this murine disease (Ponka, 2004). At 6 months of age, $Ireb^{-/-}$ mice display progressive neurological signs characterized by progressive ataxia, vestibular dysfunction, tremor, bradykinesia, and postural abnormalities. $Ireb2^{+/-}$ mice exhibit an intermediate degree of neurological impairment. Serum ferritin levels were significantly elevated in 6-month-old $Ireb2^{-/-}$ mice whereas serum iron levels were reportedly normal or only mildly increased. Iron concentrations in the liver and duodenum were increased respectively by 70% and 50% percent in these animals, although liver function tests were unremarkable (LaVaute et al., 2001). In addition to the elevated ferritin levels, the $Ireb2^{-/-}$ mice showed enhanced expression of DMT1, which transports $Fe^{2+}$ across apical cell membranes, and ferroportin, which exports iron from enterocytes to the circulation. Interestingly, IRP1 was incapable of repressing ferritin mRNA translation in the absence of IRP2. Degradation of IRP2 in a macrophage-like cell line was similarly shown by one of the current authors (Ponka) to stimulate ferritin synthesis in the face of highly active IRP1 (Kim & Ponka, 2002). In the IRP2-deficient mice, prominent deposits of iron were detected in cerebellar white matter, caudate-putamen, thalamus, and tectum (LaVaute et al., 2001). In the affected neural tissues, the co-registration of iron deposits and augmented ferritin immunoreactivity was an early event, arising prior to overt perikaryal or axonal degeneration. Yet, LaVaute et al. (2001) have argued that pathological iron deposition per se may not be directly responsible for neuronal damage in IRP2-deficient mice. These authors postulated, rather, that functional iron *deficiency* resulting from ferritin and ferroportin 1 over-expression might compromise essential iron-dependent neurochemical pathways in these animals.

Although not appreciated initially, Rouault's group subsequently reported the development of microcytic anemia in their $IRP2^{-/-}$ mice, in spite of normal or even slightly elevated serum iron concentrations and enhanced transferrin saturation (Cooperman et al., 2005). A similar observation was made in $IRP2^{-/-}$ mice generated independently in Hentze's laboratory (Galy et al., 2005). Cooperman et al. (2005) found that transferrin receptor protein levels were markedly diminished in erythroid cells isolated from $IRP2^{-/-}$ mice relative to wild-type mice. Commensurate with this finding, Galy et al. (2005) demonstrated that transferrin receptor mRNA and protein levels were significantly reduced in bone marrow cells of $IRP2^{-/-}$ animals. Both groups considered the likelihood that absent IRP2 binding to transferrin receptor mRNA in these animals downregulates transferrin receptor expression in erythroid cells, resulting in inefficient hemoglobinization and hypochromic microcytic anemia. Excessive ferritin in erythroblasts may further exacerbate the anemia by sequestering iron that would normally be destined for heme biosynthesis in the mitochondrial compartment (Schranzhofer et al., 2007).

### *15.2.7. Differential Diagnosis*

In patients with aceruloplasminemia, the systemic abnormalities of iron metabolism may be recognized before neurological symptoms become obvious. Such individuals may be misdiagnosed as type 1 hereditary hemochromatosis and subjected to inappropriate serial phlebotomies that might exacerbate the anemia. These two diseases can be distinguished by ascertainment of plasma transferrin saturation, which is elevated in hemochromatosis but low in aceruloplasminemia (Nittis & Gitlin, 2002). Patients with Wilson disease also display symptoms referable to the basal ganglia and depressed serum ceruloplasmin levels. However, in contrast to Wilson disease, patients with aceruloplasminemia do not exhibit increased hepatic and urinary copper levels or Kaiser-Fleischer rings (corneal copper deposition) on slit-lamp examination (Nittis & Gitlin, 2002). PKAN and neuroferritinopathy also present with extrapyramidal dysfunction and iron accumulation in basal ganglia. The absence of systemic iron overload in these conditions, and possible hypoferritinemia in neuroferritinopathy, distinguishes these forms of NBIA from aceruloplasminemia (Curtis et al., 2001; Nittis & Gitlin, 2002). Cerebellar atrophy and dysfunction may predominate in Friedreich's ataxia, hypoceruloplasminemia, and X-linked sideroblastic anemia with ataxia. These conditions may be differentiated by their mode of inheritance (autosomal recessive in the former two conditions; X-linked in the latter), dorsal column and cardiac involvement in Friedreich ataxia, diminished serum ceruloplasmin and absent ring sideroblasts in hypoceruloplasminemia, and elevated erythrocyte protoporphyrin levels in XLSA/A. The cerebellar impairment in XLSA/A occurs in childhood and remains static until mid-life when it may show slow progression (Hellier, Hatchwell, Duncombe, Kew, & Hammans, 2001). Cerebellar dysfunction in hypoceruloplasminemia manifests in adulthood and is progressive (Miyajima et al., 2001; Pagon et al., 1985).

## 15.3. HEMOCHROMATOSIS AND THE CNS

### *15.3.1. General Considerations*

Hereditary hemochromatosis (HH) affects approximately 0.5% of people of European origin, and is the most common autosomal recessive disorder in Caucasians (Merryweather-Clarke, Pointon, Shearman, & Robson, 1997). HH features excessive absorption of dietary iron, increased serum iron and transferrin saturation, elevated serum ferritin levels, and toxic deposition of the metal in liver, heart, pancreas, and pituitary gland (Jazwinska, 1998; Lyon & Frank, 2001). The majority of HH cases result from two missense mutations in the *HFE* gene located on chromosome 6p: (i) a guanine to adenine transition at nucleotide position 845 (G845A) causing a cysteine to tyrosine substitution at amino acid position 282 (C282Y) of the HFE protein and (ii) a cytosine to guanine transversion at nucleotide 187 (C187G) resulting in a histidine to aspartate substitution at amino acid 63 (H63D) (Feder et al., 1996). The prevalence of these mutations worldwide is estimated at 1.9% for the more penetrant C282Y mutation and 8.1% for the less penetrant H63D mutation (Merryweather-Clarke et al., 1997). Although the precise function of the normal HFE protein remains incompletely understood, there is evidence suggesting that the mutant protein may interact with the transferrin receptor (Feder et al., 1998) somehow promoting excessive tissue iron sequestration and cellular damage.

### *15.3.2. Mutant HFE and Alzheimer's Disease*

Alzheimer's disease (AD) is a dementing illness characterized by progressive neuronal degeneration, gliosis, and the accumulation of intracellular inclusions (neurofibrillary tangles) and extracellular deposits of amyloid (senile plaques) in discrete regions of the basal forebrain, hippocampus, and association cortices (Selkoe, 1991). The excessive sequestration of redox-active tissue iron, augmented levels of oxidative stress, and mitochondrial insufficiency have been consistently demonstrated in AD-affected neural tissues (Schipper, 2004; and see Chapter 7). Of note, regional concentrations of transferrin-binding sites remain unchanged or vary inversely with the elevated iron stores, suggesting that the transferrin receptor pathway of iron acquisition, important for normal iron delivery to most peripheral tissues, contributes little to pathological iron trapping in AD brain (Schipper, 2004). In normal human brain, immunoreactive HFE protein localizes to capillaries, choroid plexus, and ependymocytes. In AD brain, HFE immunostaining occurs additionally in the vicinity of neuritic plaques and in perivascular astrocytes (Connor et al., 2001).

Moalem et al. (2000) reported that the presence of mutant *HFE* alleles may place apolipoprotein E4 (apoE4)-negative men at increased risk for manifesting familial AD. In the following year, Sampietro et al. (2001) presented evidence that AD patients possessing one or two copies of the H63D allele develop AD 5 years earlier, on average, than those with wild-type HFE. The authors of these studies concluded that, in individuals with AD, HFE mutations may exacerbate pathological brain iron deposition and thereby predispose to earlier or more robust disease. If confirmed, this observation could have enormous clinical implications in so far as serial phlebotomies or chelation therapy might attenuate disease progression in patients with early AD and mild cognitive impairment (MCI; a frequent harbinger of AD) who screen positive for mutant HFE. To explore this further, we (Schipper laboratory) genotyped 213 sporadic AD, 106 MCI, and 63 normal elderly control (NEC) individuals for the H63D and C282Y HFE mutations by polymerase chain reaction (PCR)/restriction fragment length polymorphism (RFLP) analysis and determined the relationship of these mutations to the demographic, clinical, and neuropsychological attributes of our cohorts (Berlin et al., 2004). In our study, we could not demonstrate the impact of H63D or C282Y heterozygosity on age at AD diagnosis, age at onset of cognitive symptoms (AD and MCI combined), rates of MCI-to-AD conversion, or specific neuropsychological deficits. Neither did we discern any interactions between *HFE* zygosity and apoE status. Individuals *homozygous* for H63D (non-penetrant) showed trends toward accelerated MCI–AD conversion rates, and a subset of younger individuals (aged 55–75) exhibited earlier onset of cognitive symptoms relative to wild-type HFE and H63D heterozygotes. In contrast to earlier reports (Moalem et al., 2000; Sampietro et al., 2001), our findings do not implicate heterozygosity for the common HFE mutations as a genetic modifier of sporadic AD and MCI. As such, iron removal therapy cannot be currently advocated for AD/MCI individuals heterozygous for H63D or C282Y. The trend we observed toward accelerated cognitive dysfunction in H63D *homozygotes* warrants further study. The scientific basis underlying any such interaction would still require explanation, given that (i) HFE protein is thought to attenuate cellular iron uptake at the level of the transferrin receptor (Feder et al., 1998) and (ii) pathological brain iron deposition in AD has largely implicated non-transferrin pathways (Schipper, 2004).

### *15.3.3. Mutant HFE and Parkinson's Disease*

Idiopathic Parkinson disease (PD) is an extrapyramidal disorder featuring gradual loss of dopaminergic neurons in the substantia nigra pars compacta, formation of intraneuronal fibrillar inclusions (Lewy bodies) in this cell population, and variable depletion of noradrenaline and serotonin in other brain stem nuclei (Fahn, 2003). Neuropathological and MRI studies have implicated augmented iron deposition in the basal ganglia of PD patients relative to age-matched control values (Bartzokis, Tishler, Shin, Lu, & Cummings, 2004; Graham, Paley, Grunewald, Hoggard, & Griffiths, 2000; Jellinger, Paulus, Grundke-Iqbal, Riederer, & Youdim, 1990; Mondino, Filippi, Magliola, & Duca, 2002; Morris & Edwardson, 1994; Olanow, 1992; Schipper, 2004; Youdim, 1994).

In light of the perceived importance of iron in the pathogenesis of PD, investigators have examined the possibility of an association between mutant HFE and the prevalence of this neurodegenerative condition. Nielsen, Jensen, and Krabbe (1995) reported a patient with HH who developed a syndrome of dementia, dysarthria, progressive gait disturbance, rigidity, bradykinesia, tremor, and MRI evidence of excessive iron accumulation in the basal ganglia. Costello, Walsh, Harrington, and Walsh (2004) described four subjects with concurrent HH and PD. The Nielsen and Costello teams argued that augmented subcortical iron deposition related to HH may have played a causative role in the development of the extrapyramidal disorder in their subjects. However, this position remains tenuous given the small number of reported patients manifesting both conditions concurrently, and the rarity of frank CNS involvement in patients with HH. In an initial series of 137 patients with idiopathic PD and 47 with other parkinsonian syndromes, Dekker et al. (2003) found that PD patients were significantly more often homozygous for the C282Y mutation than controls ($P = 0.03$). In this analysis, and in a second case series involving 60 patients with PD and 25 with non-PD extrapyramidal symptoms, subjects with the non-PD movement disorders were significantly more likely than controls to carry a C282Y mutation ($P = 0.009$ and $P = 0.006$, respectively). Along similar lines, in a Portuguese study of 132 patients with idiopathic PD, 130 with AD, 55 with MCI, and 115 healthy age-matched controls, Guerreiro et al. (2006) noted a statistically significant association of PD (but not AD or MCI) with the C282Y allele. On the other hand, Aamodt et al. (2007) queried the possible relationship between heterozygosity for the common HFE mutations (C282Y, H63D and S65C) and the prevalence of PD in a Norwegian population and disclosed no increased susceptibility to PD in carriers of HFE gene mutations. Similarly, Akbas et al. (2006) did not detect over-representation of the C282Y or H63D mutation in 278 PD patients exhibiting enhanced substantia nigra iron by transcranial sonography. To confuse matters further, Buchanan and co-investigators (Buchanan, Silburn, Chalk, Le Couteur, & Mellick, 2002) found significant *under-representation* of the C282Y mutation in 438 Australian PD relative to 485 control subjects (odds ratio for C282Y possession 0.61; 95% confidence interval 0.42–0.90; $P = 0.011$) and concluded that carriage of the C282Y allele may confer *protection* against idiopathic PD. In light of these highly conflicting reports, additional large-scale studies of ethnically diverse populations should be conducted to ascertain whether heterozygosity for the common HFE mutations represents a risk factor, protective factor, or has no bearing on the pathogenesis of idiopathic PD and other extrapyramidal disorders.

### *15.3.4. Mutant HFE and Amyotrophic Lateral Sclerosis*

Amyotrophic lateral sclerosis (ALS) is a fatal, aging-related neurodegenerative disorder characterized by progressive upper and lower motor neuron loss and weakness of skeletal (voluntary) muscles of the head, neck, trunk, and limbs. As in the case of AD and PD, pathological iron homeostasis and free radical injury have been implicated in the CNS of ALS victims (Carri, Ferri, Cozzolino, Calabrese, & Rotilio, 2003). Wang et al. (2004) reported that 31% of study subjects with sporadic ALS carried a mutation in the *HFE* gene, in comparison with 14% of individuals with other or no neuromuscular disease ($P < 0.005$). The authors also demonstrated that transfection of a human neuronal cell line with mutant HFE disrupts the expression of cytoskeletal proteins and copper–zinc superoxide dismutase, abnormalities linked to motor neuron dysfunction in some forms of ALS. These observations were regarded as compelling evidence for a role of mutant HFE in the etiopathogenesis of this neurodegenerative disorder. Strikingly disparate results were published by Yen and colleagues in the same year (Yen, Simpson, Henkel, Beers, & Appel, 2004). These investigators noted virtually no differences in the prevalence of the C282Y and H63D mutations between 51 ALS patients and 47 normal controls. Neither did the presence of either mutation influence significantly disease age of onset or rate of progression in the ALS cohort. In two independent populations of patients with sporadic ALS (total $n = 379$) and controls (total $n = 400$), Goodall and co-investigators (2005) found over-representation of the H63D mutation in the ALS group (odds ratio 1.85, CI 1.35–2.54). Ellervik, Birgens, Tybjaerg-Hansen, and Nordestgaard (2007) performed a meta-analysis involving 202 studies (66,263 cases and 226,515 controls) to delineate possible associations between mutant hemochromatosis genotypes and the prevalence of various medical and neurological conditions. For ALS, this analysis revealed an odds ratio of 3.9 (CI 1.2–13) for H63D/H63D versus wild type/wild type, but no impact of H63D heterozygosity or the C282Y lesion on this condition.

### *15.3.5. Mutant HFE and Ischemic Stroke*

As described above, data concerning the relationship of HFE polymorphisms to human neurodegenerative disorders are conflicting. In contrast, at least four studies assessing for linkage between C282Y or H63D and ischemic stroke (atherothrombotic cerebral infarction) were consistently negative (Ellervik et al., 2007; Hruskovicova et al., 2005; Njajou et al., 2002; Saleheen, Farooq, & Frossard, 2005), although the possibility that HFE mutations may modify the relationship between smoking and stroke was raised in one of the studies (Njajou et al., 2002).

## 15.4. CONCLUDING REMARKS

Heritable perturbations in iron homeostasis and pathological deposition of this redox-active metal in the CNS have been implicated in a number of adult and pediatric neurodegenerative afflictions. Prominent among the latter are aceruloplasminemia, neuroferritinopathy, Friedreich's ataxia, pantothenate kinase-2-associated neurodegeneration, and possibly X-linked sideroblastic anemia with ataxia. It is anticipated that more genetically based NBIA conditions will come to light in the near future given the accelerated pace of discovery of novel proteins mediating the absorption, transport, valence configuration, export, and storage of this vital transition metal. Iron-regulatory protein-2 (IRP2) deficiency in mice results in iron mishandling in the gut and brain, and a degenerative movement disorder characterized by progressive extrapyramidal and cerebellar impairment. Although human cases of IRP2 deficiency have hitherto not been described, it may be worthwhile to consider this eventuality in patients with movement disorders and NBIA of uncertain etiology, especially in the context of concurrent microcytic anemia. Gene mutations responsible for hereditary hemochromatosis, a disorder of systemic iron homeostasis, have been touted as risk factors or modulators of several common human neurodegenerative disorders (Alzheimer's disease, Parkinson's disease, amyotrophic lateral sclerosis). Proof of such relationships could have important clinical implications insofar as serial phlebotomies or chelation therapy might attenuate a component of iron-related neurotoxicity in affected individuals. However, the epidemiological data on this subject are highly conflicting, and management based on depleting brain iron stores in these patients cannot be justified at this juncture.

**Acknowledgments** This work was supported, in part, by grants from the Canadian Institutes of Health Research to HMS and PP. The authors thank Drs. David Koeller and Alex Sheftel for helpful discussions, and Adrienne Liberman, Miriam Rosenzweig, and Rhona Rosenzweig for editorial assistance.

## REFERENCES

Aamodt, A. H., Stovner, L. J., Thorstensen, K., Lydersen, S., White, L. R., & Aasly, J. O. (2007). Prevalence of haemochromatosis gene mutations in Parkinson's disease. *Journal of Neurology, Neurosurgery and Psychiatry, 78*(3), 315–317.

Abboud, S., & Haile, D. J. (2000). A novel mammalian iron-regulated protein involved in intracellular iron metabolism. *Journal of Biological Chemistry, 275*(26), 19906–19912.

Aisen, P., Enns, C., & Wessling-Resnick, M. (2001). Chemistry and biology of eukaryotic iron metabolism. *International Journal of Biochemistry and Cell Biology, 33*(10), 940–959.

Akbas, N., Hochstrasser, H., Deplazes, J., Tomiuk, J., Bauer, P., Walter, U., et al. (2006). Screening for mutations of the HFE gene in Parkinson's disease patients with hyperechogenicity of the substantia nigra. *Neuroscience Letters, 407*(1), 16–19.

Allikmets, R., Raskind, W. H., Hutchinson, A., Schueck, N. D., Dean, M., & Koeller, D. M. (1999). Mutation of a putative mitochondrial iron transporter gene (ABC7) in X-linked sideroblastic anemia and ataxia (XLSA/A). *Human Molecular Genetics, 8*(5), 743–749.

Arosio, P., & Levi, S. (2002). Ferritin, iron homeostasis, and oxidative damage. *Free Radical Biology and Medicine, 33*(4), 457–463.

Askwith, C., Eide, D., Van Ho, A., Bernard, P. S., Li, L., Davis-Kaplan, S., et al. (1994). The FET3 gene of S. cerevisiae encodes a multicopper oxidase required for ferrous iron uptake. *Cell, 76*(2), 403–410.

Babady, N. E., Carelle, N., Wells, R. D., Rouault, T. A., Hirano, M., Lynch, D. R., et al. (2007). Advancements in the pathophysiology of Friedreich's Ataxia and new prospects for treatments. *Molecular Genetics and Metabolism, 92*(1–2), 23–35.

Babcock, M., de Silva, D., Oaks, R., Davis-Kaplan, S., Jiralerspong, S., Montermini, L., et al. (1997). Regulation of mitochondrial iron accumulation by Yfh1p, a putative homolog of frataxin. *Science, 276*(5319), 1709–1712.

Balsinde, J., & Balboa, M. A. (2005). Cellular regulation and proposed biological functions of group VIA calcium-independent phospholipase A2 in activated cells. *Cell Signal, 17*(9), 1052–1062.

Bartzokis, G., Tishler, T. A., Shin, I. S., Lu, P. H., & Cummings, J. L. (2004). Brain ferritin iron as a risk factor for age at onset in neurodegenerative diseases. *Annals of the New York Academy of Sciences, 1012*, 224–236.

Becker, E., & Richardson, D. R. (2001). Frataxin: Its role in iron metabolism and the pathogenesis of Friedreich's ataxia. *The International Journal of Biochemistry and Cell Biology, 33*(1), 1–10.

Becker, E. M., Greer, J. M., Ponka, P., & Richardson, D. R. (2002). Erythroid differentiation and protoporphyrin IX down-regulate frataxin expression in Friend cells: Characterization of frataxin expression compared to molecules involved in iron metabolism and hemoglobinization. *Blood, 99*(10), 3813–3822.

Bekri, S., Kispal, G., Lange, H., Fitzsimons, E., Tolmie, J., Lill, R., et al. (2000). Human ABC7 transporter: Gene structure and mutation causing X-linked sideroblastic anemia with ataxia with disruption of cytosolic iron-sulfur protein maturation. *Blood, 96*(9), 3256–3264.

Berg, D., & Hochstrasser, H. (2006). Iron metabolism in Parkinsonian syndromes. *Movement Disorders, 21*(9), 1299–1310.

Berlin, D., Chong, G., Chertkow, H., Bergman, H., Phillips, N. A., & Schipper, H. M. (2004). Evaluation of HFE (hemochromatosis) mutations as genetic modifiers in sporadic AD and MCI. *Neurobiology of Aging, 25*(4), 465–474.

Boddaert, N., Le Quan Sang, K. H., Rotig, A., Leroy-Willig, A., Gallet, S., Brunelle, F., et al. (2007). Selective iron chelation in Friedreich ataxia: Biologic and clinical implications. *Blood, 110*(1), 401–408.

Bottomley, S. S. (2006). Congenital sideroblastic anemias. *Current Hematology Reports, 5*(1), 41–49.

Buchanan, D. D., Silburn, P. A., Chalk, J. B., Le Couteur, D. G., & Mellick, G. D. (2002). The Cys282Tyr polymorphism in the HFE gene in Australian Parkinson's disease patients. *Neuroscience Letters, 327*(2), 91–94.

Burdo, J. R., & Connor, J. R. (2003). Brain iron uptake and homeostatic mechanisms: An overview. *Biometals, 16*(1), 63–75.

Burn, J., & Chinnery, P. F. (2006). Neuroferritinopathy. *Seminars in Pediatric Neurology, 13*(3), 176–181.

Cairo, G., & Pietrangelo, A. (2000). Iron regulatory proteins in pathobiology. *Biochemical Journal, 352*(Pt 2), 241–250.

Carri, M. T., Ferri, A., Cozzolino, M., Calabrese, L., & Rotilio, G. (2003). Neurodegeneration in amyotrophic lateral sclerosis: The role of oxidative stress and altered homeostasis of metals. *Brain Research Bulletin, 61*(4), 365–374.

Castelnau, P., Zilbovicius, M., Ribeiro, M. J., Hertz-Pannier, L., Ogier, H., & Evrard, P. (2001). Striatal and pontocerebellar hypoperfusion in Hallervorden-Spatz syndrome. *Pediatric Neurology, 25*(2), 170–174.

Chinnery, P. F., Crompton, D. E., Birchall, D., Jackson, M. J., Coulthard, A., Lombes, A., et al. (2007). Clinical features and natural history of neuroferritinopathy caused by the FTL1 460InsA mutation. *Brain, 130*(Pt 1), 110–119.

Chinnery, P. F., Curtis, A. R., Fey, C., Coulthard, A., Crompton, D., Curtis, A., et al. (2003). Neuroferritinopathy in a French family with late onset dominant dystonia. *Journal of Medical Genetics, 40*(5), e69.

Chretien, F., Servan, J., Mikol, J., Trierweiller, M., Elghozi, D., & Gray, F. (2006). A 70-year-old man with extrapyramidal symptoms, dementia and hemosiderosis. *Brain Pathology, 16*(3), 235–236.

Connor, J. R. (2003). Iron transport proteins in the diseased brain. *Journal of the Neurological Sciences, 207*(1–2), 112–113.

Connor, J. R., Milward, E. A., Moalem, S., Sampietro, M., Boyer, P., Percy, M. E., et al. (2001). Is hemochromatosis a risk factor for Alzheimer's disease? *Journal of the Alzheimer's Disease, 3*(5), 471–477.

Cooperman, S. S., Meyron-Holtz, E. G., Olivierre-Wilson, H., Ghosh, M. C., McConnell, J. P., & Rouault, T. A. (2005). Microcytic anemia, erythropoietic protoporphyria, and neurodegeneration in mice with targeted deletion of iron-regulatory protein 2. *Blood, 106*(3), 1084–1091.

Costello, D. J., Walsh, S. L., Harrington, H. J., & Walsh, C. H. (2004). Concurrent hereditary haemochromatosis and idiopathic Parkinson's disease: A case report series. *Journal of Neurology Neurosurgery and Psychiatry, 75*(4), 631–633.

Csere, P., Lill, R., & Kispal, G. (1998). Identification of a human mitochondrial ABC transporter, the functional orthologue of yeast Atm1p. *Federation of European Biochemical Societies Letters, 441*(2), 266–270.

Curtis, A. R., Fey, C., Morris, C. M., Bindoff, L. A., Ince, P. G., Chinnery, P. F., et al. (2001). Mutation in the gene encoding ferritin light polypeptide causes dominant adult-onset basal ganglia disease. *Nature Genetics, 28*(4), 350–354.

Daimon, M., Kato, T., Kawanami, T., Tominaga, M., Igarashi, M., Yamatani, K., et al. (1995). A nonsense mutation of the ceruloplasmin gene in hereditary ceruloplasmin deficiency with diabetes mellitus. *Biochemical Biophysical Research Communications, 217*(1), 89–95.

De Domenico, I., McVey Ward, D., & Kaplan, J. (2008). Regulation of iron acquisition and storage: Consequences for iron-linked disorders. *Nature Reviews Molecular Cell Biology, 9*(1), 72–81.

Dekker, M. C., Giesbergen, P. C., Njajou, O. T., van Swieten, J. C., Hofman, A., Breteler, M. M., et al. (2003). Mutations in the hemochromatosis gene (HFE), Parkinson's disease and parkinsonism. *Neuroscience Letters, 348*(2), 117–119.

Donovan, A., Brownlie, A., Zhou, Y., Shepard, J., Pratt, S. J., Moynihan, J., et al. (2000). Positional cloning of zebrafish ferroportin1 identifies a conserved vertebrate iron exporter. *Nature, 403*(6771), 776–781.

Ellervik, C., Birgens, H., Tybjaerg-Hansen, A., & Nordestgaard, B. G. (2007). Hemochromatosis genotypes and risk of 31 disease endpoints: Meta-analyses including 66,000 cases and 226,000 controls. *Hepatology, 46*(4), 1071–1080.

Fahn, S. (2003). Description of Parkinson's disease as a clinical syndrome. *Annals of the New York Academy of Sciences, 991*, 1–14.

Feder, J. N., Gnirke, A., Thomas, W., Tsuchihashi, Z., Ruddy, D. A., Basava, A., et al. (1996). A novel MHC class I-like gene is mutated in patients with hereditary haemochromatosis. *Nature Genetics, 13*(4), 399–408.

Feder, J. N., Penny, D. M., Irrinki, A., Lee, V. K., Lebron, J. A., Watson, N., et al. (1998). The hemochromatosis gene product complexes with the transferrin receptor and lowers its affinity for ligand binding. *Proceedings of the National Academy of Sciences United States of America, 95*(4), 1472–1477.

Fitzsimons, E. J., & May, A. (1996). The molecular basis of the sideroblastic anemias. *Current Opinion in Hematology, 3*(2), 167–172.

Fleming, M. D., Trenor, C. C., 3rd, Su, M. A., Foernzler, D., Beier, D. R., Dietrich, W. F., et al. (1997). Microcytic anaemia mice have a mutation in Nramp2, a candidate iron transporter gene. *Nature Genetics, 16*(4), 383–386.

Galy, B., Ferring, D., Minana, B., Bell, O., Janser, H. G., Muckenthaler, M., et al. (2005). Altered body iron distribution and microcytosis in mice deficient in iron regulatory protein 2 (IRP2). *Blood, 106*(7), 2580–2589.

Gerber, J., Muhlenhoff, U., & Lill, R. (2003). An interaction between frataxin and Isu1/Nfs1 that is crucial for Fe/S cluster synthesis on Isu1. *The European Molecular Biology Organization Reports, 4*(9), 906–911.

Goodall, E. F., Greenway, M. J., van Marion, I., Carroll, C. B., Hardiman, O., & Morrison, K. E. (2005). Association of the H63D polymorphism in the hemochromatosis gene with sporadic ALS. *Neurology, 65*(6), 934–937.

Graham, J. M., Paley, M. N., Grunewald, R. A., Hoggard, N., & Griffiths, P. D. (2000). Brain iron deposition in Parkinson's disease imaged using the PRIME magnetic resonance sequence. *Brain, 123*(Pt 12), 2423–2431.

Grasbeck, R., Majuri, R., Kouvonen, I., & Tenhunen, R. (1982). Spectral and other studies on the intestinal haem receptor of the pig. *Biochimica et Biophysica Acta, 700*(2), 137–142.

Grimes, D. A., Lang, A. E., & Bergeron, C. (2000). Late adult onset chorea with typical pathology of Hallervorden-Spatz syndrome. *Journal of Neurology, Neurosurgery and Psychiatry, 69*(3), 392–395.

Guerreiro, R. J., Bras, J. M., Santana, I., Januario, C., Santiago, B., Morgadinho, A. S., et al. (2006). Association of HFE common mutations with Parkinson's disease, Alzheimer's disease and mild cognitive impairment in a Portuguese cohort. *BioMed Central Neurology, 6*, 24.

Gunshin, H., Mackenzie, B., Berger, U. V., Gunshin, Y., Romero, M. F., Boron, W. F., et al. (1997). Cloning and characterization of a mammalian proton-coupled metal-ion transporter. *Nature, 388*(6641), 482–488.

Halliwell, B. (2001). Role of free radicals in the neurodegenerative diseases: Therapeutic implications for antioxidant treatment. *Drugs and Aging, 18*(9), 685–716.

Harris, Z. L., Durley, A. P., Man, T. K., & Gitlin, J. D. (1999). Targeted gene disruption reveals an essential role for ceruloplasmin in cellular iron efflux. *Proceedings of the National Academy of Sciences United States of America, 96*(19), 10812–10817.

Harris, Z. L., Takahashi, Y., Miyajima, H., Serizawa, M., MacGillivray, R. T., & Gitlin, J. D. (1995). Aceruloplasminemia: Molecular characterization of this disorder of iron metabolism. *Proceedings of the National Academy of Sciences United States of America, 92*(7), 2539–2543.

Hart, P. E., Lodi, R., Rajagopalan, B., Bradley, J. L., Crilley, J. G., Turner, C., et al. (2005). Antioxidant treatment of patients with Friedreich ataxia: Four-year follow-up. *Archives of Neurology, 62*(4), 621–626.

Hayflick, S. J. (2003). Unraveling the Hallervorden-Spatz syndrome: Pantothenate kinase-associated neurodegeneration is the name. *Current Opinion in Pediatrics, 15*(6), 572–577.

Hayflick, S. J. (2006). Neurodegeneration with brain iron accumulation: From genes to pathogenesis. *Seminars in Pediatric Neurology, 13*(3), 182–185.

Hellier, K. D., Hatchwell, E., Duncombe, A. S., Kew, J., & Hammans, S. R. (2001). X-linked sideroblastic anaemia with ataxia: Another mitochondrial disease? *Journal of Neurology, Neurosurgery and Psychiatry, 70*(1), 65–69.

Hellman, N. E., & Gitlin, J. D. (2002). Ceruloplasmin metabolism and function. *Annual Review of Nutrition, 22*, 439–458.

Hentze, M. W., & Kuhn, L. C. (1996). Molecular control of vertebrate iron metabolism: mRNA-based regulatory circuits operated by iron, nitric oxide, and oxidative stress. *Proceedings of the National Academy of Sciences United States of America, 93*(16), 8175–8182.

Hentze, M. W., Muckenthaler, M. U., & Andrews, N. C. (2004). Balancing acts: Molecular control of mammalian iron metabolism. *Cell, 117*(3), 285–297.

Hruskovicova, H., Milanez, T., Kobal, J., Potisk, K. P., Petrovic, D., & Peterlin, B. (2005). Hemochromatosis-causing mutations C282Y and H63D are not risk factors for atherothrombotic cerebral infarction. *Medical Science Monitor, 11*(7), BR248–BR252.

Jazwinska, E. C. (1998). Hemochromatosis: A genetic defect in iron metabolism. *Bioessays, 20*(7), 562–568.

Jellinger, K., Paulus, W., Grundke-Iqbal, I., Riederer, P., & Youdim, M. B. (1990). Brain iron and ferritin in Parkinson's and Alzheimer's diseases. *Journal of Neural Transmission, Parkinson's Disease and Dementia Section, 2*(4), 327–340.

Jeong, S. Y., & David, S. (2003). Glycosylphosphatidylinositol-anchored ceruloplasmin is required for iron efflux from cells in the central nervous system. *Journal of Biological Chemistry, 278*(29), 27144–27148.

Jeong, S. Y., & David, S. (2006). Age-related changes in iron homeostasis and cell death in the cerebellum of ceruloplasmin-deficient mice. *The Journal of Neuroscience, 26*(38), 9810–9819.

Johnson, M. A., Kuo, Y. M., Westaway, S. K., Parker, S. M., Ching, K. H., Gitschier, J., et al. (2004). Mitochondrial localization of human PANK2 and hypotheses of secondary iron accumulation in pantothenate kinase-associated neurodegeneration. *Annals of the New York Academy of Sciences, 1012*, 282–298.

Justesen, C. R., Penn, R. D., Kroin, J. S., & Egel, R. T. (1999). Stereotactic pallidotomy in a child with Hallervorden-Spatz disease. Case report. *Journal of Neurosurgery, 90*(3), 551–554.

Kim, S., & Ponka, P. (2000). Effects of interferon-gamma and lipopolysaccharide on macrophage iron metabolism are mediated by nitric oxide-induced degradation of iron regulatory protein 2. *Journal of Biological Chemistry, 275*(9), 6220–6226.

Kim, S., & Ponka, P. (2002). Nitrogen monoxide-mediated control of ferritin synthesis: Implications for macrophage iron homeostasis. *The Proceedings of the National Academy of Sciences United States of America, 99*(19), 12214–12219.

Kispal, G., Csere, P., Guiard, B., & Lill, R. (1997). The ABC transporter Atm1p is required for mitochondrial iron homeostasis. *Federation of European Biochemical Sciences Letters, 418*(3), 346–350.

Klomp, L. W., Farhangrazi, Z. S., Dugan, L. L., & Gitlin, J. D. (1996). Ceruloplasmin gene expression in the murine central nervous system. *The Journal of Clinical Investigation, 98*(1), 207–215.

Koeppen, A. H., & Dickson, A. C. (2001). Iron in the Hallervorden-Spatz syndrome. *Pediatric Neurology, 25*(2), 148–155.

Lamarche, J. B., Cote, M., & Lemieux, B. (1980). The cardiomyopathy of Friedreich's ataxia morphological observations in 3 cases. *Canadian Journal of Neurological Sciences, 7*(4), 389–396.

LaVaute, T., Smith, S., Cooperman, S., Iwai, K., Land, W., Meyron-Holtz, E., et al. (2001). Targeted deletion of the gene encoding iron regulatory protein-2 causes misregulation of iron metabolism and neurodegenerative disease in mice. *Nature Genetics, 27*(2), 209–214.

Levi, S., Cozzi, A., & Arosio, P. (2005). Neuroferritinopathy: A neurodegenerative disorder associated with L-ferritin mutation. *Best Practice and Research Clinical Haematology, 18*(2), 265–276.

Lill, R., & Muhlenhoff, U. (2006). Iron-sulfur protein biogenesis in eukaryotes: Components and mechanisms. *Annual Review of Cell and Developmental Biology, 22*, 457–486.

Lyon, E., & Frank, E. L. (2001). Hereditary hemochromatosis since discovery of the HFE gene. *Clinical Chemistry, 47*(7), 1147–1156.

Maciel, P., Cruz, V. T., Constante, M., Iniesta, I., Costa, M. C., Gallati, S., et al. (2005). Neuroferritinopathy: Missense mutation in FTL causing early-onset bilateral pallidal involvement. *Neurology, 65*(4), 603–605.

Maguire, A., Hellier, K., Hammans, S., & May, A. (2001). X-linked cerebellar ataxia and sideroblastic anaemia associated with a missense mutation in the ABC7 gene predicting V411L. *British Journal of Haematology, 115*(4), 910–917.

Maines, M. D. (1997). The heme oxygenase system: A regulator of second messenger gases. *Annual Review of Pharmacology and Toxicology, 37*, 517–554.

Mancuso, M., Davidzon, G., Kurlan, R. M., Tawil, R., Bonilla, E., Di Mauro, S., et al. (2005). Hereditary ferritinopathy: A novel mutation, its cellular pathology, and pathogenetic insights. *Journal of Neuropathology and Experimental Neurology, 64*(4), 280–294.

Martelli, A., Wattenhofer-Donze, M., Schmucker, S., Bouvet, S., Reutenauer, L., & Puccio, H. (2007). Frataxin is essential for extramitochondrial Fe-S cluster proteins in mammalian tissues. *Human Molecular Genetics, 16*(22), 2651–2658.

McCord, J. M. (1998). Iron, free radicals, and oxidative injury. *Seminars in Hematology, 35*(1), 5–12.

McKie, A. T., Barrow, D., Latunde-Dada, G. O., Rolfs, A., Sager, G., Mudaly, E., et al. (2001). An iron-regulated ferric reductase associated with the absorption of dietary iron. *Science, 291*(5509), 1755–1759.

McKie, A. T., Marciani, P., Rolfs, A., Brennan, K., Wehr, K., Barrow, D., et al. (2000). A novel duodenal iron-regulated transporter, IREG1, implicated in the basolateral transfer of iron to the circulation. *Molecular Cell, 5*(2), 299–309.

Merryweather-Clarke, A. T., Pointon, J. J., Shearman, J. D., & Robson, K. J. (1997). Global prevalence of putative haemochromatosis mutations. *Journal of Medical Genetics, 34*(4), 275–278.

Mikulits, W., Schranzhofer, M., Beug, H., & Mullner, E. W. (1999). Post-transcriptional control via iron-responsive elements: The impact of aberrations in hereditary disease. *Mutation Research, 437*(3), 219–230.

Miret, S., Simpson, R. J., & McKie, A. T. (2003). Physiology and molecular biology of dietary iron absorption. *Annual Review of Nutrition, 23*, 283–301.

Miyajima, H., Kono, S., Takahashi, Y., Sugimoto, M., Sakamoto, M., & Sakai, N. (2001). Cerebellar ataxia associated with heteroallelic ceruloplasmin gene mutation. *Neurology, 57*(12), 2205–2210.

Miyajima, H., Nishimura, Y., Mizoguchi, K., Sakamoto, M., Shimizu, T., & Honda, N. (1987). Familial apoceruloplasmin deficiency associated with blepharospasm and retinal degeneration. *Neurology, 37*(5), 761–767.

Moalem, S., Percy, M. E., Andrews, D. F., Kruck, T. P., Wong, S., Dalton, A. J., et al. (2000). Are hereditary hemochromatosis mutations involved in Alzheimer disease? *American Journal of Medical Genetics, 93*(1), 58–66.

Mondino, F., Filippi, P., Magliola, U., & Duca, S. (2002). Magnetic resonance relaxometry in Parkinson's disease. *Neurological Science, 23*(Supplement 2), S87–S88.

Moos, T., Rosengren Nielsen, T., Skjorringe, T., & Morgan, E. H. (2007). Iron trafficking inside the brain. *Journal of Neurochemistry, 103*(5), 1730–1740.

Morgan, E. H., & Moos, T. (2002). Mechanism and developmental changes in iron transport across the blood-brain barrier. *Developmental Neuroscience, 24*(2–3), 106–113.

Morgan, N. V., Westaway, S. K., Morton, J. E., Gregory, A., Gissen, P., Sonek, S., et al. (2006). PLA2G6, encoding a phospholipase A2, is mutated in neurodegenerative disorders with high brain iron. *Nature Genetics, 38*(7), 752–754.

Morris, C. M., & Edwardson, J. A. (1994). Iron histochemistry of the substantia nigra in Parkinson's disease. *Neurodegeneration, 3*(4), 277–282.

Muhlenhoff, U., Gerber, J., Richhardt, N., & Lill, R. (2003). Components involved in assembly and dislocation of iron-sulfur clusters on the scaffold protein Isu1p. *The European Molecular Biology Organization Journal, 22*(18), 4815–4825.

Napier, I., Ponka, P., & Richardson, D. R. (2005). Iron trafficking in the mitochondrion: Novel pathways revealed by disease. *Blood, 105*(5), 1867–1874.

Nielsen, J. E., Jensen, L. N., & Krabbe, K. (1995). Hereditary haemochromatosis: A case of iron accumulation in the basal ganglia associated with a parkinsonian syndrome. *Journal of Neurology, Neurosurgery and Psychiatry, 59*(3), 318–321.

Nittis, T., & Gitlin, J. D. (2002). The copper-iron connection: Hereditary aceruloplasminemia. *Seminars in Hematology, 39*(4), 282–289.

Njajou, O. T., Hollander, M., Koudstaal, P. J., Hofman, A., Witteman, J. C., Breteler, M. M., et al. (2002). Mutations in the hemochromatosis gene (HFE) and stroke. *Stroke, 33*(10), 2363–2366.

Ohgami, R. S., Campagna, D. R., Greer, E. L., Antiochos, B., McDonald, A., Chen, J., et al. (2005). Identification of a ferrireductase required for efficient transferrin-dependent iron uptake in erythroid cells. *Nature Genetics, 37*(11), 1264–1269.

Okamoto, N., Wada, S., Oga, T., Kawabata, Y., Baba, Y., Habu, D., et al. (1996). Hereditary ceruloplasmin deficiency with hemosiderosis. *Human Genetics, 97*(6), 755–758.

Olanow, C. W. (1992). Magnetic resonance imaging in parkinsonism. *Clinical Neurology, 10*(2), 405–420.

Osaki, S., Johnson, D. A., & Frieden, E. (1971). The mobilization of iron from the perfused mammalian liver by a serum copper enzyme, ferroxidase I. *Journal of Biological Chemistry, 246*(9), 3018–3023.

Pagon, R. A., Bird, T. D., Detter, J. C., & Pierce, I. (1985). Hereditary sideroblastic anaemia and ataxia: An X linked recessive disorder. *Journal of Medical Genetics, 22*(4), 267–273.

Pandolfo, M. (1999). Friedreich's ataxia: Clinical aspects and pathogenesis. *Seminars in Neurology, 19*(3), 311–321.

Pantopoulos, K., Weiss, G., & Hentze, M. W. (1996). Nitric oxide and oxidative stress (H2O2) control mammalian iron metabolism by different pathways. *Molecular and Cellular Biology, 16*(7), 3781–3788.

Patel, B. N., & David, S. (1997). A novel glycosylphosphatidylinositol-anchored form of ceruloplasmin is expressed by mammalian astrocytes. *Journal of Biological Chemistry, 272*(32), 20185–20190.

Patel, B. N., Dunn, R. J., & David, S. (2000). Alternative RNA splicing generates a glycosylphosphatidylinositol-anchored form of ceruloplasmin in mammalian brain. *Journal of Biological Chemistry, 275*(6), 4305–4310.

Patel, B. N., Dunn, R. J., Jeong, S. Y., Zhu, Q., Julien, J. P., & David, S. (2002). Ceruloplasmin regulates iron levels in the CNS and prevents free radical injury. *The Journal of Neuroscience, 22*(15), 6578–6586.

Perry, T. L., Norman, M. G., Yong, V. W., Whiting, S., Crichton, J. U., Hansen, S., et al. (1985). Hallervorden-Spatz disease: Cysteine accumulation and cysteine dioxygenase deficiency in the globus pallidus. *Annals of Neurology, 18*(4), 482–489.

Pondarre, C., Campagna, D. R., Antiochos, B., Sikorski, L., Mulhern, H., & Fleming, M. D. (2007). Abcb7, the gene responsible for X-linked sideroblastic anemia with ataxia, is essential for hematopoiesis. *Blood, 109*(8), 3567–3569.

Ponka, P. (1997). Tissue-specific regulation of iron metabolism and heme synthesis: Distinct control mechanisms in erythroid cells. *Blood, 89*(1), 1–25.

Ponka, P. (2004). Hereditary causes of disturbed iron homeostasis in the central nervous system. *Annals of the New York Academy of Sciences, 1012*, 267–281.

Ponka, P., Beaumont, C., & Richardson, D. R. (1998). Function and regulation of transferrin and ferritin. *Seminars in Hematology, 35*(1), 35–54.

Ponka, P., Wilczynska, A., & Schulman, H. M. (1982). Iron utilization in rabbit reticulocytes. A study using succinylacetone as an inhibitor or heme synthesis. *Biochimica et Biophysica Acta, 720*(1), 96–105.

Puccio, H., Simon, D., Cossee, M., Criqui-Filipe, P., Tiziano, F., Melki, J., et al. (2001). Mouse models for Friedreich ataxia exhibit cardiomyopathy, sensory nerve defect and Fe-S enzyme deficiency followed by intramitochondrial iron deposits. *Nature Genetics, 27*(2), 181–186.

Radisky, D. C., Babcock, M. C., & Kaplan, J. (1999). The yeast frataxin homologue mediates mitochondrial iron efflux. Evidence for a mitochondrial iron cycle. *Journal of Biological Chemistry, 274*(8), 4497–4499.

Richardson, D. R., & Ponka, P. (1997). The molecular mechanisms of the metabolism and transport of iron in normal and neoplastic cells. *Biochimica et Biophysica Acta, 1331*(1), 1–40.

Rouault, T. A. (2001). Iron on the brain. *Nature Genetics, 28*(4), 299–300.

Saleheen, D., Farooq, U., & Frossard, P. (2005). A lack of association of variants in Hemochromatosis gene with ischemic stroke. *Medical Science Monitor, 11*(9), LE9.

Sampietro, M., Caputo, L., Casatta, A., Meregalli, M., Pellagatti, A., Tagliabue, J., et al. (2001). The hemochromatosis gene affects the age of onset of sporadic Alzheimer's disease. *Neurobiology of Aging, 22*(4), 563–568.

Savoiardo, M., Halliday, W. C., Nardocci, N., Strada, L., D'Incerti, L., Angelini, L., et al. (1993). Hallervorden-Spatz disease: MR and pathologic findings. *American Journal of Neuroradiology, 14*(1), 155–162.

Schipper, H. M. (2004). Brain iron deposition and the free radical-mitochondrial theory of ageing. *Ageing Research Reviews, 3*, 265–301.

Schranzhofer, M., Schifrer, M., Galy, B., Hentze, M., Ponka, P., & Muellner, E. W. (2007). Low cytosolic non-heme iron levels in erythroid cells prevent IRP2-mediated ferritin upregulation during differentiation. *Experimental Hematology, 35*, 108–109.

Schroder, J. M. (2005). Ferritinopathy: Diagnosis by muscle or nerve biopsy, with a note on other nuclear inclusion body diseases. *Acta Neuropathologica, 109*(1), 109–114.

Selkoe, D. J. (1991). The molecular pathology of Alzheimer's disease. *Neuron, 6*(4), 487–498.

Stearman, R., Yuan, D. S., Yamaguchi-Iwai, Y., Klausner, R. D., & Dancis, A. (1996). A permease-oxidase complex involved in high-affinity iron uptake in yeast. *Science, 271*(5255), 1552–1557.

Stehling, O., Elsasser, H. P., Bruckel, B., Muhlenhoff, U., & Lill, R. (2004). Iron-sulfur protein maturation in human cells: Evidence for a function of frataxin. *Human Molecular Genetics, 13*(23), 3007–3015.

Swaiman, K. F. (2001). Hallervorden-Spatz syndrome. *Pediatric Neurology, 25*(2), 102–108.

Swaiman, K. F., Smith, S. A., Trock, G. L., & Siddiqui, A. R. (1983). Sea-blue histiocytes, lymphocytic cytosomes, movement disorder and 59Fe-uptake in basal ganglia: Hallervorden-Spatz disease or ceroid storage disease with abnormal isotope scan? *Neurology, 33*(3), 301–305.

Vidal, R., Ghetti, B., Takao, M., Brefel-Courbon, C., Uro-Coste, E., Glazier, B. S., et al. (2004). Intracellular ferritin accumulation in neural and extraneural tissue characterizes a neurodegenerative disease associated with a mutation in the ferritin light polypeptide gene. *Journal of Neuropathology and Experimental Neurology, 63*(4), 363–380.

Vidal, R., Miravalle, L., Gao, X., Barbeito, A. G., Baraibar, M. A., Hekmatyar, S. K., et al. (2008). Expression of a mutant form of the ferritin light chain gene induces neurodegeneration and iron overload in transgenic mice. *The Journal of Neuroscience, 28*(1), 60–67.

Vulpe, C. D., Kuo, Y. M., Murphy, T. L., Cowley, L., Askwith, C., Libina, N., et al. (1999). Hephaestin, a ceruloplasmin homologue implicated in intestinal iron transport, is defective in the sla mouse. *Nature Genetics, 21*(2), 195–199.

Wang, X. S., Lee, S., Simmons, Z., Boyer, P., Scott, K., Liu, W., et al. (2004). Increased incidence of the Hfe mutation in amyotrophic lateral sclerosis and related cellular consequences. *The Journal of Neuroscience, 227*(1), 27–33.

Welch, J. J., Watts, J. A., Vakoc, C. R., Yao, Y., Wang, H., Hardison, R. C., et al. (2004). Global regulation of erythroid gene expression by transcription factor GATA-1. *Blood, 104*(10), 3136–3147.

Worthington, M. T., Cohn, S. M., Miller, S. K., Luo, R. Q., & Berg, C. L. (2001). Characterization of a human plasma membrane heme transporter in intestinal and hepatocyte cell lines. *American Journal of Physiology Gastrointestinal and Liver Physiology, 280*(6), G1172–G1177.

Yen, A. A., Simpson, E. P., Henkel, J. S., Beers, D. R., & Appel, S. H. (2004). HFE mutations are not strongly associated with sporadic ALS. *Neurology, 62*(9), 1611–1612.

Yonekawa, M., Okabe, T., Asamoto, Y., & Ohta, M. (1999). A case of hereditary ceruloplasmin deficiency with iron deposition in the brain associated with chorea, dementia, diabetes mellitus and retinal pigmentation: Administration of fresh-frozen human plasma. *European Neurology, 42*(3), 157–162.

Yoon, S. J., Koh, Y. H., Floyd, R. A., & Park, J. W. (2000). Copper, zinc superoxide dismutase enhances DNA damage and mutagenicity induced by cysteine/iron. *Mutation Research, 448*(1), 97–104.

Yoshida, K., Furihata, K., Takeda, S., Nakamura, A., Yamamoto, K., Morita, H., et al. (1995). A mutation in the ceruloplasmin gene is associated with systemic hemosiderosis in humans. *Nature Genetics, 9*(3), 267–272.

Youdim, M. (1994). Inorganic neurotoxins in neurodegenerative disorders without primary dementia. In D. B. Calne (Ed.), *Neurodegenerative Diseases* (pp. 251–276). Philadelphia: Saunders, W.B.

Zanella, I., Derosas, M., Corrado, M., Cocco, E., Cavadini, P., Biasiotto, G., et al. (2008). The effects of frataxin silencing in HeLa cells are rescued by the expression of human mitochondrial ferritin. *Biochimica et Biophysica Acta, 1782*(2), 90–98.

Zhou, B., Westaway, S. K., Levinson, B., Johnson, M. A., Gitschier, J., & Hayflick, S. J. (2001). A novel pantothenate kinase gene (PANK2) is defective in Hallervorden-Spatz syndrome. *Nature Genetics, 28*(4), 345–349.

Zimmerman, E. A., & Schenck, J. F. (2007). Neurodegeneration with brain iron accumulation. *MedLink Neurology*, from http://www.medlink.com/cip.asp?UID=mlt002h8&src=Search&ref=19850753

Zlokovic, B. V. (2008). The blood-brain barrier in health and chronic neurodegenerative disorders. *Neuron, 57*(2), 178–201.

Zupanc, M. L., Chun, R. W., & Gilbert-Barness, E. F. (1990). Osmiophilic deposits in cytosomes in Hallervorden-Spatz syndrome. *Pediatric Neurology, 6*(5), 349–352.

# IV Public Health Issues

# 16 Iron and Heart Disease: A Review of the Epidemiologic Data

*Christopher T. Sempos, Anne C. Looker, Daniel L. McGee, and Jürgen Rehm*

**Summary**

- In 1981, Dr. Jerome Sullivan proposed the hypothesis that the risk of coronary heart disease (CHD) increases in a positive fashion as body iron stores increase.
- Serum ferritin and other less precise measures of body iron stores have been used in those studies to test the hypothesis.
- Serum ferritin was *not* significantly related to risk of developing CHD in the vast majority of the observational cohort studies, case-control, or cross-sectional studies.
- In an underpowered clinical trial, those receiving phlebotomy to lower body stores of iron did not have a significantly lower risk of death from all causes (primary endpoint) or of death plus non-fatal heart attack or stroke compared to controls.
- The presence of the Cys282Tyr mutation, which accounts for most of the cases of hemochromatosis, was not found to be associated with CHD risk in two meta-analysis studies.
- At present, the vast majority of the epidemiological data does not support the hypothesis that body iron stores are directly related to the risk of developing CHD.

**Key Words:** Iron; ferritin; CHD; heart disease; hemochromatosis; epidemiology

## 1. INTRODUCTION

Dr. Jerome Sullivan (1981) proposed a new theory to explain the differences in coronary heart disease (CHD) incidence and mortality between men and women. He noticed that as men and women age, the gaps between them in heart disease incidence and in body iron stores both decrease (Sullivan, 1983, 1989). Lower stores of iron levels in women are due mostly to menstrual blood loss, and with menopause the differences in iron stores decrease. As a result, he theorized that body iron stores are directly or positively related to CHD risk, i.e., the higher your body iron

The findings and conclusions in this chapter are those of the authors and do not necessarily represent the views of the Centers for Disease Control and Prevention, the National Institutes of Health, or the US Department of Health and Human Services.

From: *Nutrition and Health: Iron Deficiency and Overload*
Edited by: S. Yehuda and D.I. Mostofsky, DOI 10.1007/978-1-59745-462-9_16

stores the greater your CHD risk. Until the publication of results from Finland by Salonen et al. (1992) showing that men with serum ferritin levels, a measure of body iron stores, at or above 200 μg/L had double the risk of having a heart attack, the hypothesis was largely ignored. Since then, however, there has been an intense interest in this topic. It is thought that iron might promote the atherosclerosis leading to CHD by catalyzing the oxidation of low-density lipoprotein (LDL) cholesterol (Halliwell & Chirico, 1993; Reaven & Wiztum, 1996; Steinberg, 1997; Yuan & Brunk, 1998; Heinecke, 1998).

The purpose of this chapter is to examine and update the recent epidemiologic data which are directly related to Dr. Sullivan's hypothesis (Danesh & Appleby, 1999; Sempos, Looker, & Gillum, 1996; Sempos, Gillum, & Looker, 1997). Important related topics, e.g., the relationship of antioxidant nutrients, oral contraceptives, estrogen replacement therapy and menopause to CHD risk, and iron and myocardial reperfusion injury, are not discussed.

## 2. SERUM MEASURES OF BODY IRON STORES

Serum ferritin is currently the best measure of body iron stores that is feasible to use in epidemiologic studies (Expert Scientific Working Group, 1985). It is a fairly sensitive indicator of changes in body iron stores as you move along the stages of iron status from deficient to replete to iron overload in healthy individuals, e.g., not suffering from an infection, inflammation, or cancer. Less direct and sensitive measures of body iron stores are serum iron, total iron-binding capacity (TIBC), and transferrin saturation (TS), which is calculated as the ratio of serum iron to total iron binding capacity. TS is the best measure of circulating iron available to tissues and is considered to be a better measure of iron stores than serum iron or TIBC, but not as good as serum ferritin. Other common iron status measures are even less directly related to body iron stores, e.g., hemoglobin, hematocrit, and erythrocyte protoporphyrin. Hemoglobin and hematocrit are measures of the oxygen-carrying capacity of blood and viscosity.

As body iron stores increase so do serum ferritin levels (Bothwell, Charlton, Cook, & Finch, 1979; Herbert, 1992). As a result, serum ferritin can be useful in detecting iron deficiency and overload. A serum ferritin level of <15 μg/L has been used as an indicator of iron deficiency in both men and women (Custer, Finch, Sobel, & Zettner, 1995). Separate upper limits have been suggested for adult men (400 μg/L), menstruating women (200 μg/L), and postmenopausal women (300 μg/L) (Custer et al., 1995).

TS and serum iron levels also tend to increase as stores increase over the normal range, while TIBC levels tend to decrease as stores increase. The opposite trends occur as body iron stores decrease. At very high levels of body iron stores as in homozygous hemochromatosis (TS > 60%), or at depleted levels (TS < 16%), i.e., iron deficiency, TS is considered to be a good measure of body iron stores. Within the normal range of TS, i.e., 20–60%, it is not clear how well TS reflects body iron stores. Data from the third National Health and Nutrition Examination Survey or NHANES III (Table 1), conducted during the years 1988–1994, show that there does appear to be a positive correlation, albeit low, between the two measurements, with the result that with increasing levels of TS mean levels of serum ferritin tend to rise as well, especially in women. The correlation between log transformed serum ferritin and TS for men and women 45–74 years of age was $r = 0.22$ overall and $r = 0.14$ for men and $r = 0.25$ for women.

Serum iron status measures are also affected by inflammation, cancer, and infection. Serum ferritin levels tend to increase in response to inflammation (Bothwell et al., 1979; Herbert, 1992; Custer et al., 1995; Hulthén, Lindstedt, Lundberg, & Hallberg, 1998) while TS, TIBC, and serum iron levels decrease (Yip & Dallman, 1988). For example, in response to a heart attack, ferritin

**Table 1**
**Geometric[a] Mean Serum Ferritin by Serum Transferrin Saturation Level[b]**

| | *Men* | | *Women* | |
|---|---|---|---|---|
| *Transferrin Saturation(%)*[c] | *N* | *Ferritin (μg/L)* | *N* | *Ferritin (μg/L)* |
| <16% | 492 | 93 | 974 | 49 |
| 16–19% | 567 | 119 | 789 | 66 |
| 20–29% | 1,513 | 145 | 1,638 | 87 |
| 30–44% | 1,101 | 161 | 714 | 99 |
| 45–59% | 183 | 186 | 104 | 117 |
| ≥60% | 53 | 269 | 17 | 220 |
| Total | 3,909 | 142 | 4,236 | 75 |

[a] Within each transferrin saturation group, the serum ferritin data were transformed using natural logarithms. The antilog of the mean of the log transformed distribution is the geometric mean value shown in the table.
[b] US men and women aged 45 years and older.
[c] Calculated as the ratio of serum iron (μmol/L) divided by total iron-binding capacity (μmol/L).
Source: CDC/NCHS: Unpublished data from the third National Health and Nutrition Examination Survey, conducted in 1988–1994.

levels are initially raised while TS, TIBC, and serum iron levels decrease (Birgegård, Hälgren, Venge, & Wilde, 1979; Griffiths et al., 1985). In the study by Schouw et al. (1990) serum ferritin levels returned to control levels 6 weeks after the heart attack while TS and serum iron levels continued to be depressed.

The distribution of serum TS and ferritin by age and sex from the NHANES III are shown in Table 2. The important issues in monitoring iron status measures over time in the national surveys have been discussed by Zacharski, Ornstein, Woloshin, and Schwartz (2000) and Looker, Gunter, and Johnson (1995), with the latter giving more details on iron status data from NHANES III.

**Table 2**
**Mean Levels of Serum Transferrin Saturation[a] and Geometric[b] Mean Serum Ferritin by Age and Sex[c]**

| | *Serum Transferrin (%)* | | *Geometric Serum Ferritin (μg/L)* | |
|---|---|---|---|---|
| *Age group* | *Men (n = 7,529)* | *Women (n = 8,533)* | *Men (n = 7,529)* | *Women (n = 8,533)* |
| 20+ | 29 | 24 | 135 | 49 |
| 20–29 | 31 | 25 | 110 | 33 |
| 30–39 | 30 | 24 | 147 | 37 |
| 40–49 | 28 | 23 | 146 | 38 |
| 50–59 | 28 | 23 | 148 | 73 |
| 69–69 | 28 | 24 | 146 | 95 |
| 70+ | 27 | 24 | 128 | 89 |

[a] Calculated as the ratio of serum iron (μmol/L) divided by total iron-binding capacity (μmol/L).
[b] Within each age and sex group, the serum ferritin data were transformed using natural logarithms. The antilog of the mean of the log transformed distribution is the geometric mean value shown in the table.
[c] US men and women aged 20 years and older.
Source: CDC/NCHS: Unpublished data from the third National Health and Nutrition Examination Survey, conducted in 1988–1994.

There are no published data from the Centers for Disease Control and Prevention (CDC) on more recent trends in iron status measures from the NHANES. [Parenthetically, Cusick et al. (2008) have published data on the trends in anemia between NHANES III and NHANES 1999–2002.]

## 3. BODY IRON STORES AND RISK OF HEART DISEASE: THE EPIDEMIOLOGIC DATA

### *3.1. Cohort Studies Based on Serum Ferritin*

Cohort studies are referred to also as prospective, incidence, follow-up, and longitudinal studies. The question being asked in cohort studies is, Do persons with the risk factor develop or die from the disease more frequently or sooner than those who do not have the risk factor? For example, are persons who have high serum ferritin levels more likely to develop CHD in the future than are persons who do not? Because risk factor exposure is measured prior to the onset of clinically apparent disease, cohort studies are considered to be the strongest observational study design in epidemiology (Beaglehole, Bonita, & Kjellström, 1993; Gordis, 2008). Using various measures of body iron stores, a number of researchers have attempted to assess the hypothesis that CHD risk increases with body iron stores (Table 3).

As stated earlier, the theory was largely ignored until the publication of results from the Finnish Kuopio Ischemic Heart Disease Risk Factor Study (KIHD) (Salonen et al., 1992). The study consisted of 1,931 randomly selected men who were 42, 48, 54, or 60 years of age and who were free of clinical symptoms of CHD at baseline. During an average of 3 years of follow-up, 46 men had either a definite or possible heart attack as defined by ECG or enzyme criteria. Five additional men who were admitted to the hospital for prolonged chest pain did not meet the criteria. The authors reported that the results were not changed substantively by including those men and the published results were based on 51 heart attacks.

Salonen et al. (1992) reported finding a statistically significant linear association between serum ferritin level and the risk of heart attack ($z = 2.64$, $p < 0.01$) after adjusting for possible confounding. Thus, as serum ferritin levels increased so did the risk of heart attack. The more surprising finding was, however, that men with a serum ferritin ≥200 μg/L had a greater than twofold higher risk of heart attack compared to those with lower serum ferritin values. The difference was statistically significant (relative risk = 2.2, 95% CI 1.2–4.0, $p < 0.01$). Again the results were adjusted for possible confounding in a multivariate model. Additionally, they reported finding that compared to men with serum ferritin levels <200 μg/L, men with a ferritin of 200–399 μg/L had a nearly identical risk of heart attack as did men with ferritin levels ≥400 μg/L (Salonen et al., 1992).

The study by Salonen et al. (1992), although based on a small number of heart attacks, was a well-conducted study. [In a letter to the editor, they presented data to indicate that the relationship was still significant after an average of 5 years of follow-up and 83 heart attacks – relative risk = 2.0, 95% CI = 1.2–3.1, $p = 0.004$ (Salonen, Nyyssönen, & Salonen, 1994).] They have been criticized, however, for not having adequately adjusted for inflammation (Weiss, Fuchs, & Wachter, 1993) and because there was a negative correlation between age and serum ferritin (MacDonald, 1993). But neither criticism appears to be entirely justified (Salonen et al., 1993a, 1993b). The authors reported that they found no correlation between serum ferritin and plasma fibrinogen (an acute-phase protein) in the whole sample or with C-reactive protein in a subsample (Salonen et al., 1992, 1993a, 1993b). Moreover, the authors adjusted for blood leukocyte count in their analyses (Salonen et al., 1992). More importantly, the association between serum ferritin and heart attack was not attenuated when the analysis was repeated after removing heart attacks

**Table 3**
**Serum Ferritin and Heart Disease: Cohort Studies**

| *Study (Reference)* | *Sex* | *Sample Size* | *Association* |
|---|---|---|---|
| *Kuopio Ischemic Heart Disease Risk Factor Study (KIHD)*[a] | | | |
| Salonen et al. (1992) | M | 1,931 | + |
| Salonen et al. (1994) | M | 1,931 | + |
| Tuomainen et al. (1998) | M | 197[b] | + |
| Magnusson et al. (1994) | M | 990 | None |
| | W | 1,046 | None |
| Stampfer et al. (1993) | M | 476[b] | None |
| Mänttäri et al. (1994) | M | 268[b] | None |
| Kiechl et al. (1997) | M/W | 826 | + |
| Sempos (2000) | M/W | 1,376 | None |
| Knuiman et al. (2003) | M/W | 1,612 | None |
| Galan et al. (2006) | M | 3,223 | None |
| | W | 6,694 | None |
| van der A, Marx, Grobee, Kamphius, Georgiou, & van Kats-Renaud (2006) | W | 1,319[b] | None |
| Sun et al. (2008) | W | 725[b] | None |
| Frey and Krider (1994) | M | 298[c] | None |
| Aronow and Ahn (1996) | M/W | 577[c] | None |

[a] All three studies are from the same cohort – *Kuopio Ischemic Heart Disease Risk Factor Study (KIHD)*. The difference between the two papers by Salonen et al. (1992, 1994) is that the first consisted of the results after 3-year follow-up and the second after a 5-year follow-up of the same individuals. The third paper is a study on a subset of the cohort in the first two studies looking at the transferrin/ferritin ratio and risk of heart attack.

[b] Nested case-control study, i.e., a case-control or retrospective study, which is "nested" within a cohort or cohort study (Clayton & Hills, 1993). Serum transferrin/ferritin ratio (Tuomainen et al. (1998); Sun et al., 2008) or ferritin (Stampfer et al., 1993; Mänttäri et al., 1994; Sun et al., 2008) were determined on frozen sera collected at the beginning of the study. Cases accrued during the follow-up period, and controls were selected from the pool of individuals who were at risk of having CHD at the time a case was diagnosed. Because of the efficient sample design, only small sample sizes are required (Clayton & Hills, 1993). The study by van der A, Marx et al. (2006) was a case-cohort study, which is similar to a nested case-control study.

[c] Reports appear to be based on a case-series from a clinical practice rather than from traditional cohort studies.

which occurred within the first 6 months following blood collection. As was stated earlier, serum ferritin levels go up after a heart attack but return to baseline levels within 6 months after the heart attack (Schouw et al., 1990).

In a subsample of their cohort, the Salonen research group also reported that the ratio of transferrin to ferritin was positively related to CHD risk (Tuomainen, Punnonen, Nyyssönen, & Salonen, 1998). This is not surprising given the strong finding in the larger cohort. Moreover, because the three studies by their group were based on the same set of individuals from the KIHD cohort, we have considered them as one study supporting the Sullivan hypothesis (Table 3).

The results from 11 other cohort studies on the association between serum ferritin and CHD have been reported (Table 3). Only one of them found an association between serum ferritin and

CHD (Kiechl, Willeit, Egger, Poewe, & Oberholenzer, 1997). In that study, it was reported that the 5-year progression of carotid stenosis was significantly related to serum ferritin levels. The study consisted of 826 men and women aged 40–79 years who were randomly selected from the population Bruneck, Italy. Carotid atherosclerosis was assessed by repeated carotid ultrasound evaluation. The authors further reported that changes in iron stores were associated with changes in the progression of carotid atherosclerosis in that lowering of stores was associated with a decreased risk of progression while increases in stores were associated with an increased risk. We can find no reports where these interesting results have been replicated.

Of the studies which found no association between serum ferritin and CHD (Table 3), two appear to be based on case-series (Frey & Krider, 1994; Aronow & Ahn 1996) rather than a true cohort. The studies by Magnusson et al. (1994), Stampfer, Grodstein, Rosenberg, Willett, & Hennekens (1993), Mänttäri et al. (1994), Sempos et al. (2000), Knuiman, Divitini, Olynyk, Cullen, and Batholomew (2003), Galan et al. (2006), van der A, Marx et al. (2006), and Sun et al. (2008) while based on a traditional cohort design, all used slightly different procedures to analyze their results and address different aspects of the iron hypothesis.

In the study by Magnusson et al. (1994), 2,036 Icelandic men and women aged 25–74 years were followed for an average of 8.5 years. During that time 81 participants (63 men and 18 women) had a heart attack. In their multivariate models, Magnusson et al. included both serum ferritin, in the normal units or log transformed, and serum TIBC as *continuous* variables to test if a statistically significant linear association exists between serum ferritin and risk of heart attack. Neither serum ferritin (RR = 0.999, 95% CI 0.997–1.001) nor log ferritin (RR = 0.781, 95% CI 0.540–1.129) were significantly associated with the risk of heart attack. In contrast with Salonen et al.'s (1994) results, those results indicated that body iron stores as measured by serum ferritin were not associated with the risk of having a heart attack.

The interesting finding was that TIBC was shown to have a significant negative association with risk of heart attack (RR = 0.95, 95% CI 0.92–0.98). That is, those with higher TIBC levels had a lower risk of heart attack. Their interpretation of the results for TIBC was very interesting. As we have said TIBC levels are inversely related to body iron stores, but compared to ferritin it is a relatively weak index of stores. However, TIBC is also known to have antioxidant properties (Dormandy, 1978). Given the recent results concerning the oxidative modification of LDL cholesterol and the reported protective effects of antioxidant nutrients, Magnusson et al. postulated that "If iron increases the risk of coronary artery disease by oxidizing LDL, as has been postulated, a critical step in its pathogenic pathway would be the accumulation of free iron in the subendothelial space. The serum iron binding capacity might be a more reliable indicator of this accumulation of free iron in the vessel wall than the total iron stores (Magnusson et al., 1994, p. 107)." Additionally, they felt that their results "support the concept that iron being an important transition metal might contribute to atherogenesis along with other classic risk factors, although arguing against the recent hypothesis that iron stores per se increase risk (Magnusson et al., 1994, p. 107)."

Sempos et al. (2000) directly addressed the issue of a threshold at 200 μg/L. The data were based on the mortality follow-up of 1,376 white men and women who participated in the second National Health and Nutrition Examination Survey (NHANES II). The NHANES II was conducted in 1976–1980, with mortality follow-up through December 31, 1992. Serum ferritin levels were divided into four categories: (1) <50 μg/L; (2) 50–99 μg/L [reference level]; (3) 100–199 μg/L; and (4) ≥200 μg/L. For white men and women, serum ferritin levels ≥200 μg/L were not associated with increased risk of death from all cardiovascular diseases (men: RR = 0.7, 95% CI 0.3–1.6; women: RR = 2.0, 95% CI 0.6–7.3), or CHD (men: RR = 1.2, 95% CI 0.5–2.9;

women: RR = 1.2, 95% CI 0.3–4.9) compared with the reference level. Furthermore, there was no association with heart attack death in white men (RR = 0.5, 95% CI 0.2–1.2); there were not a sufficient number of heart attack deaths to test the hypothesis in white women ($n = 13$).

The study by Stampfer et al. (1993) also directly addressed the issue of a threshold at 200 μg/L. Using a nested case-control design (Clayton & Hill, 1993), 238 men participating in the US Physicians Study had a heart attack during the period after the 1982 baseline. Stored serum for those men and for 238 controls matched for age and smoking status were analyzed for serum ferritin concentrations. And after adjustment for other CHD risk factors, men with serum ferritin levels ≥200 μg/L were not found to have a higher risk of heart attack (RR = 1.1, 95% CI 0.7–1.6).

Similar results were found also in another nested case-control study by Mänttäri et al. (1994). The participants in this study were a subset of men from the Finnish Helsinki Heart Study – a randomized clinical trial of the lipid-lowering drug gemfibrozil. In that study, the authors looked to see if the threshold for ferritin occurs at much lower levels than the 200 μg/L cutoff used by Salonen et al. (1992). Mänttäri et al. (1994) looked at the risk of developing CHD in two groups of men with serum ferritin levels of 43–84 μg/L or ≥85 μg/L compared with men with serum ferritin levels of ≤42 μg/L and found that it was not different.

In a 17-year follow-up of a cohort from Busselton, Western Australia, no association was found between serum ferritin and risk of CHD or stroke (Knuiman et al., 2003). The cohort included 1,612 men and women who participated in the 1981 Busselton Heath Survey. The association was assessed with ferritin divided up into sex specific tertiles or as a continuous variable. The tertiles were men – ≤126 μg/L [reference], >126 – ≤233 μg/L, >233 μg/L; women – ≤49 μg/L [reference], >49 – ≤122 μg/L, and >122 μg/L. The results for women, therefore, do not directly address the 200 μg/L cutoff. The results for the association between serum ferritin, as a continuous variable, and CHD were: men – RR = 0.944, 95% CI 0.71 – 1.25; women – RR = 0.849, 95% CI 0.60–1.2.

Three additional reports by Galan et al. (2006), van der A, Marx et al. (2006), and Sun et al. (2008) found no association between serum ferritin and coronary heart disease. The study by van der A, Marx et al. (2006) directly addressed the 200 μg/L cutoff while neither of the other two did. However, in that study there were relatively few CHD events – only 9 – in those with a serum ferritin ≥ 200 μg/L. Galan et al. (2006) used serum ferritin groups of <31 μg/L, 31–70 μg/L, 71–160 μg/L, and >160 μg/L while Sun et al. (2008) quartile. Sun et al. (2008) also evaluated the association between the ratio of transferrin receptor to ferritin (see, Skikine, 2008) and CHD risk and, again, found no association.

In case series studies, patients who receive a particular test or procedure are followed over time using cohort study methods in order to evaluate the association between the test result and an outcome. The information from such a study may be very useful in suggesting hypotheses or testing a current one. But because the test or procedure was ordered for a particular medical reason which may be favorably or unfavorably related to the outcome of interest, the results from those studies may be biased and thus cannot be considered as rigorous as the data from a standard cohort study (Hennekens & Buring, 1987). The study by Frey and Krider (1994) was based on clinical case series of 298 men with serum ferritin measurements taken at some point over a 10-year period (mean 5.2 years) in a West Virginia medical practice. Over that follow-up period, 32 men had a heart attack. The authors reported finding no difference in mean serum ferritin levels between patients who had or did not have a heart attack. Nor was there any association between risk of heart attack and having a serum ferritin level above 200 μg/L. Unfortunately, none of the results appeared to have been adjusted for age or for other CHD risk factors. Finally, in a small study (it is not clear if it is a defined cohort or a case series) of 577 men and women aged 62 years of age and older, no association was found between serum ferritin and incident CHD based on 3 years of follow-up (Aronow & Ahn, 1996).

### 3.2. Cohort Studies Based on TS

The association between TS (Sempos, Looker, Gillum, & Makuc, 1994; Liao, Cooper, & McGee, 1994; Baer, Tekawa, & Hurley, 1994; Reunanen, Takkunen, Knekt, Sappänen, & Aromaa, 1995; Asperen IA van, Feskens, Bowels, & Kromhout, 1995; van der A, Marx et al., 2006; Wells et al., 2004), serum iron (Liao et al., 1994; Baer et al., 1994; Morrison, Semenciw, Mao, & Wigle, 1994; Corti et al., 1997, van der A, Marx et al., 2006) or TIBC (Magnusson et al., 1994; Liao et al., 1994; Reunanen et al., 1995; Asperen IA van et al., 1995), and CHD risk has been investigated in nine different cohorts (Table 4). Only the studies by Wells et al. (2004) and Morrison et al. (1994) reported finding a significant positive association. Wells et al. (51) took the interesting approach of looking at the combined effect of both low-density lipoprotein (LDL) cholesterol and TS on all causes and CVD mortality using data from the NHANES II Mortality Study. [Sempos et al. (2000) previously reported finding no association between serum ferritin and mortality in the NHANES II Mortality Study.] Participants ($n = 3{,}410$) in this more recent analysis of the NHANES II data were divided into four groups: [1] LDL $< 160$ mg/dL and TS $<$ 55% (reference group), [2] LDL $< 160$ mg/dL and TS $\geq 55\%$, [3] LDL $\geq 160$ mg/dL and TS $<$ 55% and [4] LDL $\geq 160$ mg/dL and TS $\geq 55\%$. Only those persons in the fourth group had a significantly greater RR compared to the first group for all causes mortality, i.e., RR = 3.53 95% CI 1.08–11.58, and for CVD mortality, i.e., RR = 5.74 95% CI 1.04–31.54. However, in our

**Table 4**
**Serum TS and Heart Disease: Cohort Studies**

| *Study (Reference)* | *Sex* | *Sample Size* | *Association* |
|---|---|---|---|
| *NHANES I Follow-Up Study*[a] | | | |
| Sempos et al. (1994) | M | 1,345 | None |
| | W | 1,750 | None |
| Liao et al. (1994) | M | 1,827 | None |
| | W | 2,410 | None |
| Baer et al. (1994) | M | 15,167 | None |
| | W | 31,765 | None |
| Reunanen et al. (1995) | M | 6,068 | None |
| | W | 6,102 | None |
| Asperen IA van et al. (1995) | M | 129 | None |
| | W | 131 | None |
| van der A, Marx et al. (2006) | W | 1,319[b] | None |
| Wells et al. (2004)[b] | M/W | 3,410 | + |
| Morrison et al. (1994) (serum iron) | M | ? | + |
| | W | ? | + |
| Magnusson et al. (1994) (TIBC) | M | 990 | – |
| | W | 1,046 | None |
| Corti et al. (1997) (serum iron) | M | 1,385 | – |
| | W | 2,551 | – |

[a] The studies by Sempos et al. (1994) and Liao et al. (1994) are from the same cohort – The NHANES I Epidemiologic Follow-up study. Because cases within the first 3 years of follow-up were deleted in the paper by Sempos et al., the sample size in their paper is smaller than the sample size reported by Liao et al.

[b] The studies by Sempos et al. (2000) and Wells et al. (2004) are from the same cohort – The NHANES II Mortality Study.

attempt to replicate those findings we discovered that there were at most eight participants and only four deaths in the fourth group (data not shown). As a result, the reported association is questionable until the results can be replicated with more deaths and/or CHD events.

In the study by Morrison et al. (1994), 9,920 men and women 35–79 years of age were followed for approximately 16 years. During that time, 141 men and 83 women died of an acute myocardial infarction (MI) or heart attack. Persons with a serum iron level ≥175 ug/L compared to those with a value <120 ug/L were found to have a significantly higher risk of dying of an acute MI (men: RR = 2.18, 95% CI 1.01–4.74; women: RR = 5.53, 95% CI 1.69–18.12). However, as with the paper by Wells et al., there were relatively few deaths in the highest category, i.e., only seven deaths among the men and three among the women. Therefore, although the results are consistent with those from Finland, the small numbers of events in the highest category tend to make their results less certain. In contrast, Corti et al. (1997) reported finding a significant inverse association between serum iron and CHD and cardiovascular death (CVD), i.e., the higher a person's serum iron level the lower their risk of death from CHD or CVD.

The supporters of the "iron" hypothesis have been curiously contradictory about whether or not TS is an indicator of body iron stores. The papers that found no association between iron status and CHD have been criticized for using TS as a measure of body iron stores (Salonen et al., 1994; Ascherio & Willett, 1994; Sullivan, 1996) and for using the lowest levels of TS as the comparison group. However, while criticizing the heart disease studies which have not found an association, the proponents of the iron hypothesis have cited studies finding an association between TS and risk of cancer (Sullivan, 1996; Salonen et al., 1995) or serum iron and risk of CHD (Salonen et al., 1995) as evidence that high body iron stores generally increase the risk of both heart disease and cancer. Clearly, if TS or serum iron are indicators of body iron stores in one setting, they must also be in the other.

Because persons with very low TS levels (<16%) as well as those with very high levels (>60%) are probably sick individuals, we agree that persons with the lowest TS levels may not be the most appropriate comparison group. To explore the effects of using the lowest TS levels as the comparison group, we have reanalyzed the relationship between TS and risk of CHD (Sempos et al., 1997) using the methods previously described (Sempos et al., 1997) and where TS was divided into six categories (<16%, 16–19%, 20–29%, 30–44%, 45–59%, and ≥60%). For those new analyses, the TS category of 20–29% was used as the reference category. A TS <16% is used to indicate iron deficiency, and a TS between 16% and 29% is at the low end of the normal range. The relative risk of CHD for TS <16%, 16–19%, 30–44% 45–59% and the ≥60% categories was 1.09, 1.09, 1.01, 0.75, and 0.76, respectively, for men and 1.28, 1.18, 0.84, 0.97, and 0.86, respectively, for women. None of the estimates were significantly different ($p > 0.05$) than the risk of CHD in the 20–29% TS category. Persons with TS levels between 16% and 19% appeared to be at equal or higher risk of CHD while persons between 30% and 60% appeared to be possibly at lower risk of CHD than those with a TS of 20–29%. As a result, changing the comparison group for TS does not appear to change the conclusion that those data do not support the hypothesis that body iron stores are positively related to CHD risk.

There have also been a few cohort studies that used TS to look at the association between iron status and risk of stroke and all causes mortality. A u-shaped association between TS and stroke was reported for white women (Gillum, Sempos, Looker, & Chien, 1996) where those with a TS < 29% and a TS ≥ 44% had a significantly higher risk of stroke compared to those with a TS of 30–36%. However, no association was found for white men or blacks. Additionally, no association has been found between TS and all causes mortality (Sempos et al., 1997; Corti et al., 1997; Takkunen, Reunanen, Knekt, & Aromaa, 1989).

### 3.3. Case-Control or Cross-Sectional Studies

There have been a number of studies ( Duthie et al., 1994; Rengström, Tonrvall, Kallner, Nilsson, & Hamsten, 1994; Moore, Folsom, Barnes, & Eckfeldt, 1995; van der Schouw, Verbeek, & Ruijs, 1992; Eichner, Qi, Moorre, & Schechter, 1998; Endbergs et al., 1998; Aronow, 1993; Solymoss et al., 1994; Rauramaa et al., 1994; Kiechl et al., 1994) that have used a case-control or cross-sectional study design (Table 5). All of the studies used serum ferritin as the measure of body iron stores. Only one (Kiechl et al., 1994) of the studies reported finding a significant positive association between serum ferritin and CHD and then in only the youngest of two age groups examined, i.e., aged 40–59 years.

**Table 5**
**Serum Ferritin and Heart Disease: Case-Control and Cross-Sectional Studies**

| *Study (Reference)* | *Sex* | *Sample Size* | *Association* |
|---|---|---|---|
| *Case-Control Studies* | | | |
| Duthie et al. (1994) | M/W | 225 | None |
| Rengström et al. (1994) | M | 194 | None |
| Moore et al. (1995) | M/W | 730 | None |
| Van der Schouw et al. (1992) | M/W | 162 | None |
| Eichner et al. (1998) | M | 457 | None |
| | W | 114 | None |
| Endbergs et al. (1998) | M | 208 | None |
| | W | 67 | None |
| *Cross-Sectional Studies* | | | |
| Aronow (1993) | M | 171 | None |
| | W | 406 | None |
| Solymoss et al. (1994) | M | 225 | None |
| | W | 74 | None |
| Rauramaa et al. (1994) | M | 206 | None |
| Kiechl et al. (1994) | M/W | 431 | + (Aged 40–59) |
| | | 416 | None (Aged 60–79) |

Case-control and cross-sectional studies are not generally considered to be as rigorous an observational study design as cohort studies (Beaglehole et al., 1993; Gordis, 2008, Kahn & Sempos, 1989). The problem with both types of studies is that both disease status, e.g., heart disease, and risk factor exposure, e.g., serum ferritin, are measured at the same time so that it is impossible to tell if risk factor exposure preceded the disease or was a consequence of it. For example, the disease itself may alter body iron stores or serum ferritin levels. Additionally, people who already know they are sick may change their behavior so as to alter their levels of body iron stores. As a result, it is difficult to establish if the exposure lead to the disease or vice versa with those experimental designs.

Because serum ferritin levels rise in response to inflammation, infection, cancer, and heart attack, clinically apparent CHD should increase serum ferritin levels so that more often than not a false positive association would be found between ferritin and CHD. The fact that only one of the studies in this category found an association is then a somewhat stronger argument against the hypothesis. On the other hand, including persons with CHD in these studies who have changed their diets to lower their serum cholesterol levels would tend to produce false negative results, since a reduction in the intake of meat and animal products may also, over time, reduce their levels of body iron stores and, as a result, their serum ferritin levels. One way to evaluate this possibility is to assess the association between serum total and LDL cholesterol and CHD concurrently with the serum ferritin and CHD assessments. In six of the nine studies that found no association between serum ferritin and CHD (Duthie et al., 1994; Rengström et al., 1994; Endbergs et al., 1998; Solymoss et al., 1994; Rauramaa et al., 1994) and in the one study that found a positive association (Kiechl et al., 1994), LDL cholesterol was positively associated with having CHD, suggesting that it is less likely that changes in behavior have produced false negative results.

### *3.4. Dietary Iron and CHD Risk*

Salonen et al. (1992) also reported that dietary iron intake was positively associated with the risk of having a heart attack. Other researchers have not been able to corroborate this finding (Sempos et al., 1997; Liao et al., 1994; Reunanen et al., 1995; Morrison et al., 1994; Moore et al., 1995; Rauramaa et al., 1994; Ascherio, Willett, Rimm, Giovannucci, & Stampfer, 1994; Klipstein-Grobusch et al., 1999), and to date only two other studies (Tzonou, Lagiou, Trichopoulou, Tsoutsos, & Trichopoulos, 1998, Lee, Folsom, & Jacobs, 2005) have found a positive association between dietary iron intake and CHD risk.

Three papers have reported finding an association between heme iron intake and risk of heart attack (Ascherio et al., 1994; Klipstein-Grobusch et al., 1999; Lee et al., 2005) while a fourth found no association (Reunanen et al., 1995). In any event, it is not clear what a relationship between dietary heme iron and CHD would mean in the context of a discussion of the association between body iron stores and CHD risk. Dietary intake methods do not adequately capture long-term dietary patterns (Sempos, Liu, & Ernst, 1999), nor do they reflect the effect of menopausal status on body iron stores all of which are important factors in determining body iron stores. Additionally, an association between dietary iron and CHD risk may be a marker for a high-fat, high-cholesterol diet, or something totally unrelated to body iron stores. For example, in the paper by Klipstein-Grobusch et al. (1999), heme iron intake was positively correlated with hypercholesterolemia, a clear marker for a diet high in saturated fatty acids and cholesterol, as well as with hypertension, current cigarette smoking, and diabetes.

To help reduce the potential for confounding, epidemiologists use multivariate models to simulate an experiment (Clayton & Hills, 1993, pp. 271–281) as did the authors of the papers on heme iron intake and CHD risk. By using multivariate models that adjust for possible confounding factors, it is possible to evaluate the association between the exposure of interest and the outcome variable while holding all other variables in the model constant (Kahn & Sempos, 1988). But there are limits to modeling. The sad fact is that confounding due to correlation in intakes or metabolism simply cannot be reduced or eliminated by statistical modeling (Gordon, 1974; McGee, Reed, & Yano, 1984; Sempos et al., 1999).

### *3.5. Blood Donor Studies and Iron and Oxidized LDL Cholesterol*

Blood donation has been hypothesized as a way to decreasing body iron stores to reduce the risk of heart disease (Sullivan, 1991, 1992). Clearly, frequent blood donation will reduce body iron stores and serum ferritin levels (Finch, Cook, Labbe, & Culala, 1977). But while there has been no direct evidence that blood donation will lead to a reduction in CHD risk, two approaches have been used to address this issue.

An indirect way to test the hypothesis is to look at the risk of CHD in voluntary blood donors and non-donors in existing epidemiologic studies. There have been three such studies (Meyers et al., 1997; Tuomainen, Salonen, Nyyssönen, & Salonen, 1997; Salonen, Tuomainen, Salonen, Lakka, & Nyyssönen, 1998; Ascherio, Rimm, Giovannucci, Willett, & Stampfer, 2001) [The paper by Salonen et al. (1998) is an expanded version of the earlier paper by Tuomainen et al. (1997) and not a separate study.] as well as a study looking at the effects of blood donation on cancer incidence (Merk et al., 1990). The results were mixed. Meyers et al. (1997) reported that blood donation was associated with a reduced risk of CHD in non-smoking men but not in male smokers or in women, while Salonen et al. (Tuomainen et al., 1997; Salonen et al., 1998) reported a significant reduction in risk of heart attack in the cohort of Finnish men from the KIHD Study that originally reported an association between serum ferritin and risk of heart attack. Ascherio et al. (2001) found no association between the history of blood donation and the incident heart attack or fatal CHD.

There are several concerns about theses interesting studies. The principal one is that volunteers for blood donation are healthier than non-donors and that any association may be a result of some unmeasured selection bias (Ford, 1997; Gillum, 1997). The data from both studies do clearly indicate that the volunteers were healthier. For example, in contrast to the usual practice in cohort studies, Salonen et al. (Tuomainen et al., 1997; Salonen et al., 1998) did *not* eliminate persons with pre-existing clinical CHD at baseline from their analyses as they had done in their previous papers (Salonen et al., 1992). In their study, over a quarter of the 2,529 non-donors (26.3%) had pre-existing disease compared to 8.5% in the 153 voluntary donors. As a result, not only were blood donors healthier, because participants with pre-existing CHD were not excluded from the analyses, but it is impossible to determine whether voluntary blood donation was influenced by the presence of heart disease. Moreover, as stated earlier, that bias cannot be completely removed or eliminated by statistical analysis (Gordon, 1974; McGee et al., 1984; Sempos et al., 1999).

The paper by Ascherio et al. (2001) examined the issue using 38,244 men in the Health Professionals Study who were free of CHD at baseline. During 4 years of follow-up there were 328 non-fatal heart attacks and 131CHD deaths among the cohort. In the 1992 questionnaire, the participants were asked to report the number of times they had donated blood over the past 30 years. The categories for lifetime blood donation in the analyses were: 0, 1–4, 5–9, 10–19, 20–29, and $\geq 30$ times. In order to validate the self-reported history of lifetime blood donation, the authors measured serum ferritin levels in stored blood samples, which were collected in 1986 from a random sample of 123 men in the study. The authors found that there was a negative association between the number of times blood was donated and their level of serum ferritin. That finding supports the general accuracy of the blood donation questionnaire. In addition, no association was found between blood donation with non-fatal heart attack or fatal CHD.

In what might be a more direct test of the hypothesis, Salonen et al. (1995) used a Latin Squares design to look at the effects of donating 500 mL of blood three times over a 14-week period in 14 men who were heavy smokers on measures of non-HDL (very low-density lipoprotein [VLDL] plus LDL) cholesterol oxidizability. The authors reported finding that serum ferritin levels were reduced by 44% while the maximal oxidation velocity was decreased by 20% and the lag time to start oxidation was lengthened by 33%. In addition, frequent blood donors have been shown to have decreased oxidative stress and enhanced vascular function compared to those who donate blood infrequently (Zheng, Cable, Spencer, Votto, & Katz, 2005).

While interesting, the results of Salonen et al. (1995) even if replicated are uncertain (Weintraub, Wenger, Parthasaranthy, & Brown, 1996). The LDL oxidation theory is interesting and increasingly accepted (Heinecke, 1998). However, a problem lies in the measurement of LDL oxidation itself (Halliwell & Chirico, 1993). LDL oxidizability is usually measured by using LDL and exposing it to oxidative stress. The question is whether such a marker of LDL oxidizability corresponds to the extent of oxidation in vivo and whether it predicts risk of CHD (Zock & Katan, 1998).

The results of the few epidemiological studies which have looked at the association between LDL oxidizability and markers of atherosclerosis or CHD risk are mixed (Iribarren et al., 1997; van de Vijver et al., 1998; Halevy et al., 1997; Yoshida et al., 2004). There are also mixed results concerning the association between autoantibodies against oxidized LDL and atherosclerosis (Zheng et al., 2005). "Thus the available markers for oxidized LDL cannot yet be regarded as valid predictors of CAD [*coronary artery disease*] risk in humans (Zock & Katan, 1998)."

Putting aside the possible problems with the measurement of oxidized LDL, several observational studies have looked at the association between serum ferritin and LDL oxidizability (Halevy et al, 1997; Uusitupa et al., 1996; Iribarren, Sempos, Echfelt, & Folsom, 1998, Craig et al., 1995). No association was found in any of the studies. In fact, Craig et al. (1995) reported that serum ferritin accounted for about 1.6% of the variability in measures of LDL oxidizability while serum copper accounted for 21% of that variability. Serum copper also is considered as a possible catalyst for the oxidation of LDL (Sempos et al., 1996; Ferns, Lamb, & Taylor, 1997).

The results from two human feeding studies appear to be at variance with the with the hypothesis that there is a positive association between body iron stores and the susceptibility of LDL to oxidation (Derstine et al., 2003; Binoski, Kris-Etherton, & Beard, 2004). In the first study, Derstine et al. (2003) tested the oxidizability of the LDL cholesterol in the plasma samples of 77 men and women aged 20–65 years of age who were participating in one of three feeding studies. No association was found between serum ferritin and the measures of LDL oxidizability. In the second study by Binoski et al. (2004), 26 women aged 19–47 with low hemoglobin and serum ferritin levels, i.e., low iron status, participated in a randomized double-blind two-period crossover study). Participants were randomized to an iron supplement (50 mg elemental iron per day) or placebo. They were then randomly assigned to an "average American diet" or a low-fat diet known as the Step 2 Diet (Expert Panel on Detection, Evaluation, and Treatment of High Blood Cholesterol in Adults, 1993). The average American diet contained 36% of the energy intake, i.e., kcals, as fat with 15% of the total kcals from saturated fatty acids. The Step 2 diet contained 26% of energy from fat and 7% from saturated fatty acids. Both diets contained about 25 g of fiber per day. Each diet was consumed for 3 weeks with a 2-week "washout" period. While iron supplementation resulted in an increase in serum ferritin levels ($p = 0.008$), there was no association between iron supplementation and LDL oxidative susceptibility as measured by the rate of oxidation or total dienes.

## 4. CLINICAL TRIALS: REDUCATION OF IRON STORES AND CVD RISK

There has been one reported trial testing the impact of reduction of iron stores on Cardiovascular Disease (CVD) risk (Zacharski et al., 2007). The study was a 6-year multi-center single-blind clinical trial testing the effect of phlebotomy to remove defined levels of blood at 6-month intervals to maintain serum ferritin levels between 25 and 60 μg/L in Veteran's Administration (VA) patients – primarily men (99%) – with peripheral arterial disease. The treatment group contained 636 participants and the control group contained 641 or 1,277 total participants. The primary endpoint was death from any cause and the secondary endpoint was death plus non-fatal heart attack or stroke. At the end of 6 years of follow-up there were 148 deaths in the control group and 125 in the treatment group (RR = 0.85, 95% CI = 0.67–1.08, $p = 0.17$). In addition, there were 205 secondary events in the control group and 180 such events in the phlebotomy group (RR = 0.88, 95% CI = 0.72–1.07, $p = 0.20$).

In a letter to the Editor, Dr. Sullivan (2007) suggested that a reason why the study was unsuccessful was that it did not eliminate body iron stores as measured by serum ferritin levels. A more serious limitation of the study may be that the study was underpowered (Zacharski et al., 2007; Hu, 2007). Given that fewer veterans were recruited into the study than initially thought to be necessary, the results of this study are very difficult to interpret. In fact, the results do tantalizingly suggest that lowering serum ferritin levels may actually reduce death from all causes and the combination of death and non-fatal heart attack and stroke. However, there were questions about the success of the intervention and the suitability of the participants and the overall generalizability of the results to the general population (Hu, 2007). In his editorial accompanying the paper, Dr. Hu (2007) suggested that a larger trial in postmenopausal women may help to shed light on the issue. He also pointed out that even though there were so many problems with the trial, the results are consistent with the large body of negative results from observational epidemiology; that is, there is no association between body iron stores and the risk of CHD.

## 5. IRON OVERLOAD AND CHD RISK

Hemochromatosis is a genetic disorder which in the homozygous state leads to iron overload, serious illness, and early death usually from liver cancer, other liver diseases, cardiomyopathy, or diabetes (Yang, McDonnell, Khoury, Cono, & Parrish , 1998). Persons with the heterozygous form of hemochromatosis are unlikely to develop iron overload. The concern is that, while iron overload is uncommon, heterozygotes tend to have higher levels of body iron stores, as indicated by higher serum ferritin and TS levels, than do persons without the condition and because the heterozygous form of the disease is relatively common, i.e., a prevalence of 10–15% (Bulaj, Griffen, Jorde, Edwards, &, Kushner, 1996; McLaren et al., 1995; Steinberg et al., 2001). Given that, if the iron hypothesis were to be correct, then heterozygotes would form a substantial pool of persons at increased risk of CHD.

The cysteine-to-tyrosine substitution on the hemochromatosis gene (Cys282Tyr mutation) is thought to account for most of the cases of hemochromatosis. There have been a number of studies looking at the association between the presence of the Cys282Tyr mutation as well as other mutations in an individual and the risk of heart disease. In a recent meta-analysis including 66,000 individuals with hemochromatosis and 226,000 controls, it was found that hemochromatosis genotypes were not associated with increased risk of heart disease or stroke (Ellervik, Birgens, Tybjærg-Hansen, & Nordestgaard 2007). Note carefully that the papers on this topic have looked at the association between the presence or the absence of a mutation and CHD risk and not whether serum ferritin or some other marker of body iron stores was related to risk.

In a meta-analysis of prospective or cohort studies, van der A, Peeters, Grobbee, Roest, Marx, & Voorbij (2006) reported that men and women who were carriers of the C282Y allele compared to non-carriers were not at higher risk of developing CHD (RR = 1.02, 95% CI 0.94–1.11). Similarly, they reported that carriers of the H63D allele were not at higher risk of developing CHD compared to non-carriers (RR = 1.03, 95% CI 0.96–1.11)

## 6. SUMMARY

In 1981, Dr. Jerome Sullivan proposed that body iron stores are directly or positively related to CHD risk, i.e., the higher your body iron stores the greater your CHD risk. Until the publication of results from Finland by Salonen et al. (1992) showing a positive relationship between serum ferritin levels and risk of heart attack in men, the hypothesis was largely ignored. While a plausible hypothesis was proposed by Dr. Sullivan to define a role for iron in the development of CHD, possibly by catalyzing the free radical oxidation of LDL cholesterol, the vast majority of the epidemiologic results published since the study by Salonen et al. (1992) have failed to support the original hypothesis. Whether looking at the direct relationship between serum ferritin and CHD risk, serum ferritin and measures of atherosclerosis, serum TS and CHD risk, iron intake and CHD risk, serum ferritin and measures of LDL oxidizability, or iron overload and CHD risk, the results are the same: the data do *not* consistently support the hypothesis that body iron stores are a risk factor for CHD. Additionally, there does not appear to be a relationship between hemochromatosis and the risk of CHD. However, the effects of blood donation on serum levels of oxidized LDL and on all causes mortality or CVD risk remain open questions.

## 7. RECOMMENDATIONS

Sound clinical guidance and public health recommendations must be based on reasonably solid evidence that what is being recommended is both safe and effective. To date the vast majority of the results do not support the iron hypothesis (Hu, 2007; Sempos, 2002; Yuan & Li, 2003; Kalantar-Zadeh, Kalantar-Zadeh, & Lee, 2006).

Finally, it must be remembered that currently there are a number of proven CHD risk factors including high blood cholesterol, high blood pressure, cigarette smoking, obesity, diabetes, and lack of exercise for which there are proven and effective guidelines and measures for decreasing CHD risk (Expert Panel on Detection, Evaluation, and Treatment of High Blood Cholesterol in Adults, 2001, Tomkin et al., 2001; De Backer et al., 2003; Grundy et al., 2004). Until other measures are proven and established, it is our recommendation that we should focus on the proven measures rather than on unproven ones.

## REFERENCES


Aronow, W. S. (1993). Serum ferritin is not a risk factor for coronary artery disease in men and women aged $\geq$ 62 years. *American Journal of Cardiology, 72*, 347–348.

Aronow, W. S., & Ahn, C. (1996). Three-year follow-up shows no association of serum ferritin levels with incidence of new coronary events in 577 persons aged $\geq$ 62 years. *American Journal of Cardiology, 78*, 678–679.

Ascherio, A., Rimm, E. B., Giovannucci, E., Willett, W. C., & Stampfer, M. J. (2001). Blood donations and risk of coronary heart disease in men. *Circulation, 103*, 52–57.

Ascherio, A., & Willett, W. C. (1994). Are body iron stores related to risk of coronary heart disease? *New England Journal of Medicine, 330*, 1152–1153. (editorial).

Ascherio, A., Willett, W. C., Rimm, E. B., Giovannucci, E. L., & Stampfer, M. J. (1994). Dietary iron and risk of coronary heart disease among men. *Circulation, 89*, 969–974.

Asperen, I. A. van, Feskens, E. J. M., Bowels, C. H., & Kromhout, D. (1995). Body iron stores and mortality due to cancer and ischemic heart disease: A 17-year follow-up study of elderly men and women. *International Journal of Epidemiology, 24*, 665–670.

Baer, D. M., Tekawa, I. S., & Hurley, L. B. (1994). Iron stores are not associated with acute myocardial infarction. *Circulation, 89*, 2915–2918.

Beaglehole, R., Bonita, R., & Kjellström, T. (1993). *Basic epidemiology*. Geneva, Switzerland: World Health Organization.

Binoski, A. E., Kris-Etherton, P. M., & Beard, J. L. (2004). Iron supplementation does not affect the susceptibility of LDL to oxidative modification in women with low iron status. *Journal of Nutrition, 134*, 99–103.

Birgegård, G., Hällgren, R., Venge, P., & Wide, L. (1979). Serum ferritin during inflammation. A study on myocardial infarction. *Acta Medica Scandinavica, 206*, 361–366.

Bothwell, T., Charlton, R., Cook, J., & Finch, C. (1979). *Iron metabolism in man*. Oxford: Blackwell Scientific.

Bulaj, Z. J., Griffen, L. M., Jorde, L. B., Edwards, C. Q., & Kushner, J. P. (1996). Clinical and biochemical abnormalities in people heterozygous for hemochromatosis. *New England Journal of Medicine, 335*, 1799–1805.

Clayton, D., & Hills, M. (1993). *Statistical models in epidemiology*. Oxford: Oxford University Press.

Corti, M. C., Guralnik, J. M., Salvie, M. E., Ferrucci, L., Pahor, M., Wallace, R. B., et al. (1997). Serum iron level, coronary artery disease, and all cause mortality in older men and women. *American Journal of Cardiology, 79*, 120–127.

Craig, W.Y., Poulin S. E., Palomaki, G. E., Neveux, L. M., Ritchie, R. F., & Ledue, T. B. (1995). Oxidation-related analytes and lipid and lipoprotein concentrations in adults. *Arteriosclerosis, Thrombosis, and Vascular Biology, 15*, 733–739.

Cusick, S. E., Mei, Z., Freedman, D. S., Looker, A. C., Ogden, C. L., & Gunter, E. (2008) Unexplained decline in prevalence of anemia among US children and women between 1988–1994 and 1999–2002. *American Journal of Clinical Nutrition, 88*, 1611–1617.

Custer, E. M., Finch, C. A., Sobel, R. E., & Zettner, A. (1995). Populations norms for serum ferritin. *Journal of Laboratory and Clinical Medicine, 126*, 88–94.

Danesh, J., & Appleby, P. (1999). Coronary heart disease and iron status. Meta-analysis of prospective studies. *Circulation, 99*, 852–854.

De Backer, G., Ambrosioni, E., Borch-Johnsen, K., Brotons, C., Cifkova, R., Dallongeville, J., et al. (2003). European guidelines on cardiovascular disease prevention in clinical practice. Third Joint Task Force of European and other Societies on Cardiovascular Disease Prevention in Clinical Practice. *European Heart Journal, 24*, 1601–1610.

Derstine, J. L., Murray-Kolb, L. E., Yu-Poth, S., Hargrove, R. L., Kris-Etherton, P., & Beard, J. L. (2003). Iron status in association with cardiovascular disease risk in three controlled feeding studies. *American Journal of Clinical Nutrition, 77*, 56–62.

Dormandy, T. L. (1978). Free-radical oxidation and antioxidants. *The Lancet, 311*(8065), 647–650.

Duthie, G. G., Beattie, J. A. G., Arthur, J. R., Franklin, M., Morrice, P. C., & James, W. P. T. (1994). Blood antioxidants and indices of lipid peroxidation in subjects with stable angina. *Nutrition, 10*, 313–306.

Eichner, J. E., Qi, H., Moorre, W. E., & Schechter, E. (1998). Iron measures in coronary angiography patients. *Atherosclerosis, 136*, 241–245.

Ellervik, C., Birgens, H., Tybjærg-Hansen, A., & Nordestgaard, B. G. (2007). Hemochromatosis gentoypes and risk of 31 disease endpoints: Meta-Analysis including 66,000 cases and 226,000 controls. *Hepatology, 46*, 1071–1080.

Endbergs, A., Dorzewski, A., Luft, M., Mönnig, G., Kleemann, A., Schulte, H., et al. (1998). Failure to confirm ferritin and ceruloplasmin as risk factors for the angiographic extent of coronary atherosclerosis. *Coronary Artery Disease, 9*, 119–124.

Expert Panel on Detection, Evaluation, and Treatment of High Blood Cholesterol in Adults. (1993). Summary of the second report of the National Cholesterol Education Program (NCEP) expert panel on detection, evaluation, and treatment of high blood cholesterol in adults (Adult Treatment Panel II). *Journal of the American Medical Association, 269*, 3015–3023.

Expert Panel on Detection, Evaluation, and Treatment of High Blood Cholesterol in Adults. (2001). Executive summary of the third report of the National Cholesterol Education Program (NCEP) expert panel on detection, evaluation, and treatment of high blood cholesterol in adults (Adult Treatment Panel III). *Journal of the American Medical Association, 285*, 2486–2497.

Expert Scientific Working Group. (1985). Summary of a report on assessment of the iron nutritional status of the United States population. *American Journal of Clinical Nutrition, 42*, 1318–1330.

Ferns, G. A. A., Lamb, D. J., & Taylor, A. (1997). The possible role of copper ions in atherosclerosis: the Blue Janus. *Atherosclerosis, 133*, 130–152.

Finch, C. A., Cook, J. D., Labbe, R. F., & Culala, M. (1977). Effect of blood donation on iron stores as evaluated by serum ferritin. *Blood, 50*, 441–447.

Ford, I. (1997). Is blood donation good for the donor [Editorial]. *Heart, 78*, 107.

Frey, G. H., & Krider, D. W. (1994). Serum ferritin and myocardial infarct. *The West Virginia Medical Journal, 90*, 13–15.

Galan, P., Noisette, N., Czernichow, S., Mennen, L., Renversez, J.-C., Briançon, S., et al. (2006). Serum ferritin, cardiovascular risk factors and ischaemic heart diseases: A prospective analysis in the SU.VI.Max (SUpplementation en VItamines et Minéraux AntioXydants) cohort. *Public Health Nutrition, 9*, 70–74.

Gillum, R. F. (1997). Body iron stores and atherosclerosis [Editorial]. *Circulation, 96*, 3261–3263.

Gillum, R. F., Sempos, C. T., Looker, A. C., & Chien, C. Y. (1996). Serum transferrin saturation and stroke incidence and mortality in men and women: The NHANES I Epidemiologic Follow-up Study. *American Journal of Epidemiology, 144*, 59–68.

Gordis, L. (2008). *Epidemiology* (4th ed.). Philadelphia: WB Saunders Co.

Gordon, T. (1974). Hazards in the use of the logistic function with special reference to data from prospective cardiovascular disease studies. *Journal of Chronic Diseases, 27,* 97–102.

Griffiths, J. D., Campbell, L. J., Woodruff, I. W., Cruickshank, D., Mathews, Y. B., Hunt, D., et al. (1985). Acute changes in iron metabolism following myocardial infarction. *American Journal of Clinical Pathology, 84,* 649–654.

Grundy, S. M., Cleeman, J. I., Bairey Merz, N., Brewar, B., Clark, L. T., Hunninghake, D. B., et al. (2004). Implications of recent clinical trials for the National Cholesterol Education Program Adult Treatment Panel III Guidelines. *Circulation, 110,* 227–239.

Halevy, D., Thiery, J., Nagel, D., Arnold, S., Erdmann, E., Höfling, B., et al. (1997). Increased oxidation of LDL in patients with coronary artery disease is independent from dietary vitamins E and C. *Arteriosclerosis, Thrombosis, and Vascular Biology, 17,* 1432–1437.

Halliwell, B., & Chirico, S. (1993). Lipid peroxidation: Its mechanism, measurement and significance. *American Journal of Clinical Nutrition, 57,* 715s–725s.

Heinecke, J. W. (1998). Oxidants and antioxidants in the pathogenesis of atherosclerosis: Implications for the oxidized low density lipoprotein hypothesis. *Atherosclerosis, 141,* 1–5.

Hennekens, D. G., & Buring, B. G. (1987). *Epidemiology in medicine.* Boston: Little Brown & Co.

Herbert, V. (1992). Everyone should be tested for iron disorders. *Journal of the American Dietetic Association, 92,* 1502–1509.

Hu, F. B. (2007). The iron-heart hypothesis: Search for the ironclad evidence. *Journal of the American Medical Association, 297,* 639–641.

Hulthén, L, Lindstedt, G., Lundberg, P.-A., & Hallberg, L. (1998). Effect of a mild infection on serum ferritin concentration – clinical and epidemiological implications. *European Journal of Clinical Nutrition, 52,* 376–379.

Kiechl, S., Willeit, J., Egger, G., Poewe, W., & Oberholenzer, F. (1996). Body iron stores and the risk of carotid atherosclerosis. *Circulation, 96,* 3300–3307.

Iribarren, C., Folsom, A. R., Jacobs, D. R., Gross, M. D., Belcher, J. D., & Eckfeldt, J. H. (1997). Association of serum vitamin levels, LDL susceptibility to oxidation, and autoantibodies against MDA-LDL with carotid atherosclerosis. *Arteriosclerosis, Thrombosis, and Vascular Biology, 17,* 1171–1177.

Iribarren, C., Sempos, C. T., Eckfeldt, J. H., & Folsom, A. (1998). Lack of association between ferritin level and measures of LDL oxidation. The ARIC Study. *Atherosclerosis, 139,* 189–195.

Kahn, H. A., & Sempos, C. T. (1988). *Statistical methods in epidemiology.* New York:. Oxford University Press.

Kalantar-Zadeh, K., Kalantar-Zadeh, K., & Lee, G. H. (2006).The fascinating but deceptive ferritin: To measure it or not to measure it in chronic kidney disease. *Clinical Journal of the American Society of Nephrology, 1,* S9–S18.

Kiechl, S., Aichner, F., Gerstenbrand, F., Egger, G., Mair, A., Rungger, G., et al. (1994). Body iron stores and presence of carotid atherosclerosis. Results from the Bruneck Study. *Arteriosclerosis and Thrombosis, 14,* 1625–1630.

Kiechl, S., Willeit, J., Egger, G., Poewe, W., & Oberholenzer, F. (1997). Body iron stores and the risk of carotid atherosclerosis. *Circulation, 96,* 3300–3307.

Klipstein-Grobusch, K., Grobbee, D. E., den Breejien, J. H., Boeing, H., Hofman, A., & Witterman, J. C. M. (1999). Dietary iron and risk of myocardial infarction in the Rotterdam Study. *American Journal of Epidemiology, 149,* 421–428.

Knuiman, M. W., Divitini, M. L., Olynyk, J. K., Cullen, D. J., & Batholomew, H. C. (2003). Serum ferritin and cardiovascular disease: A 17-year follow-up in Busselton, Western Australia. *American Journal of Epidemiology, 58,* 144–149.

Lee, D. H., Folsom, A. R., & Jacobs, D. R., Jr. (2005). Iron, zinc, and alcohol consumption and mortality from cardiovascular diseases: the Iowa Women's Health Study. *American Journal of Clinical Nutrition, 81,* 787–791.

Liao, Y., Cooper, R. S., & McGee, D. L. (1994). Iron status and coronary heart disease: Negative findings from the NHANES I Epidemiologic Follow-up Study. *American Journal of Epidemiology, 139,* 704–712.

Looker, A. C., Gunter, A. W., & Johnson, C. L. (1995). Methods to assess iron status in various NHANES Surveys. *Nutrition Reviews, 53,* 246–254.

MacDonald, H. B. (1993). High stored iron levels are associated with excess risk of myocardial infarction in Eastern Finnish Men. [Letter] *Circulation, 87,* 2063.

Magnusson, M. K., Sigfusson, N., Sigvaldason, H., Johannesson, G. M., Magnusson, S, & Thorgeirsson, G. (1994). Low iron-binding capacity as a risk factor for myocardial infarction. *Circulation, 89,* 102–108.

Mänttäri, M., Manninen, V., Huttunen, J. K., Palosuo, T., Ehnholm, C., Heinonen, P. O., et al. (1994). Serum ferritin and ceruloplasmin as coronary risk factors. *European Heart Journal, 15,* 1599–1603.

McGee, D., Reed, D., & Yano, K. (1984). The results of logistic regression analyses when the variables are highly correlated: An empirical example using diet and CHD incidence. *Journal of Chronic Diseases, 37*, 713–719.

McLaren, C. E., Gordeuk, V. R., Looker, A. C., Hasselblad, V., Edwards, C. Q., Griffen, L. M., et al. (1995). Prevalence of heterozygotes for hemochromatosis in the white population of the United States. *Blood, 86*, 2021–2027.

Merk, K., Mattsson, B., Mettsson, A., Holm, G., Gullbring, B., & Björkholm, M. (1990). The incidence of cancer among blood donors. *International Journal of Epidemiology, 19*, 505–509.

Meyers, D. G., Strickland, D., Maloley, P. A., Seburg, J. J., Wilson, J. E., & McManus, B. F. (1997). Possible association of a reduction in cardiovascular events with blood donation. *Heart, 78*, 188–193.

Moore, M., Folsom, A. R., Barnes, R. W., & Eckfeldt, J. H. (1995). No association between serum ferritin and asymptomatic carotid atherosclerosis. . The Atherosclerosis Risk in Communities (ARIC) Study. *American Journal of Epidemiology, 141*, 719–723.

Morrison, H. I., Semenciw, R. M., Mao, Y., & Wigle, D.T. (1994). Serum iron and fatal acute myocardial infarction. *Epidemiology, 5*, 243–246.

Rauramaa, R., Väisänen, S., Mercuri, M., Rankinen, T., Penttila, I., & Bond, M.G. (1994). Association of risk factors and body iron status to carotid atherosclerosis in middle-aged Eastern Finnish men. *European Heart Journal, 15*, 1020–1027.

Reaven, P. D., & Wiztum, J. L. (1996). Oxidized low density lipoproteins in atherogenesis: Role of dietary modification. *Annual Review of Nutrition, 16*, 51–71.

Rengström, J., Tonrvall, P., Kallner, A., Nilsson, J., & Hamsten, A. (1994). Stored iron levels and myocardial infarction at a young age. *Atherosclerosis, 106*, 123–125.

Reunanen, A., Takkunen, H., Knekt, P., Sappänen, R., & Aromaa, A. (1995). Body iron stores, dietary iron intake and coronary heart disease mortality. *Journal of Internal Medicine, 238*, 223–230.

Salonen, J. T., Korpela, H., Nyyssönen, K., Porkkala, E., Toumainen, T. P., Belcher, J. D., et al. (1995). Lowering of body iron stores by blood letting and oxidation resistance of serum lipoproteins: a randomized cross-over trial in male smokers. *Journal of Internal Medicine, 237*, 161–168.

Salonen, J. T., Nyyssönen, K., Korpela, H., Salonen, R., Tuomilehto, J., & Seppänen, R. (1993a). High stored iron levels and the risk of myocardial infarction. [Reply] *Circulation, 87*, 1425–1426.

Salonen, J. T., Nyyssönen, K., Korpela, H., Salonen, R., Tuomilehto, J., & Seppänen, R. (1993b). High stored iron levels are associated with excess risk of myocardial infarction in Eastern Finnish Men. [Reply] *Circulation, 87*, 2063–2064.

Salonen, J. T., Nyyssönen, K., Korpela, H., Tuomilehto, J., Seppänen, R., & Salonen R. (1992). High stored iron levels are associated with excess risk of myocardial infarction in eastern Finnish men. *Circulation, 86*, 803–811.

Salonen, J. T., Nyyssönen, K., & Salonen, R. (1994). Body iron stores and the risk of coronary heart disease. [Letter]. *New England Journal of Medicine, 331*, 1159.

Salonen, J. T., Tuomainen, T.-P., Salonen, R., Lakka, T. A., & Nyyssönen K. (1998). Donation of blood is associated with reduced risk of myocardial infarction. *American Journal of Epidemiology, 148*, 445–451.

Schouw, Y. T. van der, Veeken, P. M. W. C. van der, Kok, F. J., Koster, J. F., Schouten, E. G., & Hofman, A. (1990). Iron status in the acute phase and six weeks after myocardial infarction. *Free Radical Biology and Medicine, 8*, 47–53.

Sempos, C. T. (2002). Do body iron stores increase the risk of coronary heart disease? *American Journal of clinical Nutrition, 76*, 501–503.

Sempos, C. T., Gillum, R. F., & Looker, A. C. (1997). Iron and heart disease: A review of the epidemiologic data. Chapter 10. In A. Bendich & R. J. Deckelbaum (eds.), *Preventive nutrition: The comprehensive guide for health professionals*. Totowa, NJ: Humana Press Inc.

Sempos, C. T., Liu, K., & Ernst, N. D. (1999). Food and nutrient exposures: What to consider when evaluating epidemiologic evidence. *American Journal of Clinical Nutrition, 69*,1330s–1338s.

Sempos, C. T., Looker, A. C., & Gillum, R. F. (1996). Iron and heart disease: The epidemiologic data. *Nutrition Reviews, 54*(3), 73–84.

Sempos, C. T., Looker, A. C., Gillum, R. F., & Makuc, D. M. (1994). Body iron stores and the risk of coronary heart disease. *New England Journal of Medicine, 330*, 1119–1124.

Sempos, C. T., Looker, A. C., Gillum, R. F., McGee, D. L., Vuong, C. V., & Johnson, C. L. (2000). Serum ferritin and risk of death from all causes, and cardiovascular disease. The NHANES II Mortality Study. *Annals of Epidemiology, 10*, 441–448.

Skikine, B. S. (2008). Serum transferring receptor. *American Journal of Hematology, 83*, 872–875.

Solymoss, B. C., Marcil, M., Gilfix, B. M., Gelinas, F., Poitras, A. M., & Campeau, L. (1994). The place of ferritin among risk factors associated with coronary artery disease. *Coronary Artery Disease, 5*, 231–235.
Stampfer, M. J., Grodstein, F., Rosenberg, I., Willett, W., & Hennekens, C. (1993). A prospective study of plasma ferritin and risk of myocardial infarction in US physicians [Abstract]. *Circulation, 87*, 688.
Steinberg D. (1997). Oxidative modification of LDL and atherogenesis. *Circulation, 95*, 1062–1071.
Steinberg, K. K., Cogswell, M. E., Chang, J. C., Caudill, S. P., McQuillan, G. M., Bowman, B. A., et al. (2001). Prevalence of C282Y and H63D mutations in the hemochromatosis (HFE) gene in the United States. *Journal of the American Medical Association, 285*, 2216–2222.
Sullivan, J. L. (1981). Iron and the sex difference in heart disease risk. *The Lancet, 317*(8233), 1293–1294.
Sullivan, J. L. (1983). The sex difference in ischemic heart disease. *Perspectives in Biology and Medicine, 26*, 657–671.
Sullivan, J. L. (1989). The iron paradigm of ischemic heart disease. *American Heart Journal, 117*, 1177–1188.
Sullivan, J. L. (1991). Blood donation may be good for the donor. *Vox Sanguinis, 61*, 161–164.
Sullivan, J. L. (1992). Stored iron and ischemic heart disease. Empirical support for the new paradigm. *Circulation, 86*, 1036–1037.
Sullivan, J. L. (1996). Iron versus cholesterol – perspectives on the iron heart disease debate. *Journal of Clinical Epidemiology, 49*, 1345–1352.
Sullivan, J. L. (2007). Iron reduction and cardiovascular outcomes [Letter]. *Journal of the American Medical Association, 297*, 2075.
Sun, Q., Ma, J., Rifai, N., Franco, O. H., Rexrode, K. M., & Hu, F. B. (2008). Excessive body iron stores are not associated with risk of coronary heart disease in women. *Journal of Nutrition, 138*, 2436–2441.
Takkunen, H., Reunanen, A., Knekt, P., & Aromaa, A. (1989). Body iron stores and the risk of cancer [Letter]. *New England Journal of Medicine, 320*, 1013–1014.
Tomkin, A., Barter, P., Best, J., Boyden, A., Cooper, C., Sheerin, N., et al. (2001). Lipid management guidelines – 2001. *Medical Journal of Australia, 175*, S57–S88.
Tuomainen, T.-P., Punnonen, K., Nyyssönen, K., & Salonen, J. T. (1998). Association between body iron stores and the risk of acute myocardial infarction. *Circulation, 97*, 1461–1466.
Tuomainen, T.-P., Salonen, R., Nyyssönen, K., & Salonen, J. T. (1997). Cohort study of relation between donating blood and risk of myocardial infarction in 2,682 men in eastern Finland. *British Medical Journal, 314*, 793–794.
Tzonou, A., Lagiou, P., Trichopoulou, A., Tsoutsos, V., & Trichopoulos, D. (1998). Dietary iron and coronary heart disease risk: A study from Greece. *American Journal of Epidemiology, 147*, 161–166.
van der A, D. L, Marx, J. J. M., Grobee, D. E., Kamphuis, M. H., Georgiou, N. A., van Kats-Renaud, J. H., et al. (2006). Non-transferrin-bound iron and risk of coronary heart disease in postmenopausal women. *Circulation, 113*, 1942–1949.
van der A, D. L., Peeters, P. H. M., Grobbee, D. E., Roest, M., Marx, J. J. M., Voorbij, H. M., et al. (2006). HFE mutations and the risk of coronary heart disease in middle-aged women. *European Journal of Clinical Investigation, 36*, 682–690.
van der Schouw, Y. T., Verbeek, A., & Ruijs, J. (1992). ROC curves for the initial assessment of new diagnostic tests. *Family Practice, 9*, 506–511.
van de Vijver, L. P. L., Kardinaal, A. F. M., van Duyvenvoorde, W., Kruijssen, D. A. C. M., Grobee, D. E., van Poppel, G., et al. (1998). LDL oxidation and extent of coronary atherosclerosis. *Arteriosclerosis, Thrombosis, and Vascular Biology, 18*, 193–199.
Uusitupa, M. I. J., Niskanen, L., Luoma, J., Vilja, P., Mercuri, M., Rauramaa, R., et al. (1996). Autoantibodies against oxidized LDL do not predict atherosclerotic vascular disease in non-insulin dependent diabetes. *Arteriosclerosis, Thrombosis, and Vascular Biology, 16*, 1236–1242.
Weintraub, W. S., Wenger, N. K., Parthasaranthy, S., & Brown, W. V. (1996). Hyperlipidemia versus iron overload and coronary heart disease: Yet more arguments on the cholesterol debate. *Journal of Clinical Epidemiology, 49*, 1353–13568.
Weiss, G., Fuchs, D., & Wachter, H. (1993). High stored iron levels and the risk of myocardial infarction. [Letter] *Circulation, 87*, 1425.
Wells, B. J., Mainous, A. G., King, D. E., Gill, J. M., Carek, P. J., & Geesey, M. E. (2004). The combined effect of transferrin saturation and low density lipoprotein on mortality. *Family Medicine, 36*, 324–329.
Yang, Q., McDonnell, S. M., Khoury, M. J., Cono, J., & Parrish, R. G. (1998). Hemochromatosis-associated mortality in the United States from 1979 to 1992: An analysis of multiple-cause mortality data. *Annals of Internal Medicine, 129*, 946–953.

Yip, R., & Dallman, P. R. (1988). The roles of inflammation and iron deficiency as causes of anemia. *American Journal of Clinical Nutrition, 48*, 1295–1300.

Yoshida, H., Sasaki, K., Hirowatari, Y., Kurosawa, H., Sato, N., Furutani, N., et al. (2004). Increased serum iron may contribute to enhanced oxidation of low-density lipoprotein in smokers in part through changes in lipoxygenase and catalase. *Clinica Chimica Acta, 345*, 161–170.

Yuan, X.-M., & Brunk, U. T. (1998). Iron and LDL-oxidation in atherogenesis. *Acta Pathalogica Microbiologica et Immunologica Scandinavica, 106*, 825–842.

Yuan, X.-M., & Li, W. (2003). The iron hypothesis of atherosclerosis and its clinical impact. *Annals of Medicine, 35*, 578–591.

Zacharski, L. R., Chow, B. K., Howes, P. S., Shamayeva, G., Baron, J. A., Dalman, R. L., et al. (2007). Reduction of iron stores and cardiovascular outcomes in patients with peripheral arterial disease. *Journal of the American Medical Association, 297*, 603–610.

Zacharski, L. R., Ornstein, D. L., Woloshin, S., & Schwartz, L. M. (2000). Association of age, sex, and race with body iron stores in adults: Analysis of NHANES III data. *American Heart Journal, 140*, 98–104.

Zheng, H., Cable, R., Spencer, B., Votto, N., & Katz, S. D. (2005). Iron stores and vascular function in voluntary blood donors. *Circulation, 25*, 1577–1583.

Zock, P. L., & Katan, M. B. (1998). Diet, LDL oxidation, and coronary artery disease [Editorial]. *American Journal of Clinical Nutrition, 68*, 759–760.

# 17 Global Concept of Iron Deficiency

*S.M. Lewis and J.C. Emmanuel*

**Summary**

- World Health Organization has been concerned with nutritional anaemias for 50 years.
- Management strategies have been developed by WHO and other international organizations, but burden of disease remains a serious problem with 2 billion persons affected globally, mainly in developing countries but also in industrialized countries.
- Highest incidence of iron deficiency occurs in pregnancy and in children.
- Iron deficiency causes impaired mental development in children and decreased work capacity in adults. In this respect latent iron deficiency without anaemia can be as serious as the anaemic phase, and specific laboratory tests are essential for diagnosis and clinical management.

**Key Words:** Incidence; effects on populations; WHO programmes; management strategies

Since 1958 the World Health Organization (WHO) has been interested in nutritional anaemias when a statistical study by De Maeyer and Adiels-Tegman (1985) indicated it to be the most common and widespread nutritional disorder in the world, affecting a large number of children and women in developing countries as well as having a significant prevalence in virtually all industrialized countries. In the 1960 s, WHO established a scientific group to study the deleterious effects of anaemia, iron deficiency and folate deficiency as a global problem (Patwardhan, 1966; WHO, 1968).

Subsequently, the minimum requirements of dietary iron (and also folate and vitamin $B_{12}$) were proposed by WHO in collaboration with Food and Agriculture Organization (FAO) (WHO, 1970). The need for food fortifications to prevent anaemia was recognized, but its practicability was considered to be debatable as "the factors that inhibit iron absorption may greatly inhibit the effectiveness of fortification programmes unless they could all be identified and eliminated or neutralized".

An important contribution came from a joint meeting of WHO with the International Atomic Energy Agency and the United States Agency for International Development (WHO, 1975a). Their report, with 197 bibliographic references to publications from many countries in a 10-year period, highlighted the fact that iron deficiency was by far the commonest nutritional disorder and the commonest cause of anaemia, with folate deficiency being the next common cause, whilst vitamin $B_{12}$ and protein deficiency played a less important part in the pathogenesis of the anaemia. They noted that nutritional anaemia was a worldwide problem but with highest

From: *Nutrition and Health: Iron Deficiency and Overload*
Edited by: S. Yehuda and D.I. Mostofsky, DOI 10.1007/978-1-59745-462-9_17

incidence in developing countries, occurring in people of all age groups but especially amongst pregnant women and young children. And they recognized the detrimental effects of anaemia on maternal morbidity and mortality, on work capacity and on resistance to infection. They proposed a scheme of action, which noted the importance of assessing the iron status of different populations by measurement of serum iron and ferritin; they advocated standardization of the methods for their assay.

A standardized method for measuring serum iron was established by the International Council for Standardization in Haematology (ICSH, 1978), followed by a serum ferritin standard which was adopted as a WHO International reference preparation (ICSH, 1985).

The extent and consequences of anaemia in pregnancy have been studied extensively (van den Broek, 1998). It was reported that each year half a million women, almost all in developing countries, died from pregnancy-related causes, with anaemia, especially iron deficiency anaemia, being a major factor (WHO, 1991, 1992).

In 1992, a resolution of the World Health Assembly (WHA 45.33) urged all member states to establish as part of their health systems "a micronutrient monitoring and evaluation system capable of assessing the magnitude of iodine, vitamin A and iron deficiency disorders and monitor the implementation and impact of control programmes." This led 90 countries to develop national programmes, particularly iron supplementation for pregnant women. Although many of these programmes were not systematically implemented, the health authorities became increasingly aware of the immediate health problems associated with iron deficiency, and also of the serious socio-economic implications for their populations.

Programmes were increasingly being devised by various international authorities. In WHO a number of different departments and units are concerned with various aspects of anaemia. In an attempt to co-ordinate these with relevant professional bodies, a series of meetings were organized by WHO in collaboration with the International Society of Hematology, International Society of Blood Transfusion and the International Council for Standardization in Haematology. WHO participants included representatives from the following units:

Nutrition for Health and Development
Parasitic Diseases and Vector Control
Reproductive Health and Research
Making Pregnancy Safer
Child and Adolescent Health and Development
Essential Health Technology
Blood Transfusion Safety

The WHO Regional offices have also established working groups on nutrition and anaemia, and there is active collaboration with other international organizations, *inter alia*, UNICEF, International Nutritional Anaemia Consultative Group (INACG), Food and Agriculture Organization (FAO). The reports of these and other publications from WHO, including those from the regional offices, are to be found on the WHO website which lists 2,500 items under *Iron deficiency anaemia*.

WHO has established a Statistical Information System (WHOSIS) that includes a global database on anaemia, through the network of its regional and country offices in close collaboration with national health authorities; the aims are to assess the magnitude of malnutrition, to monitor and evaluate the impact of treatments for prevention and control and to track related events over time (see www.Micronutrient *Deficiency Information System*).

There are also abundant independent reports of national and regional studies of nutritional anaemias in general and iron deficiency in particular. In the United States, *National Health and Nutrition Examination Survey* (NHANES) is a government-based activity of the CDC National Center for Health Statistics; fact sheets and published reports are published on their website. In Britain, the government-based Food Standards Agency is responsible for *National Diet and Nutrition Surveys* (e.g. Gregory, Collins, Davies, Hughes, & Clarke, 1995). In European Union, the profession-based *Eurogrowth Iron Study Group* provides journal publications (e.g. van't Hof & Haschke, 2000; Male et al, 2001). A *Google* request for "nutritional surveys" identifies almost 1.2 million items in general; and when the search is restricted to scientific articles, *Google Scholar* yields 60,000 titles on nutritional surveys and 150,000 references for "iron deficiency"!

Inevitably, there is repetition in the many different reports, but no fundamental disagreement as to the widespread occurrence of iron deficiency anaemia, its effects and the importance of diagnosis, management and prevention. A comprehensive review with extensive bibliography has been provided for WHO by its Department of Nutrition for Health and Development (NHD) in collaboration with UNICEF and the United Nations University (UNU) (WHO, 1998a, 2001). These documents describe methods for assessing, monitoring and preventing the occurrence of iron deficiency, taking account of scientific advances in understanding of the physiological process and the pathology of body iron.

Within individual countries, community-based surveys with cluster sampling identify prevalence of anaemia and delineate the specific contribution of iron deficiency, in order to provide insight into appropriate preventative and control strategies (Schellenberg et al, 2003). These various projects have shown or further confirmed that in developing countries severe anaemia with a variable degree of iron deficiency is found in conditions associated with (1) blood loss (schistosomiasis, hookworm infestation, childbirth haemorrhage, trauma); (2) deficiency of other nutrients (vitamin $B_{12}$, vitamin C, folic acid); (3) infectious diseases, notably tuberculosis and puerperal sepsis. Morbidity from infectious diseases may be increased in iron-deficient populations because of the adverse effect of the iron deficiency on the immune system, with reduced activity of leucocytes and decreased ability of lymphocytes to replicate. However, there is some debate on this, as in certain conditions iron repletion may have an adverse effect on the course of infection. In one study of Somali nomads, this occurred in subjects with tuberculosis, hepatitis, brucellosis, pneumonia, and also malaria (Murray, Murray, Murray, Murray, 1978). Other studies have also implicated iron overload as a risk factor for bacterial infection, with alteration in chemotactic and phagocytic properties of neutrophils and replication and dissemination of bacterial pathogens that use iron as a growth factor (Hoen, 1999) – see also below.

## 1. PREGNANCY AND THE NEWBORN

Anaemia during pregnancy is associated with increased stillbirths, perinatal death, prematurity and low birth weight babies. After birth, iron deficiency gives rise to impaired failure of infants and children to thrive; there is impairment of mental development and retarded physical growth in the pre-school and school-age children, as well as decreased physical capacity and work performance in adolescents and adults. Thus, when personal health and self-fulfilment are impaired by iron deficiency, national socio-economic development is unsustainable, with economic implications and the likelihood of continuing nutritional deficiencies in the next generation (WHO, 2001); An extreme example of this process is the "inherited" iron deficiency syndrome, when pregnant women, who are iron depleted and perhaps concomitantly suffer from other nutrient deficiencies, give birth to physically malformed babies (Reimann & Erdogan, 1976; Black, 2001).

## 2. MALARIA

There is debate about the management of iron deficiency associated with malaria. It has been shown that improved nutritional status lessens the severity of malaria episodes, resulting in fewer deaths due to malaria, whereas deficiencies in micronutrients, including iron, are responsible for a substantial proportion of malaria morbidity and mortality (Caulfield, Richard, & Black, 2004). Thus, it is generally perceived wisdom that iron deficiency associated with malaria requires treatment for both conditions, with the nutrition programs being integrated into existing malaria intervention programs (e.g. Alonzo Gonzalez et al., 2000). In an extensive WHO/UNICEF study of children in Zanzibar, in a community where there is a high year-round incidence of *Plasmodium falciparum*, it was found that routine low-dose daily iron supplementation did not affect the prevalence of malaria infection or parasite density, nor the clinical outcome (Mebrahtu et al., 2004).

On the other hand, a subsequent randomized placebo-controlled study of children under 3 years of age was carried out by Sazawal et al. (2006) in Pemba (Zanzibar), where there is a similar high incidence of malaria and other infections. The children were assigned to one of three groups: (a) iron + folic acid, (b) iron + folic acid + zinc, (c) placebo; those with clinical malaria also received treatment with sulphadoxine/pyrimethamine as per standardized local guidelines. It was found that in the children who were not iron-deficient, but whose diet was supplemented with iron and folic acid, there was significant risk of serious adverse reaction to infection even when they received appropriate specific treatment for malaria and other infections. By contrast, no such adverse reactions occurred in the children who were initially iron-deficient. It was concluded that routine supplementation with iron (and folic acid) in non-anaemic children might be harmful, and that it should be a safer approach to identify those with iron deficiency anaemia and treat them specifically, rather than adopt the programme of universal supplementation with iron and folic acid, at least in areas endemic for malaria. This approach supports the view that iron excess favours the pathogens, possibly by inhibiting absorption of zinc, thus compromising the immune response to infection. In this context it is of interest to note an experimental study by Koka et al. (2007) on mice infected with *Plasmodium berghei*, demonstrating that iron deficiency accelerates suicidal erythrocyte death with subsequent rapid clearance of infected cells from circulation, thus favourably influencing the course of the malaria and significantly enhancing the survival of the infected mice. Conversely, in an experimental study on mice in which iron *overload* was induced together with infection by *Plasmodium yoelli*, there was rapid penetration and development of the plasmodium in the hepatocytes (Goma, Renia, Miltgen, & Mazier, 1996).

## 3. LATENT IRON DEFICIENCY

A limitation in many of the reports and published papers has been failure to distinguish between degrees of severity of the anaemia: i.e. whether "mild", "moderate", "severe" or "critical", on the basis of either haemoglobin measurement or any other laboratory tests. Another cause of confusion is the fact that the terms *iron deficiency* (ID) and *iron deficiency anaemia* (IDA) are sometimes used interchangeably. It is important to appreciate that iron deficiency anaemia is a subset of iron deficiency, and that tissues are functionally impaired by iron deficiency, even when the deficiency is not severe enough to have led to anaemia (Yip, 1989). The extent of overlap between ID and IDA varies between populations, occurring especially in populations in which dietary iron absorbability is low or blood loss is common, as, for example, in hookworm infestation or bilharzia.

To plan effective interventions, there is need to obtain data on the iron status of the population as well as to record clinical features and to measure haemoglobin concentration in the individuals. A recent WHO-CDC consultation noted that despite many efforts to treat and prevent anaemia and iron deficiency over the past two decades, this remains a major problem. It was concluded that most programmes have been based on assuming iron deficiency anaemia as the essential feature and underestimating the role of infectious diseases or deficiencies of other micronutrients (WHO, 2005a). Furthermore, they have not recognized that latent iron deficiency per se, without anaemia, is a major and common health problem, affecting people of all ages, but especially women of child-bearing age and children. And it is also a problem in industrialized countries: thus, for example, in one study in the United States on a set of apparently healthy infants under 1 year of age it was found that 3% were anaemic, whilst a sensitive screening test (reticulocyte haemoglobin content, see below) indicated that a further 11% of the infants had iron deficiency without anaemia and, in a subsequent follow-up 1 year later, were then found to have developed anaemia (Ulrich et al., 2005).

The effects of ID on children's mental and physical development and reduced productivity of manual workers are as serious as with IDA. Accordingly, the WHO-CDC consultation recommended that, in population studies, iron deficiency should be assessed by a combination of five indicators, namely Hb concentration, zinc protoporphyrin, mean red-cell volume (MCV), transferrin receptors in serum and serum ferritin (WHO, 2005a). To assess the potential utility of these indicators to detect change in iron status as a result of interventions, iron was added to the diet as supplements or as food fortified with iron for periods of 4–18 months to infants, pre-school children, school children, pregnant women and non-pregnant women. From this study it was concluded that serum ferritin or transferrin receptor, together with haemoglobin, was the best indicator to judge the effectiveness of the procedure. The importance of ferritin measurement in differential diagnosis was also apparent by a study showing that if iron deficiency is the major cause of the anaemia, haemoglobin may improve more rapidly than the serum ferritin, whereas if serum ferritin improves but haemoglobin does not, factors in addition to iron are likely to be the cause of anaemia (Cook, Flowers, & Skikne, 2003). However, it should be noted that ferritin may be misleading as it is also an acute-phase protein, so that a deficiency of less than 12–15 μg may not be valid as an assessment of iron deficiency, so that in the presence of infection the level should be adjusted to threshold of less than 30 μg; and it is advisable to use a second indicator of acute-phase reaction such as CRP or alpha-1-antichymotrypsin (ACT) or alpha-1-acid glycoprotein (AGP) (WHO, 2005a). The use and utility of erythrocyte sedimentation rate (ESR) was not mentioned in this document, although it is a simple and reliable screening test for infections and inflammations (Osei-Bimpong, Meek, & Lewis, 2007). Serum iron assay is no longer included on the list of recommended tests as it provides little useful clinical information, because there is considerable diurnal variation from hour to hour in normal subjects and as low concentrations are found in inflammations and infections, low serum iron concentration does not necessarily indicate an absence of storage iron.

As mentioned earlier, laboratories with appropriate automated blood count analyzers can also determine the reticulocyte cell haemoglobin (CHr); this is a reliable parameter for detecting functional iron deficiency and absence of iron store before the onset of anaemia, and for distinguishing IDA from the anaemia of chronic disease (Brugnara, 2003). However, the utility of these various tests will obviously depend on their availability in different situations, especially in developing countries.

## 4. MANAGEMENT STRATEGIES

Current management strategies have been described in the WHO Nutrition for Health and Development review (WHO, 2001), whilst a booklet by Stoltzfus and Dreyfuss (1998) for INACG, WHO and UNICEF provides guidelines for use of iron supplements. The latter includes a useful list of addresses and websites of international agencies engaged in the control of iron deficiency. The prevention strategy (Table 1) must take account of the fact that iron deficiency may occur despite adequate or the provision of dietary supplements, as absorption is often inhibited by the high phytate content of many of the grain-based diets in the tropics as well as tropical sprue, parasitic enteropathies and enteropathy as a result of HIV infection (van den Broek, White, & Neilson et al, 1998).

**Table 1**
**Strategies for Management of Iron Deficiency in a Population**

| |
|---|
| *Dietary Improvement* |
| Animal meat, organs of fowl and fish |
| Green leafy vegetables |
| *Enhance Absorption* |
| Vitamin C-rich foods – Fruit, juices, potatoes |
| Fermented foods and condiments – Soy sauce, sauerkraut |
| *Avoid Absorption Inhibitors at Mealtimes** |
| Phytates and high inositol content – cereal bran and grains, high-extract flour, legumes, nuts and seeds |
| Tannins – tea, coffee, herbal infusions |
| Calcium – milk and dairy products |
| *Food Fortifications* |
| Ferrous sulphate |
| Iron – EDTA |
| For young children from 6 months of age: |
| Ferrous sulphate in cow's milk or modified infant formula |
| Metallic iron in infant cereals |
| Other iron-rich complementary foods |
| *Control Secondary Causes* |
| Hookworm, schistosomiasis, malaria (see text) |

* But can be taken at other times of the day.
Compiled from WHO (2001)

In intestinal helminth infection, the administration of antihelminthic agents results in a marginal increase in haemoglobin of *c* 1.7 g/L (Gulani, Nagpal, Osmond, & Sachdev, 2007). In countries with a high prevalence of intestinal helminthiasis, dietary malnutrition is generally a far greater factor in the anaemia that occurs, and deworming has little impact on the incidence of anaemia unless combined with iron therapy. However, given the low cost of deworming together with iron supplementation, in appropriate populations this combination should be encouraged in young people (Partnership for child development, 1999) and also in pregnant women (Bundy, Chan, & Savioli, 1995).

It is important to differentiate between supplementation that aims at preventing IDA by correcting iron deficiency before anaemia is manifest and therapy that aims to correct the haemoglobin concentration in established IDA. When iron-deficient anaemia is established, appropriate treatment is required according to standard medical practice.

Account must be taken of failure to take the prescribed iron supplements because of their side effects, and efforts should be made to use iron preparations that have fewer side effects than ferrous sulphate, even if they are more expensive, as this may ultimately be more cost-effective if it improves adherence to the regimen (Ekstrom et al., 1996).

Iron supplementation should be linked to other food supplementation programmes. The NHD recommendations (WHO, 2001) noted the value of integrating the iron supplementation programme with micronutrient programmes for folic acid, vitamin C and vitamin A, especially when intended for infants, children, and pregnant or lactating women. Multiple micronutrient-fortified food preparations would also be valuable for supervised feeding programmes in schools and in emergency situations. Combination of iron and folate supplementation in pregnancy is also proposed as a standard procedure for Integrated Management of Pregnancy and Childbirth (IMPAC). It is recommended that all pregnant women should routinely receive iron and folate supplements, 60 mg iron and 400 μg folic acid daily for 6 months of pregnancy and continuing for 3-months postpartum, but if this period cannot be achieved the dose of iron should be increased to 120 mg iron during pregnancy. Available sources of vitamin C should also be included in the diet (WHO, 2003a; 2006).

Iron cooking pots are commonly used in many countries in Africa. This has been recognized as a potential way to increase the iron content of food (Geerligs, Brabin, & Omari, 2003), and thus to achieve a significant improvement in haemoglobin (Geerligs Brabin, Mkumbwa, Broadhead, & Cuevas, 2003), It has been suggested that iron pots should be provided to all families in rural communities as the estimated cost would be significantly lower than the cost of iron fortification (Adish, Esrey, Gyorkos, Jean-Baptiste, & Rojhani, 1999). It has been suggested that in an iron-replete population there may be a potentially toxic effect, especially when there is present a genetic determinant of increased absorption. However, no ill effects have been shown in long-term oral iron supplementation in young children (Mitra, Akramuzzaman, Fuchs, Rahman, & Mahalanabis, 1997).

## 5. BURDEN OF DISEASE IN A POPULATION

In 1998, it was calculated that 2 billion people globally were affected by iron deficiency (Stoltzfus and Dreyfus, 1998). Despite many meetings of expert groups, workshops, population studies, clinical trials and advice on treatments, progress is slow, and anaemia, predominantly IDA, remains one of the world's most serious global health problems (WHO, 2004a; 2005b). It affects nearly half of the pregnant women in the world, especially in developing countries where inadequate nutrition is compounded by parasitic and bacterial infections contributing to depletion of iron reserves as discussed above. As the greatest burden of anaemia falls on the most "hard to reach" women and children aged 6–24 months, WHO has targeted this in its Millenium Development Goals relating to maternal and childhood mortality (WHO, 2003b; 2004b).

The seriousness has been highlighted by the WHO data given in the 2004 Report on mortality and also on burden of disease (see below). In this record 0.24% of all deaths in the world were attributed directly to iron deficiency anaemia; the distribution of the deaths between regions is shown in Table 2. As mentioned earlier, the limitation of these statistics and other various studies is that no distinction is made between degrees of severity of anaemia based on haemoglobin values.

Table 2
**Death Rate from Iron Deficiency Anaemia***

| *Region* | *Total No. of Deaths* ($\times 10^6$) | *Iron Deficiency Deaths* ($\times 10^3$) | *Incidence (%)* |
|---|---|---|---|
| Southeast Asia | 14.66 | 80 | 0.54 |
| Western Pacific | 11.94 | 9 | 0.08 |
| Africa | 10.66 | 17 | 0.16 |
| Europe | 9.56 | 6 | 0.06 |
| America | 5.96 | 15 | 0.25 |
| Eastern Mediterranean | 4.15 | 10 | 0.24 |
| Total | 57.0 | 137 | 0.24 |

*Based on data (rounded off) from WHO (2004a).

The assessment of the public health importance of various factors in prevention and control of a specified disease was hampered in the past by lack of common methods to investigate and measure the global burden of the disease. The Global Burden of Disease Study now provides a standardized approach to epidemiology, using a standard unit termed "disability-adjusted life years" (DALY) in order to aid comparisons (Murray & Lopis, 1997; see also WHO website – search: *DALY*). This is obtained by calculating YLL + YLD, where YLL is the potential years of life lost due to premature death and YLD is the equivalent of healthy life lost by virtue of poor health or disability in the context of the specified disease. Thus, DALY combines these two factors in one measure and one DALY equates to one lost year of healthy life. The burden of disease is a measurement of the gap between the current health status of a population and an ideal standard life expectancy where every person in the population would live into old age, free of disease and disability

The DALY data for 2004 showed a total burden of 12,209 years, with variation in the burden between regions (Table 3). As high DALY is likely to impair individuals, family and community as well as overall socio-economic development, interventions, if competently carried out, are likely to be highly cost-effective and sustainable. There is thus an obligation to carry out appropriate measures at local, regional and national level, with the ultimate goal of promoting developing countries into thriving industrialized communities.

Table 3
**Burden of Disease from Iron Deficiency Anaemia, Expressed by Disability Adjusted Life Years (DALY)**

| *Region* | *DALY* | *Percentage of Total* |
|---|---|---|
| Southeast Asia | 4,850 | 39.7 |
| Western Pacific | 2,277 | 18.7 |
| Africa | 2,064 | 16.9 |
| Europe | 768 | 6.3 |
| America | 988 | 8.1 |
| Eastern Mediterranean | 1,262 | 10.3 |
| Total | 12,209 | 100 |

Data from WHO (2004a).

The results in Tables 2 and 3, and other studies, have shown clear-cut regional differences in the burden of iron deficiency anaemia. Whilst iron deficiency is generally considered to be essentially a problem of developing countries, it is also an important public health problem in industrialized countries. In the United Kingdom, 12% of a nationally representative sample of children at 1½ and 2½ years of age had haemoglobins below 110 g/L (Gregory et al, 1995), but in a more recent study in one major city with a large number of children from ethnic minorities, the prevalence of IDA was estimated to be 18% for Caucasian and 27% for Asian young children, increasing to as much as 45% of children with haemoglobins as low as 60 g/L in some inner city clinics (Moy, 2006). A study of early infant nutrition in eleven European centres showed an incidence of IDA of only 2.3%, but 7.2% were iron-deficient (Male et al, 2001). In the United States, Looker, Dallman, Carroll, Gunter, and Johnson (1997) recorded iron deficiency in 9% and IDA in 3% of 1–2 year old toddlers, whilst iron deficiency was present in 9–11% of adolescent girls and women of child-bearing age and IDA in 2–5%. However, when the population was subdivided for the analysis, children in families living below the poverty line, especially those from Black or Hispanic racial groups, had a higher prevalence of iron deficiency (18%) and IDA (5%).

In Japan, a nutrition survey in two metropolitan areas ($n = 13{,}147$) revealed that 17.3% of healthy young women had anaemia, with severe IDA (Hb $<$ 100 g/l) in 3.3%. In women over 50 years old anaemia was present in 22.3%, with severe IDA in 1.6% of the selected population (Kusumi, Shoji, Endou, Kishi, Shibata, 2006). It was noted that in Japan there is no nationwide preventive policy aimed at iron deficiency.

In conclusion, the global problem of iron deficiency and its complex causes continue to stimulate studies and publication of papers that describe the introduction and effectiveness of the preventive and therapeutic control strategies adopted in various countries. But the problem persists and the websites of WHO, UNICEF and INACG provide updated reports of these various activities. The present situation has been comprehensively described in a 400-page report of a recent Nutritional Anaemia workshop in Barcelona, with 44 internationally recognized experts; this has been published (Kraemer & Zimmermann, 2007) and can be accessed in full at www.sightandlife.org/pdf/NAbook.pdf

## 6. EFFECT ON BLOOD TRANSFUSION SERVICES

The global prevalence of anaemia, especially iron deficiency anaemia, results in a problem for blood transfusion services in many countries. For the past 50 years blood donors have generally been accepted with haemoglobins of at least 135 g/L for men and 125 g/L for women. More recently, this limitation has been reduced in some countries – in the United Kingdom to 130 g/L for men and 120 g/L for women (Boulton, 1999), and in Canada to 125 g/L for men and 120 g/L for women (Ali, McAvoy, Ali, & Goldsmith, 1985).

But in many developing countries even these reduced criteria would exclude many potential blood donors, so that blood transfusion is often limited to life-saving situations for children with severe malaria, pregnant women with haemorrhage and for severe trauma. As some national authorities are now promoting blood donation from youth in the age range of 16–25 years, it is important to give such donors recommendations on diet and food, possibly a course of ferrous sulphate and a haemoglobin recheck after 3–6 months. The Haemoglobin Colour Scale (described below) is a useful method for selecting acceptable blood donors as it provides a reliable cutoff point at the critical level of 12 g/dL (120 g/L) (Lewis & Emmanuel, 2001).

## 7. TESTS IN UNDER-RESOURCED COUNTRIES

The role of laboratory tests that are relevant for diagnosis and management of iron deficiency and IDA are summarized in Table 4. Details of methods for the various tests are described in *Dacie and Lewis Practical Haematology* by Worwood (2006). The main problem in under-resourced countries concerns the limited facilities that may be available for population studies and for clinical management of individual patients outside the main towns. The network of laboratory services that are usually available in these countries are listed in Table 5, and the recommended technical methods are described in *Dacie and Lewis Practical Haematology* by Bates and Mendelow (2006). A parallel document from WHO (1998b) describes the limited laboratory services that might be expected for field studies and at primary health centres; the only tests that are usually available in those situations for investigating iron deficiency are haemoglobin measurement and ESR, the latter to exclude infections as a possible factor. District hospital laboratories may have automated analyzers that can measure packed cell volume (PCV), mean cell volume (MCV), mean cell haemoglobin (MCH) and mean cell haemoglobin concentration (MCHC), while more sophisticated analyzers, usually available only in central reference laboratories, can also measure reticulocyte haemoglobin concentration.

**Table 4**
**Measurements of Iron Status**

| | *Early Fe Deficient* | *Fe Depletion* | *Fe-Deficient Erythropoiesis* | *Anaemia* |
|---|---|---|---|---|
| Hb | N | N | N | ↓ |
| Blood count values (MCV/MCH/MCHC) | N | N | ↓ | ↓ |
| Hypochromic cell morphology | <5% | <5% | <5% | ↑ >5% |
| Serum ferritin | ↓ | ↓ | ↓ | ↓ |
| Serum iron | N | N | ↓++ | ↓+++ |
| Total iron-binding capacity | N | N | ↑+ | ↑++ |
| Serum Tf receptors | ↑± | ↑+ | ↑+++ | ↑+++ |
| RBC Zinc protoporphyrin | N | N | ↑++ | ↑+++ |
| Bone marrow Fe | +→± | 0 | 0 | 0 |

In general, if an individual in a peripheral locality is found to be severely anaemic, a decision must be made whether to treat locally on the probability of iron deficiency or to refer the patient to a district hospital, although this often requires a long and difficult journey. This is especially a problem during late pregnancy or if there are clinical signs of respiratory distress or oedema. Thus, primary health clinics should have at least the facility for assessing the presence and severity of anaemia, and there is urgent need for development of simple quantitative screening tests for transferrin receptors, zinc protoporphyrin and ferritin. As microscopes are often available in peripheral health centres for diagnosing malaria infection, examination of stained blood films may help in making a diagnosis of iron-deficient anaemia from the characteristic morphological

Table 5
**Haematology Laboratory Services in Under-Resourced Countries**

| *Level of Laboratory* | *Haematology Services Performed* |
|---|---|
| Field studies – on site | Haemoglobin screening by simple method |
| Health centres | Simple haemoglobinometry |
| | Erythrocyte sedimentation rate (ESR) |
| | Screening for malaria (usually thick and thin blood films microscopy – possibly dipstick or slide screen test if available) |
| | HIV serology |
| District hospitals | Haemoglobin measurement |
| | Blood count and RBC parameters if automated analyzer is available |
| | Blood film morphology |
| | Screening for sickle cell haemoglobin |
| | Malaria screening by thick and thin blood films; also rapid immunological test |
| Central/regional hospitals | |
| | Blood count and RBC parameters |
| | Reticulocyte count |
| | G6PD screen and assay |
| | Haemoglobin electrophoresis |
| | Bone marrow aspirates (including staining for estimation of iron status) |
| | Serum ferritin |
| | Serum iron |
| | Total iron-binding capacity |
| | Serum transferring receptors |
| | Red cell zinc protoporphyrin |

Based on Bates and Mendelow (2006).

features of microcytic hypochromic red cells – and also some other causes of anaemia from their different morphologies, as illustrated in the WHO *Bench-Aid for Morphological Diagnosis of Anaemia* (Lewis, Bain, & Swirsky, 2001).

## 8. HAEMOGLOBINOMETRY

Haemoglobin measurement must be sufficiently reliable for its intended purpose – i.e. for research, field surveys, clinical diagnosis or therapeutic management. WHO had recognized the need for a simple method to measure haemoglobin infield surveys and in peripheral health centres in developing countries with limited resources. They required a device that would be cheap and robust, portable, capable of being used reliably by health workers with minimal training, often in the absence of electricity (WHO, 1975b).

A recent study on several commonly used methods by Medina Lara, Mundy, Kandulu, Chisuwo, and Bates (2005) concluded that the HemoCue haemoglobinometer was the method of choice, providing the most reliable and clinically useful results, but also the most expensive because of the relatively high cost of the disposable cuvettes. In an attempt to reduce the cost HemoCue has now developed a modified version named *HemoCue 301*, with disposable cuvettes that contain no reagents, do not deteriorate in adverse climates, and are considerably cheaper, thus making the method more feasible within the limited budgets of many health authorities. An independent evaluation has shown it to give reliable measurements of haemoglobin, conforming to the requirements of CLIA'88 regulations (Morris, Osei-Bimpong, McKeown, Roper, & Lewis, 2007).

However, considering the financial limitations of the health services in the poorest countries, the WHO Haemoglobin Colour Scale was developed for use as a semi-quantitative screening method for anaemia, costing less than 2 US cents per test (Stott & Lewis, 1995; Lewis, Stott, Wynn , 1998). A drop of blood on a test strip is compared with a set of colours on the scale that identify six levels of haemoglobin between 40 and 140 g/l, as well as intermediate levels of ±10 g/l between two colours. These represent normal and five clinical levels of anaemia, i.e. mild, moderate, marked, severe, critical. The technique is simple; readings are easy (even for colour-blind individuals who read the colours as shades of grey). There have been variable results by some users (Critchley & Bates, 2005), but in general it has been shown to be more reliable than clinical assessment of anaemia and, where there is no laboratory, it can provide a useful point-of-care screening method for diagnosing anaemia and for following response to its clinical management (Montresor et al., 2000; Ingram & Lewis, 2000; also WHO website: *Haemoglobin colour scale information leaflet*).

## REFERENCES*


Adish, A. A., Esrey, S. A., Gyorkos, T. W., Jean-Baptiste, J., & Rojhani, A. (1999). Effect of consumption of food cooked in iron pots on iron status and growth of young children: A randomised trial. *Lancet, 353, 712–716.*

Ali, A. M., McAvoy, A. T., Ali, M. A., & Goldsmith, C. H. (1985). An approach to determine objectively minimum hemoglobin standards for blood donors. *Transfusion 25*, 286–288.

Alonzo Gonzalez, M., Menendes, C., Font, F., Kahigwa, E., Kimario, J., Mshinda, H., et al. (2000). Cost-effectiveness of iron supplementation and malaria chemoprophylaxis in the prevention of anaemia and malaria among Tanzanian infants. *Bulletin of the World Health Organization, 78*, 97–107.

Bates, I., & Mendelow, B. (2006). Haematology in under-resourced laboratories. In *Dacie & Lewis Practical Haematology 10E* (Chapter 27, pp. 673–688). London: Churchill Livingstone-Elsevier.

Black, R. E. (2001). Micronutrients in pregnancy. *British Journal of Nutrition, 85*(Suppl 2), S193–S197.

Boulton, F. (1999). Threshold Concentration of Haemoglobin in Donor Blood. *Vox Sanguinis, 77*, 108–109.

Brugnara, C. (2003). Iron deficiency and erythropoiesis: New diagnostic approaches. *Clinical Chemistry, 49*, 1573–1578.

Bundy, D. A. P., Chan, M. S., & Savioli, L. (1995). Hookworm infection in pregnancy. *Transactions of Royal Society of Tropical Medicine and Hygiene, 89*, 521–522.

Caulfield, L. E., Richard, S. E., & Black, R. E. (2004). Undernutrition as an underlying cause of malaria norbidity and mortality in children less than five years old. *American Journal of Tropical Medicine and Hygeine, 71*(suppl 2), 55–63.

Cook, J. D., Flowers, C. H., & Skikne, B. S. (2003). The quantitative assessment of body iron. *Blood, 101*, 3359–3364.

Critchley, J., & Bates, I. (2005). Haemoglobin colour scale for anaemia diagnosis where there is no laboratory: A systematic review. *International Journal of Epidemiology, 34*, 1425–1434.

De Maeyer, E. M., & Adiels-Tegman, M. (1985). The prevalence of anaemia in the world. *World Health Statistical Quarterly, 38*, 302–316.

Ekstrom, E. C., Kavishe, F. P., Habicht, J. P., Frongillo, E. A., Rasmussen, K. P., & Hemed, L. (1996). Adherence to iron supplementation during pregnancy in Tanzania determinants and hematologic consequences. *American Journal of Clinical Nutrition, 64*, 368–374.

Geerligs, P. P., Brabin, B., Mkumbwa, A., Broadhead, R., & Cuevas, L. E. (2003). The effect on haemoglobin of the use of iron cooking pots in rural Malawian households in an area with high malaria prevalence: A randomized trial. *Tropical Medicine & International Health, 8*, 310–315.


*Murray and Lopez is one of a series of four papers in consecutive issues: Part 1.Mortality by cause for eight regions of the world (1269–1276); Part 3. Global mortality, disability and the contribution of risk factors (1436–1442); Part 4. Alternative projections of mortality and disability by cause 1990–2020 (2498–1504).

Geerligs, P. D., Brabin, B. J., & Omari, A. A. (2003). Food prepared in iron cooking pots as an intervention for reducing iron deficiency anaemia in developing countries: A systematic review.*Journal of Human Nutrition & Dietetics*, ***16***, 275–281.

Goma, J., Renia, L., Miltgen, F., & Mazier, D. (1996). Iron overload increases hepatic development of Plasmodium yoelli in mice. *Parasitology, 112*, 165–168.

Gregory, J. R., Collins, D. L., Davies, P. S. W., Hughes, J. M., & Clarke, P. C. (1995). *National diet and nutrition survey: Children aged 1 to 4 years*. Report of the Diet and Nutrition Survey. London: HMSO.

Gulani, A., Nagpal, J., Osmond, C., & Sachdev, H. P. S. (2007). Effect of administration of intestinal anthelminthic drugs on haemoglobin: Systematic review of randomised controlled trials. *British Medical Journal, 334*, 1095–1097.

Hoen, B. (1999). Iron and infection: Clinical experience. *American Journal of Kidney Disease, 34*(4 Suppl 2), 30–34.

Ingram, C. F., & Lewis, S. M. (2000). Clinical use of WHO haemoglobin colour scale: Validation and critique. *Journal of Clinical Pathology, 53*, 933–937.

ICSH: International Committee for Standardization in Haematology. (1978). Recommendations for measurement of serum iron in human blood. *British Journal of Haematology, 38*, 291–294.

ICSH: International Committee for Standardization in Haematology. (1985). Proposed international standard of human ferritin for the serum ferritin assay. *British Journal of Hamatology, 61*, 61–63.

Koka, S, Foller, M., Lamprecht, G., Boini, K. M., Lang, C., Huber, S. M., et al. (2007). Iron deficiency influences the course of malaria in Plasmodium berghei infected mice. *Biochemistry and Biophysics Research Communication, 357*, 608–614.

Kraemer, K., & Zimmermann, M. B. (Eds.). (2007). ***Nutritional anemia.*** Basel: Sight and Life Press. Retrieved from www.sightandlife.org; e-mail: info@sightandlife.org

Kusumi, E., Shoji, M., Endou, S., Kishi, Y., & Shibata, T. (2006). Prevalence of anemia among healthy women in 2 metropolitan areas of Japan. *International Journal of Hematology, 84*, 217–219.

Lewis, S. M., & Emmanuel, J. (2001). Validity of the haemoglobin colour scale in blood donor screening. *Vox Sanguinis, 80*, 28–33.

Lewis, S. M., Bain, B. J., & Swirsky, D. M. (2001). *WHO bench aids for the morphological diagnosis of anaemia*. Geneva: WHO, , ISBN 92 4 154532 1.

Lewis, S. M., Stott, G. J., & Wynn, K. J. (1998). An inexpensive and reliable new haemoglobin colour scale for assessing anaemia. *Journal of Clinical Pathology, 51*, 21–24.

Looker, A. C., Dallman, P. R., Carroll, M. D., Gunter, E. W., & Johnson, C. L. (1997). Prevalence of iron deficiency in the United States. *Journal of the American Medical Association, 277*, 973–976.

Male, C., Persson, L. A., Freeman, V., Guerra, A., van't Hof, M. A., & Haschke, F. (2001). Prevalence of iron deficiency in 12 month old infants from 11 European areas and influence of dietary factors on iron status (European-Growth study). *Acta paediatrica, 90*, 492–498.

Mebrahtu, T., Stoltzfus, R. J., Chwaya, H. M., Jape, K. J., Savioli, L., Montresor, M., et al. (2004). Low-dose daily iron supplementation for 12 months does not increase the prevalence of malarial infection or density of parasites in young Zanzibari children. *Journal of Nutrition, 134*, 3037–3041.

Medina Lara, A., Mundy, C., Kandulu, J., Chisuwo, L., & Bates, I. (2005). Evaluation and costs of different haemoglobin methods for use in district hospitals in Malawi. *Journal of Clinical Pathology, 58*, 56–60.

Mitra, A. K., Akramuzzaman, S. M., Fuchs, G. I., Rahman, M. M., & Mahalanabis, D. (1997). Long term oral supplementation with iron is not harmful for young children in a poor community of Bangladesh. *Journal of Nutrition, 127*, 1451–1455.

Montresor, A., Albonico, M., Khalfan, N., Stoltzfus, R. J., Tielsch, J. M., Chwaya, H. M., et al. (2000). Field trial of a haemoglobin colour scale: An effective tool to detect anaemia in preschool children. *Tropical Medicine and International Health, 5*, 129–133.

Morris, L. D., Osei-Bimpong, A., McKeown, D., Roper, D., & Lewis, S. M. (2007). Evaluation of the clinical utility of the Hemocue 301 haemoglobinometer for blood donor screening. *Vox Sanguinis, 93*, 64–69.

Moy, R. J. D. (2006). Prevalence, consequences and prevention of childhood nutritional iron deficiency: A child public health perspective. *Clinical and Laboratory Haematology, 28*, 291–298.

Murray, C. J. L., & Lopez, A. D. (1997). Global burden of disease study: Part 2. Regional patterns of disability-free life expectancy and disability-adjusted life expectancy. *Lancet, 349*, 1347–1352.

Murray, M. J., Murray, A. B., Murray, M. B., & Murray, C. J. (1978). The adverse effect of iron repletion on the course of certain infections. *British Medical Journal, 2*, 1113–1115.

Osei-Bimpong, A., Meek, J., & Lewis, S. M. (2007). ESR or CRP? A comparison of their clinical utility. *Hematology, 12*, 353–357.

Partnership for child development. (1999). The cost of large-scale school health programmes which deliver antihelminthics to children in Ghana and Tanzania. *Acta Tropica, 73*, 183–284.

Patwardhan, V. N. (1966). Nutritional anaemias – WHO research program. Early developments and progress report of collaborative studies. *American Journal of Clinical Nutrition, 19*, 63–71.

Reimann, F., & Erdogan, G. (1976). Missbildungen, Anomalien und Variationen bei Patienten mit schwerer Eisenmangelkrankheit [Malformations, anomalies and variations in patients with severe iron deficiency] *Blut, 32*, 423–432.

Sazawal, S., Black, R. E., Ramsan, M., Chwaya, H. M., Stoltzfus, R. J., Dutta, A., et al. (2006). Effects of routine prophylactic supplementation with iron and folic acid on admission to hospital and mortality in preschool children in a high malaria transmission setting: Community-based, randomised, placebo-controlled trial. *Lancet, 367*, 133–143.

Schellenberg, D., Armstrong Schellenberg, J. R. M., Mushi, A., de Savigny, D., Mgalula, L., Mbuya, C., et al. (2003). The silent burden of anaemia in Tanzanian children: A community-based study. *Bulletin of the World Health Organization, 81*, 581–590.

Stoltzfus, R. J., & Dreyfus, M. L. (1998). Guidelines for the use of iron supplements to prevent and treat iron deficiency anemia (INACG, WHO, UNICEF). ILSI Press, International Life Science Institute, Washington, DC 20036–4810

Stott, G. J., & Lewis, S. M. (1995). A simple and reliable method for estimating haemoglobin. *Bulletin of the World Health Organization, 73*, 369–373.

Ulrich, C., Wu, A., Armsby, C., Rieber, S., Wingerter, S., Brugnara, C., et al. (2005). Screening healthy infants for iron deficiency using reticulocyte hemoglobin content. *Journal of American Medical Association, 294*, 924–930.

van den Broek, N. (1998). Anaemia in pregnancy in developing countries. *British Journal of Obstetrics and Gynaecology, 105*, 385–390.

van den Broek, N. R., White, S. A., & Neilson, J. P. (1998). The relationship between asymptomatic human immunodeficiency virus infection and the prevalence and severity of anaemia in pregnant Malawian women. *American Journal of Tropical Medicine and Hygiene, 59*, 1004–1007.

van't Hof, M. A., & Haschke, F. (2000). The Euro-growth study: Why, who, and how. *Journal of Pediatric Gastroenterology and Nutrition 31*(Suppl 1), S3–S13

World Health Organization. (1968). Scientific group on Nutritional anaemias. *WHO Technical Report Series No.405.*

World Health Organization. (1970). Joint FAO/WHO Expert group on requirements of ascorbic acid, vitamin D, vitamin B12, folate and iron. *WHO Technical report series No. 452*

World Health Organization. (1975a). Control of nutritional anaemia with special reference to iron deficiency. Report of an IAEA/USAID/WHO Joint Meeting. *WHO Technical report series No. 580.*

World Health Organization. (1975b). Report of consultation on standardization in haematology. *Document LAB/75.3.*

World Health Organization. (1991). Maternal mortality ratio and rates. *Document WHO/MCH/MSM/91.6.*

World Health Organization. (1992). The prevalence of anaemia in women: A tabulation of available information. *Document WHO/MCH/MCM/92.2.*

World Health Organization. (1998a). *WHO, UNICEF and UNU 1998 Iron deficiency anaemia: Prevention, assessment and control.* Report of a joint WHO/UNICEF/UNU Consultation. Geneva: WHO

World Health Organization. (1998b). Laboratory services for primary health care: Requirements for essential clinical laboratory tests. *Document LAB/98.1.*

World Health Organization. (2001). Iron deficiency anaemia Assessment, prevention and control. A guide for programme managers. *Document WHO /NHD/01.3.*

World Health Organization. (2003a). Pregnancy childbirth, postpartum and newborn care: A guide for essential practice. Geneva Guidelines for management of IDA. *Joint document WHO, INACG and UNICEF.*

World Health Organization. (2003b). *Managing complications in pregnancy and childbirth.* Geneva: WHO.

World Health Organization. (2004a). *The world health report: Changing history.* Geneva: WHO.

World Health Organization. (2004b). *Pregnancy, childbirth, postpartum, and newborn care (PCNC).* Geneva: A guide for essential practice WHO.

World Health Organization. (2005a). Assessing the iron status of populations WHO (NHD) and Centers for Disease control and prevention. *Technical Consultation, Geneva ISBN 92 4 159315 6.*

World Health Organization. (2005b). *The world health report: Make every mother and child count.* Geneva: WHO.

World Health Organization. (2006). Department of Making pregnancy safer: Integrated management of pregnancy and childbirth: Standards for maternal and neonatal care. Section 1.8: Iron and folate supplementation.

Worwood, M. (2006). Iron deficient anaemia and iron overload. In *Dacie & Lewis Practical Haematology 10E* (Chapter 7, pp. 131–160). Churchill Livingstone – Elsevier, London.

Yip, R. (1989). Iron nutritional status defined. In I. J. Filer (ed.),*Dietary iron: Birth to two years* (pp. 19–36). New York: Raven Press.

# 18 Nutritional Iron Deficiency in Early Childhood

*Robert J.D. Moy*

**Summary**

- The true prevalence of nutritional iron deficiency (ID) in childhood is unclear because of the uncertainty over its definition and the insensitivity of markers of ID.
- The major cause in developed countries is likely to be the excessive and early use of cow's milk and a diet poor in haem iron.
- Recent neuro-physiological observations support the many field studies correlating ID with cognitive and motor developmental delay in young children, although proof of causality has not been established because of environmental confounding.
- Population iron supplementation is a potentially effective means of prevention of ID but is limited by poor compliance and the risk of increased morbidity and mortality in malarious regions.
- Fortification of milk and essential infant foods is likely to be the most cost-effective means of improving the iron status of child populations.

**Key Words:** Risk factors; psychomotor development; iron supplementation and fortification; anaemia screening

## 1. INTRODUCTION

Anaemia (defined as a haemoglobin level of less than 110 g/L) affects 47% or 293 million of the world's pre-school children (World Health Organisation Vitamin and Mineral Nutrition System http://who.int.vmnis) and may be due to increased physiological requirements for iron during rapid growth in infancy and adolescence, inadequate dietary intake of iron, malabsorption of iron due to small bowel pathology and chronic blood loss usually from the gastrointestinal or urinary tracts or due to menorrhagia in adolescent girls. Worldwide, intestinal blood loss due to parasites and urinary schistosomiasis are particularly important contributors to a low haemoglobin level as is malaria (World Health Organisation, 2001). Other causes of a hypochromic, microcytic anaemia with low mean cell volume are the genetic haemoglobinopathies which may account for the apparently high prevalence of iron deficiency anaemia (IDA) in some communities (Thurlow et al., 2005). Additional nutritional deficiencies such as vitamin C that reduces iron absorption in the small bowel and vitamin A that may decrease mobilization of iron from stores in the body also contribute to the high prevalence and severity of IDA.

From: *Nutrition and Health: Iron Deficiency and Overload*
Edited by: S. Yehuda and D.I. Mostofsky, DOI 10.1007/978-1-59745-462-9_18

Surveys from Europe and the United States indicate that nutritional iron deficiency is still an important public health problem but do report a wide range of prevalence reflecting the variable nature of the population samples and differing definitions of iron deficiency (ID) and iron deficiency anaemia. Indeed, anaemia is often taken as being synonymous with iron deficiency, and population surveys to determine the prevalence of iron deficiency may then measure this parameter alone.

## 2. DEFINING THE PREVALENCE OF IRON DEFICIENCY

The United Kingdom National Diet and Nutrition survey identified that 12% of a nationally representative sample of children between 1½ and 2½ years had a Hb < 110 g/L (Gregory, Collins, Davies, Hughes, & Clarke, 1995). This has then commonly been accepted as representing the extent of the problem of severe iron deficiency in the UK children, yet it has been subsequently estimated that only 3.4% of these anaemic children had an abnormally low level of ferritin as an indicator of low iron stores (Thane, Walmsley, Bates, Prentice, & Cole, 2000), thereby questioning whether the low Hb was due to iron deficiency alone.

The American National Health and Nutrition Examination Survey III (NHANES III), a multi-stage, stratified population survey of US children aged 12–35 months, found a much lower prevalence of IDA of only 3% using a panel of indicators of iron deficiency (two or more of ferritin <10 μg/L, transferrin saturation <10%, erythrocyte protoporphyrin >1.42 μmol/L red blood cells and Hb <110 g/L) (Looker, Dallman, Carroll, Gunter, & Johnson, 1997). Nine percent of this population had iron deficiency with at least two of the iron indicators being abnormal but with normal Hb. However, a recent analysis of this data indicates that anaemia (defined as Hb <110 g/L) is an insensitive marker of iron deficiency with a low predictive value of 29% and sensitivity of 30%; that is, most anaemic toddlers in this US sample do not have ID, and most toddlers with ID are not anaemic (White, 2005). A similarly low sensitivity of 23% for a low Hb as a predictor of ID was found in a study of children attending Special Supplemental Nutrition Program for Women, Infants and Children (WIC) clinics in California, where the prevalence of anaemia was 11% (using a similar panel of indicators of ID namely two or more abnormal levels of ferritin ≤8.7 μg/L, transferrin receptors ≥8.4 μg/mL or transferring saturation ≤13.2%) (Schneider et al., 2005).

Similar conclusions can be derived from the Euro-Growth study of early infant growth and nutrition conducted across 11 European study centres (Male et al., 2001). Using multiple indicators of iron status similar to those in the NHANES III survey, the prevalence of anaemia in 12-month-old infants was found to be 9.4%, whilst that of ID was 7.2% and only 2.3% had IDA. Forty-one percent of infants with low Hb had no abnormal indicators of iron deficiency. In 75% of these infants, there was a history of recent infection, which is also a very common cause of anaemia (Yip, & Dallman, 1988). Acute infection and inflammation can depress Hb, serum iron and transferrin saturation, although it will also elevate ferritin as an acute-phase protein. These data suggest that IDA and anaemia of infection frequently co-exist and are difficult to discriminate by iron indicators alone. Population screening for IDA should, therefore, include the indicators of recent infection and inflammation such as C-reactive protein or erythrocyte sedimentation rate to correct for the effect of infection on iron status.

There is no 'gold standard' test to determine the presence of ID apart from bone marrow iron estimation. Other indicators are not specific for ID and estimate different aspects of iron absorption, transport and metabolism that are affected by factors such as infection, inflammation, time of day and a recent meal. There is a marked overlap in the values of these indicators between healthy and iron-deficient subjects, so making their interpretation difficult (Oski, 1993). A therapeutic response of Hb level to iron treatment could, therefore, be a better indicator of the presence of ID (Wright, Kelly, Trail, Parkinson, & Summerfield, 2004).

This argument does, however, centre around the use of the cut of Hb <110 g/L to define anaemia in young children. The Avon Longitudinal Study of Pregnancy and Childhood (ALSPAC) birth cohort study from the United Kingdom has collected blood specimens from 1,500 children to define the population distribution of Hb at various ages. Hb was found to follow a normal distribution at 8, 12, and 18 months (Emond, Hawkins, Pennock, Golding, & The ALSPAC Children in Focus Team, 1996, Sherriff, Emond, Hawkins, Golding, & The ALSPAC Children in Focus Team, 1999). Taking the 5th centile of this distribution, cut offs of Hb <97 g/L at 8 months and <100 g/L at 12 and 18 months (which correlated with adverse biological effects on child development) were used to define anaemia in this population, whereas 23% at 8 months and 18% at 12 and 18 months of these other healthy young children would have been deemed to be anaemic using the WHO cutoff of <110 g/L, suggesting that this cutoff overestimates the true prevalence. Furthermore, surveys of IDA prevalence based on the measurement of Hb alone should be viewed with caution (Aggett et al., 2002).

Even though the true prevalence of ID and IDA may be difficult to determine, the proportion of young children with ID is significantly higher in certain at-risk groups and is the cause for concern. The latest US National Center for Health Statistics survey (NHANES IV) identified significant racial and ethnic differences in the prevalence of ID. Twelve percent of Hispanic young children had ID compared to 6% of white and 65 of black children. Additionally, there was a higher prevalence in those children whose parents were non-English speakers (14%) and in those toddlers not in day care (10%), which may reflect the importance of poor parental education and the protective effect of better nutrition offered in day care settings among the poorer Hispanic community (Brotanek, Gosz, Weltzman, & Flores, 2007). In UK hospital and clinic-based samples, young children from particular socio-economic or racial groups have been found to have much higher numbers with anaemia generally presumed to be due to ID. In Birmingham city, renown for its considerable social inequalities and large number of children from South Asian ethnic minorities, the prevalence of anaemia in poor Caucasian and Asian young children has been estimated to be 18% and 27%, respectively, increasing to as much as 45% in certain clinic populations where pale children with Hb of 60 g/L, ferritin of 2 µmol/L and MCV of 52 are still commonplace (Moy, Aukett, 2000).

## 3. RISK FACTORS FOR IRON DEFICIENCY IN EARLY CHILDHOOD

Low birth weight and premature delivery are well-established risk factors for early infant ID because of limited time to develop foetal iron stores sufficient to last the first 6 months of life. Small premature babies are therefore routinely offered iron supplements. However, the relationship between significant maternal iron deficiency during pregnancy and the subsequent iron status of the infant is less clear. Notwithstanding the difficulty in defining iron status and normal haemoglobin during pregnancy, the prevalence of IDA in pregnant women worldwide can be 50% or higher. Yet, it is generally accepted that 'the foetus is an effective parasite for iron', and that there is no relationship between maternal iron status in pregnancy and that of the foetus, newborn or infant (Hussain, Gaafar, Laulicht, & Hoffebrand, 1997). However, a few prospective studies with follow up of the infants up to 1 year of age have identified significant positive associations. In one such study from Spain, the odds ratio for anaemia in pregnancy being associated with infant iron deficiency at age 1 year was 6.57 (95% CI 1.81, 25.97) (Colomer et al., 1990). In a similarly designed study of Palestinian refugees living in Jordan where the prevalence of anaemia in pregnancy was as high as 65%, this relationship was confirmed in 1-year-old term infants despite similar iron endowment in cord blood samples from both anaemic and non-anaemic women (Kilbride et al., 1999). In both studies the relationship was not explained by differences in environmental risk factors or feeding practices. Analysis of a public health data set from Indonesia found a correlation between low Hb level at 3–5 months of age in healthy breast-fed term babies and maternal anaemia (OR 1.81, 95% CI 1.34, 2.43) (De Pee, Bloem, Sari, Kleiss, & Yip, 2002). Furthermore, 9-month infants whose low-income American mothers were anaemic during pregnancy were 2.15 times more likely (95% CI 1.14, 4.07) to have abnormal iron status (Geltman et al., 2004). These studies all suggest that the prevention and treatment of maternal anaemia during pregnancy may be an important approach to the prevention of ID among high-risk children as well as reducing adverse pregnancy outcomes (Scholl, 2005).

The obstetric practice of immediate clamping of the umbilical cord after birth as part of the active management of labour potentially deprives the newborn of a transfusion of up to 40 mL/kg body weight of haematopoietic stem cells containing in the placental circulation, providing up to 75 mg of iron to boost iron stores. A recent trial in Mexico of delayed (2 minutes or more) clamping of the umbilical cord compared to immediate clamping found significantly higher mean corpuscular volume, serum ferritin and total body iron in infants at the age of 6 months (Chaparro, Neufeld, Alavez, Cedillo, & Dewey, 2006). A meta-analysis of this and 14 other trials confirms that early cord clamping can be a major cause of anaemia in early infancy, and that delayed clamping consistently improves iron status up to 6 months of age without adverse risks to the newborn (Hutton, & Hassan, 2007).

Iron requirements increase substantially to about 0.1 mg/kg body weight daily after the age of 6 months as blood volume increases with growth and foetal stores of iron are exhausted. The requirement is higher per kg body weight than at any other time in life. Exogenous iron is provided through breast milk which contains iron low in content (0.6 mg/l) but uniquely well absorbed and utilised. However, prolonged breastfeeding after 6 months of age can lead to ID if there are insufficient additional sources of iron in the weaning diet. Formula milk is fortified with iron (commonly 6 mg/L in the United Kingdom) and so formula-fed infants are unlikely to become iron-deficient in the first 12 months of life (Moy, 2000).

However, the inadvisable early introduction of large quantities of cow's milk as the major milk source at around the age of 6 months is commonplace in some communities in the United Kingdom and is associated with a significant risk of developing ID. In a study of infant-feeding practices in an inner city housing estate in Birmingham, infants who had already been started on cow's milk by their mothers before the age of 6 months were randomly allocated to either continue consuming cow's milk or to receive an iron-fortified formula containing 12 mg/L of iron. At 18 months 31% of the cow's milk group compared to only 2% of the formula-fed group were anaemic, and at 2 years 26% of the cow's milk group were anaemic whilst none of the formula-fed group were (Daly et al., 1996). Similar results come from the Euro-Growth study where the mean age of introduction of cow's milk was 10 months. The duration of feeding of cow's milk had the strongest and most consistent negative influence on Hb and iron status indicators at the age of 12 months. For every month of cow's milk feeding, there was an average decrease of 2 g/L in Hb (Male et al., 2001).

After the age of 12 months, a greater proportion of the daily iron requirement will be met by the weaning diet, usually from non-haem iron sources such as iron-fortified breakfast cereals and iron-fortified flours made into breads and from vegetable sources. Commercially prepared baby foods are not required by law to be fortified with iron, and children at this age are unlikely to be consuming much in the way of meat-based foods containing haem iron. Analysis of the typical Birmingham toddler's weaning diet indicates its particularly low iron content with over 80% of these young children failing to meet the reference nutrient intake (RNI) for iron of 7.8 mg/day. In addition to the large volume of cow's milk in these children's diets, tea was also frequently administered from an early age in the feeding bottle (Daly, MacDonald, & Booth, 1998). Tannins in tea bind iron and reduces its bioavailability, and so is a risk factor for ID in children already eating diets of marginal iron content (Temme, & Hoydonock, 2002).

## 4. IRON DEFICIENCY AND DEFICITS IN PSYCHOMOTOR DEVELOPMENT

Animal model studies have demonstrated that iron is required for normal myelination of nerves, neuronal metabolic activity and the formation of neurotransmitters such as dopamine, serotonin and GABA (Beard, Connor, & Jones, 1993). Irreversible changes in brain iron distribution can occur in iron-deficient rats even after prolonged iron repletion if the ID occurs during a critical phase of early brain development (Felt, & Lozoff, 1996). The relevance of these findings in often severely iron-deficient rat models to the human infant has been demonstrated by the finding of abnormal auditory and visual system functioning in children who had suffered earlier IDA in infancy.

Auditory brainstem responses (ABR) and visual evoked potentials (VEP) provide non-invasive measures of nerve transmission and CNS functioning and normally show dramatic changes during infancy as a result of progressive myelination of these systems. Significant delays in the waveform of ABR and VEP have been demonstrated in 4-year-old children who had IDA in infancy compared to non-anaemic controls (Roncagliolo, Garrido, Walter, Peirano, & Lozoff, 1998, Algarin, Peirano, Garrido, Pizarro, & Lozoff, 2003). This suggests that impaired myelination due to ID during this period of brain development leads to longlasting effects on auditory and visual system functioning. These alterations could also contribute to the specific cognitive and behavioural outcomes in children with IDA, and impaired myelination could also affect the development of motor function (Angulo-Kinzler et al., 2002).

Many reports have shown an association between IDA and impaired cognitive and psychomotor development in infants and young children (Walker et al., 2007). Yet proof of causality remains unproven because of many confounding factors. Children with IDA usually come from the poorer segments of society where other factors such as low birth weight, environmental deprivation, lack of stimulation, poor maternal IQ and education, social stress and other nutritional deficits may be the cause of both the ID and the developmental deficits (Logan, Martins, & Gilbert, 2001, Grantham-McGregor, & Ani, 2001, McCann, & Ames, 2007).

Two key questions have emerged, namely (a) does prevention of iron deficiency through iron supplementation lead to improved developmental outcome, and (b) does treatment of IDA reverse any established deficits. The former requires preventative trials where young infants who are randomised to groups receiving various levels of iron intake including no supplementation or placebo (either by iron-fortified formula milks or weaning foods of differing iron content or by the administration of iron supplements) are assessed for developmental outcome according to their subsequent iron status. The latter requires treatment trials where children with ID or IDA are randomised to receive iron or placebo for varying durations, and subsequent changes in developmental scores are measured after treatment. Such studies are subject to considerable ethical dilemmas about withholding a potentially beneficial intervention from developing young children and do not rule out the presence of a causal link between ID and developmental deficits, as this deficit may be irreversible as suggested by the neuro-physiological studies.

Despite a considerable number of these sorts of studies having already been conducted, no definite conclusions are possible because of methodological problems, inconsistencies between studies and residual environmental confounding (Logan, 1999). Most studies have utilised the Bayley Scales of Infant Development which are the standard measures of global development in early childhood and are divided into two age-stratified sub-scales, Motor Development Index (MDI) and Psychomotor Development Index (PDI), as their main outcome. Yet global measures of child development such as the Bayley scores may be inappropriate for measuring the more subtle effects of iron deficiency on behaviour, attention and sociability. Recent research on the effect of iron supplementation in pre-school Greek children has emphasised the importance of measuring the speed of information processing, accuracy of discrimination and conceptual learning to get a better understanding of the effects of ID on cognitive function (Metallinos-Katsaras et al., 2004).

Cross-sectional baseline data from an iron intervention study in young children in Costa Rica showed that those with mild IDA (Hb < 105 g/L) or moderate IDA (Hb < 100 g/L) have significantly lower MDI and PDI scores compared to children with ID but not IDA and non-iron-deficient children (Lozoff, Brittenham, & Wolf, 1987). Long-term follow-up of these children to age 19 years has revealed that those children who had moderate IDA in early children continued to display deficits in cognitive skills throughout their school years compared to non-anaemic children, despite having had corrective iron therapy in infancy (Lozoff, Jiminez, & Wolf, 1991; Lozoff, Jiminez, Hagen, Mollen, & Wolf, 2000; Lozoff, Jiminez, & Smith, 2006). At 19 years, previously anaemic of low socio-economic status demonstrated a widening gap in cognitive scores compared to those from middle socio-economic background. Whilst these findings might reflect the neurophysiological findings of an irreversible effect of iron deficiency on a critical early phase of brain development, the results might still be due to uncontrolled environmental confounders.

Preventative trials of iron fortification or supplementation are difficult to conduct because of the large number of subjects required to demonstrate an effect, loss to follow-up and uncertainty that the preventative intervention has been followed and have yielded inconclusive results on the question of whether iron deficiency has a causal link to developmental deficits. Canadian infants randomised to receive iron-fortified rather than unfortified formula had superior psychomotor development at 9 and 12 months, but the benefit had disappeared by 15 months (Moffatt, Longstaffe, Besant, & Dureski, 1994). Anaemic infants in Birmingham (Hb <110 g/L) randomised to be fed on iron-fortified formula rather than continuing on cow's milk were found to have better scores on the Griffiths' scales of Infant Development at the age of 2 years (Williams et al., 1999). Yet another UK trial of the consumption of iron-fortified formula compared to cows' milk between the ages of 9 to 18 months showed no significant difference in development despite an improvement in iron status (Morley et al., 1999). In Chile, a preventative trial involving different levels of iron fortification of formulas given to nearly 2,000 infants found no difference in global Bayley scores between those who developed IDA (Hb <100 g/L) (22.6% of the unsupplemented group compared to 3.1% of the supplemented). There were, however, a number of more subtle differences in motor functioning, tremulousness, social behaviour, and fearfulness in the anaemic children which would be congruent with current understanding of the effects of ID on the developing brain (Lozoff et al., 2003).

Various large-scale preventative trials of iron supplementation of pre-school children have all shown benefit in promoting motor, social, cognitive and language development. In Zanzibar, iron supplementation of children aged 6–59 months improved language and motor development in those whose Hb was less than 90 g/L, although in this study children were also treated with antihelminthics that also had an independent positive effect on motor and language skills (Stoltzfus, & Dreyfuss, 2001). In Bangladesh, a trial of weekly combined supplementation of infants up to the age of 1 year with iron, zinc and other micronutrients demonstrated a beneficial effect on motor development (Black et al., 2004). However, a similar trial with Indonesian infants found that daily supplementation with iron and zinc had no effect on psychomotor development whilst supplementation with iron alone was effective, indicating possible competition for absorptive pathways (Lind et al., 2004).

Treatment trials of children with IDA show no convincing evidence of any effect on improving psychomotor development in the short term (Grantham-McGregor, & Ani, 2001), and the effect of longer-term treatment remains unclear although the limited data would be compatible with a clinically significant effect. A 2-month-long controlled trial of iron versus placebo in anaemic young children in Birmingham ($Hb < 110$ g/L) found that treated children increased their level of Hb and their number of new developmental skills on the Denver Developmental Screening test (Aukett, Parks, Scott, & Wharton, 1986). Substantially greater effects were reported from a 4-month long RCT in anaemic children in Indonesia ($Hb < 105$ g/L) in which the difference in pre- to post-treatment change in Bayley PDI and MDI scores between the iron-treated and placebo groups was 18.4 and 18.8, respectively (Idjradinata, & Pollitt, 1993).

There has been debate as to whether ID without anaemia could have a significant adverse effect on development, but there is very little data to support this contention or evidence of a linear dose effect (McCann, & Ames, 2007). The previously cited cross-sectional data on iron status and developmental scores (Lozoff et al., 1987) suggest that only ID sufficiently severe to cause IDA would have this effect supporting earlier observations of no difference in MDI scores between young children with ID and those who were iron-replete (Oski, Honig, Helu, & Howanitz, 1983).

## 5. IRON DEFICIENCY AND SUSCEPTIBILITY TO INFECTION

There is a common perception that iron-deficient anaemic children are more prone to infections and which may be alleviated by iron supplementation (MacKay, 1928). In vitro studies do demonstrate that iron deficiency may depress aspects of cell-mediated immunity (reduced polymorph neutrophil function, depression of T-lymphocyte numbers, defective T-lymphocyte-induced proliferative response, impaired natural killer cell activity, impaired interleukin-2 production, reduced production of macrophage migration inhibition factor, impairment of delayed cutaneous hypersensitivity) but not humoral immunity (Oppenheimer, 2001). Alternatively, ID has been said to provide 'nutritional immunity' to infection by reducing iron-binding proteins (transferrin and lactoferrin) and blocking tissue release of iron, thereby making iron unavailable for bacterial growth (Weinburg, 1978).

Field studies of the effect of ID on morbidity from infection are very scanty and come mostly from Third World settings where they are confounded by other nutritional deficits and social deprivation ultimately resulting from poverty. Uncontrolled observations have noted that anaemia may be more common in children admitted to hospital, with infections such as chronic mucocutaneous candidiasis and staphylococcal skin infections, although the infection might be the cause of the anaemia rather than vice versa. On the other hand, it was found that Somali nomads in refugee camps had fewer infections if iron-deficient compared to those with normal iron status, and in Papua New Guinea, anaemic children were less likely to be admitted to hospital with malaria and other infections (Oppenheimer, 2001). The lack of evidence of a significant effect of ID on increasing morbidity from infections is perhaps not surprising as the degree of impairment of cell-mediated immunity in ID is relatively mild compared to that associated with congenital or acquired immune deficiency syndromes.

## 6. PREVENTION OF IRON DEFICIENCY IN CHILDHOOD

There are various public health approaches to the prevention of ID, namely dietary improvement through nutritional education, supplementation with iron medicine, fortification of milk or food with iron and screening for ID or IDA and treatment (secondary prevention).

### *6.1. Dietary Education*

The nutritional messages for the prevention of ID are clear, i.e. promotion of breastfeeding for the first 6 months of life, avoidance of cow's milk in the first year, provision of iron-fortified formula, provision of iron-rich weaning foods such as meat, oily fish, breakfast cereals, pulses and green vegetables, provision of vitamin C to enhance absorption of iron and avoidance of tea and high-fibre foods that inhibit its absorption.

However, putting these messages into practice is easier said than done! A primary care team in Bristol, UK, with a predominantly Afro-Caribbean population found a prevalence of IDA of 25% in young children aged 14 months. A programme of dietary education delivered by public health nurses during pregnancy and the first year of life about the use of iron-fortified formula and weaning foods successfully reduced the prevalence to 8% over 2 years, but after the initial enthusiasm this was difficult to sustain (James, Lawson, Male, & Oakhill, 1989, James, Laing, Logan, & Rossadle, 1997). A large-scale randomised controlled trial involving 1,000 infants in inner city Birmingham, UK, sought to compare the effect of an intensive programme of dietary education consisting of three monthly home visits to mothers by public health nurses supplied with leaflets and audio-taped dietary messages in various languages compared to routine child health clinic-based dietary advice (Childs, Aukett, Darbyshire, Ilett, & Livera, 1997). Unfortunately, this trial failed to show any benefit of the intensive intervention compared to the controls. A third of both groups were anaemic at 18 months and there was no improvement in the iron content of their diets. One might speculate about why this dietary education intervention failed. The advice offered might not have been feasible for mothers to implement because of expense or poor availability or it might have been culturally inappropriate. An approach utilising community participation rather than being health professional-led might have been more appropriate.

### *6.2. Iron Supplementation*

International bodies have recommended that universal oral supplementation with 2 mg/kg body weight of iron daily in the form of ferrous sulphate or ferrous gluconate should be given to children aged 6–24 months at significant risk of dietary ID or where the anaemia prevalence is greater than 40% (Stoltzfus, & Dreyfuss, 1998), although few countries have adopted this approach. It is therefore important to consider the benefits and risks of this public health approach as iron supplementation may have adverse effects such as the generation of free radicals that impair cellular functions and suppress enzyme activity, chronic iron overload and haemochromatosis in genetically susceptible individuals, impaired absorption of other nutrients such as zinc and increased morbidity from infections.

The Ministry of Health of Israel and of the Palestinian National Authority provide all infants with iron syrup supplements since 1985 to overcome a high prevalence of IDA (30–60%) due to short duration of breastfeeding and early use of cow's milk (Palti, Adler, Hurvitz, Tamir, &

Freier, 1987). However, compliance with oral iron is low with only 26% continuing to give iron at 9 months of age because of unpleasant taste or gastro-intestinal side effects such as nausea, vomiting, epigastric discomfort, black diarrhoea and stained teeth (Amsel, Boaz, Ballin, Filk, & Ore, 2002). Subsequently, the high prevalence of IDA persists (Kaluski et al., 2000). Additionally, there is also the increased risk of potentially fatal accidental acute iron toxicity if bottles of iron are to be found in every household.

Furthermore, in vitro studies have demonstrated that microbes proliferate with increasing iron content of the culture medium. Concerns were first raised about the safety of iron supplementation following a report of increased risk of *Escherichia coli* sepsis in newborns given parenteral iron injections (Barry, & Reeve, 1977). Subsequently, further reports (mostly from tropical countries) suggested an increased risk of respiratory infections, diarrhoea and malaria in subjects receiving oral iron supplements (Oppenheimer, 2001). Although a systematic review of 28 randomised controlled trials had identified no harmful effects of oral or parenteral iron supplementation or iron-fortified formula and cereals on the overall risk of infection in children (Gera, & Sachdev, 2002), a recent community-based trial of the impact of iron, zinc and folic acid supplementation on morbidity and mortality in young children in Zanzibar where malaria transmission is intense found an increased risk of hospitalisation and mortality from malaria (Sazawal et al., 2006), although not in a similar trial in Nepal where exposure to malaria is low (Tielsch et al., 2006).

A recent review of the benefits and risks has concluded that community iron status and neurobehavioural development are certainly improved by supplementation of all young children. There was no effect on growth in children with ID, but optimal height and weight gain can be jeopardised in non-ID children. The review concluded that iron supplementation should be targeted towards iron-deficient children rather than the whole population (Iannotti, Tielsch, Black, & Black, 2006).

### 6.3. *Iron Fortification of Food*

Fortification of food vehicles with absorbable iron is probably the most cost-effective primary prevention strategy to prevent ID, but does depend upon there being a suitable milk or staple food that is consumed in adequate quantities by all in within a community (Zimmerman, & Hurrell, 1997). Fortification of formula feeds (Moy, 2000), commercially prepared weaning foods, bread flour, breakfast cereals and condiments such as salt, sugar and curry powder have all been tried. However, the effectiveness of food fortification is limited by bioavailability of iron in cereal-based foods, the ability of the gut to absorb increasing concentrations of iron and by the adverse effects of iron on the food vehicle such as fat oxidation that limits shelf-life and causes discolouration and metallic taste. Many foods contain inhibitors of iron absorption such as phytic acid and polyphenols in cereals and legumes, and calcium and casein in milk products. However, the absorption of fortification iron can be enhanced by the addition of vitamin C, dried red blood cells or the chelating agent Sodium Iron EDTA that prevents iron from binding with cereal inhibitors (Hurrell, 1997). Safety aspects of iron fortification of food also have to be acknowledged. Some individuals who consume large amounts of the fortified food may receive an excess exposure whilst those with smaller appetites may receive inadequate amounts to prevent ID. However, in field trials adverse effects such as an increased incidence of diarrhoea or respiratory illness have not been found (Heresi et al., 1995).

One programme of iron fortification that has been effective in reducing the prevalence of IDA is the WIC (Special Supplemental Food Program for Women, Infants and Children) in the United States. This federally funded programme of nutritional supplementation of low-income pregnant and lactating women and young children at risk of nutritional deficiency was started in the 1970s and continues to reach around 3 million people. The programme provides enrolled infants with iron-fortified formula (12 mg iron/L), iron-fortified cereal and vitamin C-fortified juice. Evaluations of state programmes all show a decrease over time in the prevalence of IDA. In a New Haven inner city black and Hispanic community, the prevalence of severe IDA (defined as Hb <98 g/L) in young children fell from 23% to 1% between 1971 and 1984 (Vazquez-Seoane, Windom, & Pearson, 1985). More recent reports from the US Center for Disease Control Pediatric Nutrition Surveillance system indicate that the prevalence of IDA in US children continues to decline (Sherry, Mei, & Yip, 2001).

Elsewhere, however, population-based iron fortification programmes have had little impact on the overall prevalence of ID in small children often due to problems of sustainability of a food fortification programme and poor availability and affordability of the iron-fortified food (Yip, 2002). A novel approach of home fortification using single-dose sachets of lipid-encapsulated iron and other nutrients in the form of 'Sprinkles' that can be added directly to food on the plate has shown promise in decreasing the prevalence of IDA in young (Zlotkin et al., 2005).

### *6.4. Screening for Anaemia*

Blood test screening offers an opportunity for secondary prevention of IDA by identifying anaemic individuals and then offering treatment along with dietary advice. A relatively simple and cheap estimation of Hb or haematocrit can be performed from a capillary blood sample in a clinic or paediatric office setting. The American Academy of Pediatrics recommends universal screening with Hb or Hct once between ages 9 and 12 months and again 6 months later in communities with a high prevalence of IDA, and selective screening for children at risk of ID (e.g. low birth weight or premature infants, those being breastfed for longer periods and those consuming an excessive amount of cows milk) from lower prevalence communities. Usually, no further investigation of a low Hb level is undertaken unless there is a poor response to iron therapy. Subsequently, many million children are screened and re-tested each year as part of standard paediatric office practice in the United States.

An anaemia screening programme has been in operation for the past 15 years in community child health clinics in central Birmingham, which serve predominantly Asian immigrant and economically disadvantaged White families who had previously been shown to be at risk of ID. All children who attended a routine universal Child Health Surveillance appointment with a public health nurse at the age of 21 months were offered an Hb screening test. About 30–40% were found to have a Hb <110 reading on the HemoCue haemoglobinometer. An evaluation of this screening programme, however, found that it did not fulfil the criteria for a justifiable population screening programme (Moy, Aukett, 2000). Population coverage was limited to those that attended the clinic appointment; the test was acceptable but often inaccurate due to the difficulties in obtaining a good capillary specimen of blood from young children, 31% were non-compliant with treatment and the age at which the screening was done was probably not optimal to affect any improvement on impaired psychomotor development. On the other hand, the public health nurses found that performing the screening test did enhance the importance of the dietary messages they sought to communicate to parents.

## 7. CONCLUSIONS

Iron deficiency remains a common problem in young children not only in developing countries but also from poor and ethnic minority communities in developed countries. However, haemoglobin level that is often measured in nutritional surveys is an insensitive marker of ID and can lead to an overestimation of the true prevalence. Furthermore, recent population-based survey of haemoglobin distribution suggests that a cutoff lower than the conventional 110 g/L would better correlate with the biological effects of iron deficiency anaemia. The inappropriate early introduction of cow's milk as the major nutrient source and the low iron content of typical weaning diets are the key risk factors for the development of ID. Recent neurophysiological studies have demonstrated abnormalities in central nervous system functioning in iron-deficient young children that support the many observations of an association between ID and possible irreversible impairment of their psychomotor development. However, a causal relationship, whilst the justification for public health programmes to improve iron nutrition, remains unproven because of environmental confounding. Whilst ID can depress aspects of cell-mediated immunity and thereby increase susceptibility to infection, clinical relevance remains unclear. Various approaches to the primary and secondary prevention of ID exist, but their public health impact has been variable. The most promising approach to the eradication of ID at the population level would be iron supplementation of essential food items.

## REFERENCES


Aggett, P., Agostoni, C., Axelsson, I., Bresson, J.-L., Goulet, O., Hernell, O., et al. (2002). Iron metabolism and requirements in early childhood: Do we know enough? A commentary by the ESPGHAN Committee on Nutrition. *Journal of Pediatric Gastroenterology and Nutrition, 34*, 337–345.

Algarin, C., Peirano, P., Garrido, M., Pizarro, F., & Lozoff, B. (2003). Iron deficiency anemia in infancy: Long-lasting effects on auditory and visual system functioning. *Pediatric Research, 53*, 217–223.

Amsel, S., Boaz, M., Ballin, A., Filk, D., & Ore, N. (2002). Low compliance of iron supplementation and relation to socio-economic status in Israel. *Pediatrics, 110*, 410–411.

Angulo-Kinzler, R., Periano, P., Lin, E., Algarin, C., Garrido M., & Lozoff, B. (2002). Twenty four hour motor activity in human infants with and without iron deficiency anaemia. *Early Human Development, 70*, 85–101.

Aukett, M., Parks, Y., Scott, P., & Wharton, B. (1986). Treatment with iron increases weight gain and psychomotor development. *Archives of Disease in Childhood, 61*, 849–857.

Barry, D., & Reeve, A. (1977). Increased incidence of gram-negative neonatal sepsis with intramuscular iron administration. *Pediatrics, 60*, 908–912.

Beard, J., Connor, J., & Jones, B. (1993). Iron in the brain. *Nutrition Reviews, 51*, 157–170.

Black, M., Baqui, A., Zaman, K., Persson, L., El Artifeen, S., Le, K., et al. (2004). Iron and zinc supplementation promote motor development and exploratory behaviour among Bangladeshi Infants. *American Journal of Clinical Nutrition, 80*, 903–910.

Brotanek, J., Gosz, J., Weltzman, M., & Flores, G. (2007). Iron deficiency in early childhood in the United States: Risk factors and racial/ethnic disparities. *Pediatrics, 120*, 568–575.

Chaparro, C., Neufeld, L., Alavez, G., Cedillo, R., & Dewey, K. (2006). Effect of timing of umbilical cord clamping on iron status in Mexican infants: A randomised controlled trial. *Lancet, 367*, 1997–2004.

Childs, F., Aukett, A., Darbyshire, P. Ilett, S., & Livera, L. (1997). Dietary education and iron deficiency anaemia in the inner city. *Archives of Disease in Childhood, 76*, 144–147.

Colomer, J., Colomer, C., Gutierrez, D., Jubert, A., Nolasco, A., Donat, J., et al. (1990). Anaemia during pregnancy as a risk factor for infant iron deficiency: Report from the Valencia Infant Aneamia Cohort (VIAC) study. *Paediatric and Perinatal Epidemiology, 4*, 196–204.

Daly, A., MacDonald, A., Aukett, A., Williams, J., Davidson, J., & Booth, I. (1996). Prevention of anaemia in inner city toddlers by an iron supplemented cows' milk formula. *Archives of Disease in Childhood, 75*, 9–16.

Daly, A., MacDonald, A., & Booth, I. (1998). Diet and disadvantage; observations on infant feeding from an inner city. *Journal of Human Nutrition and Dietetics 1998, 11*, 381–389.

De Pee, S., Bloem, M., Sari, M., Kleiss, L., & Yip, R. (2002). The high prevalence of low hemoglobin concentration among Indonesian infants ages 3–5 months is related to maternal anemia. *Journal of Nutrition, 132*, 2215–2221.

Emond, A. M., Hawkins, N., Pennock, C. Golding, J., & the ALSPAC Children in Focus Team. (1996). Haemoglobin and ferritin concentrations in infants at 8 months of age. *Archives of Disease in Childhood, 74*, 36–39.

Felt, B., & Lozoff, B. (1996). Brain iron and behaviour of rats are not normalised by treatment of iron deficiency anemia during early development. *Journal of Nutrition, 126*, 693–701.

Geltman, P., Meyers, A., Mehta, S., Brugnara, C., Villon, I., Wu, Y., et al. (2004). Daily multivitamins with iron to prevent anemia in high-risk infants: A randomised clinical trial. *Pediatrics, 114*, 86–93.

Gera, T., & Sachdev, H. (2002). Effect of iron supplementation on incidence of infectious illness in children: Systematic review. *British Medical Journal, 325*, 1142–1144.

Grantham-McGregor, S., & Ani, C. (2001). A review of studies on the effect of iron deficiency on cognitive development in children. *Journal of Nutrition, 131*, 649S–666S.

Gregory, J., Collins, D., Davies, P., Hughes, J., & Clarke, P. (1995). *National Diet and Nutrition Survey: Children aged 1½ to 4½ years* (Vol. 1). Report of the diet and nutrition survey. London: HMSO.

Heresi, G., Pizarro, F., Olivares, M., Cayasso, M., Hertrampf, E., Walter, T., et al. (1995). Effect of supplementation with an iron-fortified milk on incidence of diarrhea and respiratory infection in urban-resident infants. *Scandinavian Journal of Infectious Diseases, 27*, 385–389.

Hurrell, R. (1997). Prevention of iron deficiency through food fortification. *Nutrition Reviews, 55*, 210–222.

Hussain, M., Gaafar, T., Laulicht, M., & Hoffebrand, A. (1997). Relation of maternal and cord serum ferritin. *Archives of Disease in Childhood, 52*, 782–784.

Hutton, E., & Hassan, E. (2007). Late vs early clamping of the umbilical cord in full-term neonates: Systematic review and meta-analysis of controlled trials. *Journal of American Medical Association, 297*, 1241–1252.

Idjradinata, P., & Pollitt, E. (1993). Reversal of developmental delays in iron deficient anemic infants treated with iron. *Lancet, 341*, 1–4.

Iannotti, L., Tielsch, J., Black, M., & Black, R. (2006). Iron supplementation in early childhood: Health benefits and risks. *American Journal of Clinical Nutrition, 84*, 1261–1276.

James, J., Lawson, P., Male, P., & Oakhill, A. (1989). Preventing iron deficiency anaemia in pre-school children by implementing an educational and screening programme in an inner city practice. *British Medical Journal, 299*, 838–840.

James, J., Laing, G., Logan, S., & Rossadle, M. (1997). Feasibility of screening for iron deficiency anaemia in general practice. *British Medical Journal, 315*, 102–103.

Kaluski, D., Leventhal, A., Averbuch, Y., Rishpon, S., Cohen-Dar, M., Habib, S., et al. (2001). Five decades of trends in anemia in Israeli infants: Implications for food fortification policy. *European Journal of Clinical Nutrition, 55*, 82–87.

Kilbride, J., Baker, T., Parapia, L., Khoury, S., Shuqaidef, S., & Jerwood, D. (1999). Anaemia during pregnancy as a risk factor for iron deficiency in infancy: Case-control study in Jordan. *International Journal of Epidemiology, 28*, 461–468.

Lind, T., Lonnerdal, B., Stenlund, H., Gumayanti, I., Ismail, D., Seswandhana, R., et al. (2004). A community-based randomised controlled trial of iron and zinc supplementation in Indonesian infants; effects on growth and development. *American Journal of Clinical Nutrition, 80*, 729–736.

Logan, S. (1999). Iron deficiency and developmental deficit: The jury is still out. *British Medical Journal, 318*, 697–698.

Logan, S., Martins, S., & Gilbert, R. (2001). Iron therapy for improving psychomotor development and cognitive function in children under the age of three with iron deficiency anaemia (Cochrane Review). In *The Cochrane Library* (Issue 2). Oxford: Update Software.

Looker, A., Dallman, P., Carroll, M., Gunter, E., & Johnson, C. (1997). Prevalence of iron deficiency in the United States. *Journal of the American Medical Association, 277*, 973–976.

Lozoff, B., Brittenham, G., & Wolf, A. (1987). Iron deficiency anemia and iron therapy: Effects on infant developmental test performance. *Pediatrics, 79*, 981–995.

Lozoff, B., Jiminez, E., & Wolf, A. (1991). Long-term developmental outcome of infants with iron deficiency. *New England Journal of Medicine, 325*, 687–694.

Lozoff, B., Jiminez, E., Hagen, J., Mollen, E., & Wolf, A. (2000). Poorer behavioural and developmental outcome more than 10 years after treatment for iron deficiency in infancy. *Pediatrics, 105*, E51.

Lozoff, B., De Andraca, I., Castillo, M., Smith, J., Walter, T., & Pino, P. (2003). Behavioural and developmental effects of preventing iron deficiency anemia in healthy full-term infants. *Pediatrics, 112*, 846–854.

Lozoff, B., Jiminez, E., & Smith, J. (2006). Double burden of iron deficiency in infancy and low socioeconomic status. *Archives of Pediatric and Adolescent Medicine, 160*, 1108–1113.

MacKay, H. (1928). Anaemia in infancy; its prevalence and prevention. *Archives of Disease in Childhood, 3*, 117–147.

Male, C., Persson, L., Freeman, V., Guerra, A., van't Hof, M., Haschke, F., et al. (2001). Prevalence of iron deficiency in 12 month old infants from 11 European areas and influence of dietary factors on iron status (Euro-Growth study). *Acta Paediatrica, 90*, 492–498.

McCann, J., & Ames, B. (2007). An overview of evidence for a causal relation between iron deficiency during development and deficits in cognitive or behavioural function. *American Journal of Clinical Nutrition, 85*, 931–945.

Metallinos-Katsaras, E., Valassi-Adam, E., Dewey, K. G. Lonnerdal, B., Stamoulakatou, A., & Pollitt, E. (2004). Effect of iron supplementation on cognition in Greek preschoolers. *European Journal of Clinical Nutrition, 58*, 1532–1542.

Moffatt, M., Longstaffe, S., Besant, J., & Dureski, C. (1994). Prevention of iron deficiency and psychomotor decline in high risk infants through use of iron-fortified infant formula: A randomised clinical trial. *Journal of Pediatrics, 125*, 527–533.

Morley, R., Abbott, R., Fairweather-Tate, S., MacFadyen, U., Stephenson, T., & Lucas, A. (1999). Iron fortified follow on formula from 9 to 18 months improves iron status but not development or growth: A randomised trial. *Archives of Disease in Childhood, 81*, 247–252.

Moy, R. (2000). Iron fortification of infant formula. *Nutrition Research Reviews, 13*, 215–227.

Moy, R., & Aukett, A. (2000). Population screening for anaemia in the inner city. *Ambulatory Child Health, 6*, 11–18.

Oppenheimer, S. (2001). Iron and its relation to immunity and infectious disease. *Journal of Nutrition, 131*, 616S–635S.

Oski, F., Honig, A., Helu, B., & Howanitz, P. (1983). Effect of iron therapy on behaviour performance in non-anemic iron-deficient infants. *Pediatrics, 71*, 877–880.

Oski, F. (1993). Iron deficiency in infancy and childhood. *New England Journal of Medicine, 329*, 190–193.

Palti, H., Adler, B., Hurvitz, J., Tamir, D., & Freier, S. (1987). Use of iron supplements in infancy: A field trial. *Bulletin of the World Health Organisation, 65*, 87–94.

Roncagliolo, M., Garrido, M., Walter, T., Peirano, P., & Lozoff, B. (1998). Evidence of altered central nervous system development in infants with iron deficiency anemia at 6 months: Delayed maturation of auditory brainstem responses. *American Journal of Clinical Nutrition, 68*, 683–690.

Sazawal, S., Black, R., Ramsan, M., Chwaya, H., Stoltzfus, R., Dutta, A., et al. (2006). Effect of routine prophylactic supplementation with iron and folic acid on admission to hospital and mortality in preschool children in a high malaria transmission setting: A community-based, randomised, placebo-controlled trial. *Lancet, 367*, 133–143.

Scholl, T. (2005). Iron status during pregnancy: Setting the stage for mother and infant. *American Journal of Clinical Nutrition, 81*, 1218S–1222S.

Schneider, J., Fuyii, M., Lamp, C., Lonnerdal, B., Dewey, K., & Zidenberg-Cherr, S. (2005). Anemia, iron deficiency, and iron deficiency anemia in 12–36 month old children from low-income families. *American Journal of Clinical Nutrition, 82*, 1269–1275.

Sherriff, A., Emond, A., Hawkins, N., Golding, J., & the ALSPAC Children in Focus Team. (1999). Haemoglobin and ferritin concentrations in children aged 12 and 18 months. *Archives of Disease in Childhood, 80*, 153–157.

Sherry, B., Mei, Z., & Yip, R. (2001). Continuation of the decline in prevalence of anemia in low income infants and children in five states. *Pediatrics, 107*, 677–682.

Stoltzfus, R., & Dreyfuss, M. (1998). Guidelines for the use of iron supplements to prevent and treat iron deficiency anemia. Washington, DC: The International Nutritional Anemia Consultative Group, the World Health Organisation and the United Nations Children's Fund.

Temme, E., & Hoydonock, P. (2002). Tea consumption and iron status. *European Journal of Clinical Nutrition, 56*, 379–386.

Thane, C., Walmsley, C., Bates, C., Prentice, A., & Cole, T. (2000). Risk factors for poor iron status in British toddlers: Further analysis of data from the National Diet and Nutrition Survey of children aged 1½ to 4½ years. *Public Health Nutrition, 3*, 433–440.

Thurlow, R., Winichagoon, P., Green, T., Wasantwisut, E., Pongcharoen, T., Bailey, K., et al. (2005). Only a small proportion of anemia in northeast Thai schoolchildren is associated with iron deficiency. *American Journal of Clinical Nutrition, 82*, 380–387.

Tielsch, J., Khatry, S., Stoltzfus, R., Katz, J., LeClerq, S., Adhikan, R., et al. (2006). Effect of routine prophylactic supplementation with iron and folic acid on preschool child mortality in Southern Nepal: Community-based, cluster-randomised, placebo-controlled trial. *Lancet, 367*, 144–152.

Vazquez-Seoane, P., Windom, R., & Pearson, H. (1985). Disappearance of iron deficiency anemia in a high risk infant population given supplemental iron. *New England Journal of Medicine, 313*, 1239–1240.

Walker, S., Wachs, T., Gardner, J., Lozoff, B., Wasserman, G., Pollitt, E., et al. (2007). Child development; risk factors for adverse outcomes in developing countries. *Lancet, 369*, 145–157.

Weinburg, E. (1978). Iron and infection. *Microbiology Reviews, 42*, 45–66.

White, K. (2005). Anemia is a poor predictor of iron deficiency among toddlers in the United States: For heme the bell tolls. *Pediatrics, 115*, 315–320.

Williams, J., Wolff, A., Daly, A., MacDonald, A., Aukett, A., & Booth, I. (1999). Iron supplemented formula milk related to reduction in psychomotor decline in infants from inner city areas: Randomised study. *British Medical Journal, 318*, 693–698.

World Health Organisation/United Nations University/UNICEF. (2001). Iron deficiency anaemia, assessment, prevention and control: A guide for programme managers. Geneva: WHO.

Wright, C., Kelly, J., Trail, A., Parkinson, K., & Summerfield, G. (2004). The diagnosis of borderline iron deficiency: Results of a therapeutic trial. *Archives of Disease in Childhood, 89*, 1028–1031.

Yip, R., & Dallman, P. R. (1988). The roles of inflammation and iron deficiency as causes of anemia. *American Journal of Clinical Nutrition, 48*, 1295–1300.

Yip, R. (2002). Prevention and control of iron deficiency; policy and strategic issues. *Journal of Nutrition, 132*, 802S–805S.

Zimmerman, M., & Hurrell, R. (2007). Nutritional iron deficiency. *Lancet, 370*, 511–520.

Zlotkin, S., Schauer, C., Christofides, A., Sharieff, W., Tondeur, M., & Ziauddin Hyder, S. (2005). Micronutrient Spinkles to control childhood anemia. *PLoS Medicine, 2*:e1 DOI:10.1371/journal.pmed.00200001.g001

# 19 Iron and Women's Health

*Adrianne Bendich and Ronit Zilberboim*

**Summary**

- Iron is an essential mineral required for transport of oxygen throughout the body and for the optimal development of the fetal brain.
- Iron-intake requirements are regulated by the size of body iron stores. Lifestyle factors that often influence iron status in women include amount of iron consumed, use of oral contraceptives, use of hormone replacement therapy, vegetarianism, intestinal parasites, blood donation, and regular intense exercise.
- Iron-deficiency prevalence, defined by direct measurement of tissue iron, is about 30% in adult women in developed countries; in contrast, iron deficiency defined by indirect measures such as in NHANES suggests a prevalence of about 10%. Iron deficiency is associated with impaired physical work performance, developmental delay, depressed immune function, and cognitive impairment.
- Women are more at risk for iron deficiency and anemia due to iron losses through menstruation, pregnancy, and lactation and/or inadequate dietary iron intake.
- During pregnancy, indices of iron status are in constant flux; however, iron deficiency anemia in the first trimester is consistently associated with premature delivery, low birth weight, perinatal infant and maternal mortality.
- Iron requirements decrease by about 50% after menopause; however, iron is one of the nutrients that are often deficient in the diets of many older adults.
- Adverse effects associated with genetically inherited disease characterized by high iron body stores, namely hemochromatosis, may include the development of diabetes, cancer, cardiovascular disease, and low bone mineral density.

**Key Words:** Iron deficiency anemia; transferrin; ferritin; hemochromatosis; pregnancy; lactation; osteoporosis; diabetes; fertility

## 1. INTRODUCTION

The objective of this chapter is to provide an overview of the role of iron in women during their adult lives beginning with menstruation. Particular emphasis is placed on the iron requirements during pregnancy and lactation. Other areas reviewed include the association of low iron status and decreased fertility, and the effects of low iron status on the risk of diabetes and osteoporosis.

Iron (chemical symbol: Fe) is an essential element with atomic number 26 and atomic weight 55.8. It is the fourth most common element on earth. The average iron content of the human body

From: *Nutrition and Health: Iron Deficiency and Overload*
Edited by: S. Yehuda and D.I. Mostofsky, DOI 10.1007/978-1-59745-462-9_19

is 3–4 g. The majority of the iron, almost 2/3 (~2 g), is found in hemoglobin in circulating red blood cells (RBC), 25% in iron stores, and most of the remaining iron, about 15%, is found in myoglobin in muscle and in a variety of enzymes. Women have a smaller RBC mass and iron stores than men. An average adult woman's body contains about 35–50 mg iron/kg body weight (bw) while men's contains about 40–50 mg iron/kg bw (Wood & Ronnenberg, 2006; Brody, 1999; IOM, 2001).

The recommended daily iron intakes for women of childbearing potential (Table 1) ranges between 18 and 27 mg/d depending upon age and/or pregnancy/lactation status. The actual intakes of women of childbearing age (Table 2) indicate clearly that the vast majority of women do not consume the recommended level of iron daily. Table 2 also indicates that the intakes are skewed (the average (mean intake) is greater than the midpoint level (median intake) of consumption) and is indicative of a population in which there are a few women with high iron intakes, but the majority of women consume significantly less iron than even the average intake level.

**Table 1**
**Estimated Average Requirement (EAR) and Recommended Daily Intakes (RDA) of Iron for Women of Childbearing Years and During Pregnancy and Lactation**

| | *Child Bearing* | | *Pregnancy* | | *Lactation* | |
|---|---|---|---|---|---|---|
| *Age years*[1] | *EAR mg/d* | *RDA mg/d* | *EAR mg/d* | *RDA mg/d* | *EAR mg/d* | *RDA mg/d* |
| 9–13 | 5.7 | 8[2] | N/A | N/A | N/A | N/A |
| 14–18 | 7.9 | 15[2] | 23 | 27 | 7 | 10 |
| 19–30 | 8.1 | 18 | 22 | 27 | 6.5 | 9 |
| 31–50 | 8.1 | 18 | 22 | 27 | 6.5 | 9 |
| 51–70 | 5 | 8 | N/A | N/A | N/A | N/A |
| >70 | 5 | 8 | N/A | N/A | N/A | N/A |

[1]Vegetarians 32 mg/d.
[2]+ 1.1 mg for growth spurt + 2.5 mg for menstruation before 14 years.
IOM (2001).

**Table 2**
**NHANES Dietary Intake of Iron in Women of Childbearing Years, data from 1999 to 2000**

| *Age (years)* | *Mean Intake (mg)* | *Median Intake (mg)* |
|---|---|---|
| 12–19 | 13.4 | 11.7 |
| 20–39 | 13.7 | 11.6 |
| 40–59 | 13.6 | 11.6 |

Ervin et al. (2004).

Recent data from NHANES III confirm that about 59% of premenopausal and 23% of postmenapusal women had an average iron intake at or below recommended levels (Blanck, Cogswell, Gillespie, & Reyes, 2005). Iron deficiency (as defined by serum indices) in the United States, using data from NHANES (1999–2000), was found in 16% of girls and women 12–49 years (Looker, Cogswell, & Gunter, 2002), and the severest classification of iron deficiency, iron deficiency anemia, was seen in 4% of US women 20–49 years (Wood & Ronnenberg, 2006). Similar levels of iron deficiency as well as iron deficiency anemia have been reported in France, the United Kingdom, and recently in Sweden, following the discontinuation of iron fortification of wheat flour (Zimmermann & Hurrell, 2007).

## 2. BASIC BIOCHEMICAL FUNCTIONS

Iron exists in several oxidative states in the environment varying from −2 to +6; however, for biological functions only the ferrous ($Fe^{+2}$), ferric ($Fe^{+3}$), and ferryl ($Fe^{+4}$) forms are present. Ferrous iron is the most soluble form reaching a solubility of about 0.1 M at neutral pH, while ferric iron solubility only reaches $10^{-18}$ M. Nearly all iron in the body is protein-bound rather than free; ferric iron is not soluble in aqueous media and free ferrous iron can be toxic.

There are four major classes of iron-containing proteins in the body. These include iron-containing heme proteins such as hemoglobin, myoglobin, cytochromes, coenzymes (that contain one atom of tightly bound iron such as catalase and peroxidase); iron–sulfur enzymes (flavoproteins, hemeflavoproteins); proteins for iron storage and transport (transferrin, lactoferrin, ferritin, hemosiderin); and other iron-containing or activated enzymes (sulfur, nonheme enzymes) (Brody, 1999).

### *2.1. Major Heme Proteins*

Hemoglobin (Hb), the major heme protein in RBC, is composed of four subunits, each containing an iron atom attached to a heme group. Each ferrous (reduced form) iron atom attaches to one oxygen molecule and carries oxygen from the environment to all cells and tissues in the body. The affinity of Hb to oxygen is dependent upon both the pH and the oxygen concentration of the environment (bloodstream). In the lungs, where there is a high concentration of oxygen (less acidic, higher pH), Hb binds oxygen avidly. In contrast, in the relatively more acidic pH that is found in the capillary beds, there is a decrease in the affinity of Hb for oxygen and the oxygen molecule is released and delivered to the surrounding cells (IOM, 2001; Wood & Ronnenberg, 2006; Brody, 1999).

Myoglobin, the major oxygen carrying protein in muscle cytoplasm, also serves as a short-term storage site for oxygen. It binds oxygen more tightly than Hb, and this higher oxygen affinity permits an increased rate of diffusion of oxygen from RBC to the surrounding muscle cytoplasm and within cells into the mitochondria. The rate of oxygen release increases when the environment contains very low levels of oxygen (Brody, 1999; IOM, 2001).

Cytochromes are membrane-bound heme proteins that are located in mitochondria and endoplasmic reticulum and act as electron carriers (IOM, 2001).

## 3. METABOLISM

Iron homeostasis is maintained by regulation of iron absorption from dietary sources including supplements. Absorption is related to iron stored in ferritin such that absorption is inversely proportional to serum ferritin concentrations. Absorption of iron is also dependent upon other factors including the chemical form of iron in the diet and the presence of foods that may either enhance or reduce the absorption of iron when consumed concomitantly (Hallberg, 2001; Brody, 1999; IOM, 2001). Importantly, there is a limited capacity to excrete iron and excess is stored mainly in the liver, spleen, and bone marrow (Hurrell, 1997; IOM, 2001).

### 3.1. Chemical Forms and Absorption of Iron

Iron absorption is highly regulated and is primarily dependent upon the level of iron stores and erythropoietic activity. For a constant diet, daily iron absorption is linearly directly associated with the log of the serum ferritin level. An individual's rate of iron absorption remains relatively constant once iron stores are saturated. The exceptions would be individuals with inherited disorders of iron absorption (discussed below). An important corollary to the finding that iron absorption is highly controlled once iron stores are replete is that it would not be possible to induce iron overload by consuming diets that are very high in iron even in the most bioavailable form such as heme iron.

The regulatory factors at the absorptive surface of the intestine and at the cellular level have not been completely elucidated. An intestinal heme iron transporter protein has been identified and is responsive to iron deficiency. There is a separate transporter protein for nonheme iron, and the ferric form requires reduction to the ferrous form before it can be transported across the intestinal lumen and absorbed (Zimmermann & Hurrell, 2007). Even though there are feedback mechanisms to increase the synthesis of iron carrier proteins, if the diet contains insufficient iron to meet requirements iron deficiency will develop.

It is well known that the iron in the diet can be divided into two forms: heme and nonheme. The heme iron is in the ferrous form attached to the porphyrin ring, whereas most of the nonheme iron is in the ferric form and only a small portion is in the ferrous form. Heme iron is only slightly influenced by dietary factors and relatively unaffected by the high pH of the upper intestine, making it overall highly bioavailable, at about 30%. The major source of heme iron in the diet is red meat and it provides approximately 15% of the dietary iron consumed/day. In contrast, nonheme iron contributes about 85% of the daily dietary iron intake, but is not absorbed as well as the heme iron. Nonheme iron absorption is dependent upon its solubility and interactions with other meal components. Gastric acid is needed to maintain nonheme iron in solution, and therefore decreased stomach acid may lead to impaired iron absorption. Some nonheme iron can be found in meats where it is about 20% bioavailable, whereas when it is found in plant foods is only about 10% bioavailable. The most bioavailable form of iron is found in human milk with a bioavailability of 50% (Brody, 1999; IOM, 2001; Hallberg, 2001).

Several food components enhance the absorption of nonheme iron. For example, ascorbic acid (vitamin C) increases iron absorption twofold when a small amount (25 mg) is consumed with foods, and further absorption is enhanced 3–6 fold with 50 mg/meal of ascorbic acid. The mechanism by which ascorbic acid increases iron bioavailability is related to iron's oxidation state, i.e., reduction of ferric iron to the ferrous form (Hurrell, Reddy, Juillerat, & Cook, 2006). Other organic acids, such as citric, lactic, and malic acid also enhance iron absorption from nonheme sources. It has been suggested that animal tissues increase nonheme iron absorption independent of their contribution via the heme portion. However, Reddy et al. suggested that higher iron status associated with the consumption of an omnivorous diet including animal tissues is due more to the intake of heme iron than to its enhancing effect of nonheme iron absorption (Reddy, Hurrell, & Cook, 2006).

Inhibitors of nonheme iron absorption include phytates found in legumes, rice, and grains, and the tannic acid found in tea and certain vegetable proteins. Unfortunately, foods that contain the inhibitors are also often the major potential sources of iron in the food supply, especially in developing countries. Certain minerals such as calcium also have the potential to compete for iron's absorption in the gastrointestinal tract; however, the data on the biological consequences of this interaction are not consistent (Bendich, 2001).

The level of gastric acid in the stomach also affects the potential to absorb iron; achlorhydria has been associated with increased risk of iron deficiency and is seen most frequently in the elderly. Other conditions that affect the absorptive surface of the GI tract, such as celiac disease, can also result in impaired iron (as well as other nutrients) absorption (Zimmermann & Hurrell, 2007).

### *3.2. Transport*

Transferrin, the plasma protein responsible for iron transport, is mainly synthesized in the liver and its principal function is to transport ionic iron to the liver, spleen, and bone marrow. Transferrin levels rise with iron deficiency and fall with high iron stores. Transferrin carries iron in the plasma that has been either absorbed from the intestine or released from macrophages during RBC breakdown as ferric iron. The movement of iron from the plasma into cells is regulated by the concentration of transferrin receptors on the cell membrane promoting uptake of iron. Most (70–90%) of iron on transferrin is delivered to the bone marrow for Hb synthesis in RBC precursors. The remainder of circulating iron is taken up by other tissues for synthesis of iron-containing compounds such as myoglobin, cytochromes, and iron-containing enzymes (Wood & Ronnenberg, 2006).

### *3.3. Storage*

Iron is stored in the cells and tissues of the body in the form of ferritin or when ample iron is available for storage as a condensed form of ferritin called hemosiderin. Although all cells can store iron, the primary sites for iron storage are the liver, spleen, and bone marrow. In adults, each 1 μg/L of serum ferritin is considered to represent 8 mg of stored iron (IOM, 2001). Women usually have lower iron stores than men; data from NHANES III indicate that the median serum ferritin concentration for adult menstruating women is 36–40 μg/L (Blanck et al., 2005). Women in industrialized countries have an even lower median serum ferritin concentration that lies close to 25–30 μg/L (Rangan, Blight, & Binns, 1998). In comparison, US adult men have average serum ferritin levels of about 125 μg/L (Wood & Ronnenberg, 2006). Iron status as reflected by the amount of iron stored is critical for pregnancy, and adequate iron reserves of about 500 mg are needed to meet the physiologic requirements for reproductive purposes. Unfortunately, these requirements can not be met through dietary iron alone, and therefore Milman suggested a particular scale for prophylaxis iron supplementation based on iron status (Milman, 2006b). Serum ferritin >70 μg/L is indicative of ample iron stores while levels of <30 μg/L are indicative of small iron reserves, and iron supplementation may be recommended for these individuals. When serum ferritin values are below 12 μg/L, iron stores are depleted and iron deficiency anemia is seen (IOM, 2001). Very high serum ferritin levels (>400 μg/L in men and >300 μg/L in women) are associated with the genetic defect, hemochromatosis /iron overload disease (discussed further below).

### *3.4. Excretion*

The body's iron concentration is normally highly conserved. Iron that is bound to transferrin is normally not lost in the urine due to its size. In the absence of bleeding from wounds and/or menstruation or pregnancy, only a small amount of iron is excreted daily. In non-menstruating women, daily basal iron losses are between 0.9 and 1.02 mg: the majority is lost in the feces (0.6 mg), skin (0.2–0.3 mg), and urine (0.08 mg). Menstruating women lose approximately 1.5 mg/d and during pregnancy the loss increases to 4–5 mg/d (IOM, 2001). Normal menstrual flow is about 35 ml per menstrual period, which contains about 18 mg of iron, as blood contains 0.5 mg of iron per milliliter. Excessive menstrual blood loss is the most common cause of iron deficiency in women (Brody, 1999).

## 4. CLINICAL VALUES OF IRON STATUS

Hematological tests to assess iron status include RBC characteristics such as Hb concentration and hematocrit. Biochemical tests such as serum ferritin concentration and transferrin saturation can detect earlier changes in iron status (Yip et al., 1998). Clinical measures that are frequently used to describe the iron status of women include Hb, serum ferritin, and transferrin saturation. The normal range of Hb in adult non-pregnant females is 120–160 g/L or 7.4–9.9 mmol/L; serum ferritin's normal range is from 10 to 200 μg/L and transferrin saturation is normally between 20% and 45% (Wood & Ronnenberg, 2006).

### *4.1. Iron Deficiency*

Iron deficiency is widespread, affecting all ethnic groups and thus a major global problem. It is considered the most prevalent nutrient deficiency in the world affecting about 2 billion people. Most of the burden of iron deficiency is seen in developing countries where overall its prevalence is about 50%, while in the developed world about 10% of the population is affected (Denic & Agarwal, 2007; Matkovic, Badenhop, & Ilich, 2000).

No single test is accepted for diagnosis of iron deficiency; therefore, iron deficiency is defined by the Centers for Disease Control (CDC) when two or more of the following indices of iron status are not in the normal range: serum ferritin $\leq$12 μg/L; free erythrocyte protoporphyrin is $>$1.24 μmol/L; serum transferrin saturation is $<$14% for 12–15 year olds or $<$15% for 16–39 year olds (Yip et al., 1998). Iron deficiency occurs as iron stores decline and when there is also a decrease in iron transport to all tissues including the RBC. Hb and/or hematocrit levels may be normal even though the individual has iron deficiency; therefore, these measurements do not accurately reflect total iron status. Further, a wide variation exists in Hb values in iron-replete women (from 120 to 160 g/L); there may be a 25% decrease in Hb value while it is still considered in the normal range. As deficiency progresses, there is also an increase in serum transferrin receptors lacking iron, indicating that newly forming RBCs are not getting sufficient iron to fill nearly all of the receptors (Denic & Agarwal, 2007). Hallberg argues that a hemopoetic index of iron deficiency is representative of iron deficiency for all cells in the body that require iron; and thus even though it may not be possible to measure physiological adverse effects in, for instance, muscle, there are negative effects of iron deficiency that would be ongoing in that tissue (Hallberg, 2001).

In the United States, iron deficiency is seen in over 11 million infants, children, adolescents, and adult women. According to NHANES III, 7.8 million adolescent girls and women of childbearing age have non-anemic iron deficiency (Looker, Orwoll, et al., 1997). In developed countries, iron deficiency is often seen in individuals who donate blood frequently. A single annual donation of 0.5 L of blood is equivalent to a loss of 200–250 mg of iron. This concentration of iron is equivalent to a daily loss of ~0.6–0.7 mg/d every day for 1 year. Because blood donation triggers the formation of new RBC, the concentration of stored iron is decreased as indicated by the lower serum ferritin concentration seen in blood donors. Another at-risk group is elite athletes who engage in regular intense exercise and have been shown to have increased blood loss. To compensate somewhat for the increased blood loss of elite athletes, the Institute of Medicine recommends about 30–70% higher intake of iron for those who engage in regular intense exercise (Wood & Ronnenberg, 2006). Female athletes often under-consume calories, making it likely that they will not consume adequate dietary iron. Female athletes may have increased requirements for iron because of increased losses in sweat, feces, and urine, intravascular hemolysis, and impaired absorption (Akabas & Dolins, 2005). In contrast, in developing countries iron deficiency is often linked to the presence of intestinal parasites that cause blood loss for prolonged periods of time.

### *4.2. Iron Deficiency Anemia*

Individuals with CDC defined iron deficiency and a low hemoglobin value are considered to have iron deficiency anemia (IDA). As the synthesis of iron-containing proteins, such as Hb, become compromised to the point at which values fall below specified cutoffs such as <118 g/L for females 12–14 years old and <120 g/L for non-pregnant females 15–39 years, IDA occurs (Looker, Dallman, Carroll, Gunter, & Johnson, 1997). The cutoffs in Hb levels used for the definition of IDA are based on the differences of the mean of the population and two standard deviations, which has no biological meaning; and negative effects in certain tissues may be observed before Hb reaches the definition values (Hallberg, 2001).

Iron deficiency and IDA continue to be critical issues in women who enroll in the US Armed Services even though they appear physically fit. McClung et al. looked at the prevalence of iron deficiency and IDA in 1,216 US female military personnel. They report that the prevalence of iron deficiency was greater in the basic combat training group (32.8%) compared to values at initial entry to the army (13.4%) or following at least 6 months of permanent assignment (9.6%). The prevalence of IDA was also greater in the basic combat training group (20.9%) than following the initial entry to the army (5.8%) or following at least 6 months of permanent assignment (4.8%) (McClung, Marchitelli, Friedl, & Young, 2006). Both iron deficiency and IDA were greater in Hispanic and African-American personnel than in Caucasians. Frith-Terhune et al. also found, in NHANES III, that 6.2% of Mexican-American women aged 12–39 had iron deficiency anemia compared to 2.3% of age-matched non-Hispanic white women (Frith-Terhune, Cogswell, Khan, Will, & Ramakrishnan, 2000). NHANES II data showed that obese and overweight children and teens were 2.3 times more likely to be iron-deficient compared to age-matched normal weight children (Nead, Halterman, Kaczorowski, Auinger, & Weitzman, 2004).

### *4.3. Iron Supplementation and Fortification*

In developed countries where fortification of food has been common in the past 3–4 decades, there has been an overall reduction in the prevalence of IDA. Still there are segments of the population that remain iron-deficient, illustrating the difficulties in maintaining a positive iron balance (Denic & Agarwal, 2007). It is important to note that the strict control of iron absorption appears to apply to dietary iron and not to iron supplements (Hallberg, 2001). Peterson et al. reported that iron supplements increase serum ferritin concentrations more quickly than dietary interventions, in their randomized controlled trial of 44 iron-deficient women who received either iron supplementation or a high-iron diet for 12 weeks with a 6 month follow-up (Patterson, Brown, Roberts, & Seldon, 2001). However, Blanck et al. analyzed data from NHANES III and found that healthy adults ($n = 5{,}948$) who took supplements containing average daily amounts of iron at $\leq$3 X RDA did not have significantly higher iron transport or stores than did those who did not take supplements (Blanck et al., 2005).

### *4.4. Iron and Ovulation*

Several essential nutrients have been associated with fertility in men and women. There do not appear to be controlled intervention studies that have examined the potential for iron to affect fertility in women. There is, however, one publication that examined the association of the use of supplements containing iron and decreased risk of ovulatory infertility (Chavarro, Rich-Edwards, Rosner, & Willett, 2006). This prospective survey study examined the pregnancy events between 1991 and 1999. The cohort included women who did not have a history of infertility, were married and had also provided dietary information, and were enrolled in the Nurses' Health Study II. The women were asked if they had tried to become pregnant for more than 1 year without success and were queried every 2 years about their pregnancy status and other medical information concerning fertility. Use of dietary supplements containing any concentration of iron was associated with a significant 50% reduction in risk of ovulatory infertility. Use of iron supplements containing >41 mg of iron/day had a significant 70% reduction in ovulatory infertility risk.

Interestingly, this study also found an increased risk of infertility associated with the highest intake of heme iron when the data were adjusted for age and energy intake; the risk was no longer significant when the multivariable analysis was performed. The authors point out that there are a number of lifestyle characteristics that differ between women who use supplements and those that do not; also women who consume diets high in heme iron, principally from red meats, had lifestyle factors, including smoking, that were significantly different than women with low heme iron intakes. A possible role of iron in the function of the ovum has been suggested based upon the finding of transferrin receptors and transferrin in this cell. Iron may also be important in the development of the ovarian follicle (Chavarro et al., 2006).

### *4.5. Iron Overload*

As discussed above, iron absorption is highly regulated and iron losses are relatively small under most circumstances. There are certain genctic defects that result in hereditary hemochromatosis. Most of the genetic defects are autosomal and recessive and affect about 1 in 250 persons. Five genes that increase the absorption of iron without also increasing iron excretion have been identified (Denic & Agarwal, 2007). Iron overload is characterized by increased absorption of iron and the progressive depositing of iron in hepatocytes and in cells of the heart, pancreas, and joints. The serious consequences of this genetic defect are seen mainly in middle age when iron deposits have accumulated over the lifetime and reach a level associated with heart valve and muscle defects, arthritic pain in joints, and liver damage. The most common treatment for hemochromatosis is blood donation several times per year. Rarely, iron deposits result from chronic consumption of excessive levels of iron and/or repeated blood transfusions (Brody, 1999). The Institute of Medicine had derived a tolerable upper intake level of iron for adults (including pregnant and lactating women) of 45 mg/d (IOM, 2001).

### *4.6. Lifestyle Factors That Can Affect Women's Iron Status*

Women who use oral contraceptives often have a decrease in their menstrual blood losses, which results in a lower iron requirement than menstruating women who do not use oral contraceptives. In contrast, peri- and post-menopausal women who use hormone replacement therapy may continue to menstruate, and therefore iron requirement is higher than post-menopausal women who have completely stopped menstruating. Vegetarians usually consume diets that are rich in foods which contain plant phytates and lack heme iron. Vegetarian diets contain food sources of iron with decreased bioavailability compared to diets containing meat. The bioavailability of iron from mainly vegetables in the diet is about 10% rather than 18% when diets contain more bioavailable sources such as heme iron. The consequence is that vegetarians need to consume more foods with nonheme iron or consume an iron supplement to maintain their iron balance. The iron RDA for vegetarians is 32 mg/d which is almost twice that for non-vegetarians (Akabas & Dolins, 2005).

## 5. PREGNANCY AND LACTATION

Pregnancy results in many physiological changes including an increase in blood volume of about 40% with a concomitant increase in RBC mass of 15–20%. The result of the expanded blood volume compared to expanded red cells is that the hemoglobin and hematocrit levels are relatively decreased and are usually the lowest during the second trimester and begin to rise in the third trimester (Picciano, 2003). The increased maternal RBC combined with the needs of the growing fetus as well as the need to be able to compensate for iron losses at delivery explain much of the increased iron requirements during pregnancy (Allen, 2000).

### *5.1. Iron Requirements*

While energy needs increase during pregnancy by 14–18%, nutrient needs of pregnant women increase the most for iron (50%), folate (50%), iodine (47%), vitamin B6 (46%), zinc (38%), and protein (38%) (Turner, 2006). The average concentration of absorbed iron required during pregnancy to maintain the woman's iron status is ~4.4 mg/d for the entire gestation, gradually increasing from 0.8 mg/d in the first trimester to 7.5 mg/d in the third trimester, as iron transfer to the fetus occurs mainly in the third trimester (Milman, 2006a). Iron requirements continuously increase from 6.4 mg/day in the first trimester to 18.8 mg/day in the second trimester to 22.4 mg/day in the third trimester. While gross total iron requirements are estimated to be about 1,250 mg, net maternal iron loss due to pregnancy is estimated at 600–800 mg. These are calculated based upon basal losses of 250 mg, fetal and placental deposition of 320 mg, increase in hemoglobin mass of 500 mg, and blood loss at delivery of 200 mg (Turner, 2006; Milman, 2006a). The net maternal iron requirement during pregnancy is about 1 g, which is equivalent to the amount of iron contained in 4 units of blood (Zimmermann & Hurrell, 2007).

Iron is rapidly mobilized from maternal tissue stores (ferritin) to both expand the blood volume of the mother and for the synthesis of placental and fetal tissues during early pregnancy, and thus ferritin levels may drop from a normal value of 60 μg/L to about 15 μg/L during the first 2 months of pregnancy. Serum transferrin levels increase during pregnancy and may serve to facilitate iron transport from mother to fetus (Picciano, 2003).

Iron bioavailability increases throughout pregnancy, with the most pronounced increase to 25% after 20–30 weeks of gestation (Milman, 2006a), the time of most rapid fetal growth. Despite this increase, it appears that fetal iron requirements in the first trimester are met at the expense of maternal iron stores (Turner, 2006). Furthermore, even though iron absorption efficiency increases during pregnancy, and even if the dietary sources are from heme iron and other highly bioavailable sources, Hallberg clearly states that the iron needs during pregnancy for women in developed as well as developing countries cannot be met by diet alone, especially during the latter part of the second and the third trimesters (Hallberg, 2001). Overall, the drop in serum ferritin in early pregnancy cannot be completely reversed with dietary iron supplements (Brody, 1999). The need for supplemental iron is especially critical in teen pregnancy where the teen may not have completed her full growth.

The newborn's iron status is dependent on maternal iron status during pregnancy as well as on their birth weight. At a low birth weight of ~2,500 g the iron content of the newborn is ~200 mg; at a normal birth weight of ~3,500 g the iron content is ~270 mg. Most of the iron transferred to the fetus occurs after week 30 of gestation, and therefore pre-term infants may not receive optimal levels of iron (Milman, 2006a). When maternal iron status is poor, the number of placental transferrin receptors increases so that more iron is taken up by the placenta into the fetus (Allen, 2000). If the mother is anemic (see below), there are lower iron stores in the neonate.

### 5.2. *Iron Deficiency Anemia*

Pregnancy-associated anemia is diagnosed by trimester using the following cutoff values: a pregnant woman has a hemoglobin concentration that is less than 110 g/L in the first trimester, 105 g/L in the second trimester, and 110 g/L in the third trimester she is considered anemic. Maternal anemia diagnosed before week 20 is associated with an increased risk of preterm delivery; diagnosis in the third trimester is usually reflective of the normal expansion of the maternal plasma volume and is therefore not an accurate index of iron status. Specifically, anemia and iron deficiencies are associated with over a twofold increased risk of low birth weight and preterm delivery (Scholl & Reilly, 2000b). Severe anemia, and even moderate IDA are also associated with a twofold higher risk of maternal death (Turner, 2006), possibly because of heart failure, hemorrhage, and/or infection (IOM, 2001). Of importance, high hemoglobin and/or high ferritin levels in the third trimester are associated with increased risk of preterm delivery (Scholl & Reilly, 2000a).

The World Health Organization estimates that 35–75% (56% on average) of pregnant women in developing countries and 18% of women from industrialized countries are anemic during some point in their pregnancies, with many already anemic at the time of conception (Allen, 2000). Anemia in pregnant women is associated with several factors: insufficient intake; increased requirement for maternal tissue accumulation in early gestation; expansion and dilution of blood volume; the transfer of iron (3–4 mg/day) to the fetus during the last trimester of gestation (Scholl & Reilly, 2000b).

The relationship curve between maternal hemoglobin levels and pregnancy outcome is "U" shaped, with low hemoglobin probably reflecting the combination of true and physiologic anemia and high hemoglobin reflecting failure of the plasma volume to expand and/or possibly maternal infection. Both high (above 130 g/L) and very low Hb (below 90 g/L) concentrations at delivery are associated with adverse pregnancy outcomes. High serum ferritin during the third trimester of pregnancy is a marker of an increased risk for preterm delivery, and high levels of hemoglobin or hematocrit late in pregnancy are also associated with increased risk of preterm delivery (Scholl & Reilly, 2000b).

### 5.3. *Iron Supplementation*

As indicated above, iron absorption efficiency as well as recommended intakes increases during pregnancy. However, if actual iron intakes remain in the range consumed in early pregnancy, the increased efficiency of absorption cannot compensate for the lack of sufficient dietary iron. Moreover, if iron status is low at the initiation of pregnancy, it will be difficult to make up for this deficit and also fulfill the increased needs especially during the later half of pregnancy

(Milman, 2006a; Bodnar, Cogswell, & McDonald, 2005). Thus, there may be a need for iron supplementation in a significant proportion of pregnant women in Western, developed countries. As iron deficiency anemia is a major public health problem in fertile women in developing countries, the decision about supplementation during pregnancy in developing countries may be moot.

Although a significant proportion of women of childbearing potential may have low iron status during their pregnancy, there is a continuing debate about the need for iron supplementation during pregnancy in many Western countries (Milman, 2006b). Further, there are limited data in pregnant women who are initially iron-replete and not anemic. Fortunately, well-controlled intervention studies in both women with low and normal iron status in the first trimester have shown that iron supplementation could enhance maternal iron status as well as neonatal iron status, reduce the risk of preterm delivery, and lead to significantly higher birth weights in full-term infants (Cogswell, Parvanta, Ickes, Yip, & Brittenham, 2003) . In one placebo-controlled intervention study in non-anemic US women with normal iron stores, only 1 out of 86 women in the placebo group remained non-anemic and iron-replete throughout her pregnancy. Of interest, provision of 30 mg of supplemental iron beginning at 20 week gestation was insufficient to prevent loss of iron stores in more than half of the cohort, and these women were given 60 mg/day of iron from the 28th week until delivery (Scholl & Reilly, 2000a). It is therefore understandable that if women enter pregnancy with low iron stores, iron supplements may fail to prevent postpartum iron deficiency (Milman, 2006a). In a recent placebo-controlled, double-blind intervention study with initially iron-replete pregnant women, 30 mg of iron given as part of a multivitamin-mineral supplement compared to the supplement without iron given during the second trimester, followed by 30 mg of iron for all women for the remainder of their pregnancies, resulted in a significant increase in birth weight in the offspring of the iron-supplemented women and a significant decrease in the incidence of preterm delivery (Siega-Riz et al., 2006).

Iron supplementation to prevent anemia is recommended for all pregnant women in the US by both the Centers for Disease Control (recommend 30 mg/d beginning at first prenatal visit) and the American College of Obstetricians and Gynecologists (Yip et al., 1998, ACOG, 2007). A recent Cochrane meta-analysis confirmed the benefit of iron supplementation during pregnancy in maintaining maternal iron status during pregnancy and post-natally (Pena-Rosas & Viteri, 2006). Data from NHANES III (1988–1994) indicate that only about 72% of pregnant women were taking an iron supplement even though the median iron intake among pregnant women was only 15 mg/d. The average iron concentration in the supplement used during pregnancy was about 58 mg/d (Cogswell et al., 2003).

There is a lack of consensus concerning the timing of iron supplementation (Rioux & LeBlanc, 2007). Several recommendations indicate that all pregnant women should be given iron supplements during the second and third trimesters. Others recommend supplementation throughout pregnancy and others only if there is evidence of low iron stores in the first trimester (Allen, 2000). In addition to a lack of consensus about initiating iron supplementation, there is also debate concerning the dosage of iron, whether it should be taken daily or weekly, as well as the type of iron (Viteri & Berger, 2005). However, there appears to be agreement that the concentration of iron in a standard multivitamin (18 mg, which is equivalent to 100% of the US daily value) is not sufficient to prevent iron deficiency in most pregnant women in developed countries (Allen, 2000). Milman recommends a dose of 40 mg of ferrous iron as a general iron prophylaxis dose, and that dosing should begin no later than 20 week of gestation (Milman, 2006b). Table 3 provides a synopsis of the recommended levels of supplementation found to prevent reduction in iron stores of Danish women who were iron-replete at 18 weeks gestation. Milman et al.

Table 3
Recommendations for Iron Supplementation During Pregnancy

| *Iron reserves status* | *Serum ferritin μg/L* | *Recommendation mg/d Ferrous Iron* |
|---|---|---|
| Full reserve >500 mg in first trimester | >70 | No supplementation needed |
| Limited reserves | 31–70 | 40 |
| Small reserves | <30 | 80–100 |
| Depleted (iron deficiency) | <12 | 80–100 |
| Depleted and hemoglobin <5th percentile | <12 | 80–100 |

Based upon Milman et al. (2005).

(2005) conducted a placebo-controlled, double-blind randomized trial in 301 Danish women and provided either placebo, 20, 40, 60, or 80 mg/d of ferrous iron from 18 weeks gestation and found the level of iron needed to maintain iron stores was dependent upon ferritin levels as well as serum transferrin receptor levels when supplementation was initiated. A daily dose of 40 mg of ferrous iron from 18 weeks of gestation was adequate to prevent iron deficiency in 90% of women and iron deficiency anemia in 95% of women during pregnancy and postpartum (Milman et al., 2005). Based upon this study, general recommendations for levels of supplementation were either 40 mg/d or 80–100 mg/d depending upon iron stores.

### *5.4. Maternal Iron Supplementation, Pregnancy Outcomes, and Infant Iron Status*

Well-controlled clinical studies have shown that neonates born to mothers who have taken iron supplements during gestation have higher cord blood serum ferritin and, therefore, most likely have higher body iron stores than children of mothers who have taken a placebo. Children of iron-supplemented mothers have a lower risk for becoming iron deficient during infancy and early childhood (Milman, 2006b). Maternal iron supplementation of 30–60 mg/d in the US study described above led to a significantly higher birth weight ($206 \pm 565$ g, $p = 0.010$), a significantly lower incidence of low-birth-weight infants (4% in the supplemented vs. 17% in placebo group, $p = 0.003$), and a significantly lower incidence of preterm low-birth-weight infants (3% vs. 10% in the placebo group, $p = 0.017$) (Cogswell et al., 2003).

### *5.5. Maternal Post-pregnancy Iron Status*

The immediate postpartum period is usually considered as the time of lowest risk of iron deficiency for women of childbearing potential. Under most circumstances, iron status improves following delivery as the expanded maternal RBC mass contracts and there is no longer the loss of iron to the developing fetus. Also, if lactation is begun, the significantly decreased menstrual flow or complete cessation of menstruation also contributes to the increase in iron stores. As discussed below, breast milk iron levels are relatively low compared to maternal supply of iron to the growing fetus.

There are, however, conditions that can compromise maternal iron status following pregnancy. There could be an unexpectedly great loss of blood during delivery, which could significantly reduce maternal iron status. If the woman began pregnancy with a low iron status or anemia and did not take iron supplements, her iron status would be expected to be significantly lower at term birth. The prevalence and risk factors for postpartum iron deficiency reported based on NHANES data from 1988 to 1994 showed that about 13% of US women 20–40 years of age who were 0–6 months postpartum had iron deficiency and about 4% had IDA. Importantly, in this cohort, those women in the poverty category had three to four times higher prevalence, about 30% iron deficiency and about 10% IDA (Bodnar, Cogswell, & Scanlon, 2002). Data from the WIC program indicate that up to 48% of Black women 4–26 weeks postpartum were anemic (not defined in terms of iron deficiency or IDA) (Bodnar, Scanlon, Freedman, Siega-Riz, & Cogswell, 2001).

High pre-pregnancy body mass index is a significant risk factor for postpartum anemia. Anemia risk is doubled for women with a body mass index (BMI) of 28 compared to those with a BMI of 20, and anemia is three times more prevalent with a BMI of 38. Anemia in obese pregnant women following birth may be due to the greater risk of blood loss and other complications during delivery (Bodnar, Siega-Riz, Arab, Chantala, & McDonald, 2004).

Women who deliver multiple fetuses are also at increased risk for postpartum low iron status and anemia (Yip et al., 1998). There is a greater expansion of the maternal blood supply with multiple fetuses as well as an increased need for iron for more than one fetus. There can also be a greater risk of blood loss at delivery.

The consequences of low iron status following pregnancy can include decreased endurance, impaired fitness, and decreased work efficiency – all of which can adversely affect the mother's ability to care for the neonate as well as herself and other family members. Brain function and mood may also be adversely affected by low iron status as iron is an essential co-factor for certain enzymes in the brain. Low concentrations of iron in the brain are associated with decreased neurotransmitter function, reduced thyroid hormone metabolism, and altered cellular and oxidative processes. It is possible that iron status may be a contributing factor in postpartum depression (Bodnar et al., 2005).

The effects of maternal postpartum iron status on infant developmental skills and maternal–infant interactions were studied in a prospective, randomized placebo-controlled intervention study with South African women (Perez et al., 2005). Mothers aged 18–30, whose infants were >38 weeks gestational age and had a birth weight >2,500 g and were breastfeeding, were requested to join the study at 6-week postpartum. Iron status was determined and women found to be iron-deficient and with a hemoglobin between 90 and 115 g/L and two other indices of iron deficiency were divided into two supplement intervention groups: either 25 mg of vitamin C and 10 mg of folic acid ($n = 21$ completed the study) or 25 mg of vitamin C, 10 mg of folic acid, and 125 mg of ferrous sulfate ($n = 30$). A third group of non-anemic postpartum women were not given any supplement ($n = 30$). Data from these 81 mothers who completed the 7.5 month intervention study indicate that the anemic mothers not given iron had poorer maternal–infant interactions than the other two groups whose responses were similar. At 9 months of age, the children born to non-anemic mothers scored significantly higher on tests of developmental skills.

The CDC/IOM have developed a risk assessment algorithm for screening women for postpartum iron status that includes supplementation from delivery through 6 weeks (without biochemical measures) if there was excessive bleeding, multiple births, or anemia in the third trimester. It is recommended that the women should be screened during the postpartum visit to assess their current iron status. Bodnar et al. have identified three other risk factors for postpartum iron deficiency anemia, pre-pregnancy obesity, not exclusive breastfeeding and multiparity, and suggest that these be added to those proposed by CDC/IOM (Bodnar et al., 2005). In fact, they recommend universal screening of women postpartum as iron deficiency has many adverse consequences that can be easily avoided with proper identification of those women with low iron status following delivery.

### *5.6. Lactation*

Breastfeeding is currently recommended by the US Centers for Disease Control for term infants for the first 4–6 months of life (Yip et al., 1998). With regard to iron, breast milk contains the most bioavailable source of iron with a bioavailability of about 50% compared to about a 10% bioavailability for iron from cow milk (Brody, 1999). The iron in human breast milk is contained within a specialized protein called lactoferrin, which is responsible for enhanced absorption.

Although the bioavailability is high, the actual concentration of iron in breast milk is about 20 times lower than that found in cow's milk–based infant formulas. Human milk contains about 0.5 mg/L of iron during the first month of lactation and falls to about 0.3 mg/L by 4–6 months (Brody, 1999). Cow milk–based formulas contains 12 mg/L of iron. Therefore, it is recommended that breast-fed infants be given an iron supplement containing ~7 mg/d to maintain infant's stores during the first 6 months and to ensure growth thereafter. Because of marginal supply of breast milk iron, preterm infants usually receive iron supplements beginning at 2 months of age (Wood & Ronnenberg, 2006).

NHANES III data indicate that about 57% of lactating women use iron supplements (Cogswell et al., 2003). Lactation is not considered an important source of net iron loss in women (Wood & Ronnenberg, 2006). Typical milk volumes of 0.78 L/day produced during lactation are associated with an additional 0.27 mg/day of maternal iron loss. However, the cessation of menstruation often associated with lactation serves to offset this additional iron loss in women who are breastfeeding (Wood & Ronnenberg, 2006).

## 6. MENOPAUSE

Menopause is characterized by a cessation of menstrual bleeding and consequently a reduction in loss of iron from the body. Iron requirements are thus decreased by about 50% after menopause compared to premenopausal requirements. Even though requirements are halved, iron is one of the nutrients that is often deficient in the diets of many older adults and so there still may be a risk for iron deficiency as well as iron deficiency anemia in post-menopausal women (Chernoff, 2000).

### *6.1. Intake*

NHANES data from 1999 to 2000 reports that the mean daily intake of iron in women 40–59 was 13.6 mg and intake for those women 60 years and older was 12.8 mg. The median intakes were 11.6 and 10.8, respectively, which suggests that most women over 60 have intakes near the recommended level of 8 mg/d (Ervin, Wang, Wright, & Kennedy-Stephenson, 2004). Under normal dietary intakes, with the change in the physiological need for iron, there is usually an increase in iron stores with advancing age and average iron stores increase from about 300 to 800 mg in the decade after menopause (Chernoff, 2000).

A recent analysis of essential nutrient intakes of US adults aged 51 and older from the 1994–1996 Continuing Survey of Food Intakes by Individuals (CSFII) indicates that multivitamin-mineral supplement use is a major contributor to iron intakes. Approximately 41% of women in this survey used a multivitamin-mineral supplement daily. A separate iron supplement was taken by 5% or less of the women. Because the estimated average requirement (EAR) for iron is 6 mg/d for adults 51+, <3% of women consumed less than the EAR. Daily iron intakes were similar between those 51–70 years of age and those aged 71 + and were about 11 mg/day from food and about 29 mg/day from food and supplements (Sebastian, Cleveland, Goldman, & Moshfegh, 2007). The consistency of these intakes with the data from NHANES (Ervin et al., 2004) strengthens the contention that iron intakes are adequate for most women 51+ in the United States.

### *6.2. Iron Deficiency and Iron Overload in Older Women*

The prevalence of iron deficiency in the women 51 years and older is about 5%. Confirmation that anemia in the elderly is actually iron deficiency anemia requires both a low hemoglobin level (<120 g/L) as well as a low ferritin level (<12–15 μg/L). Overt signs and symptoms may not be obvious, especially in advanced age with the exception of conjunctival pallor (Smith, 2000).

In contrast to younger age groups, the majority of anemia cases in older adults are not typically due to iron deficiency. Rather, many cases are due to chronic infectious or inflammatory processes that result in "anemia of chronic disease" (Seaverson et al., 2007). Anemia is common in elderly who are hospitalized, institutionalized, and homebound. The most common cause of iron deficiency anemia in elderly is blood loss from the gastro-intestinal tract (Chernoff, 2000).

Garry et al. conducted two studies – a 10-year longitudinal study (48 men and 77 women) and a 1-year cross-sectional study (165 men and 226 women) in healthy white seniors who were aged 60 or over when enrolled in the New Mexico Aging Process Study (Garry, Hunt, & Baumgartner, 2000). The median age of the cohort was 72 years. In the longitudinal study, they found that iron stores were normally distributed in both men and women, with a geometric mean of 113 μg/L for the men and 96 μg/L for the women. Over the 10 years, there was no meaningful change in iron stores. Use of supplemental iron increased iron stores, but the increase was not significant. In the cross-sectional study, there was a significant negative association between male BMI and serum ferritin; in women, there was a significant positive effect of age and supplemental iron on serum ferritin. Garry et al. also report that increasing heme iron intake did not effectively increase iron stores in the elderly (Garry et al., 2000).

Several researchers have commented on the potential for a set point for serum ferritin that is not attained until later life. Once reached, however, it appears that it is difficult to increase iron stores. One caveat is genetic factors that enhance iron storage even in the heterozygote. Another factor in women is the use of hormone replacement therapy (HRT). HRT could delay reaching steady-state iron levels due to continued menstrual blood loss. Also, compared to men, not enough time may have passed for postmenopausal women to reach steady-state levels of iron stores resulting in continued increases in iron absorption with age (Garry et al., 2000). Liu et al. using blood samples from 620 healthy postmenopausal women aged 44–69 who participated in the Nurses' Health Study measured serum ferritin levels to determine if there was a setpoint for iron. They showed that plasma ferritin concentrations increased with age until ~60 year and then reached a plateau (Liu et al., 2003). It is of interest that in this population about 3% were iron-depleted (serum ferritin <12 μg/L) and almost 10% had elevated serum ferritin levels (>200 μg/L). Predictors of elevated ferritin levels included age >60, body mass index (BMI) >25 and higher heme-iron and alcohol intakes.

As discussed above, certain genetic mutations increase the risk of iron overload during aging. A major mutation is found in populations with European origin, and Cade et al. prospectively investigated the iron status, diet, and genetics of over 6,700 UK women aged 35–69 (Cade et al., 2005). The cohort that was selected had about 1/3 vegetarians, 1/3 who ate fish but no meat, and

1/3 that ate meat. DNA was extracted from cheek cells and blood cells, and women who were either homozygous or heterozygous for iron-overload genes were asked to provide dietary information. This subsample included 1,745 who did not carry the genes, 713 were heterozygous, and 31 were homozygous (1.2%). Similar to the finding in the Nurses' Health Study, age and BMI as well as heme iron intakes were highly positively correlated with serum ferritin levels. Of interest, and in line with the data that risk of hemochromatosis increases with age, heme iron affected ferritin levels only in post-menopausal women who were homozygotes and not premenopausal homozygotes. Overall, independent of genetic status, heme iron, and not nonheme iron or iron from dietary supplements, was positively associated with serum ferritin levels.

Virtually all of the data discussed above involved Caucasian women. As indicated above, young Hispanic women have lower iron status than age-matched Caucasians. Seaverson et al. analyzed data from 604 Hispanic and 153 non-Hispanic white adults residing in the same neighborhoods (59–91 years) from the Massachusetts Hispanic Elders Study. They hypothesized that cultural variations in diet (having a more plant-based diet) may influence iron availability and body iron stores and contribute to an increased risk for iron deficiency anemia among some Hispanic older adults (Seaverson et al., 2007). In this population, Hispanics had significantly lower geometric mean serum ferritin levels (74.1 μg/L vs. 100 μg/L, $p < 0.001$), lower hemoglobin concentrations ($137 \pm 13$ vs. $140 \pm 12$ g/L, $p < 0.01$), higher prevalence of anemia (11.5 vs. 7.3%, $p < 0.05$), and a significantly greater percentage of women with suboptimal Hb concentrations (<125 g/L) compared to age-matched Caucasian women (21.4 vs. 13.3%, $p < 0.05$). The percentage of women with iron deficiency anemia was higher (7.2% vs. 2.3%, $p < 0.05$) in older Hispanic women and similar to the percentage seen in younger Hispanic women reported by Frith-Terhune et al. (2000) from NHANES data. Seaverson et al. documented that the older Hispanic women had a 43% lower mean total dietary iron intakes and 31% lower total vitamin C intakes compared to the matched group (Seaverson et al., 2007). The reduced dietary intake of iron as well as vitamin C that can enhance nonheme iron absorption may be the critical factors in the lowered iron status of older Hispanic women.

### 6.3. *Iron Supplement Use in Postmenopausal Women*

Blanck et al., using the NHANES III database, reported that about 22% of post-menopausal women consumed supplements containing iron in the past month. For this analysis, iron supplement use was defined as the consumption of any supplement that contained iron; however, about 95% of these women obtained their supplemental iron from multivitamin/mineral supplements (Blanck et al., 2005). The proportion of supplement users whose average iron intake was below the RDA was about 23% for post-menopausal women. Almost 90% of the sample was Caucasian and BMI averaged about 27 (overweight). Serum ferritin levels were marginally increased in post-menopausal women who consumed more than four times the RDA of iron/day.

## 7. DISEASES RELATED TO IRON STATUS

### 7.1. *Metabolic Syndrome and Type 2 Diabetes*

Based on data from NHANES 1999–2002, 8.2% of women 20 or older had either diagnosed or undiagnosed diabetes while 15.9% of women 65 or older had diagnosed diabetes (Cowie et al., 2006). The mean age at diagnosis of Type 2 diabetes for the total NHANES population (men and women) was 46 years (Koopman, Mainous, Diaz, & Geesey, 2005).

The association of impaired glucose metabolism, metabolic syndrome, and Type 2 diabetes mellitus with high iron status is based upon the findings that these conditions/diseases are common clinical manifestations of iron overload in patients with hemochromatosis. Even moderately elevated iron stores associated with hemochromatosis have been associated with diabetes. Type 2 diabetes occurs in 25–75% of patients with hereditary hemochromatosis (Jehn et al., 2007).

The metabolic syndrome is considered a major risk factor for the development of Type 2 diabetes. The question of whether higher serum ferritin levels are associated with increased risk of the metabolic syndrome was investigated by Jehn et al. using cross-sectional data from NHANES III (Jehn, Clark, & Guallar, 2004). They included 6,044 males and pre- and post-menopausal women >20 years old and classified them as having the metabolic syndrome with respect to their anthropomorphic and biochemical analyses. The average serum ferritin level in pre-menopausal women was 33.6 μg/L, for post-menopausal women it was 93.4 μg/L, and for males it was 139.9 μg/L. The prevalence of the metabolic syndrome was 10.2, 27.8, and 17.5%, respectively, in these groups. When individuals were divided into quintiles based upon their serum ferritin levels, those with metabolic syndrome were over two times more likely to be in the highest quintile of ferritin levels. This was a consistent finding for males as well as both pre- and post-menopausal women. However, the median concentration of serum ferritin associated with these increased risks was 89 μg/L in pre-menopausal women compared to 212 μg/L in post-menopausal women, and was 318 μg/L in the men. In an analysis that did not include individuals with diabetes, insulin resistance increased with increasing serum ferritin levels, but was not linear for post-menopausal women. As these data were from a cross-sectional study, it is unclear if higher serum ferritin levels are predictive of metabolic syndrome.

Vari et al. followed a cohort of men and women for 6 years who did not have a diagnosis of metabolic syndrome at baseline and examined the association of serum ferritin and transferrin levels and the risk of developing the metabolic syndrome (Vari et al., 2007). This publication extends the data already published from their 3-year longitudinal study of the same cohort. At 3 years, they reported that the baseline ferritin and transferrin levels and C-reactive protein (men only), but not serum iron, were independent predictors of the development of hyperglycemia over the 3 years in both men and women (Fumeron et al., 2006). With regard to the 6-year study, the cohort included 278 pre-menopausal women with an average age of 41 and 197 postmenopausal women with an average age of 57. Serum ferritin levels at baseline were in the normal range for the women; however, these were about 1/3 higher in the post- compared to the pre-menopausal women; transferrin levels were similar. In both groups of women, those who had serum ferritin and transferrin levels in the upper tertile had over a fourfold increased risk of incident metabolic syndrome. As indicated above, normally, serum ferritin and transferrin levels are inversely related, and therefore, it appears that in this study, there is a perturbation of iron handling that may be a factor in the increased risk of the metabolic syndrome (Vari et al., 2007).

Jiang et al. prospectively identified a cohort of 698 women participants (43–68 years old) in the Nurses' Health Study who were free of diabetes in 1989–1990 and had developed diabetes by 2000. They age-matched the cases with controls with no diabetes and attempted to match the obese diabetics with BMI-matched controls. When they looked back at the baseline levels of fasting insulin and hemoglobin A1C, in both cases and controls, these were significantly higher in the cases. The cases also were heavier, had family histories of diabetes, and exercised less often than controls. Although total iron intakes were very similar, the cases consumed more heme iron, and total calories at baseline and serum ferritin levels were significantly higher in the cases than controls. No information was provided about the serum ferritin levels in pre- vs. post-menopausal women. They also found that the ratio of transferrin receptors to ferritin were significantly lower in the cases at baseline. Based upon these factors, the relative risk of developing diabetes was over

3 in the pre-menopausal cases and over 2 in the post-menopausal women. Thus these two indices of iron storage were predictive of diabetes development independent of other well-recognized risk factors for diabetes (Jiang et al., 2004).

In a separate study, Jehn et al. examined the association of plasma ferritin and risk of Type 2 diabetes using a case-control study design and included a random sample of 576 cases of diabetes and 690 matched controls from the US-based Atherosclerosis Risk in Communities (ARIC) study. Their study included both pre- and post-menopausal women who were primarily Caucasian. In the entire cohort baseline, plasma ferritin levels were significantly higher in cases vs. controls. Post-menopausal women had 2/3 higher ferritin levels than pre-menopausal women, and showed a trend of increased diabetes with increasing plasma ferritin levels. When the analysis was restricted to Caucasian women, there was a non-significant small increase in diabetes risk associated with a fivefold increase in ferritin levels (Jehn et al., 2007). Even though there was an increase in diabetes risk as plasma ferritin levels increased in the entire cohort, the association disappeared when it was adjusted for components of the metabolic syndrome. In contrast to the findings of Jiang et al. (2004), the authors concluded that plasma ferritin did not predict risk of diabetes beyond established risk factors. Further, as ferritin levels can be increased by other factors such as inflammation (also increased in metabolic syndrome and diabetes) and these increases were relatively modest compared to those seen in individuals with hemochromatosis, the increased ferritin may not be directly reflective of a change in iron stores. Thus, from these data, it remains unclear whether higher iron stores are involved in causing diabetes or if higher ferritin levels is another consequence of the metabolic syndrome. No data were provided concerning serum transferrin levels.

A second recent survey study examined the association of elevated serum ferritin levels (below the range for hemochromatosis) and risk of Type 2 diabetes in a UK population of men and women (Forouhi et al., 2007). In this case-control study of 360 cases and 758 matched controls, the cohort was older and heavier and had a greater percentage of men than that from the ARIC study. Results were not presented separately for men and women. In this study, the risk of developing diabetes was significantly increased sevenfold for the individuals with the highest serum ferritin levels.

### *7.2. Osteoporosis*

Iron has been shown to be required for the synthesis of collagen, a critical component of bone. Iron is also a co-factor in the conversion of serum 25-OH vitamin D (the indicator of vitamin D status) to serum 1,25 dihydroxy vitamin D (the active form of vitamin D). Certain laboratory animal studies have found that iron deficiency results in weaker bones (Harris et al., 2003).

The association of iron status and bone mineral density stems from the findings that about 15–66% of individuals with hemochromatosis often are found to have osteoporosis (Shapiro, 2001; Weinberg, 2006). The first case study was described in 1960 by Delbarre, and other reports have substantiated that the diagnosis of hemochromatosis often follows a bone fracture at a young age, especially in men (Schneider & Shane, 2001). As men with hemochromatosis often also have testicular atrophy, the bone loss may be secondary to the iron overload, and in certain cases where men were treated with phlebotomy and testosterone injections, there were improvements in bone indices, but not always (Angelopoulos, Goula, Papanikolaou, & Tolis, 2006).

Survey data from US postmenopausal women without hemochromatosis showed that iron status was directly related to bone mineral density (BMD) and that calcium status modulated this relationship. Specifically, Harris et al. reported that daily iron intakes of >20 mg were associated with increased BMD in women consuming 800–1,200 mg of calcium daily (Harris et al., 2003). If calcium intakes were less or greater, the iron/BMD association was no longer significant. This study confirmed other survey data associating low iron status with decreased BMD.

The cross-sectional survey data from Harris et al. was extended and included a 1-year intervention with 800 mg/d of calcium in postmenopausal women, half of whom were taking hormone replacement therapy (HRT). Iron intakes were calculated based upon dietary recall. In this study, both total calcium intake and use of HRT affected the association of iron and BMD. In women with the lowest calcium intakes, and using HRT, BMD in the femur increased with increasing iron intake up to 32 mg/d. In contrast, without HRT, only women in the highest tertile of calcium intake showed increases in femur BMD as iron intakes increased (Maurer et al., 2005).

Abraham et al. in 2006 also examined the association of iron and BMD changes in postmenopausal women who were not using HRT (Abraham et al., 2006). Detailed information about dietary intakes was collected over 2.5 years, and the rate of loss of bone at the spine was calculated with the objective of examining the dietary practices that were associated with a slowing of bone loss. For several nutrients, the greater the intake of fat, carbohydrate, and protein, the greater was the loss of bone. The only nutrient found to be directly associated with a preservation of bone mass was iron. The range of intakes was 6.2–24 mg/d of total iron intake that included iron from supplements. These findings remained significant independent of body mass index.

The question of whether low iron status, either as iron deficiency or as iron deficiency anemia, is associated with decreased BMD and/or fracture has been examined in two studies. Cesari et al. (2005) examined the association between measures of WHO-defined anemia and hemoglobin levels and bone mass as determined by peripheral quantitative computerized tomography (pQCT) in 101 men and women whose average age was 75. They found a significant increased risk of lower bone density (especially cortical bone) as hemoglobin levels decreased. About 10% of the women were found to be anemic. Of importance, they report that women with lower hemoglobin levels have greater bone losses than seen in men.

A recent abstract from the Women's Health Initiative (WHI) observational study looked at the association of hemoglobin levels measured in over 91,000 post-menopausal women with risk of hip fractures and total fractures (Chen, Arendell, Thomson, & Bassford, 2006). At baseline, over 6% of the women were anemic. Anemia at baseline was associated with a significant 70% increased risk of hip fracture and a 7% significant increased risk of total fractures. As this was a preliminary report, it will be of great interest to see further publications in this area, as it may well be that anemia is an independent risk factor for fracture in postmenopausal women.

## 8. CONCLUSIONS

Iron is an element and therefore is an essential nutrient as it cannot be synthesized by humans or any living organism. Iron is the mineral found in hemoglobin and is responsible for delivering oxygen to all tissues of the human body. There are a number of other critical proteins that have iron as a co-factor, and thus iron has several functions in the body in addition to transfer of oxygen in blood.

Iron status is best defined by the level of iron stores as well as the concentration of hemoglobin and transferrin saturation. Iron deficiency anemia is the end stage of progression from normal iron status to frank deficiency. Iron deficiency anemia is preventable with optimal intakes of iron over the lifetime. The stages of iron status and the recommended intakes during pregnancy (the most at-risk period for iron deficiency anemia in women) are outlined in Table 4. The CDC and WHO have defined the cutoffs for the stages of deficiency in non-pregnant women.

Table 4
**Women in Developed Countries who are at Increased Risk of Iron Deficiency (ID), Iron Deficiency Anemia (IDA)[1] or Modified Iron Needs**

| *Population* | *Database Used* | *ID/IDA/Modified Iron Needs* | *References* |
|---|---|---|---|
| Pre-pregnancy BMI | Women who participated in the Iron Supplementation Study | Postpartum anemia[1] risk doubled (BMI of 28 relative to 20); Risk tripled (BMI of 38 relative to 20) | Bodnar et al. (2004) |
| Overall pregnant women aged 20–40 who were 0–6 months post partum | NHANES III 1994–1998 | ID 13%<br>IDA 4.2% | Bodnar et al. (2002) |
| Overall pregnant women aged 20–40 who were 0–6 months postpartum who are at poverty level | NHANES III 1994–1998 | ID 22%<br>IDA 10% | Bodnar et al. (2002) |
| Parity comparison of 0–1 to 2–3 to >4 | NHANES III 1994–1998 | ID for parity of 2–3 was about double that of 0–1 (about 15%) and for >4 ID was three times that of 0–1 (about 22%) | Looker, Dallman, et al. (1997) |
| Delivery of multiple fetuses | | Based on iron needs for pregnancy | Yip et al. (1998) |
| Black postpartum | WIC participants | Anemia[1] 48% | Bodnar et al. (2001) |
| Female (12–15) | NHANES III 1994–1998 | ID 9%<br>IDA 2% | Looker, Dallman, (1997) |
| Female (16–19) | NHANES III 1994–1998 | ID 11%<br>IDA 3% | Looker, Dallman, (1997) |
| Women in basic training in the armed services | Military personnel | ID ~13% at entry up to ~33% after training<br>IDA ~ 6% at entry and ~20% after training<br>Increased ID and IDA in Hispanic and African-Americans subgroup | McClung et al. (2006) |
| Mexican American women aged 12–39 | NHANES III | IDA prevalence was 6.2% relative to 2.3% in age matched non-Hispanic white | Frith-Terhune et al. (2000) |
| Elite athletes | | Increased iron needs by 30–70% | Wood, Ronnenberg, (2006) |

(*Continued*)

Table 4
**(Continued)**

| *Population* | *Database Used* | *ID/IDA/Modified Iron Needs* | *References* |
|---|---|---|---|
| Blood donors | | Increased iron needs based on frequency of donation | Wood, Ronnenberg, (2006) |
| Post-menopausal women on HRT | | Years of menstrual blood loss continue as long as HRT continues | Wood, Ronnenberg, (2006) |
| Vegans, and vegetarians | 9113 young Australians | Diagnosed with low iron, ID, or anemia increased 1.6 fold (to 42.6%) for vegetarians relative to non vegetarians. | Baines, Powers, and Brown (2007) |
| Obese overweight children (2–11 years) and adolescents (12–16 years) | NHANES III | More than twice likely to be ID than age-matched normal weight children and adolescence (children 2.1–5.5% and for adolescence 3.5–9.1% for normal relative to obese) | Nead et al. (2004) |
| Children and adolescents (2–16) | NHANES III | Girls were about 3 times more at risk for iron deficiency (1.6 vs 4.3%) | Nead et al. (2004) |
| Women using oral contraceptive | | 60% reduction in menstrual blood loss | Wood, Ronnenberg, (2006) |

[1]Anemia data were used when there were no data for ID or IDA.

The iron status of menstruating women in developed and developing nations is often below recommended levels. The most common reasons for the low iron status are low dietary intake, loss of blood during menstruation, blood donations, and/or heavy exercise. Pregnancy puts an additional burden on a woman's iron status and it appears that it is very difficult to maintain iron balance during pregnancy without the use of iron supplements. Lactation can further reduce iron stores, especially if the woman had depleted stores during the pregnancy.

Once menstruation ceases, there is usually an increase in iron stores; however, repletion is dependent upon adequate intake of iron-rich foods with bioavailable iron. Post-menopausal women who use HRT may continue to menstruate and therefore their iron status may not improve. Even if women do not use HRT, if iron intake is low, post-menopausal women may have iron deficiency and/or iron deficiency anemia.

There are a number of genetic defects that result in increased absorption of iron without a balanced excretion of the excess. The resulting iron storage disease or hemochromatosis is often diagnosed in mid-life and causes deposition of iron in vital organs and may increase the risk of premature death. Treatment usually includes reduction in iron stores through blood donation.

Recent data links low iron status during the post-menopausal period with increased risk of Type 2 diabetes and osteoporosis. Thus, maintenance of recommended levels of iron stores throughout life can decrease the risk of several chronic diseases of aging and reduce the risk of iron deficiency and iron deficiency anemia.

## REFERENCES

*ACOG Education Pamphlet AP001 – Nutrition During Pregnancy* (2007). http://www.acog.org/publications/patient_education/bp001.cfm [On-line].

Abraham, R., Walton, J., Russell, L., Wolman, R., Wardley-Smith, B., Green, J. R. et al. (2006). Dietary determinants of post-menopausal bone loss at the lumbar spine: A possible beneficial effect of iron. *Osteoporosis International, 17*, 1165–1173.

Akabas, S. R., & Dolins, K. R. (2005). Micronutrient requirements of physically active women: What can we learn from iron? *The American Journal of Clinical Nutrition, 81*, 1246S–1251S.

Allen, L. H. (2000). Anemia and iron deficiency: Effects on pregnancy outcome. *The American Journal of Clinical Nutrition, 71*, 1280S–1284S.

Angelopoulos, N. G., Goula, A. K., Papanikolaou, G., & Tolis, G. (2006). Osteoporosis in HFE2 juvenile hemochromatosis. A case report and review of the literature. *Osteoporosis International, 17*, 150–155.

Baines, S., Powers, J., & Brown, W. J. (2007). How does the health and well-being of young Australian vegetarian and semi-vegetarian women compare with non-vegetarians? *Public Health Nutrition, 10*, 436–442.

Bendich, A. (2001). Calcium supplementation and iron status of females. *Nutrition, 17*, 46–51.

Blanck, H. M., Cogswell, M. E., Gillespie, C., & Reyes, M. (2005). Iron supplement use and iron status among US adults: Results from the third National Health and Nutrition Examination Survey. *The American Journal of Clinical Nutrition, 82*, 1024–1031.

Bodnar, L. M., Cogswell, M. E., & McDonald, T. (2005). Have we forgotten the significance of postpartum iron deficiency? *American Journal of Obstetrics and Gynecology, 193*, 36–44.

Bodnar, L. M., Cogswell, M. E., & Scanlon, K. S. (2002). Low income postpartum women are at risk of iron deficiency. *Journal of Nutrition, 132*, 2298–2302.

Bodnar, L. M., Scanlon, K. S., Freedman, D. S., Siega-Riz, A. M., & Cogswell, M. E. (2001). High prevalence of postpartum anemia among low-income women in the United States. *American Journal of Obstetrics and Gynecology, 185*, 438–443.

Bodnar, L. M., Siega-Riz, A. M., Arab, L., Chantala, K., & McDonald, T. (2004). Predictors of pregnancy and postpartum haemoglobin concentrations in low-income women. *Public Health Nutrition, 7*, 701–711.

Brody, T. (1999). Inorganic nutrients. In *Nutritional biochemistry* (2 ed., pp. 693–878). London: Academic Press.

Cade, J. E., Moreton, J. A., O'Hara, B., Greenwood, D. C., Moor, J., Burley, V. J. et al. (2005). Diet and genetic factors associated with iron status in middle-aged women. *The American Journal of Clinical Nutrition, 82*, 813–820.

Cesari, M., Pahor, M., Lauretani, F., Penninx, B.W., Bartali, B., Russo, R. et al. (2005). Bone density and hemoglobin levels in older persons: Results from the InCHIANTI study. *Osteoporos. Int., 16*, 691–699.

Chavarro, J. E., Rich-Edwards, J. W., Rosner, B. A., & Willett, W. C. (2006). Iron intake and risk of ovulatory infertility. *Obstetrics & Gynecology, 108*, 1145–1152.

Chen, Z., Arendell, L. A., Thomson, C. A., & Bassford, T. I. Anemia and Fractures. 9-17-2006.

Chernoff, R. (2000). Trace element requirements in the elderly. In J. D. Bogden & L. M. Klevay (Eds.), *Clinical nutrition of the essential trace elements and minerals* (pp. 183–197). Totowa, NJ: Humana Press.

Cogswell, M. E., Parvanta, I., Ickes, L., Yip, R., & Brittenham, G. M. (2003). Iron supplementation during pregnancy, anemia, and birth weight: A randomized controlled trial. *The American Journal of Clinical Nutrition, 78*, 773–781.

Cowie, C. C., Rust, K. F., Byrd-Holt, D. D., Eberhardt, M. S., Flegal, K. M., Engelgau, M. M. et al. (2006). Prevalence of diabetes and impaired fasting glucose in adults in the U.S. population: National Health and Nutrition Examination Survey 1999–2002. *Diabetes Care, 29*, 1263–1268.

Denic, S., & Agarwal, M. M. (2007). Nutritional iron deficiency: An evolutionary perspective. *Nutrition, 23*, 603–614.

Ervin, R. B., Wang, C. Y., Wright, J. D., & Kennedy-Stephenson, J. (2004). Dietary intake of selected minerals for the United States population: 1999–2000. *Advance Data, Issue 341*, 1–5.

Forouhi, N. G., Harding, A. H., Allison, M., Sandhu, M. S., Welch, A., Luben, R. et al. (2007). Elevated serum ferritin levels predict new-onset type 2 diabetes: Results from the EPIC-Norfolk prospective study. *Diabetologia, 50*, 949–956.

Frith-Terhune, A. L., Cogswell, M. E., Khan, L. K., Will, J. C., & Ramakrishnan, U. (2000). Iron deficiency anemia: Higher prevalence in Mexican American than in non-Hispanic white females in the third National Health and Nutrition Examination Survey, 1988–1994. *The American Journal of Clinical Nutrition, 72*, 963–968.

Fumeron, F., Pean, F., Driss, F., Balkau, B., Tichet, J., Marre, M. et al. (2006). Ferritin and transferrin are both predictive of the onset of hyperglycemia in men and women over 3 years: The data from an epidemiological study on the Insulin Resistance Syndrome (DESIR) study. *Diabetes Care, 29*, 2090–2094.

Garry, P. J., Hunt, W. C., & Baumgartner, R. N. (2000). Effects of iron intake on iron stores in elderly men and women: Longitudinal and cross-sectional results. *Journal of the American College of Nutrition, 19*, 262–269.

Hallberg, L. (2001). Perspectives on nutritional iron deficiency. Annual Review of Nutrition, *21*, 1–21.

Harris, M. M., Houtkooper, L. B., Stanford, V. A., Parkhill, C., Weber, J. L., Flint-Wagner, H. et al. (2003). Dietary iron is associated with bone mineral density in healthy postmenopausal women. *Journal of Nutrition, 133*, 3598–3602.

Hurrell, R. F. (1997). Bioavailability of iron. European Journal of Clinical Nutrition, *51*(Suppl. 1), S4–S8.

Hurrell, R. F., Reddy, M. B., Juillerat, M., & Cook, J. D. (2006). Meat protein fractions enhance nonheme iron absorption in humans. *Journal of Nutrition, 136*, 2808–2812.

IOM (2001). Iron. In *Dietary reference intakes for vitamin A, vitamin K, arsenic, boron, chromium, copper, iodine, iron, manganese, molybdenum, nickel, silicon, vanadium, and zinc* (pp. 290–393). Washington, DC: National Academy Press.

Jehn, M., Clark, J. M., & Guallar, E. (2004). Serum ferritin and risk of the metabolic syndrome in U.S. adults. *Diabetes Care, 27*, 2422–2428.

Jehn, M. L., Guallar, E., Clark, J. M., Couper, D., Duncan, B. B., Ballantyne, C. M. et al. (2007). A prospective study of plasma ferritin level and incident diabetes: The Atherosclerosis Risk in Communities (ARIC) Study. *American Journal of Epidemiology 165(9)*, 1047–1054.

Jiang, R., Manson, J. E., Meigs, J. B., Ma, J., Rifai, N., & Hu, F. B. (2004). Body iron stores in relation to risk of type 2 diabetes in apparently healthy women. *JAMA, 291*, 711–717.

Koopman, R. J., Mainous, A. G., III, Diaz, V. A., & Geesey, M. E. (2005). Changes in age at diagnosis of type 2 diabetes mellitus in the United States, 1988 to 2000. *Annals of Family Medicine, 3*, 60–63.

Liu, J. M., Hankinson, S. E., Stampfer, M. J., Rifai, N., Willett, W. C., & Ma, J. (2003). Body iron stores and their determinants in healthy postmenopausal US women. *The American Journal of Clinical Nutrition, 78*, 1160–1167.

Looker, A. C., Cogswell, M. E., & Gunter, M. T. (2002). Iron Deficiency-United States 1999–2000 . MMWR Morb. Mortal. Wkly. Rep. [On-line]. Retrieved from http://www.cdc.gov/mmwr/preview/mmwrhtml/mm5140a1.htm

Looker, A. C., Dallman, P. R., Carroll, M. D., Gunter, E. W., & Johnson, C. L. (1997). Prevalence of iron deficiency in the United States. *JAMA, 277*, 973–976.

Looker, A. C., Orwoll, E. S., Johnston, C. C., Jr., Lindsay, R. L., Wahner, H. W., Dunn, W. L. et al. (1997). Prevalence of low femoral bone density in older U.S. adults from NHANES III. *Journal of Bone and Mineral Research, 12*, 1761–1768.

Matkovic, V., Badenhop, N. E., & Ilich, J. Z. (2000). Trace elements and minerals in adolescents. In J. D. Bogden & L. M. Klevay (Eds.), *Clinical nutrition of the essential trace elements and minerals* (pp. 153–182). Totowa, NJ: Humana Press.

Maurer, J., Harris, M. M., Stanford, V. A., Lohman, T. G., Cussler, E., Going, S. B. et al. (2005). Dietary iron positively influences bone mineral density in postmenopausal women on hormone replacement therapy. *Journal of Nutrition, 135*, 863–869.

McClung, J. P., Marchitelli, L. J., Friedl, K. E., & Young, A. J. (2006). Prevalence of iron deficiency and iron deficiency anemia among three populations of female military personnel in the US Army. *Journal of the American College of Nutrition, 25*, 64–69.

Milman, N. (2006a). Iron and pregnancy – a delicate balance. *Annals of Hematology, 85*, 559–565.

Milman, N. (2006b). Iron prophylaxis in pregnancy – general or individual and in which dose? *Annals of Hematology, 85*, 821–828.

Milman, N., Bergholt, T., Eriksen, L., Byg, K. E., Graudal, N., Pedersen, P. et al. (2005). Iron prophylaxis during pregnancy – how much iron is needed? A randomized dose- response study of 20–80 mg ferrous iron daily in pregnant women. *Acta Obstetricia Et Gynecologica Scandinavica, 84*, 238–247.

Nead, K. G., Halterman, J. S., Kaczorowski, J. M., Auinger, P., & Weitzman, M. (2004). Overweight children and adolescents: A risk group for iron deficiency. *Pediatrics, 114*, 104–108.

Patterson, A. J., Brown, W. J., Roberts, D. C., & Seldon, M. R. (2001). Dietary treatment of iron deficiency in women of childbearing age. *The American Journal of Clinical Nutrition, 74*, 650–656.

Pena-Rosas, J. P., & Viteri, F. E., (2006). Effects of routine oral iron supplementation with or without folic acid for women during pregnancy. Cochrane Database of Systematic Reveiws, *4*, 1–133.

Perez, E. M., Hendricks, M. K., Beard, J. L., Murray-Kolb, L. E., Berg, A., Tomlinson, M. et al. (2005). Mother-infant interactions and infant development are altered by maternal iron deficiency anemia. *Journal of Nutrition, 135*, 850–855.

Picciano, M. F. (2003). Pregnancy and lactation: Physiological adjustments, nutritional requirements and the role of dietary supplements. *Journal of Nutrition, 133*, 1997S–2002S.

Rangan, A. M., Blight, G. D., & Binns, C. W. (1998). Iron status and non-specific symptoms of female students. *Journal of the American College of Nutrition, 17*, 351–355.

Reddy, M. B., Hurrell, R. F., & Cook, J. D. (2006). Meat consumption in a varied diet marginally influences nonheme iron absorption in normal individuals. *Journal of Nutrition, 136*, 576–581.

Rioux, F. M., & LeBlanc, C. P. (2007). Iron supplementation during pregnancy: What are the risks and benefits of current practices? Applied Physiology, Nutrition, and Metabolism, *32*, 282–288.

Schneider, A., & Shane, E. (2001). Osteoporosis secondary to illnesses and medications. In R. Marcus, D. Feldman, & J. Kelsey (Eds.), *Osteoprosis*, (2nd ed., pp. 303–326). New York: Academic Press.

Scholl, T. O., & Reilly, T. (2000a). Anemia, iron and pregnancy outcome. *Journal of Nutrition, 130*, 443S–447S.

Scholl, T. O., & Reilly, T. M. (2000b). Trace element and mineral nutrition in human pregnancy. In J. D. Bogden & L. M. Klevay (Eds.), *Clinical nutrition of the essential trace elements and minerals* (pp. 115–138). Totowa, NJ: Humana Press.

Seaverson, E. L., Buell, J. S., Fleming, D. J., Bermudez, O. I., Potischman, N., Wood, R. J. et al. (2007). Poor iron status is more prevalent in Hispanic than in non-Hispanic white older adults in Massachusetts. *Journal of Nutrition, 137*, 414–420.

Sebastian, R. S., Cleveland, L. E., Goldman, J. D., & Moshfegh, A. J. (2007). Older adults who use vitamin/mineral supplements differ from nonusers in nutrient intake adequacy and dietary attitudes. *Journal of the American Dietetic Association, 107*, 1322–1332.

Shapiro, J. R. (2001). Osteogenesis imperfecta and other defects of bone development as occasional causes of adult osteoporosis. In R. Marcus, D. Feldman, & J. Kelsey (Eds.), *Osteoprosis*, (2nd ed., pp. 271–301). New York: Academic Press.

Siega-Riz, A. M., Hartzema, A. G., Turnbull, C., Thorp, J., McDonald, T., & Cogswell, M. E. (2006). The effects of prophylactic iron given in prenatal supplements on iron status and birth outcomes: A randomized controlled trial. *American Journal of Obstetrics and Gynecology, 194*, 512–519.

Smith, D. L. (2000). Anemia in the elderly. *American Family Physician, 62*, 1565–1572.

Turner, R. E. (2006). Nutrition during pregnancy. In M. E. Shils, M. Shike, A. C. Ross, B. Caballero, & R. J. Cousins (Eds.), *Modern nutrition in health and disease* (10 ed., pp. 771–783). Baltimore: Lippincott Williams & Wilkins.

Vari, I. S., Balkau, B., Kettaneh, A., Andre, P., Tichet, J., Fumeron, F. et al. (2007). Ferritin and transferrin are associated with metabolic syndrome abnormalities and their change over time in a general population: Data from an Epidemiological Study on the Insulin Resistance Syndrome (DESIR). *Diabetes Care, 30*, 1795–1801.

Viteri, F. E. & Berger, J. (2005). Importance of pre-pregnancy and pregnancy iron status: Can long-term weekly preventive iron and folic acid supplementation achieve desirable and safe status? *Nutrition Review, 63*, S65–S76.

Weinberg, E. D. (2006). Iron loading: A risk factor for osteoporosis. *Biometals, 19*, 633–635.

Wood, R. J., & Ronnenberg, A. G. (2006). Iron. In M. E. Shils, M. Shike, A. C. Ross, B. Caballero, & R. J. Cousins (Eds.), *Modern nutrition in health and disease* (10 ed., pp. 248–270). Baltimore: Lippincott Williams & Wilkins.

Yip, R., Parvanta, I., Cogswell, M. E., McDonnell, S. M., Bowman, B. A., Grummer-Strawn, L. M. et al. (1998). Recommendations to prevent and control iron deficiency in the United States. *Morbidity and Mortality Weekly Report, 47*, 1–36.

Zimmermann, M. B. & Hurrell, R. F. (2007). Nutritional iron deficiency. *Lancet, 370*, 511–520.

# Appendix A: *Reference Ranges for Common Laboratory Assays of Iron Metabolism*

*Anthony N. Sireci and Alexander Kratz*

## INTRODUCTORY COMMENTS

The following is a table of reference values for laboratory tests commonly used in the workup of suspected disorders of iron metabolism. In preparing the appendix, the authors have taken into account the fact that the system of international units (SI, système international d'unités) is used in many countries and in some medical journals. However, conventional units continue to be used in many areas of the world, as well as in the lay press. Therefore, both systems are provided in the table.

A variety of factors can influence reference values. Such variables include the population studied, the duration and means of specimen transport, laboratory methods and instrumentation, and even the type of container used for the collection of the specimen. The reference or "normal" ranges given in this table may therefore not be appropriate for all laboratories, and the values should only be used as general guidelines. Whenever possible, reference values provided by the laboratory performing the testing should be utilized in the interpretation of laboratory data. Values supplied in this table reflect typical reference ranges in adults. Pediatric reference ranges may vary significantly from adult values (Kratz, Pesce, & Fink, 2008).

From: *Nutrition and Health: Iron Deficiency and Overload*
Edited by: S. Yehuda and D.I. Mostofsky, DOI 10.1007/978-1-59745-462-9

| *Analyte* | *Specimen* | *Reference Range* | | *Diagnostic Notes* | *References* |
|---|---|---|---|---|---|
| | | *Conventional Units* | *SI Units* | | |
| Ferritin | S | Female: 10–150 ng/mL<br>Male: 29–248 ng/mL | Female: 10–150 μg/L<br>Male: 29–248 μg/L | Ferritin reflects total body iron stores and correlates with stainable iron in marrow. It is elevated in iron overload; however, it can also be elevated in liver disease and in inflammatory states as an acute-phase reactant. | British Nutrition Foundation (1995) |
| Hepcidin | S | 51.6–153.4 ng/mL | 51.6–153.4 μg/L | High levels of hepcidin, stimulated by IL-6 and IL-1, antagonize iron absorption. Levels are high in anemia of chronic disease and low in iron deficiency anemia as well as some forms of hereditary hemochromatosis. | Kulaksiz et al. (2004) |
| Iron | S | 41–141 μg/dL | 7–25 μmol/L | There is significant hour-to-hour and day-to-day variation in serum iron levels. Serum iron levels should therefore only be used in conjunction with other measures of iron status. | Kratz et al. (2008) |
| Mean corpuscular hemoglobin (MCH) | WB | 26.7–31.9 pg/cell | 26.7–31.9 pg/cell | Low levels indicate prolonged iron deficiency affecting erythrocytes. Represents iron status over the past 120 days. | Kratz et al. (2008) |
| Percentage of hypochromatic red cells | WB | <6% | <0.6 | A direct measure of iron deficiency, the percentage of hypochromatic red cells increases with worsening iron deficiency. | Tessitore et al. (2001) |
| Percentage of iron saturation | S | 16–60% | 0.16–0.60 | An iron saturation of <16% is considered inadequate for erythropoesis. If iron saturation is >100%, interference by non-transferrin iron (e.g., iron bound to ferritin) should be considered. | IV. NKF-K/DOQI Clinical Practice Guidelines for Anemia of Chronic Kidney Disease: Update 2000 (2001) |

| | | | | | |
|---|---|---|---|---|---|
| Red cell ferritin, basic | WB | 3–37.3 $*10^{-17}$ g/cell | 3–37.3 $*10^{-17}$ g/cell | A measure of erythroid marrow iron; elevated in thalassemia and myelodysplastic syndrome; low levels in iron deficiency anemia | Cazzola et al. (1983) |
| Reticulocyte hemoglobin content (CHr) | WB | 28–32 pg/ cell | 28–32 pg/ cell | A measure of the hemoglobin content of reticulocytes; allows a real-time assessment of the functional state of the erythroid marrow. Possibly, the best predictor of iron deficiency in children. | Fishbane, Shapiro, Dutka, Valenzuela, and Faubert (2001); Thomas and Thomas (2002) |
| RET-Y (Reticulocyte parameter available on certain cell counters) | WB | 1661–1820 arbitrary units (channel numbers) | | A forward light scatter measure corresponding to size and content of reticulocytes. Values are lower in iron deficiency. | Buttarello, Temporin, Ceravolo, Farina, and Bulian (2004) |
| Soluble transferrin receptor (sTfR) | S | <2.6 mg/L | <35.13 nmol/L | sTRF reflects the overall level of erythropoeisis. Elevated in Fe deficiency and with erythropoietin therapy. Not elevated in anemia of chronic disease. | Tessitore et al. (2001) |
| sTfR/ferritin index | S | <1.6 | <1.6 | Determined by dividing the sTfR level by the log of the serum ferritin. Increases in iron deficiency. | Thomas and Thomas, (2002) |
| Stainable iron in bone marrow | BM | Present | Present | Gold standard for diagnosis of iron deficiency when iron stain (Prussian blue) is performed on bone marrow aspirate. | Jakkunen (1973); Stuart-Smith, Hughes, and Bain (2005) |
| Total Iron-binding capacity (TIBC) or transferrin | S | 251–406 µg/dL | 45–73 µmol/L | Elevated in iron deficiency. | International Committee for Standardisation in Haematology (Iron Panel) (1978); Worwood (1997) |
| Transferrin saturation | S | 16–60% | 0.16–0.60 | Decreased in iron deficiency. | Worwood (1997) |
| Zinc protoporphyrin (ZPP) | WB | <40 µmol/mol heme | <40 µmol/ mol heme | In iron deficiency, or ferrochelatase inhibition by lead, zinc is incorporated into protoporphyrin instead of iron, leading to the generation of ZPP. The measure was originally known as free erythrocyte protoporphoryin; ZPP is elevated in iron deficiency. | Hastka, Lasserre, Schwarzbeck, Strauch, and Hehlmann (1992); Kulaksiz et al. (2004) |

S: Serum; WB: Whole Blood; BM: Bone Marrow.

## REFERENCES


British Nutrition Foundation. (1995). *Iron: Nutritional and physiologic significance*. London: Chapman and Hall.

Buttarello, M., Temporin, V., Ceravolo, R., Farina, G., & Bulian, P. (2004). The new reticulocyte parameter (RET-Y) of the Sysmex XE 2100: its use in the diagnosis and monitoring of posttreatment sideropenic anemia. *American Journal of Clinical Pathology, 121*(4), 489–495.

Cazzola, M., Dezza, L., Bergamaschi, G., Barosi, G., Bellotti, V., Caldera, D., et al. (1983). Biologic and clinical significance of red cell ferritin. *Blood, 62*(5), 1078–1087.

Fishbane, S., Shapiro, W., Dutka, P., Valenzuela, O. F., & Faubert, J. (2001). A randomized trial of iron deficiency testing strategies in hemodialysis patients. *Kidney International, 60*(6), 2406–2411.

Hastka, J., Lasserre, J. J., Schwarzbeck, A., Strauch, M., & Hehlmann, R. (1992). Washing erythrocytes to remove interferents in measurements of zinc protoporphyrin by front-face hematofluorometry. *Clinical Chemistry, 38*(11), 2184–2189.

International Committee for Standardisation in Haematology (Iron Panel). (1978). Recommendations for measurement of serum iron in human blood. *British Journal of Haematology, 38*, 291–294.

IV. NKF-K/DOQI Clinical Practice Guidelines for Anemia of Chronic Kidney Disease: Update 2000. (2001). *American Journal of Kidney Diseases, 37*(1 Suppl 1), S182–S238.

Jakkunen, H. (1973). Iron deficiency in the Finnish adult population. *Scandinavian Journal of Haematology, 25*, 1–91.

Kratz, A., Pesce, M., & Fink, D. J. (2008). Laboratory values of clinical importance. In E. B. D. L. Kasper, A. S. Fauci, S. L. Hauser, D. L. Longo, & J. L. Jameson (Eds.), *Harrison's principles of internal medicine* (17th ed., pp. A1–A18). New York: McGraw-Hill.

Kulaksiz, H., Gehrke, S. G., Janetzko, A., Rost, D., Bruckner, T., Kallinowski, B., et al. (2004). Pro-hepcidin: expression and cell specific localisation in the liver and its regulation in hereditary haemochromatosis, chronic renal insufficiency, and renal anaemia. *Gut, 53*(5), 735–743.

Stuart-Smith, S. E., Hughes, D. A., & Bain, B. J. (2005). Are routine iron stains on bone marrow trephine biopsy specimens necessary? *Journal of Clinical Pathology, 58*(3), 269–272.

Tessitore, N., Solero, G. P., Lippi, G., Bassi, A., Faccini, G. B., Bedogna, V., et al. (2001). The role of iron status markers in predicting response to intravenous iron in haemodialysis patients on maintenance erythropoietin. *Nephrology, Dialysis, Transplantation, 16*(7), 1416–1423.

Thomas, C., & Thomas, L. (2002). Biochemical markers and hematologic indices in the diagnosis of functional iron deficiency. *Clinical Chemistry, 48*(7), 1066–1076.

Worwood, M. (1997). The laboratory assessment of iron status – an update. *Clinica Chimica Acta, 259*(1–2), 3–23.

# Appendix B: *Nutritional Sources of Iron*

*Anthony N. Sireci and Alexander Kratz*

## INTRODUCTORY COMMENTS

Common food sources vary in the quantity and type of their iron content. The following table provides information on the value of some of the most common nutrients as sources of iron (Linus Pauling Institute: Micronutrient Research for Optimum Health, 2006; McKinley Health Center University of Illinois at Urbana-Champagne, 2006; National Institutes of Health Office of Dietary Supplements, 2004).

The table is divided into non-heme (A) and heme (B) sources of iron. Heme iron is present only in foods of animal origin (meat, poultry, fish) and is absorbed more easily than non-heme iron, found in plant foods.

The iron content for each food is indicated in milligram of iron per gram of food. In the United States, federal regulations require mandatory nutrition labeling of packaged foods. This nutrition information is expressed in both common household measures appropriate to the food (e.g., one slice of bread) and in the system of international units (SI, système international d'unités). The serving size reflects the amount of food customarily consumed per eating occasion. In order to convey this information, the table lists the customary serving size for each food as determined by the US Food and Drug Administration (FDA) in both common household measures and the SI system. The iron content of one serving of each food is then given in the last column.

A more exhaustive list of foods and their iron content can be found on the United States Department of Agriculture's (USDA) National Nutrient Database web site at http://www.nal.usda.gov/fnic/foodcomp/Data/SR18/nutrlist/sr18w303.pdf (U.S. Department of Agriculture: Agricultural Research Service, 2005).

**Table B 1**
**Non-Heme Sources of Iron**

| *Food* | *Iron Content (mg Iron/g of Food)* | *Serving Size in Common Household Measures* | *Weight (in g) of Serving Size* | *Iron Content (in mg) of Serving Size* |
|---|---|---|---|---|
| Almonds, raw | 0.039 | 1 oz, 23 kernels | 28.3 | 1.1 |
| Asparagus, canned | 0.018 | 4 spears | 72 | 1.3 |
| Beans, kidney, mature seeds, cooked, boiled | 0.029 | 1 cup | 177 | 5.2 |
| Beans, lima | 0.018 | 1 cup | 241 | 4.4 |
| Beans, lentil, boiled | 0.033 | 1 cup | 198 | 6.6 |
| Beans, navy | 0.024 | 1 cup | 182 | 4.3 |
| Beans, soy | 0.024 | 1 cup | 180 | 4.4 |
| Bread, wheat or white | 0.032 | 1 slice | 28 | 0.9 |
| Broccoli, florettes, raw | 0.0083 | 1 cup | 72 | 0.6 |
| Bulgar, cooked | 0.0096 | 1 cup | 182 | 1.8 |
| Cashew nuts | 0.060 | 18 nuts | 28.3 | 1.7 |
| Cereals, 100% fortified | 0.60 | ¾ cup | 30 | 18 |
| Cereals, 25% fortified | 0.15 | ¾ cup | 30 | 4.5 |
| Chickpeas, cooked | 0.029 | 1 cup | 164 | 4.7 |
| Chocolate, baking, unsweetened | 0.17 | 1 square | 28.35 | 4.8 |
| Collard greens, boiled, no salt | 0.012 | 1 cup | 190 | 2.2 |
| Cornmeal, whole grain, yellow | 0.034 | 1 cup | 122 | 4.2 |
| Grits, white, with water | 0.0062 | 1 cup | 242 | 1.5 |
| Lettuce, butterhead | 0.012 | 1 head | 163 | 2.0 |
| Oats, regular, quick and instant, unenriched, prepared with water | 0.0068 | 1 cup | 2.34 | 1.6 |
| Potato, baked | 0.011 | 1 medium | 173 | 1.9 |
| Prune juice | 0.012 | 1 cup | 256 | 3.0 |
| Raisins, seedless | 0.019 | 1 cup | 145 | 2.7 |
| Rice, brown | 0.0061 | 1 cup | 164 | 1.0 |
| Rice, white, enriched | 0.011 | 1 cup | 158 | 1.8 |
| Seeds, pumpkin, roasted | 0.148 | 1 oz | 28.3 | 4.2 |
| Soy milk | 0.011 | 1 cup | 245 | 2.7 |
| Spinach, frozen and boiled | 0.019 | 1 cup | 190 | 3.7 |
| Tofu, raw, firm | 0.016 | ¼ block | 81 | 1.3 |

Table B 2
Heme Sources of Iron

| *Food* | *Iron Content (mg Iron/ g of Food)* | *Serving Size in Common Household Measures* | *Weight (in g) of Serving Size* | *Iron Content (in mg) of Serving Size* |
|---|---|---|---|---|
| Beef, composite of trimmed retail cuts, separable lean and fat, trimmed to 1/8" fat, cooked | 0.025 | 3.0 | 85 | 2.1 |
| Chicken, dark meat , roast | 0.013 | 3.4 oz | 94 | 1.3 |
| Chicken, light meat, roast | 0.011 | 3.5 oz | 100 | 1.1 |
| Clams, canned, drained | 0.28 | 3 oz | 85 | 23.8 |
| Egg, boiled | 0.012 | 1 large egg | 50 | 0.6 |
| Halibut, cooked | 0.011 | 3.0 oz | 85 | 0.9 |
| Liver, goose, raw | 0.31 | 3.5 | 100 | 30.5 |
| Liver (pork, chicken) simmered | 0.12–0.18 | 3.5 oz | 100 | 12.0–18.0 |
| Oysters, fried | 0.033 | 6 medium | 136 | 4.5 |
| Pork, (leg, loin, shoulder, and spareribs), separable lean and fat, cooked | 0.011 | 3.0 oz | 85 | 0.9 |
| Scallops, steamed | 0.030 | 3.5 oz | 100 | 3.0 |
| Shrimp, cooked (moist heat) | 0.032 | 8 large | 44 g | 1.4 |
| Tuna, bluefin, cooked | 0.013 | 3.0 oz | 85 | 1.1 |
| Tuna, light, in water | 0.015 | 1 can | 165 | 2.5 |
| Turkey, dark meat, roasted | 0.023 | 3.5 oz | 100 | 2.3 |
| Turkey, light meat, roasted | 0.014 | 3.5 oz | 100 | 1.4 |

## REFERENCES

Linus Pauling Institute: Micronutrient Research for Optimum Health. (2006, January 6). *Micronutrient information center*. Retrieved August 2, 2008, from http://lpi.oregonstate.edu/infocenter/minerals/iron/

McKinley Health Center University of Illinois at Urbana-Champagne. (2006, December 14). *Dietary sources of iron*. Retrieved August 2, 2008, from http://www.mckinley.uiuc.edu/Handouts/dietary_sources_iron.html

National Institutes of Health Office of Dietary Supplements. (2004, August 24th, 2007). *Dietary supplement fact sheet: Iron*. Retrieved August 2, 2008, from http://ods.od.nih.gov/factsheets/iron.asp

U.S. Department of Agriculture: Agricultural Research Service. (2005, May 16, 2008). *National nutrient database for standard reference, release 18*. Retrieved August 2, 2008, from http://www.nal.usda.gov/fnic/foodcomp

# Subject Index


**A**

Aβ, *see* Amyloid β–peptide (Aβ)
ABCB7, 15, 256, 264, 265
*ABCB7* gene, mutation in, 264–265
ABCB7 protein, 264, 265
Aceruloplasminemia, 5, 33, 105, 127, 231, 259–262, 266, 269
  brain MRI of 70-year-old man with, 261
  GPI in, 260
  gross neuropathology in, 261
  treatment of, 262
Acute hypoferremia of inflammation, 58, 59
Acute iron ingestion, treatment of, 83–84
  exchange transfusion, 84
  iron chelator role in, 83–84
  whole bowel irrigation for, 83
AD, *see* Alzheimer's disease (AD)
Administration, 13, 41, 52, 78–82, 86, 101, 103, 128, 130, 131, 135, 153, 200, 209–211, 259, 260, 291, 304, 317, 355
Aging, 109, 114, 125–135, 170, 197, 227, 242, 245, 269, 341, 348
Aging CNS, 135
ALAS, *see* Amino laevulinic acid synthase (ALAS)
Alopecia, 172
ALS, *see* Amyotrophic lateral sclerosis (ALS)
ALSPAC, *see* Avon Longitudinal Study of Pregnancy and Childhood (ALSPAC)
Alzheimer's disease (AD), 96, 105, 111, 112, 113, 126, 127, 129, 132–133, 134, 189, 225, 241–246, 267–268, 270
  clinical and pathological features of, 241–242
  evidence for dysregulation of brain iron homeostasis in patient with, 243
  HO-1 and, 127, 132–133
  iron and pathogenesis of, 242–243
    experimental evidence for a pathogenic role, 243–245
    therapeutic implications of iron in, 245–246
  key features of lesions in, 242
  mutant HFE and, 267–268
  sources of oxidative stress in, 127
Amino laevulinic acid synthase (ALAS), 38, 264
Amyloid, 127, 129, 130, 132, 133, 134, 225, 241, 242, 244, 245, 267
Amyloid β–peptide (Aβ), 242
  source of ROS in AD, 244
Amyloid precursor protein (APP) gene, mutation in, 242
Amyotrophic lateral sclerosis, 126, 127, 269, 270
Amyotrophic lateral sclerosis (ALS), mutant HFE and, 269
Anaemia, 4, 5, 10, 15, 18, 55, 58, 59, 77, 78, 82, 84, 86, 99, 159, 160, 161, 162, 163, 164, 165, 166, 167, 168, 169, 170, 171, 173, 201, 202, 255, 256, 260, 264–265, 266, 269, 282, 329, 331, 333, 336, 337, 338, 339, 340, 341, 342, 345
  blood transfusion service effects, 307
  death rate, from, 306
  haemoglobinometry, 309–310
  latent iron deficiency, 302–303
  and malaria, 301
  in newborn, 301
  nutritional iron deficiency, 313–323
  during pregnancy, 301
  during pregnancy and lactation, 335
  screening, 322
  in under-resourced countries, 308–309
  in women, 335
  *See also* Iron deficiency
Anisocytosis, 166–167
Antigen-presenting cells (APC), 213
APC, *see* Antigen-presenting cells (APC)
ASS, *see* Autonomic sympathetic system (ASS)
Astrocyte, 106, 108, 128, 129, 131, 132, 134, 135, 208, 257, 260, 261, 263, 267
Atrophy of lingual papillae, 168
Attention-deficit hyperactivity disorder (ADHD), 152–153
Auditory system and iron deficiency, 202
Autoimmunity, 214, 215, 216
Autonomic sympathetic system (ASS), 207
Avon Longitudinal Study of Pregnancy and Childhood (ALSPAC), 315

## B


Bacillibactin, 68
BBB, *see* Blood–brain barrier (BBB)
BCRP/ABCG2, *see* Breast cancer resistance protein (BCRP/ABCG2)
Behavioral deficits in iron-deficient infants
  biological basis of, 141
Bendich, Adrianne, Dr., 327–348
Blood–brain barrier (BBB), 20, 207
  free passage to transferrin, ceruloplasmin, 254
  permeabilty of, 207–208
Blood donor studies, CHD risk and, 289–291
Blood-oxygenlevel-dependent (BOLD), 227
Blood transfusion service effects, and anaemia, 307
Body iron
  compartments and fluxes, 36
  loss, 40–41
  regulation of, 39–41
  stores, *see* Body iron stores
  *See also* Brain iron
Body iron stores
  CHD risk and, 282–291
    blood donor studies and iron and oxidized LDL cholesterol, 289–291
    case-control/cross-sectional studies, 288–289
    cohort studies based on serum ferritin, 282–285
    cohort studies based on TS, 286–287
    dietary iron, 289
  reducation of, clinical trials, 291–292
  serum measures of, 280–282
  TIBC in, 280–282
BOLD, *see* Blood-oxygenlevel-dependent (BOLD)
Bone mineral density (BMD), 344, 345
Bone morphogenetic protein (BMP) pathway, 55
Brain copper, biology of, 227–231
Brain hemorrhage, iron role in, 189, 227
Brain iron, 96, 97–100, 101–102, 105, 106–108, 110, 112, 113, 125–135, 142, 144, 146, 151, 195–203, 223–235, 243, 251–269, 317
  in adult rats, 196
  biology of, 227–231
  and brain dopamine, 197–198
  deposition in aging and disease, model for, 134
  forms of, 227
  imaging at 7 tesla, 234–235
  inherited neurological diseases with accumulation of, 231
  metabolism of, 97
    inborn errors of, 231
  MRI techniques for imaging, 232–234
    overview, 223–226
    pulse sequences and quantifying brain iron effects, 233
  and Parkinson's disease
    role of transition metals in, 105
  research papers published per year on, 226
  uneven distribution of, 196
  *See also* Body iron
Brain iron deficiency and opamine–endogenous opiate
  function of, 101–102
  interaction between, 101
Brain iron homeostasis
  evidence for dysregulation of, in AD patient, 243
Brain MRI
  of patient with PKAN, 257
  of 70-year-old man with aceruloplasminemia, 261
Brain neurotransmitter receptors, effect of ID on, 98–99
Breast cancer resistance protein (BCRP/ABCG2), 34


## C


CA, *see* Catecholamines (CA)
CAD risk, *see* Coronary artery disease (CAD) risk
Catecholamines (CA), 111, 143, 147, 211–214, 216
Catecholate siderophore
  enterobactin, 66–67
  salmochelin S4, 67
$CD8^+$ T cells, in MS patient, 215
$CD4^+$ Th cells, 212, 215
Cellular iron homeostasis, proteins involved in, 3–6, 9, 18, 19
Central nervous system (CNS)
  in animals, 207
  cytokines in, 211–212
  hemochromatosis and, 266–269
  iron homeostasis, genetic disorders of, *see* Genetic disorders of CNS, iron homeostasis and
  role in maintaining control of chemical microenvironment and iron, 254
  stress and, 208
Ceruloplasmin (Cp), 5, 17, 32, 33, 34, 35, 37, 105, 127, 231, 252, 253, 254, 259, 260, 261, 262, 266, 269
  GPI-linked form of, 18
  hepatic macrophages in knockout mice, 260
  role in iron release, 17–18
Ceruloplasmin knockout mice, 259–260
  hepatic macrophages in, 260
Chaperones, metal, 230
  function of, 231
CHD, *see* Coronary heart disease (CHD)
CHD risk
  and body iron stores, 282–291
    blood donor studies and iron and oxidized LDL cholesterol, 289–291
    case-control/cross-sectional studies, 288–289
    cohort studies based on serum ferritin, 282–285
    cohort studies based on TS, 286–287
    dietary iron, 289
  hemochromatosis and, 292
Cheilitis, 169, 170

Chelation, 68, 84, 85, 86, 145, 146, 148, 149, 228, 230, 245, 259, 267, 270
  deferasirox, 87
  deferiprone, 86–87
  deferoxamine, 86
Chronic iron overload
  classification of, 84
  clinical signs and symptoms of, 84–85
  measure of, 85–86
  treatment of
    chelation therapy, 86–87
    phlebotomy, 86
Chronic transfusion therapy, 85, 86
CNS, *see* Central nervous system (CNS)
Cognition, 101, 102, 126, 212
Cognitive deficits in iron-deficient infants, biological basis of, 141
Cognitive impairment, 95–113, 132, 204, 241, 245, 267
Compensatory mechanisms, 166
Coronary artery disease (CAD) risk, 284, 291
Coronary heart disease (CHD), 279, 280, 282, 283, 284, 285, 287, 288, 289, 290, 291, 292, 293
Corticotrophin-releasing hormone (CRH), 211, 212
CRH, *see* Corticotrophin-releasing hormone (CRH)
CSH-treated astroglia
  DAB-positive glial granules, 128–129
  morphological changes, 128
  non-transferrin iron sequestration in, 129
  peroxidase-positive astrocyte granules in, 128
Cysteine, in patients with PANK2 deficiency, 258–259
Cys282Tyr mutation, 292
Cytokines, 16, 19, 20, 38, 127, 129, 130, 132, 133, 134, 203, 207–216
  in CNS, 211–212
  depression associated with proinflammatory, 210–211
  effects of stress hormones on proinflammatory and anti-inflammatory, 212
  inflammatory, 209
    human disease and, 212
    stress-like effects of, 210
  interaction with HPA axis, 210–211
  as mediators of neuroimmune communication, 208–210
  peripheral, 209
  stimulation of HPA axis by, 211
Cytosol, iron regulation and, 35

D

DALY, *see* Disability-adjusted life years (DALY)
DAT expression, 146, 152
Dcytb, 4, 19, 31, 32, 34, 35, 37, 110, 252, 253
Deferasirox, 86, 87
Deferiprone, 86–87, 256
Deferoxamine, 83, 84, 86, 87, 135, 259, 262
Deferoxamine infusion, 83–84
Depression, associated with proinflammatory cytokines, 210–211
Deranged body iron homeostasis, 40
Dexamethasone
  effect on IL-4 production, 214
Diabetes, 84, 85, 212, 242, 245, 260, 263, 289, 292, 293, 327, 342, 343, 344, 348
  type 2, 342–344
Dietary education, prevention of iron deficiency, 320
Dietary iron
  and CHD risk, 289
  intestinal absorption of, 35
  types of, 33
Diferric transferrin, 4, 7, 11, 21, 40, 42, 55, 129, 130, 253, 254
Disability-adjusted life years (DALY), 306
Divalent metal-ion transporter 1 (DMT1), 4, 7, 10, 12, 13, 19, 20, 31, 32, 34, 35, 36, 37, 38, 39, 184, 185, 186, 187, 253, 254, 265
  in cellular iron acquisition, 12
  function of, 12
  human iron physiology and, 253
  knockout of, 35
  in mucosal proton-dependent uptake of divalent metals, 34
Divalent metal transporter I, 182
DMT1, *see* Divalent metal-ion transporter 1 (DMT1)
Dopamine, 97–100, 101–102, 106–109, 126, 127, 129–131, 133–135, 141, 142–147, 152, 153, 190, 196, 197–198, 199, 231, 317
  brain iron and brain, 197–198
  catabolism of, 144
  $D_2$R-DAT link, 146
  pathways in brain, 142
  receptors
    $D_1$ receptors, 144
    $D_2$ receptors, 144–145
    effects of ID on, 145
  synthesis of
    post-weaning ID in rats, 144
    TH role in, 142–144
  transport, 145
Dopamine D1 receptor, 144
Dopamine D2 receptor, 144–145
  in brains of ID rats, 99, 101–102
Dopamine-endogenous opiate and brain iron deficiency, 101–102
  function of, 101–102
  interaction between, 101
Dopamine/$H_2O_2$-mediated PC12 cell death, 135
$D_2$R-DAT communication, 146
Dysphagia, 169–170
Dyspnea, 159, 166

## E

EAR, *see* Estimated average requirement (EAR)
Early iron deficiency, 100–101, 200–201
effect on brain function
and biochemistry, 100
during erly brain development, 101
longlasting effects of, 200–201
Effects on populations, 301
Endocrine system and iron deficiency, 202
Endorphins, 101, 153
Enkephalins, 99, 101, 103
Enterobactin, 66–69, 72, 73
biosynthesis, 67
components of, 66
enzymes synthesizing, 66
glucosylated, 67–69
Enterocyte iron transport, mechanism, 34
Epidemiology, 282, 292, 306
Erythrocyte morphologies, 167
Erythroid cell, 8–10
iron metabolism in, 8
iron uptake of immature, 9–10
release of iron from, 18
Erythropoiesis, 35, 42, 55, 57, 59, 163, 308
Erythropoiesis and hepcidin synthesis, 59
*Escherichia coil*, 66–67, 70, 84
enterobactin, *see* Enterobactin
enterobactin synthesis by, 66
uropathogenic, *see* Uropathogenic *E. coli* (UPEC)
Estimated average requirement (EAR), of iron in women, 328, 341
Estrogen, 153, 280
*Eurogrowth Iron Study Group,* 301
Exchange transfusion, in acute iron ingestion, 84

## F

FA, *see* Friedreich's ataxia (FA)
FAO, *see* Food and Agriculture Organization (FAO)
Feline leukemic virus protein C (FLVCR), 34
Ferric gluconate, 81
Ferric reductase redundancy, in guinea pigs and humans, 34
Ferric siderophores, 66
Ferritin, 4, 5, 7, 9, 13–19, 31–39, 85, 86, 96, 98, 102–105, 107–113, 127, 129, 152, 163–167, 181–184, 187–190, 196, 199, 201, 225, 226, 227, 230, 231, 243, 252, 253, 254, 256, 260, 262, 263, 265, 266–286, 288–293, 300, 303, 308, 309, 314, 315, 316, 329–334, 336, 338, 341–344, 352
accumulation, defect in, 110–111
distribution in hippocampus
addition of zinc to iron therapy, 103–105
iron deficiency effects on, 102–103
MF system, 103–104
spatiotemporal trend in, 102
iron release from, 108
level within cells, 16
subunits of, 16
Ferritin-binding protein, 14
Ferroportin, 5, 17, 19, 31–41, 52–53, 58, 110, 182–184, 186, 187, 189, 252–254, 260, 265, 266
cellular iron export function of, 52
cellular regulation of, 53
internalization, 52–53
in iron efflux from cells, 32–33
regulation by hepcidin, 52–53
Ferroportin 1 (FPN), 17, 252, 266
expression, 17
Fertility, 327, 334
Finnish Kuopio Ischemic Heart Disease Risk Factor Study (KIHD), 282, 283, 290
FLVCR, *see* Feline leukemic virus protein C (FLVCR)
Food and Agriculture Organization (FAO), 299, 300
Frataxin, 5, 15, 231, 252, 254–256
*FRDA* gene, in FA, 231, 254, 255
Friedreich's ataxia (FA), 105, 111, 231, 254–256, 266, 269
erythroblasts, 255
*FRDA* gene in, 254
treatment of, 256

## G

GABA, *see* Gamma amino butyric acid (GABA)
Gamma amino butyric acid (GABA), 150, 151, 230
$GABA_A$ and $GABA_B$, 152
synthesis of, 151
Gastric lavage, 83
Gastritis, 161, 170–171
GC, *see* Glucocorticoids (GC)
Genetic disorders of CNS, iron homeostasis and, 254–266
aceruloplasminemia, 259–262
differential diagnosis, 266
IRP2 deficiency, 265–266
neuroferritinopathy, 262–263
PKAN, 257–259
XLSA/A, 264–265
Glial senescence, 128–129
and iron sequestration
cysteamine model, 128
mitochondrial precursors of, 128–129
non-transferrin iron sequestration in, 129
Globus pallidus, of patient with PKAN, 258
Glossitis, 168, 169
GLP-1, *see* Glucagon-like peptide 1 (GLP-1)
Glucagon-like peptide 1 (GLP-1), 245
Glucocorticoids (GC), 211, 212, 214, 216
inflammatory cytokines and, 212
stress and, 214
suppressive effect on Th1 cells, 214

Glutamate, 97, 104, 113, 134, 141, 150, 151, 152, 153, 200, 242, 244, 265
GABA$_A$ and GABA$_B$, 152
synthesis of, 151
Glycosylphosphatidylinositol (GPI), 18, 54, 260
GPI, *see* Glycosylphosphatidylinositol (GPI)
Gradient-recalled echo (GRE) imaging, 233
Graves' disease, 214–215
GRE imaging, *see* Gradient-recalled echo (GRE) imaging

**H**

Hallervorden-Spatz syndrome, *see* Pantothenate kinase-2-associated neurodegeneration (PKAN)
HAMP, *see* Hepcidin antimicrobial peptide (HAMP)
Haptoglobin complex, 13
HCP1, *see* Heme carrier protein 1 (HCP1)
Heart disease, 162, 279–293
Heme, 33–34
intestinal absorption of, 35
Heme carrier protein 1 (HCP1), 14, 31, 34, 37
Heme catabolic pathway, 130
Heme/hemopexin complex, 13–14
Hemeoglobinometry, 309–310
Heme oxygenase 1 (HO-1), 34, 126, 127, 129–135, 189, 230
in AD-affected neural tissues, 132–133
and human brain aging, 132
over-expression in "stressed" astroglia, 135
and Parkinson's disease
dopamine/$H_2O_2$-related killing, 134–135
iron sequestration, 133
role in glial iron homeostasis, 130–132
role in multiple sclerosis (MS), 135
upregulation of, 129
Heme proteins, 329
Heme sources, of iron, 357
Hemochromatosis, 5, 6, 11–13, 16, 17, 21, 54, 55, 56, 84, 85, 86, 110, 111, 172, 182, 266–269, 280, 292, 331, 334, 342, 343, 344, 347, 352
and CHD risk, 292
and CNS, 266–269
HFE, 56
primary, 84
secondary, 84
Hemochromatosis proteins, 54
Hemoglobin, 9, 13, 17, 20, 78, 80, 85, 86, 163, 165, 166, 167, 189, 196, 199, 201, 202, 223, 227, 236, 251, 253, 260, 266, 280, 291, 328, 329, 333
Hemojuvelin, 21, 54, 55, 57, 58, 59, 252
BMP-dependent effect of, 54
as hepcidin regulator, 54
Hemosiderin, 7, 16, 86, 163, 168, 225, 227, 230, 329, 331
Hepcidin, 5, 6, 7, 9, 18, 19, 20, 21, 31, 35, 36, 37, 38, 39, 40, 41, 42, 51–60, 165, 166, 252, 352
catabolism, 53
expression, 21
ferroportin regulation by, 52–53
as inhibitor of iron release, 20–21
in regulation of iron absorption and distribution, 41–42
structure–function analysis of, 53
synthesis regulation by erythropoietic activity, 59–60
synthesis regulation by hypoxia-inducible transcription factors
HIF-dependent mechanism, 58
hypoxia, 57
synthesis regulation by iron
BMP pathway, 55
hemochromatosis proteins, 54
HFE mutations, 56–57
holotransferrin, 56
model of, 57
TfR1 deficiency, 55
TfR2 deficiency, 56
*in vivo* iron-regulatory activity of, 52
Hepcidin antimicrobial peptide (HAMP), 41, 54
Hephaestin, 5, 18, 31–35, 371, 252, 253
Hereditary hemochromatosis (HH), 266, 268
mutant HFE in, 267–268
overview, 266–267
HFE, 6, 12, 17, 21, 37, 54, 56, 57, 110, 252, 267, 268, 269, 291, 341
HFE gene mutation, 56, 268
HFE hemochromatosis, 56, 110
HFE mutant
and Alzheimer's disease, 267–268
and amyotrophic lateral sclerosis, 269
and idiopathic Parkinson's disease, 268–269
and ischemic stroke, 269
HIF, *see* Hypoxia-inducing factor (HIF)
High-resolution MR brain imaging, at 7 tesla, 235
Hippocampus, zinc and iron interaction in
FER distribution pattern, 102
iron therapy, 103–105
MF neuro-anatomy, 102–103
Hippocampus iron metabolism, 199–200
HNE, *see* 4-hydroxynoneal (HNE)
HO-1, *see* Heme oxygenase 1 (HO-1)
Holotransferrin, 55, 56, 57, 58
Hormone replacement therapy (HRT), 334, 341, 345, 347
HPA axis, *see* Hypothalamic pituitary–adrenal (HPA) axis
HRT, *see* Hormone replacement therapy (HRT)
Human iron physiology, 251–253
Hydroxynonenal, 244, 245
4-Hydroxynoneal (HNE), 244
Hypoferremia, 58

Hypoferritinemia, 263
Hypothalamic pituitary–adrenal (HPA) axis, 207
  interaction with cytokines, 210–212
Hypoxia, 166
  effect on erythropoiesis, 57
  iron and hepcidin regulation by, 57–58
Hypoxia-inducing factor (HIF), 166, 189
  role in hepcidin suppression, 58
  subunits of, 57

I

ICSH, *see* International Council for Standardization in Hemeatology (ICSH)
ID, *see* Iron deficiency (ID)
IDA, *see* Anaemia
IL-1, effects on interstitial levels of monoamines, 210
IL-4, dexamethasone effect on production of, 214
IL-12, differentiate Thp cells to Th1, 213, 214, 215
Immune system
  and iron deficiency, 203
  stress and, 208
Immunoreactivity, transferrin, 133, 200
IMPAC, *see* Integrated Management of Pregnancy and Childbirth (IMPAC)
Inborn errors, of brain iron metabolism, 231
Incidence, 81, 87, 173, 279, 282, 290, 300, 302, 304, 306, 307, 321, 337, 338
Infection susceptibility, in iron deficiency, 319–320
Inflammation, 20, 21, 33, 41, 42, 58–59, 85, 164, 165, 203, 208, 211, 212, 214–215, 216, 227, 208, 282, 288, 303, 314, 344
  acute hypoferremia of, 58
  hemojuvelin regulation by, 59
  hepcidin and anemia of, 58
  hepcidin regulation by, 59
  role of Th17 in, 215–216
  stress and, 214–215
Inherited neurological diseases, with brain iron accumulation, 231
Integrated Management of Pregnancy and Childbirth (IMPAC), 305
International Council for Standardization in Hemeatology (ICSH), 300
Intestinal absorption, of dietary iron, 35
Intra-neuronal iron metabolism, 142
IRE, *see* Iron-responsive elements (IRE)
*Ireb*$^{-/-}$ mice, 5, 265
*Ireb2*$^{+/-}$ mice, 265
*Ireb2*$^{-/-}$ mice, 265
*IroA* cluster, 67–68
Iron, 3
  accumulation, 15, 17, 18, 39, 40, 52, 84, 96, 111, 126, 129, 182, 183, 189, 224, 225, 231, 232, 255, 257, 258, 260, 261, 266, 268
  biochemical functions, 329
  in brain, *See* Brain iron
  in cellular proteins, 7, 9
  clinical value, 332–335
  deposition in aging and degenerating CNS
    Alzheimer's disease, 127
    glial senescence and iron sequestration, 128–130
    heme-degrading enzyme, 126
    idiopathic PD, 127
    regional predilections on, 126
  "distribution map", 196
  elevated levels in bloodstream, 188
  excretion, 331–332
  GI absorption of, 78
  in hemorrhage, 189
  neuromelanin, interaction with
    iron-binding ability of, 109–110
    neuroprotectant in PD, 109–110
    in SN of patients with PD, 109
  as nutrient, 65–66
  overload, 4, 5, 6, 15, 16, 17, 32, 33, 35, 36, 38, 40, 41, 42, 52, 54, 55, 56, 60, 84, 85, 86, 129, 189, 190, 254, 255, 260, 263, 266, 280, 292, 293, 301, 302, 320, 330, 331, 334, 341, 343, 344, 352
  and ovulation, 334
  and pathogenesis of AD, 242–243
    experimental evidence for, 243–245
    therapeutic implications of, 245–246
  and pathogenic bacteria, 66
  role in myelination, 197
  salts, 78, 79, 223
  and schizophrenia, 198
  sensing, 56
  starvation, 65, 70, 71, 72
  starvation, RyhB activity during, 70–71
  supplementation and fortification, 333–334
  trafficking and regulation in cell, 7
  turnover, 42, 253
  utilization, intracellular
    mitochondrion role in, 14–15
  and women's health, 327–348
  and zinc interaction in hippocampus
    FER distribution pattern, 102
    iron therapy, 103–105
    MF neuro-anatomy, 102–103
Iron absorption, 31–43, 57, 299, 330–331, 334
  hepcidin in regulation of, 41–42
  increase in, 57
  mechanisms adjusting, 51
  mechanisms of, in mammals, 33–35
  putative functions of proteins involved in intestinal, 37
Iron chelator, in acute iron ingestion, 83–84
Iron-containing proteins, hemoglobin and myoglobin, 9, 163, 329, 333
Iron deficiency (ID)
  animal IDD model of, 198

BBB, 198
hippocampus iron metabolism, 198–199
learning paradigms, 199
transferrin immunoreactivity, 200
auditory system and, 202
BBB studies in, 101
causes of, 161–162
cerebral iron homeostasis in
developmental stages affected by, 187
myelin formation in, 188
transferrin receptor changes in, 187–188
clinical manifestations of, 159–160, 195
immune function, 173
muscular function and exercise tolerance, 173
during development, 146–147
$D_2$R-DAT link, 146
and drugs of abuse, 152
early, *see* Early iron deficiency
and endocrine system, 202
global, 299–310
high-risk group for, 195
history of, 159–160
human studies of, 200
and immune system, 203
infection susceptibility, 319–320
laboratory evaluation of
MCV and MCH, 165
reticulocyte hemoglobin content (CHr), 165
serum transferrin receptor, 165
TIBC, 164
and lactation, 340
latent iron deficiency, 302–303
lifestyle factors, in women, 334–335
long-term effects of rehabilitated infancy, 201
management strategies, 304–305
and menopause, 340–342
and myelination of neurons, 100
neuronal effects in humans, 148
nutritional, 313–323
pathogenesis of
epithelial cells and skeleton, 164
proteins and enzymes, 163–165
and pregnancy, 335–340
and pretems, 200–201
prevalence, 161, 314–315
prevention, in childhood, 320–322
psychomotor development deficits, 317–318
risk factors, in childhood, 315–317
in women, 327–348
*See also* Anaemia
Iron deficiency anaemia (IDA)
causes of, 161–162
clinical manifestations of
alopecia, 172
anisocytosis, 166–167
atrophy of lingual papillae, 168
cheilitis, 167, 168
compensatory mechanisms, 166
dysphagia, 167–168
dyspnea, 166
effects on epithelial tissues, 168
erythrocyte morphologies, 167
gastritis, 170–171
hypoxia, 166
koilonychia, 171–172
microcytic and hypochromic red cells, 168
orthopnea, 166
peripheral blood, 167
pica, 172–173
platelet count, 168
tongue and mouth, 168–169
elemental iron treatment dose for, 77–78
Iron deficiency diet (IDD)
animal model of iron deficiency, 198–200
effect on hippocampus iron metabolism, 199–200
magnitude of effect on, 201
nutritional iron deficiency by, inducing, 196
transferrin receptor immunoreactivity and, 200
Iron dextran injection
administration methods, 79–80
dose for
adults and children over 15 kg, 80–81
children 5–15 kg, 81
Iron distribution
disordered, in chronic inflammatory conditions, 38
hepcidin in regulation of, 41–42
Iron efflux, from cells, 15, 17, 32–33, 41, 52, 259
Iron fortification, 305, 318, 321–322, 329, 333
Iron homeostasis, 4, 8, 9, 10, 15, 17, 18, 19, 20, 21, 33, 40, 51–60, 69–73, 113, 125, 126, 127, 129–135, 147, 184, 186, 187, 189, 207, 211, 242, 243, 251–270, 329
in bacteria, intracellular
RyhB activity, 70–71
sRNAs and environmental stresses, 69–70
genetic disorders of CNS, 254–266
aceruloplasminemia, 259–262
differential diagnosis, 266
IRP2 deficiency, 265–266
neuroferritinopathy, 262–263
PKAN, 257–259
XLSA/A, 264–265
inherited disturbances in, 10
mitochondrial, 15
in myelin-forming cells
oligodendrocyte-derived transferrin, 186–187
uptake of iron, 186
in neural and peripheral tissues, 125
proteins in mammalian, 252
in Schwann cells, 187

Iron loss
body, 40–41
mechanisms of, in mammals, 33–35
relative size of, 40
Iron metabolism, 329–332
disorders of, 110–111
in duodenal enterocyte, 8
in erythroid cell, 8
in hepatocyte, 8
importance of, 65–66
intra-neuronal, *see* Intra-neuronal iron metabolism
in macrophage, 8
neuronal, *see* Neuronal iron metabolism
regulation of
IREs role in, 19
IRPs role in, 18–19
posttranslational, 19–20
systemic, *see* Systemic iron metabolism
Iron overload, *see* Chronic iron overload; Hemochromatosis
Iron physiology, human, 251–254, 262
Iron regulation
at body level, 39–41
at cellular level, 38–39
in cytosol, 35
hepcidin in, 41–42
putative functions of proteins involved in intestinal, 37
Iron-regulatory protein (IRP1, IRP2), 5, 18, 100, 187, 243, 254, 269
Iron regulatory protein, in iron regulation at cellular level, 31, 38–39, 100
Iron release
by cells, 32–33
liver function to control, 36
Iron requirements, during pregnancy and lactation, 327, 335–336
Iron-responsive elements (IRE), 12, 16, 17, 18, 19, 34, 38–39, 53, 185, 187–188, 254
Iron-responsive proteins (IRP), 16, 17, 18, 19, 37, 38, 39, 187, 231, 254
Iron saccharate, *see* Iron sucrose
Iron salts
elemental iron content of, 79
Iron storage
intracellular
biology of, 16–17
ferritin, 16
hemosiderin, 16
liver function to control, 36
Iron sucrose, 81
Iron–sulfur (Fe–S)-dependent enzymes, FA and, 255–256
Iron–sulfur (FeSS) clusters
biogenesis, 15
in mitochondria and cytoplasm, 15
roles in electron transport and catalysis, 9
Iron supplement
during pregnancy and lactation, 336–338
for prevention of iron deficiency, 320–321, 333
use in postmenopausal women, 342
Iron toxicity
clinical stages of, 82
measure of, 85
range of, 83
treatment of
exchange transfusion, 84
iron chelator role in, 83–84
whole bowel irrigation for, 83
Iron transport, 331
in body and tissue uptake, 35–38
cellular, in mammals, 32–33
Iron uptake
by cells, 32–33
Iron uptake, cellular
DMT1 role in, 12
by heme/hemopexin complex, 13–14
from internalized heme, 14
non-transferrin-bound, 12–13
under normal conditions, 9–10
in pathological states, 9
TfR2 role in, 11
transferrin receptor 1 role in, 10–11
IRP, *see* Iron regulatory protein (IRP)
IRP1, 5, 7, 9, 18, 31, 34, 37, 38, 100, 254, 256, 265
anaemia and, 39
loss of, 38
IRP2, 5, 7, 18, 19, 31, 34, 37, 38, 39, 100, 110, 111, 113, 251, 254, 265, 266, 269
anaemia and, 39
loss of, 38–39
IRP2 deficiency, 100, 265–266, 269–270
IRP2$^{-/-}$ mice, 266
IRPs (iron-regulatory proteins)
IRP1, 18
IRP2, 18–19
Ischemic stroke, 269
Ischemic stroke, mutant HFE and, 269

**K**

Kaiser-Fleischer rings, 266
KIHD, *see* Finnish Kuopio Ischemic Heart Disease Risk Factor Study (KIHD)
Koilonychia, 171–172

**L**

Labile iron pool (LIP), 230, 231
expansion of, 253–254
Laboratory assays, of iron metabolism, reference ranges for, 351–353

Lactation, 146, 150, 153, 162, 328, 335–340
anaemia during, 336
ID and, 339
iron supplement, 336–338
LDL cholesterol, *see* Low-density lipoprotein (LDL) cholesterol
LEAP1, *see* Liver-expressed antimicrobial peptide (LEAP1)
L-ferritin gene, 263
Lifestyle, and ID, 334–335
LIP, *see* Labile iron pool (LIP)
Liver, controls iron storage and release by ferroportin, 14, 16, 17, 36, 51, 86
Liver-expressed antimicrobial peptide (LEAP1), 41
Low-density lipoprotein (LDL) cholesterol, 278
oxidized, CHD risk and, 289–291
Lymphocytes, differentiation into Th1/Th2 cells, 213

M

Macrophage, iron metabolism in, 8, 17, 20–21, 331
Magnetic resonance imaging, 85, 107, 108, 223, 227, 256
Major histocompatibility complex (MHC) antigens, 56, 208
Mammalian iron homeostasis, proteins in, 252
Management strategies, 304
MAO blockade, *see* Monoamine oxidase (MAO) blockade
MAP, *see* Metabolically active iron pool (MAP)
Maternal iron supplementation, 338
Maternal post-pregnancy iron status, 338–339
Menopause, ID and, 279, 280, 340–342
Metabolically active iron pool (MAP), 231
Metabolic syndrome, 342–344
Metal chaperones, 230
Mfrn, *see* Mitoferrin (Mfrn)
MHC antigens, *see* Major histocompatibility complex (MHC) antigens
Mitochondria, 3, 5, 7, 9, 15, 16, 111, 112, 126, 127, 128, 129, 130, 131, 132, 133, 134, 135, 142, 228, 231, 244, 251, 252, 254, 255, 256, 264, 329
Mitochondrial ferritin (MtF), 5, 16, 252, 256
Mitochondrial iron accumulation, 15, 111, 255
Mitoferrin (Mfrn), 5, 15, 22, 252
Monoamine oxidase (MAO) blockade, 135
Monoamines
dopamine, *see* Dopamine
endorphins, 153
estrogen, 153
norepinephrine, *see* Norepinephrine
serotonin, *see* Serotonin
Mostofsky, D. I., 100, 181, 182, 195–204
Motor neuron, 182–185, 269
Mouse strains, with inherited disturbances in iron homeostasis, 10
MPTP-induced dopaminergic neurotoxicity, 112
MRI imaging techniques, for brain iron, 232–234
imaging at 7 tesla, 234–235
overview, 223–226
pulse sequences and quantifying brain iron effects, 233
MS, *see* Multiple sclerosis (MS)
MTP, 253
Multiple sclerosis (MS), 105, 111, 126, 128, 135, 215, 225, 231
Myelin, 100, 135, 141, 181, 186, 187, 187, 188, 190, 197, 230, 242
Myelination, iron role in, 187, 197, 317
Myoglobin, 9, 33, 77, 163, 328, 329, 331

N

Naïve T cells, differentiation into effector T-cell subtype induced by cytokines, 213
National Diet and Nutrition Surveys, 301, 314
National Health and Nutrition Examination Survey (NHANES), 161, 280, 281, 282, 284, 301, 314
National Health and Nutrition Examination Survey III (NHANES III), 280, 281, 282, 314, 329, 331, 332, 333, 337, 340, 342, 343, 346, 347
NBIA, *see* Neurodegeneration with brain iron accumulation (NBIA)
*Neisseria meningitidis*, gene repression pattern under Fe starvation, 72
Neural damage, in neuropathological conditions, 125–126
Neurodegeneration with brain iron accumulation (NBIA), 225, 257, 259, 266, 269, 270
Neurodegenerative diseases, 96, 105, 111, 113, 208, 223–236
Neurodegenerative diseases, localized brain ferritin and iron deposits in, 105
Neuroferritinopathy, 231, 262–263, 266, 269
molecular pathophysiology of, 263
MRI images in, 262
Neurofibrillary tangles (NFT), 127, 132, 241, 242, 243, 244, 245, 267
Neuroimmune communication, cytokines as mediators of, 208–210
Neurological diseases, inherited, with brain iron accumulation, 231
Neuromelanin
concentration of nigral, 109
interaction with iron
iron-binding ability of, 109–110
neuroprotectant in PD, 109–110
in SN of patients with PD, 109
Neuronal iron metabolism
in basal ganglia, 182–183
in cerebellum, 184
in cerebral cortex, 182, 185
in cranial nerve nuclei, 184
in pontine nucleus, 184

Neuronal iron metabolism (*Cont.*)
in red nucleus, 184
in spinal cord motor neurons, 184–185
in substantia nigra, 182–183, 185
Neurotransmitters, 97, 98, 104, 141, 142, 150, 181, 190, 210, 317
NFT, *see* Neurofibrillary tangles (NFT)
NHANES, *see* National Health and Nutrition Examination Survey (NHANES)
NHANES dietary intake, of iron in women, 328
NHANES III, *see* National Health and Nutrition Examination Survey III (NHANES III)
Non-hemeiron, 34
intestinal absorption of, 35
Non-heme sources, of iron, 356
Non-ribosomal peptide synthesis (NRPS)
activities, 66–67
protein–protein interactions within, 67
Non-transferrin-bound iron (NTBI), 9, 11, 12, 13, 20, 35, 36, 86, 186
uptake, 13
under iron-loading syndromes, 12
by liver, 13
molecular basis of, 13
Noradrenergic innervation of rodent brain, 148
Norepinephrine (NE)
degradation of, 148
signaling, 148
synthetic pathway of, 147
transport of, 148
NTBI, *see* Non-transferrin-bound iron (NTBI)
Nutritional iron deficiency (NID), 95–97, 196, 313–322
effect on brain
behavioral abnormalities, 97
brain enzymes, 97–98
CNS aminergic neurotransmitters, 97
iron distribution, uneven, 96, 97
iron transport, 96
neurotransmitter receptors, 98–99
neurochemical aspect of, 96
in rats
BBB examination, 100
brain enzyme activity, 97–98
dopamine D2 receptor, 99
neurotransmitter activities, 98
Nutritional sources, of iron, 355–357
heme sources, 357
non-heme sources, 356

**O**

Oligodendrocyte, 100, 108, 181, 184, 186–190, 200, 208, 243, 263
Oral iron preparations, 77
bioavailability of, 78
drug interactions with, 79–80
side effects of, 78–79
Oral iron therapy, drug interactions with, 80
Organum vasculosum of the laminae terminalis (OVLT), 209
Orthopnea, 166
Osteoporosis, 327, 344–345
OVLT, *see* Organum vasculosum of the laminae terminalis (OVLT)
Ovulation, and iron, 334
Oxidative stress, 96, 108, 109, 112, 113, 126, 127, 129, 130, 131, 132, 134, 135, 183, 189, 203, 242, 244, 245, 254, 267, 290, 291
soruces in AD brain, 127

**P**

PANK2, *see* Pantothenate kinase-2 (PANK2)
Pantothenate kinase-2-associated neurodegeneration (PKAN), 257–259, 269
brain MRI of patient with, 257
globus pallidus of patient with, 258
PANK2 in, 258–259
biosynthetic pathway of, 259
Parenchymal brain copper
in normal adult, 230
quantitative measurements of, 228
Parenchymal brain iron
in normal adult, 230
quantitative measurements of, 228
Parenteral iron formulations, 77, 78
ferric gluconate injection, 81
iron dextran injection
administration methods, 79–80
for adults and children over 15 kg, 80–81
for children 5–15 kg, 81
iron sucrose injection, 81
side effects of, 81–82
Parkinsonian substantia nigra, iron overload in
6-hydroxydopamine neurotoxicity, 112
MPTP-induced dopaminergic neurotoxicity, 112
protein aggregation in Lewy bodies, 111
α–synuclein
crosslinking, 111
protofibrils, 111–112
Parkinson's disease (PD), 96, 105, 107, 112, 113, 114, 126, 127, 133, 134, 183, 189, 190, 208, 225, 231, 268
and heme oxygenase-1, 133–135
dopamine/$H_2O_2$-related killing, 134–135
iron sequestration, 133
idiopathic, 127
iron in, increased levels of
MRI experiments of, 108
putamen and globus pallidus, 107
SN pars compacta, 106–107
SN pars reticulata, 108
mutant HFE and idiopathic, 268–269

neuromelanin interaction in SN of patients with, 109
neuroprotectant in, 109–110
role of transition metals in, 105
Pathogenic bacteria, 65–69, 71
salmochelin-secreting, 68
siderophores synthesized by, 66
virulence factor in
*IroA* cluster, 67–68
siderophore modification., 68
PD, *see* Parkinson's disease (PD)
Perls stain, 224, 225, 230, 231
*See also* Brain iron
Peterobactin, 68
PGE, *see* Prostaglandin E (PGE)
Phlebotomy, 16, 17, 85, 86, 291, 344
Pica, 172–173, 195
PKAN, *see* Pantothenate kinase-2-associated neurodegeneration (PKAN)
PLA2G6, 259
Plasma iron regulation, by inflammation, 58–59
*Plasmodium falciparum,* 302
*Plasmodium yoelli,* 302
Platelet count, 168
Postmenopausal women, iron supplement use in, 280, 292, 341, 342, 344, 345
Pregnancy, 21, 33, 41, 203, 300, 301, 305, 308, 315, 316, 320, 327, 328, 331, 334–339, 345–347
anaemia during, 336
ID during, 335–339
iron requirements during, 335–336
iron supplement during, 336–338
Prenatal period, 200
Presenilin-1, 242, 245
Pretems and iron deficiency, 200–201
Primary hemochromatosis, 84, 85, 86
Prostaglandin E (PGE), 209
Proteins, in mammalian iron homeostasis, 252
*Pseudomonas aeruginosa,* gene repression pattern under Fe starvation, 72
Psychomotor development, 317, 318, 319, 322
Psychomotor development deficits, ID, 317–319, 322

**R**

RDA, *see* Recommended daily intakes (RDA)
Reactive oxygen species (ROS), 243
Aβ source of, in AD, 244
Recommended daily intakes (RDA), of iron in women, 328, 334, 335, 342
Reference ranges, for laboratory assays of iron metabolism, 351–353
Restless leg syndromes, 173
Risk factors, 270, 284, 285, 293, 315, 316, 339, 344
ROS, *see* Reactive oxygen species (ROS)
RyhB, 69–72

**S**

*Saccharomyces cerevisiae,* gene repression pattern under Fe starvation, 72
Salmochelin S4, 67
Salmochelin-secreting pathogenic bacteria, 68
Schizophrenia and iron, 198
*Schizosaccharomyces pombe,* gene repression pattern under Fe starvation, 72
Schwann cells, iron homeostasis in, 181, 187
Secondary hemochromatosis, 84
Serotonin
catabolism of, 150
5-HT
receptors, 150
synthesis of, 149
transport, 149–150
Serum ferritin
CHD risk and
case-control/cross-sectional studies, 288–289
cohort studies based on, 282–285
geometric mean, 281
Serum iron measurement, 300
Serum transferrin saturation level, 281
geometric mean serum ferritin by, 281
mean, by age and sex, 281
Seven-tesla research magnet, 234
Siderophores, 66–68, 73
in *Bacillus anthracis,* 68
biosynthesis and RyhB, 72
post-synthetic modification of
enterobactin, 66–67
salmochelin S4, 67
synthesized by pathogenic bacteria, 66
Signal transduction and activator of transcription (STAT)-4, 216
Six-transmembrane, epithelial antigen of the prostate 3 (*Steap3*) gene, 253
Small regulatory RNAs, 69
sRNA RyhB
role during iron starvation
intracellular Fe levels, 71
mRNA degradation, 70
role in acid resistance, 71
role in biofilms and chemotaxis, 71
siderophore biosynthesis and, 72
*Staphylococcus aureus*
gene repression pattern under Fe starvation, 72
STAT-4, *see* Signal transduction and activator of transcription (STAT)-4
STEAP3, 4, 10, 31, 32, 36, 252
STEAP3 expression, 10
*Steap3* gene, *see* Six-transmembrane, epithelial antigen of the prostate 3 (*Steap3*) gene
Step 2 Diet, 291

Stress, 3, 17, 65, 69, 78, 79, 95, 96, 108, 109, 112, 113, 114, 126, 127, 129, 130, 131, 132, 134, 135, 148, 183, 189, 199, 203, 207–216, 242, 244, 245, 254, 267, 290, 308, 317
  and autoimmune inflammatory disease, 214–215
  characteristics of, 207–208
  CNS and immune system in, 208
  defined, 207
  depression and, 210–211
  and glucocorticoids effects on Th1/ Th2 balance, 214
  and increase in IL-6 and IL-1 secretion, 216
  and Th1/Th2 subsets, 212–213
Stress hormones, 207, 211, 212–213, 214, 215, 216
Striatal neurotransmitters
  in brains of ID rats, 98
  deficiency in rats, 100
Striatum, 97–99, 103, 108, 113, 142–145, 147, 149–151, 361
Stroke, *see* Ischemic stroke
Sullivan, Dr. Jerome, 279, 280, 287, 289, 292, 293
Synaptic dysfunction, 242
α–Synuclein, mutations in, 111
Systemic iron metabolism
  regulation of iron homeostasis
    ferroportin role in, 52
    hepcidin role in, *see* Hepcidin
    hypoxia-inducible transcription factors, 57–58
    supply of iron to plasma Tf, 20
  systemic iron transport, 20
Systemic regulation, 5, 20, 35, 53

T

Tangles, 127, 132, 241, 242–244
TfR1, *see* Transferrin receptor (TFR1)
TfR2, 6, 11, 20, 21, 32, 37, 54–57, 110, 111
  affinity for diferric Tf, 11
  deficiency and iron regulation, 56
  expression of, 11
TfR1–apoTf complex, 7
Th17 cells, role in inflammation, 215–216
T-helpers, 212, 214, 215–216
T-helper progenitor (Thp) cells, 214
Thp cells, *see* T-helper progenitor (Thp) cells
Th1/ Th2 balance, 213–214
  stress and glucocorticoids effects on, 214
Th1/Th2 cells, 212–214
  glucocorticoids suppressive effect on, 214
  and stress, 212–213
Th1/Th2 cells, differentiation of lymphocytes into, 213
TIBC, *see* Total iron-binding capacity (TIBC)
TIM-2, binding with ferritin, 14
Tissue copper concentration, in normal adult brain, 229
Tissue iron concentration, in normal adult brain, 229
Tissue uptake, and iron transport in body, 35–38
TLR, *see* Toll-like receptors (TLR)
Toll-like receptors (TLR), 213
Total iron-binding capacity (TIBC), 83, 280
  in body iron stores, 280–282
Toxicity, 82–87, 109, 112, 129, 134, 151, 185, 189, 200, 231, 242–245, 252, 270, 321
  of drug, 82–87
    acute, 82
    chronic, 84
Transferrin, 331
  in cellular iron transport, 32–33
  genetic deficiency of, 56
  receptor 1, 4, 10, 22, 37
  receptor 2, 6, 11, 37, 54
Transferrin-bound iron uptake, 12–13
  low-affinity uptake of, 11
  TfR1 role in, 10–11
Transferrin immunoreactivity, 200
Transferrin pathway of iron mobilization, 127
Transferrin receptor 1 (TfR1), 4, 10, 37
  binding with diferric Tf, 10
  homolog transferrin receptor 2, 11
  homozygous ablation of, 55
  iron regulation controlled by, 38
  iron uptake by, 10–11
Transferrin saturation (TS), 56, 163, 266, 267, 280, 281, 314, 332, 345, 353
  in body iron stores, 280–282
  cohort studies based on, CHD risk and, 286–287
$T_{reg}$, *see* T regulatory cell ($T_{reg}$)
T regulatory cell ($T_{reg}$), 215, 216
TS, *see* Transferrin saturation (TS)
Turpentine-induced inflammation, hypoferremic response to, 58
Type 2 diabetes, 342–344

U

Untranslated region (UTR), 16, 17, 19, 22, 38, 72, 244, 254
UPEC, *see* Uropathogenic *E. coli* (UPEC)
Uropathogenic *E. coli* (UPEC), 66, 67
  acute cystitis due to, 66
  chemical structures of catecholate siderophores used by, 67
UTR, *see* Untranslated region (UTR)

V

Veteran's Administration (VA) patients, serum ferritin levels in, 291

W

WHA, *see* World Health Assembly (WHA)
WHO, global iron deficiency, 299–310
Whole bowel irrigation, for acute iron ingestion, 83
WHO programmes, 96, 241, 299–310, 315, 345

WHOSIS, 300
Wilson disease, 266
World Health Assembly (WHA), 300

X

X-linked sideroblastic anemia with ataxia (XLSA/A), 256, 264, 266, 269
  differential diagnosis of, 266
  sagittal T1-weighted MR image of patient with, 264
XLSA/A, *see* X-linked sideroblastic anemia with ataxia (XLSA/A)

Y

Yehuda, Shlomo, 97, 100, 101, 102, 113, 144, 145, 153, 182, 187, 188, 196, 197, 198, 201, 203
Yfh1 mutants, 255

Z

Zinc and iron interaction in hippocampus, 102–105
  FER distribution pattern, 102
  iron therapy, 103–105
  MF neuro-anatomy, 102–103

# About the Editors

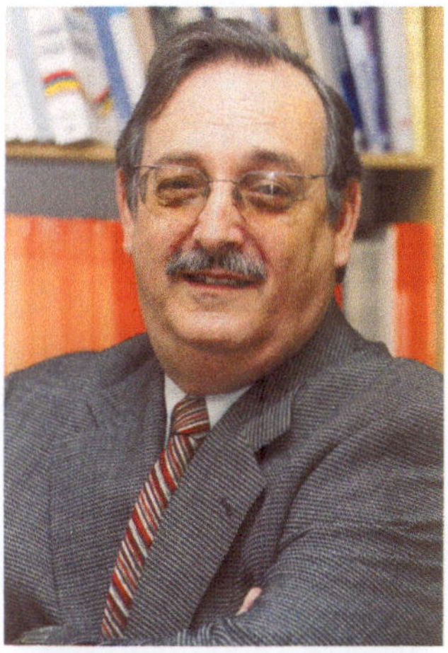

Shlomo Yehuda received his Ph.D. degree in Psychology and Brain Sciences from M.I.T. He is a Professor at the Department of Psychology and he is the Director of the Psychopharmacology Laboratory at Bar Ilan University. He is currently held the Ginsburg Chair Alzheimer Research and Farber Center. He is trained in Prof. Wurtman's laboratory at M.I.T., a visiting professor at Kastin's Peptide Laboratory (Tulane Medical School, New Orleans), and Rosenstadt Professor at Toronto Medical School – Nutrition Department. He published over 180 scientific papers and 7 books in the following fields: brain biochemistry, effects of nutrients on brain and behavior (mainly brain iron and essential fatty acids), ADHD children, and aging of the brain.

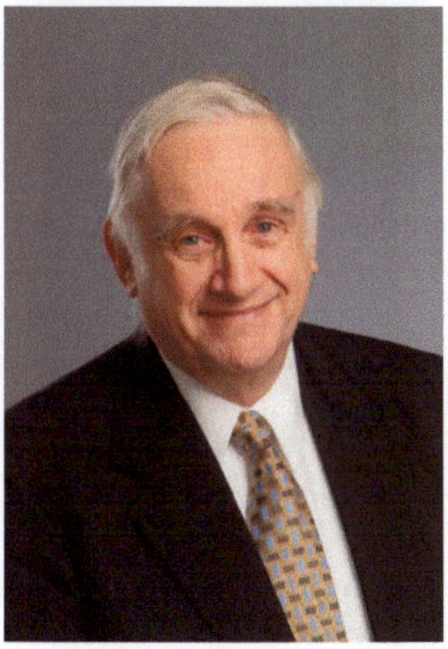

David I. Mostofsky is a Professor of Experimental Psychology and Behavioral Medicine at Boston University, and holds associate appointments at several major medical institutions in the Boston area. A Charter Fellow of the Academy for Behavioral Medicine Research, he has been involved with Behavioral Medicine and Psychopharmacology for many years. Scientific and scholarly activities during his career include research investigations with both human and animal subjects, concerning basic science experimentation as well as clinical applications. He has published numerous articles and books on a variety of topics in this area, especially with regard to epilepsy, pain, stress, essential fatty acids, and psychoneuroimmunology. He has been the recipient of many awards including, a Marshal Fund Award, Einstein Award, NIH Fogarty Fellowship, Fulbright Fellow, and is active as an invited lecturer in Europe, South America, and the Far East.

# About the Editors

# About the Series Editor

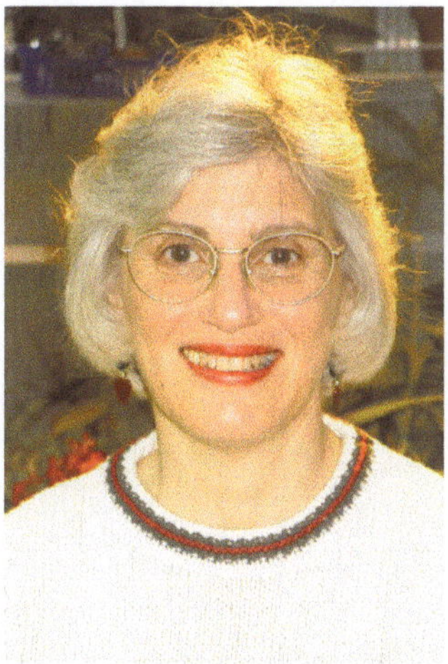

Dr. Adrianne Bendich is Clinical Director, Medical Affairs at GlaxoSmithKline (GSK) Consumer Healthcare, where she is responsible for leading the innovation and medical programs in support of many well-known brands including TUMS and Os-Cal. Dr. Bendich had primary responsibility for GSK's support for the Women's Health Initiative (WHI) intervention study. Prior to joining GSK, Dr. Bendich was at Roche Vitamins Inc. and was involved with the groundbreaking clinical studies showing that folic acid-containing multivitamins significantly reduced major classes of birth defects. Dr. Bendich has co-authored over 100 major clinical research studies in the area of preventive nutrition. Dr. Bendich is recognized as a leading authority on antioxidants, nutrition and immunity and pregnancy outcomes, vitamin safety, and the cost-effectiveness of vitamin/mineral supplementation.

Dr. Bendich is the Editor of nine books including *Preventive Nutrition: The Comprehensive Guide For Health Professionals*, co-edited with Dr. Richard Deckelbaum, and is Series Editor of *Nutrition and Health* for Humana Press with 29 published volumes including *Probiotics in Pediatric Medicine* edited by Dr. Sonia Michail and Dr. Philip Sherman; *Handbook of Nutrition and Pregnancy* edited by Dr. Carol Lammi-Keefe, Dr. Sarah Couch, and Dr. Elliot Philipson; *Nutrition and Rheumatic Disease* edited by Dr. Laura Coleman; *Nutrition and Kidney Disease* edited by Dr. Laura Byham-Grey, Dr. Jerrilynn Burrowes, and Dr. Glenn Chertow; *Nutrition and Health in Developing Countries* edited by Dr. Richard Semba and Dr. Martin Bloem; *Calcium in Human Health* edited by Dr. Robert Heaney and Dr. Connie Weaver, and *Nutrition and Bone Health* edited by Dr. Michael Holick and Dr. Bess Dawson-Hughes.

Dr. Bendich served as Associate Editor for *Nutrition, the International Journal*; served on the Editorial Board of the *Journal of Women's Health and Gender-based Medicine*, and was a member of the Board of Directors of the American College of Nutrition.

Dr. Bendich was the recipient of the Roche Research Award, is a Tribute to Women and Industry Awardee, and was a recipient of the Burroughs Wellcome Visiting Professorship in Basic Medical Sciences, 2000–2001. In 2008, Dr. Bendich was given the Council for Responsible Nutrition (CRN) Apple Award in recognition of her many contributions to the scientific understanding of dietary supplements. Dr. Bendich holds academic appointments as Adjunct Professor in the Department of Preventive Medicine and Community Health at UMDNJ, and has an adjunct appointment at the Institute of Nutrition, Columbia University P&S, and is an Adjunct Research Professor, Rutgers University, Newark Campus. She is listed in *Who's Who in American Women*.

MIX
Papier aus verantwortungsvollen Quellen
Paper from responsible sources
FSC® C105338

If you have any concerns about our products,
you can contact us on
**ProductSafety@springernature.com**

In case Publisher is established outside the EU,
the EU authorized representative is:
**Springer Nature Customer Service Center GmbH**
**Europaplatz 3, 69115 Heidelberg, Germany**

Printed by Libri Plureos GmbH
in Hamburg, Germany